- Get as fast as possible: arterial blood gas analysis, glucose, and potassium
- Carefully search for occult head trauma
- Order a cerebral CT if:
  - History of head injury *and* Glasgow coma scale < 15
  - Pupils differ in size
- Worsening of mental status while under observation
- No improvement in mental status within 3 hours after admission
- Thiamine 100 mg i.v.
- i.v. glucose 10% 500 ml or glucose 30% 100 ml
- Consider additional toxin ingestion
- Frequently assess pupils

SYMPTOMS AND SIGNS: WHOM TO SUSPECT FOR ALCOHOL INTOXICATION

Consider acute alcohol intoxication in a patient with:

- History of alcohol intake (ask accompanying persons)
- Coma
- Syncope
- Any inappropriate behavior
- Any neurologic abnormality
- Trauma
- Traffic accident
- Hypothermia

TYPICAL COMPLICATIONS AND PROBLEMS IN ACUTE ALCOHOL INTOXICATION

- Ensure dedicated care for every alcohol-intoxicated patient
- Avoid benzodiazepines
- Aggressive patients:
  - Try to listen, and talk
  - Haloperidol 10 mg p.o., i.v., i.m., or s.c.
  - Physical restraints are only a last resort
- Coingested poisons, esp. cocaine, benzodiazepines, and antidepressants
- Hypoglycemia
- Hypothermia
- Rhabdomyolysis
- Occult head injury (intracranial bleeding)
- Upper gastrointestinal bleeding
- Wernicke encephalopathy
- Methanol
- Hyponatremia

RECOMMENDED DIAGNOSTIC TESTS

Perform the following tests in all symptomatic patients:

Laboratory Parameter	Normal Range (Innsbruck University Hospital)
Glucose	70–110 mg dl^{-1}, i.e., 3.9-6.1 mmol^{-1}
Potassium	3.5–5.2 mmol l^{-1}
Sodium	135–152 mmol l^{-1}
Chloride	95–110 mmol l^{-1}
Arterial blood gas analysis:	
pH	7.35–7.45
pCO$_2$	35–45 mmHg
Bicarbonate = HCO$_3$	22–26 mmol l^{-1}
SaO$_2$	Greater than 89%
Ethanol	0 mg dl^{-1}
Creatinine	0.7–1.4 mg dl^{-1}, i.e., 62–24 µmol l^{-1}
Creatine kinase	14–108 UI^{-1}
Urea	10–50 mg dl^{-1} urea (x 0.46 = BUN in mg dl^{-1})
Serum osmolality	280–298 mosm kg^{-1}
Peripheral blood cell count:	
Hemoglobin	men: 13-18 g dl^{-1}; women:12-16 g/dl
Leukocytes	4000–10,000 /cubic millimeter
Platelets	140,000–400,000 /cubic millimeter

Handbook of alcoholism

HANDBOOK OF
ALCOHOLISM

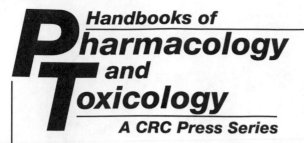

Handbooks of Pharmacology and Toxicology

A CRC Press Series

Mannfred A. Hollinger, Series Editor
University of California, Davis

Published Titles

Handbook of Pharmacokinetic and Pharmacodynamic Correlations with Computer Applications
Hartmut Derendorf and Guenther Hochhaus

Handbook of Methods in Gastrointestinal Pharmacology
Timothy S. Gaginella

Handbook of Targeted Delivery of Imaging Agents
Vladimir P. Torchilin

Handbook of Pharmacology of Aging, Second Edition
Jay Roberts, David L. Snyder, and Eitan Friedman

Handbook of Plant and Fungal Toxicants
J. P. Felix D'Mello

Handbook of Immunological Methods
Canadian Networking Toxicology Center

Handbook of Alcoholism
Gerald Zernig, Alois Saria, Martin Kurz, and Stephanie S. O' Malley

HANDBOOK OF
ALCOHOLISM

EDITED BY
Gerald Zernig, M.D.
Alois Saria, Ph.D.
Martin Kurz, M.D.
Stephanie S. O'Malley, Ph.D.

CRC Press
Boca Raton   London   New York   Washington, D.C.

Library of Congress Cataloging-in-Publication Data

Handbook of alcoholism / Gerald Zernig, editor-in-chief ; Alois Saria, Martin Kurz,
    Stephanie S. O'Malley, co-editors.
        p.   cm. — (Pharmacology and toxicology)
    Includes bibliographical references and index.
    ISBN 0-8493-7801-X (alk. paper)
    1. Alcoholism—Handbooks, manuals, etc. I. Zernig, Gerald, 1960– II. Saria, Alois.
III. Kurz, Martin, 1963– IV. O' Malley, Stephanie S. V. Pharmacology & toxicology (Boca
Raton, Fla)
    [DNLM: 1. Alcoholism—therapy. WM 274 H2355 2000]
RC565 .H245 2000
616.86¢1—dc21   99-053180
                                                         CIP

© 2000 by CRC Press LLC

No claim to original U.S. Government works
International Standard Book Number 0-8493-7801-X
Library of Congress Card Number 99-053180
Printed in the United States of America 1 2 3 4 5 6 7 8 9 0
Printed on acid-free paper

How You Can Benefit From This Handbook (... By Way of a Preface)

The overwhelming majority of problem drinkers (i.e., alcohol-abusing patients) and alcohol-dependent patients are first seen by physicians in general practice, in a primary care setting, or at nonpsychiatric inpatient facilities, such as departments of internal medicine or surgery. If you work in such a setting, this book is for you. It is my firm belief that comprehensive treatment of your alcohol-abusing or alcohol-dependent patient lies within your grasp and should, for that matter, ultimately lie in the hands of one therapist; this book will help you to acquire the necessary expertise to achieve this. You will, in all likelihood, find that you want to delegate some aspects of the medical care of your alcoholic patient to more specialized partners who might have more resources than you with respect to time, logistics, and specialized training. Still, it is you who can give crucial help to your patient who is experiencing alcohol-related problems, right from the first contact and interview. And, let's face it, you have to do it — you are the one your patient usually first contacts and not necessarily because he or she is aware of her/his alcohol problem. Not yet. With the help of this handbook, you will acquire the necessary skills to help him/her recognize the underlying alcohol problem. Two chapters (Chapter 1, First Contact and Early Intervention; Chapter 9, Psychotherapy) are dedicated to explaining which psychological problems you are most likely to encounter at every stage of the disease and how to best cope with the negative emotions that the alcohol-dependent patient — so severely affected by the disease — will most likely induce in you, his physician.

However, alcoholism is not restricted to underlying psychological problems. Alcohol damages a number of organs — and these somatic symptoms are very often those that actually bring the patient into your office. This handbook will help you to better diagnose and treat these nonpsychiatric medical disorders as well. The first section of this handbook, PATIENT CARE, describes the diagnosis and therapy of alcohol-induced somatic and psychiatric disorders.

In the second section of the handbook, RESEARCH, you will find review-like chapters on current issues in research on alcoholism. Again, emphasis is on the clinical aspects: epidemiology, comorbidity, heritability, psychometric instruments assessing treatment success, and meta-analysis of clinical trials, as well as patient-to-treatment matching. If you want to go deeper into basic science issues, this handbook offers chapters on the neurochemistry, histopathology, and behavioral pharmacology of alcoholism. Research on alcoholism, like any research into substance dependence (addiction), is jeopardized by moralizing and ideology or by ideas that are intellectually stimulating and attractive, but lack sufficient empirical evidence; thus, a chapter is dedicated to such controversial issues.

So, how many grams of alcohol to a can of beer? How much can somebody drink before exceeding the legal limit in your state? How much can someone drink before risking organ damage? What is the correct psychiatric definition of alcohol dependence? Where can that MAST test form be found for photocopying? You will find answers to these and other questions in the third and final section of this handbook, USEFUL DATA AND DEFINITIONS.

A final word on different psychotherapeutic approaches: please remember that the aim of this handbook is to help you obtain a helpful attitude toward the alcohol-dependent patient and explain his or her behavior in a way that opens new therapeutic perspectives for you. Trans-Atlantic differences in clinical traditions (i.e., the "behavioral-cognitive U.S." vs. the "psychoanalytic Central Europe") should not be of too much concern. Do not be disconcerted by skirmishes between the different psychotherapeutic "schools"; always ask yourself how you can make use of what each school has to offer. Remain open and eclectic when trying to help each patient, one at a time, each with his/her personal history and special needs. One of the great strengths of this handbook lies in the fact that both U.S. and European clinicians and researchers have contributed to it; make use of the different cultural approaches represented in this book and be flexible in adapting your own therapeutic approach to the special therapeutic setting in which you find yourself. Both "oversocialized institutionalization" and the "merciless kick 'em-out-quick" health care systems have their advantages and disadvantages. Use them in your patients' best interest.

The goal of this handbook is to provide you with everything (well, almost everything) you need in a book that you can hold in one hand. We truly hope that you like it so much that you consult it again and again. If we have forgotten something that you consider important, please let us know. My e-mail address is gerald.zernig@uibk.ac.at and my telephone number is +43-699-1714-1714. You can find my complete postal address in the contributor list. We really would like to hear from you — good or bad.

Gerald Zernig, M.D.
Editor-in-Chief

Dedication

A number of people have helped me to obtain the necessary competence to conceive and edit this handbook. Every one of them has furthered my education in her/his own special way. Dear friends, please allow me to thank you in this public way (and in temporal order). This book is dedicated to you.

My parents Horst and Gertrude, Oma, Karin (although she does not want me to) and her mother Erni; my kids Patrick and Bernhard (for having led the nomadic life with me and for being such great sons); my brother and his family, Karli and Margit Leyrer; Uncle Heri and Aunt Inge; Uncle Rudi, Uncle Herfried, and Aunt Hansi; Helmut Tritthart (for introducing me to science); Rob and Lynne MaLeod (for lifelong friendship and for introducing me to the American, sorry, Canadian way of life); Wolfgang Schreibmayer (for showing me how much fun tinkering in the lab can be, and for being Skipper Wolf); Fred Lembeck (for initiating my scientific adolescence and for watching over me in his quiet way) and the people in his lab; Rufina Schuligoi (for teaching me early on that psychology isn't bogus at all); Kypt Stoschitzky Moni and Monika (for being such great learning partners and loyal friends); Les and Sandy Bailey and Hali Hartmann; Hartmut Glossmann (for the good things he has done to me) and his crew; Alison Abbott (for being such a strict style teacher, for introducing me to a whole new world of science, scones, and everything British, and for putting up with my American accent); Ryan Huxtable (for whetting my appetite for addiction research); Hermann Dietrich (for teaching me so much about animal behavior and care); Uschi and Peter Schallert; Norbert Reider; Ruth Galvan; Gerda Topar; Martin and Thea Holtzhauer; the Mittelbauvertreter at the University of Innsbruck (for standing by me in hard times); Hans Tuppy; Sigurd Hoellinger (for seeing to it that things were done the right way in very emotional times); Hartmann Hinterhuber, W. Wolfgang Fleischhacker, and the members of the Akutstation (for allowing me to get my first whiff of psychiatric work and for many, many fruitful discussions); Sue Iversen; Jim Woods (for taking me into his lab and welcoming my family and me to the U.S., for teaching me most of what I know about behavioral pharmacology, for being such a generous supervisor, and for being a boss who came to help us to carry boxes); Gail Winger (for teaching me how to do i.v. self-admin and for being such a great style teacher); Eduardo and Kirsten Butelman (who, among other things, gave me my first subscription to *The New Yorker*); Beck Q.O.P. McLaughlin, the Woods Lab and Jim's friends — Charles France, Alice Young, Ellen Walker, Harriet deWit, Bill Woolverton, Bob Schuster; Pat Needle (for being such a great mother for us needy NIDA INVEST fellers), Ben Lucchesi and his Motley Crew, Ed Domino, Rick Neubig; Chris Fibiger (for taking me into his lab, for teaching me *in vivo* microdialysis, for very generously letting me do things that he was not really particularly interested in anymore, and for being such an excellent science, logics, and style teacher); Catriona Wilson, Matt Taber (among other things, for brewing that Hornikeivitz), Emmerich and Genevieve Ceschi (for helping us to feel right at home in Vancouver); Michael Lehofer, Norbert Kriechbaum, and Doris Hoenigl (for teaching me so much about psychotherapy, with special thanks to Norbert for his navigational skills); Hans-Georg Zapotoczky (for exposing me to psychiatric work); Konrad Schauenstein (for his support and very fruitful discussions); Regina Hutter (for being my first therapist and supervisor); Mannfred Hollinger (for picking me and whetting my appetite for this handbook); Hartmann Hinterhuber (for steering my little academic ship gently into a safe and productive harbor); the members of the Psychiatry Department at the University of Innsbruck (for taking me aboard); some officials of the University of Innsbruck (for watching over me and providing us with the operant conditioning set-up), and the members of the Saria lab for keeping up with me; Helmuth Provaznik (for showing me a whole new world); Brigitte (for her support and for being such a wonderful partner in our LATship); Lisa (for helping me to understand adolescence better); and Wuff (for tolerating the competitor for his mother's love in such a cavalier fashion). Last, but certainly not least, I would like to thank Luis and Astrid Saria, who have stood by me in very hard times, have tolerated my more expansive moods, and are such perfect hosts. Luis, thank you for talking science with me for over 20 years now and for managing the difficult task of being both my boss and my friend!

Gerald Zernig, M.D.

The Editors

Gerald Zernig, M.D., is Associate Professor in the Division of Neurochemistry, Department of Psychiatry, School of Medicine, University of Innsbruck, Austria. Born in 1960 in Hartberg, Austria, he obtained his medical degree in 1984 from the University of Graz, Austria. He worked as an Assistant Professor in the Department of Biochemical Pharmacology, University of Innsbruck, where he attended rounds at the Intensive Care Ward of the Department of Psychiatry (W. Wolfgang Fleischhacker and Hartmann Hinterhuber). He became Associate Professor in 1992. From 1992 to 1995, Dr. Zernig worked as a NIDA INVEST fellow and as an FWF Schroedinger Fellow with James H. Woods, Department of Pharmacology, University of Michigan, Ann Arbor, investigating the behavioral pharmacology of drug dependence. From 1995 to 1996, he worked with H. Christian Fibiger, Department of Psychiatry, University of British Columbia, Vancouver, Canada, on neuro-chemical and behavioral experiments on cocaine, heroin, and nicotine dependence. From 1996 to 1997, Dr. Zernig treated patients suffering from alcohol and/or other substance dependence and other psychiatric disorders at the Department of Psychiatry, University of Graz (Hans-Georg Zapotoczky). Upon his return to the University of Innsbruck, Dr. Zernig became a member of Alois Saria's Division of Neurochemistry. He contributes behavioral pharmacological experiments to the division's neurochemical investigations on neuropeptides and drugs of abuse; he is currently investigating the effect of alcohol on "Ecstasy" (MDMA) reinforcement.

Alois Saria, Ph.D., is Professor of Neurochemistry and Head of the Division of Neurochemistry, Department of Psychiatry, School of Medicine, University of Innsbruck. Born in Austria, he obtained his Ph.D. degree in 1979 from the University of Graz, Austria. He worked as Assistant Professor from 1979 to 1985 in the Department of Pharmacology and became Associate Professor in 1985. In 1987, he moved to Innsbruck to become head of the Division of Neurochemistry at the Department of Psychiatry. His research included molecular mechanisms of signal transduction with special emphasis on neuropeptides, psychoactive drugs, and narcotics. In 1993, the Institute of Scientific Information evaluated xenobiotics research (research about biological actions of exogenous compounds) and ranked Dr. Saria as number 17 of the top 50 "high-impact authors" worldwide (*Current Contents*, 3/1993, pp. 3–13) Trained as a biochemist, his clinical duties involve drug monitoring of antipsychotics and antidepressants. In 1998, Dr. Saria became full Professor of Neurochemistry. From 1982 to 1996, he carried out research at several institutions including the Karolinska Institute in Sweden, and facilities in the United States. In 1996, he was a Fulbright scholar and Burroughs Wellcome Visiting Professor at the Department of Anatomy and Neurobiology, University of Kentucky at Lexington. Dr. Saria is a member of the editorial board of the *European Journal of Pharmacology* and the *Journal of Neural Transmission.*

Martin Kurz, M.D., is Head Physician, Alcohol and Substance Dependence Therapy Unit, Department of Psychiatry, School of Medicine, University of Innsbruck. Born in 1963 in Innsbruck, Austria, he studied medicine at Graz and Innsbruck. After obtaining his medical degree in 1989, he joined the Department of Psychiatry, Innsbruck University Hospital, where he specialized in psychiatry and neurology. He was board-certified as a psychiatrist and neurologist in 1997. Dr. Kurz became a certified psychotherapist in 1997. Since 1997, he has been Head Physician at the Alcohol and Substance Dependence Therapy Unit, Innsbruck University Hospital.

Stephanie S. O'Malley, Ph.D., is Professor of Psychiatry and Director of the Division of Substance Abuse Research, Department of Psychiatry, School of Medicine, Yale University. Dr. O'Malley received her Ph.D. from Vanderbilt University and joined Yale University in 1984. Dr. O'Malley has contributed a number of seminal studies and research articles on the pharmacotherapy and psychotherapy of alcohol dependence, among them the "classic" on the combined use of psychotherapy and naltrexone (S. S. O'Malley, A. J. Jaffe, G. Chang, R. S. Schottenfeld, R. E. Meyer, and B. Rounsaville, Naltrexone and coping skills therapy for alcohol dependence. A controlled study. *Arch.Gen.Psychiatry* 49, 881–887, 1992).

Contributors

Elio Acquas, Ph.D.
Department of Toxicology
University of Cagliari and
Center for Neuropharmacology — CNR
V.le A. Diaz, 182,
I-09126 Cagliari
Italy
Tel: +39 70 303 819
Fax: +39 70 300 740
acquas@unica.it

John P. Allen, Ph.D.
Associate Director of Treatment Studies
Division of Clinical and Prevention Research
National Institute on Alcohol Abuse and
  Alcoholism (NIAAA)
6000 Executive Boulevard — Suite 505
Bethesda, MD 20892-7003
Tel: (301) 443-0633
Fax: (301) 443-8774
jallen@willco.niaaa.nih.gov

Hans J. Battista, M.D., Ph.D.
Head, Division of Chemistry and Toxicology
Department of Forensic Medicine
University of Innsbruck
Muellerstrasse 44
A-6020 Innsbruck
Austria
Tel: +43-512-507-3330
Fax: +43-512-507-2770
H-J.Battista@uibk.ac.at

Thomas Berger, M.D.
Department of Neurology
University of Innsbruck
Anichstrasse 35
A-6020 Innsbruck
Austria
Tel: +43-512-504-3860
Fax: +43-512-504-4260
thomas.berger@uibk.ac.at

Irene Berti, abs. med.
Andechsstrasse 40
A-6020 Innsbruck
Austria
irene.berti@uibk.ac.at

Lloyd Cantley, M.D.
Assistant Professor of Medicine
Beth Israel Deaconess Medical Center
Harvard Medical School
330 Brookline Avenue
Boston, MA
Tel: (617) 667-2147
Fax: (617) 667-5276
lcantley@caregroup.harvard.edu

Harriet de Wit, M.D.
Associate Professor of Psychiatry
Department of Psychiatry
University of Chicago
5841 S. Maryland Avenue MC3077
Chicago, IL 60637
Tel: (773) 702-1537
Fax: (773) 702-6454
hdew@midway.uchicago.edu

Rolf R. Engel, M.D.
Head, Division of Clinical Psychology and
  Psychophysiology
Department of Psychiatry
Ludwig-Maximilians–University of Munich
Nussbaumstrasse 7
D-80336 Munich
Germany
re@psy.med.uni-muenchen.de

Peter Fickert, M.D.
Division of Gastroenterology and Hepatology
Department of Internal Medicine
University of Graz
Auenbruggerplatz 15
A-8036 Graz
Austria
Tel: +43-316-385-2648

Hanspeter S. Fischer, Ph.D.
Division of Neurochemistry
Department of Psychiatry
University of Innsbruck
Anichstrasse 35
A-6020 Innsbruck
Austria
hanspeter.fischer@uklibk.ac.at

W. Wolfgang Fleischhacker, M.D.
Professor of Psychiatry
Head, Division of Biological Psychiatry
Department of Psychiatry
University of Innsbruck
Anichstrasse 35
A-6020 Innsbruck
Austria
Tel: +43-512-504-3669
Fax: +43-512-504-5267
wolfgang.fleischhacker@uibk.ac.at

Michael Fleming, M.D., MPH
Professor of Family Medicine
University of Wisconsin
777 S. Mills Street
Madison, WI 53715-1896
Tel: (608) 263-9953
Fax: (608) 263-5813
mfleming@smtp.fammed.wisc.edu

Richard K. Fuller, M.D.
Director, Division of Clinical and Prevention
  Research
National Institute on Alcohol Abuse and
  Alcoholism (NIAAA)
6000 Executive Boulevard — Suite 505
Bethesda, MD 20892-7003
Tel: (301) 443-0633
Fax: (301) 443-8774
rfuller@willco.niaaa.nih.gov

Alfred Grassegger, M.D.
Dermatologist (private practice)
Schubertstrasse 3
A-6020 Innsbruck
Austria
Tel./Fax: +43-512-5885570
a.grassegger@aon.at

Hartmann Hinterhuber, M.D.
Professor of Psychiatry
Chair, Department of Psychiatry
Head, Division of General Psychiatry
University of Innsbruck
Anichstrasse 35
A-6020 Innsbruck
Austria
Tel: +43-512-504-3630
Fax: +43-512-504-3644
hartmann.hinterhuber@uibk.ac.at

Sabine M. Hoelter, Ph.D.
Max-Planck-Institut fuer Psychiatrie
Kraepelinstrasse 10
D-80804 Muenchen
Germany

Michael Joannidis, M.D.
Nephrology Unit
Department of Internal Medicine
University of Innsbruck
Anichstrasse 35
A-6020 Innsbruck
Austria
michael.joannidis@uklibk.ac.at

Georg Kemmler, Ph.D.
Chief Statistician
Department of Psychiatry
University of Innsbruck
Anichstrasse 35
A-6020 Innsbruck
Austria
Tel: +43-512-504-3689
Fax: +43-512-504-3628
georg.kemmler@uklibk.ac.at

Jason R. Kilmer, Ph.D.
Postdoctoral Research Associate
Department of Psychology, Box 351525
University of Washington
Seattle, WA 98195-1525
jkilmer@u.washington.edu

Andrea C. King, Ph.D.
Assistant Professor of Psychiatry
Department of Psychiatry
University of Chicago
5841 S. Maryland Avenue, MC-3077
Chicago, IL 60637
Tel: (773) 702-6181
Fax: (773) 702-6454
aking@yoda.bsd.uchicago.edu

Guenther Konwalinka, M.D.
Associate Professor of Internal Medicine
Department of Internal Medicine
University of Innsbruck
Anichstrasse 35
A-6020 Innsbruck
Austria
guenther.konwalinka@uklibk.ac.at

Norbert Kriechbaum, M.D.
Registered Psychotherapist
Director, Adolescent Psychiatry Outpatient
  Clinic
Department of Psychiatry
University of Graz
Auenbruggerplatz 22
A-8036 Graz
Austria
Tel: +43-316-385-2188
Fax: +43-316-385-3556
norbert.kriechbaum@kfunigraz.ac.at

Suchitra Krishnan-Sarin, Ph.D.
Assistant Professor of Psychiatry
Substance Abuse Treatment Unit
Department of Psychiatry
School of Medicine
Yale University
1 Long Wharf Drive, Box 18
New Haven, CT 06511
Tel: (203) 789-6988
Fax: (203) 789-6990
suchitra.krishnan-sarin@yale.edu

Martin Kurz, M.D.
Psychoanalyst
Head Physician, Alcohol Dependence Therapy
  Unit
Therapie- und Gesundheitszentrum Mutters
Department of Psychiatry
University of Innsbruck
Nockhofweg 23
A-6162 Mutters
Austria
Tel: +43-512-548353-0
Fax: +43-512-548353-44
martin.kurz@uklibk.ac.at

Mary E. Larimer, Ph.D.
Research Assistant Professor
Associate Director, Addictive Behaviors
  Research Center
University of Washington
Department of Psychology, Box 351525
Seattle, WA 98195-1525
Tel: (206) 543-3513
larimer@u.washington.edu

Frank Majewski, M.D.
Professor
Department of Human Genetics and
  Anthropology
University of Duesseldorf
Moorenstrasse 5
D-40225 Duesseldorf
Germany
Fax: +49-211-811-2538

Linda Baier Manwell, Ph.D.
Deputy Director, UW Center for Addiction
  Research and Education
University of Wisconsin
777 S. Mills Street
Madison, WI 53715-1896
Tel: (608) 263-4550
Fax: (608) 263-5813
lmanwell@smtp.fammed.wisc.edu

Goetz Mundle, M.D.
Department of Psychiatry
Addiction Research Center
Osianderstrasse 24
72076 Tuebingen
Germany
Tel: +49 7071 29 82685
Fax: +49 7071 29 5384
goetz.mundle@uni-tuebingen.de

Barbara Obermayer-Pietsch, M.D.
Department of Endocrinology and Nuclear
  Medicine
University of Graz
Auenbruggerplatz 1
A-8036 Graz
Austria

Patrick G. O'Connor, M.D., M.P.H.
Department of Internal Medicine
Primary Care Center
Yale University School of Medicine
Suite A
333 Cedar Street
P.O. Box 208025
New Haven, CT 06520-8025
Tel: (203) 785-6532
Fax: (203) 737-4092
patrick.oconnor@yale.edu.

Stephanie S. O'Malley, Ph.D.
Professor of Psychiatry
Director, Division of Substance Abuse Research
Department of Psychiatry
Yale University School of Medicine
1 Long Wharf Box 18
New Haven, CT 06511
Tel: (203) 789-6988
Fax: (203) 789-6990
stepanie.omalley@yale.edu

Christoph Pechlaner, M.D.
Intensive Care Unit
Department of Internal Medicine
University of Innsbruck
Anichstrasse 35
A-6020 Innsbruck
Austria
christoph.pechlaner@uklibk.ac.at

Ulrich W. Preuss, M.D.
Department of Psychiatry
Ludwig-Maximilians-University of Munich
Nussbaumstrasse 7
D-80336 Munich
Germany
Tel: +49-89-5160-5740
Fax: +49-89-5160-5748
up@psy.med.uni-muenchen.de

Elisabeth Ratzenboeck, Cand. Med.
Kirchenstrasse 107
A-5723 Uttendorf
Austria
elisabethratzenboeck@hotmail.com

Norbert Reider, M.D.
Director, Allergy Outpatient Clinic
Department of Dermatology
University of Innsbruck
Anichstrasse 35
A-6020 Innsbruck
Austria
Tel: +43-512-504-2978
Fax: +43-512-504-4852
norbert.reider@uibk.ac.at

Alois Saria, D.I., Ph.D.
Professor of Neurochemistry
Head, Division of Neurochemistry
Department of Psychiatry
University of Innsbruck
Anichstrasse 35
A-6020 Innsbruck
Austria
Tel: +43-512-504-3710
Fax: +43-512-504-3716
alois.saria@uklibk.ac.at

Michael Schirmer, M.D.
Department of Internal Medicine
University of Innsbruck
Anichstrasse 35
A-6020 Innsbruck
Austria
Tel: +43-512-504-3255
Fax: +43-512-504-3415
michael.schirmer@uibk.ac.at

Claudia Schoechlin, Dipl.Psych.
Division of Clinical Psychology and
  Psychophysiology
Department of Psychiatry
Ludwig-Maximilians-University of Munich
Nussbaumstrasse 7
D-80336 Munich
Germany
Tel: +49-89-5160-3350
Fax: +49-89-5160-5562
claudia.schoechlin@psy.med.uni-muenchen.de

Rajita Sinha, Ph.D.
Associate Professor of Psychiatry
Program Director
Substance Abuse Treatment Unit
Connecticut Mental Health Center
Department of Psychiatry
Yale University
1 Long Wharf Drive, Box 18
New Haven, CT 06511
Tel: (203) 789-7387
Fax: (203) 789-6990
rajita.sinha@yale.edu

Michael Soyka, M.D.
Professor of Psychiatry
Department of Psychiatry
University of Munich
Nussbaumstrasse 7
D-80336 Muenchen
Tel: +49-89-5160-5324
Fax: +49-89-5160-5617
kyriaki@psy.med.uni-muenchen.de

Rainer Spanagel, Ph.D.
Max-Planck-Institut fuer Psychiatrie
Kraepelinstrasse 10
D-80804 Munich
Germany
Tel: +49-89-306-2228-8
Fax: +49-89-306-2256-9
spanagel@mpipsykl.mpg.de

Rudolf E. Stauber, M.D.
Associate Professor of Internal Medicine
Division of Gastroenterology and Hepatology
Chief Physician, Liver Outpatient Clinic
Department of Internal Medicine
University of Graz
Auenbruggerplatz 15
A-8036 Graz
Austria
Tel: +43-316-385-2863
Fax: +43-316-385-3062
rudolf.stauber@kfunigraz.ac.at

Friedhelm Stetter, M.D.
Associate Professor of Psychiatry and
  Psychotherapy
Chief Physician, Oberbergklinik Extertal
Brede 29
D-32699 Extertal
Germany
Tel: +49-5754-87-510
Fax: +49-5754-87-231
friedhelm.stetter@t-online.de
http://www.oberbergkliniken.de
http://www.medizin.uni-tuebingen.de/ukpp

Brigitte Stoschitzky
Registered Midwife
Suedtirolerplatz 1
A-6020 Innsbruck
Austria
Tel./Fax: +43-512-574782

Kurt Stoschitzky, M.D., FESC
Associate Professor of Cardiology
Division of Cardiology
Department of Medicine
Karl Franzens University
Auenbruggerplatz 15
A-8036 Graz
Austria
Tel: +43-316-385-2544
Fax: +43-316-385-3733
kurt.stoschitzky@kfunigraz.ac.at

Lisa Stoschitzky
Hofaeckergasse 12
A-8200 Gleisdorf
Austria

Monika Stoschitzky, M.D.
General Practitioner
Schillerstrasse 8
A-8200 Gleisdorf
Austria
Tel: +43-3112-7244

Christoph H. Stuppaeck, M.D.
Head, Department of Psychiatry 1
Christian Doppler Klinik
Ignaz-Harrerstrasse 79
A-5020 Salzburg, Austria
Tel: +43-662-4483-4300
Fax: +43-662-4483-4304
c.stuppaeck@lkasbg.gv.at

Paul C.C. Stuppaeck
Am Heuberg 26
A-5023 Salzburg
Austria

Michael Trauner, M.D.
Associate Professor of Internal Medicine
Division of Gastroenterology and Hepatology
Department of Internal Medicine
University of Graz
Auenbruggerplatz 15
A-8036 Graz
Austria
Tel: +43-316-385-2863 or 2648
Fax: +43-316-385-3062
michael.trauner@kfunigraz.ac.at

Peter A. Vanable, Ph.D.
Syracuse University
Department of Psychology
430 Huntington Hall
Syracuse, NY 13244-2340
Phone: (315) 443-1210
Fax: (315) 443-4123
pvanable@psych.syr.edu

Alexandra B. Whitworth, M.D.
Department of Psychiatry 2
Christian Doppler Klinik
Ignaz-Harrerstrasse 79
A-5020 Salzburg
Austria
Tel: +43-662-4483-0
Fax: +43-662-4483-4304
whitstup@ping.at

Christian Wiedermann, M.D.
Associate Professor of Internal Medicine
Department of Internal Medicine
University of Innsbruck
Anichstrasse 35
A-6020 Innsbruck
Austria
christian.wiedermann@uklibk.ac.at

Gail Winger, Ph.D.
Department of Pharmacology
University of Michigan
1301 Medical Science Research Building III
Ann Arbor, MI 48109
email: gwinger@umich.edu

Wie Mooi Wong, M.D.
Bad Aibling Health Clinic
Postfach 1425
D-83043 Bad Aibling
Germany
Tel: +49-8061-385791
up@psy.med.uni-muenchen.de

Kurt Zatloukal, M.D.
Division of Experimental Cell Research and
  Oncology
Department of Pathology
University of Graz
Auenbruggerplatz 25
A-8036 GRAZ
Austria
Tel: +43-316-380-4404
Fax: +43-316-384329
kurt.zatloukal@kfunigraz.ac.at

Gerald Zernig, M.D.
Associate Professor of Pharmacology
  and Toxicology
Division of Neurochemistry
Department of Psychiatry
University of Innsbruck School
  of Medicine
Anichstrasse 35
A-6020 Innsbruck
Tel: +43-699-1714-1714
Fax: +43-512-504-5866, -3716
gerald.zernig@uibk.ac.at

Table of Contents

SECTION I: PATIENT CARE

PART 1: SCREENING AND DIAGNOSIS

Chapter 1
First Contact and Early Intervention 5
Martin Kurz and Gerald Zernig

Chapter 2
Natural History 13
Mary E. Larimer and Jason R. Kilmer

Chapter 3
Laboratory Parameters 29
Alois Saria and Gerald Zernig

Chapter 4
Psychometric Screening Instruments 39
Peter A. Vanable, Andrea C. King, and Harriet de Wit

PART 2: ACUTE TREATMENT

Chapter 5
Acute Alcohol Intoxication 49
Christoph Pechlaner, Michael Joannidis, and Christian Wiedermann

Chapter 6
Alcohol Withdrawal Syndrome 65
Christoph H. Stuppaeck, Alexandra B. Whitworth, and Paul C.C. Stuppaeck

Chapter 7
Alcohol-Induced Psychotic Disorders 73
Michael Soyka

PART 3: TREATMENT OF ALCOHOL ABUSE AND DEPENDENCE

Chapter 8
Overview and Outlook 81
Stephanie S. O'Malley

Chapter 9
Psychotherapy 89
Friedhelm Stetter

Chapter 10
Pharmacotherapy..121 √
Gerald Zernig, Alois Saria, W. Wolfgang Fleischhacker, Martin Kurz, and
Hartmann Hinterhuber

Chapter 11
Adolescent Patients..129
Norbert Kriechbaum and Gerald Zernig

Chapter 12
Geriatric Patients..137
Goetz Mundle

PART 4: TREATMENT OF NON-PSYCHIATRIC ALCOHOL-RELATED DISORDERS

Chapter 13
Women..151
Rajita Sinha

Chapter 14
Primary Care Setting..165
Patrick G. O'Connor

Chapter 15
Nervous System ....173 √
Thomas Berger

Chapter 16
Liver ....183 √
Rudolf E. Stauber, Michael Trauner, and Peter Fickert

Chapter 17
Gastrointestinal System and Pancreas..195
Rudolf E. Stauber, Michael Trauner, and Peter Fickert

Chapter 18
Cardiovascular System..203 √
Kurt Stoschitzky

Chapter 19
Kidney and Electrolyte Disturbances ....209 √
Michael Joannids and Lloyd Cantley

Chapter 20

Immune System...225
Michael Schirmer, Christian Wiedermann, and Guenther Konwalinka

Chapter 21

Endocrine System 231
Michael Trauner, Barbara Obermayer-Pietsch, Peter Fickert, and Rudolf E. Stauber

Chapter 22

Vitamin Deficiencies, Zinc Deficiency, and Anaphylactic Reactions...........................239
Norbert Reider

Chapter 23

Skin...243
Alfred Grassegger

Chapter 24

Alcohol Embryopathy: Symptoms, Course, and Etiology...251
Frank Majewski

SECTION II: RESEARCH

Chapter 25

Epidemiology 271
Michael Fleming and Linda Baier Manwell

Chapter 26

Comorbidity 287
Ulrich W. Preuss and Wie Mooi Wong

Chapter 27

Heritability 305
Suchitra Krishnan-Sarin

Chapter 28

Pathogenesis of Alcoholic Liver Disease 317
Peter Fickert and Kurt Zatloukal

Chapter 29

Harmful Alcohol Consumption..325
Linda Baier Manwell and Michael Fleming

Chapter 30

Psychometric Instruments to Evaluate Outcome in Alcoholism Treatment 331
Andrea C. King, Peter A. Vanable, and Harriet de Wit

Chapter 31

Meta-analysis of Pharmacotherapeutic Trials...339

Claudia Schoechlin and Rolf R. Engel

Chapter 32

Meta-analysis Without Tears: a Step-by-Step Introduction 353

Georg Kemmler

Chapter 33

Patient-to-Treatment Matching 363

Richard K. Fuller and John P. Allen

Chapter 34

Molecular Pharmacology and Neuroanatomy 369

Elio Acquas

Chapter 35

Behavioral Pharmacology 385

Gail Winger

Chapter 36

Controversial Research Areas 401

Rainer Spanagel and Sabine M. Hoelter

SECTION III: USEFUL DATA AND DEFINITIONS

Chapter 37

Physicochemical Properties of Ethanol 417

Chapter 38

How to Calculate Maximum Blood Alcohol Levels after a Drinking Event 419

Gerald Zernig and Hans J. Battista

Chapter 39

Basic Pharmacokinetics of Alcohol...421

Gerald Zernig and Hans J. Battista

Chapter 40

Drug Interactions...425

Gerald Zernig and Hans J. Battista

Chapter 41

Definitions of a "Standard Drink"..429

Chapter 42

Harmful Daily Alcohol Consumption 431

Chapter 43

DSM-IV and ICD-10 Definitions of Alcohol Intoxication, Abuse, Dependence, and
  Withdrawal 433

Chapter 44

Alphabetical List of Psychometric Test Instruments 439

Chapter 45

Useful (Internet) Addresses 457

Chapter 46

Abbreviations Used..459

INDEX 463

Section I

Patient Care

Part 1

Screening and Diagnosis

1 First Contact and Early Intervention

Martin Kurz and Gerald Zernig

OVERVIEW

In this chapter you will find a list of patient- and illness-related data that you should gather during your first interview with the patient, as well as a short introduction on how you can motivate your patient to realize his/her problem drinking and accept treatment. Alcohol abuse and dependence distort the patient's inner life in a predictable manner. This chapter will alert you to some aspects of the patient's behavior that might be most stressful for you and will help you solve these conflicts in your daily professional life. Many of the issues in this introductory chapter will be discussed in detail in several of the following chapters. Please see the corresponding parts of this handbook for further information.

INTRODUCTION

This chapter focuses on the situation of health professionals who see themselves confronted with persons who complain about problems related to alcohol abuse or dependence for the first time in their lives. However, these patients are not aware that their problematic alcohol consumption is the cause of their complaints. Quite the contrary: often, as you will see, the patient has spent a considerable amount of mental energy to keep this realization from him/herself. Therefore, you may very often find yourself in a bad position: you must give the patient a diagnosis (i.e., substance abuse or dependence) that the patient absolutely refuses to accept for him/herself.

In the last decade, many efforts have been made to develop special intervention strategies and interview techniques aimed at reducing harm to the patient and at increasing the patient's motivation to seek specialized abstinence-oriented medical, psychological, and psychotherapeutic treatment facilities.[1] Evaluation studies showed good efficacy of these early intervention methods with respect to use of further treatment, harm reduction, and prognosis of the illness.[2-10] The psychological approach of these interventions is based on dependent behavior as a chronic illness rather than a weakness of character. Unfortunately, the belief that alcohol abuse and dependence represent a "lack of moral fiber" is still very common in our society (for detailed information, see Chapter 9 on psychotherapy). These early intervention methods have several basic attitudes and consequent communication strategies in common, which will be summarized in this chapter.

You do not need to convince your patient on the first interview. He will need time to accept his/her illness, to accept help, to realize the positive aspects of abstinence (or of a decrease in his/her alcohol consumption), and to develop the coping skills necessary to negotiate high-risk situations (e.g., social gatherings at which alcohol is repeatedly offered to him/her). The natural history of dependence disorders (see also Chapter 2 on natural history) shows that the course of the illness is very strongly linked to social and psychological developmental deficits and resources during an individual life course. The aim of every professional intervention is therefore to support the alcohol-dependent or -abusing individual in his/her personal efforts to change his/her addictive experience and behavior by strengthening his/her individual resources rather than confront the patient with his/her deficits, which the patient knows better than any of the involved health care professionals anyway. As alcohol dependence or abuse is a disorder with a strongly destructive potential in every aspect of the patient's life, it clearly makes sense to intervene as early as possible to reduce harm, even if the patient is, at the moment, unable to remain abstinent for a longer period of time. *Every* intervention in favor of a dependent individual becomes part of a positive development for this patient, even if the results are not as successful at the moment as professionals and patients might wish. Frustrations will be unavoidable on this long road to contented abstinence, but they can be minimized by knowing how to obtain and what to do with the specific information individuals provide us about their alcohol-dependence or -abuse problems.

DIAGNOSIS: MANY LEVELS OF CONCERN AT ONE GLANCE

During the initial interview, you have to be aware simultaneously of several levels of concern related to the disorder in order to get sufficient information for diagnosis. Along with questions aimed at psychiatric and alcohol-related phenomena, a somatic examination should be done. A routine laboratory investigation including red and white blood cell counts, liver enzymes, glucose, lipids and, if possible, a drug screening and CDT (carbohydrate-deficient transferrin) values are very useful to support the diagnosis (see also Chapter 3 on laboratory markers). Table 1.1 shows a summary of clinical signs indicating chronic elevated alcohol consumption in alcohol-abusing or -dependent individuals. For further informtion, please consult the respective chapters on non-psychiatric alcohol-related disorders.

Nevertheless, we would like to comment on some of the clinical signs mentioned above. There is an abundance of somatic signs of chronic alcohol abuse that you can either recognize at first glance or that the patient will report to you if asked specifically. Gastrointestinal and neurological disorders can be seen most frequently and are highly responsible for the increased mortality among patients.

Sexual dysfunctions (i.e., erectile impotence and loss of libido) are very common in alcohol-abusing patients. The patient suffers deeply from the psychological and relational consequences of these sexual dysfunctions. It may seem improper for you to ask the patient such intimate details. However, sexual dysfunctions might be perceived by the patient as a tremendous disability; it is very important for most of your patients that this severe problem is recognized and accepted as such by you.[12]

Acne rosacea (sometimes erroneously referred to as "facies ethylica," i.e., "alcoholic face") is not necessarily related to chronic abuse of alcohol (see Chapter 23 on dermatologic problems). Unfortunately, it is regarded by many clinicians as a "classical" sign of alcoholism and has thus often led to the mislabeling and stigmatization of non-alcohol-dependent patients as "alcoholics." Acne rosacea should only serve to remind you to check the patient thoroughly for other clinical signs of alcohol. It is not a proof for alcoholism. In any case, it can and should be treated properly (see Chapter 23 on skin).

Abusive or dependent behavior is the key criterion leading to diagnosis. You should also ask questions about other drug consumption; poly-drug use will complicate further treatment and is very common nowadays, especially among adolescents (see Chapter 11 on adolescent patients).

Comorbid depression is very common in alcohol-dependent individuals, especially in women. Sociophobia seems to be a specific male comorbid disorder. Suicidal behavior is very strongly associated with alcohol-related disorders. More detailed information about this very important issue is provided in Chapter 26.

Cognitive deficits[13] can lead to a kind of diffuse style of communication. Many patients suffer from feelings of stress and insufficiency that are caused by deficits in concentration and memory. These feelings, in turn, are likely to lead to alcohol intake again.

In the primary care setting, you will probably not see the more severe forms of alcohol-induced neuropsychiatric disorders (e.g., amnestic syndrome). These disorders are more likely to be encountered by the clinician in inpatient settings (e.g., departments of surgery or internal medicine). However, less severe neuropsychiatric disorders are very frequently seen.

TABLE 1.1
Summary of Common Alcohol-Specific Clinical Signs

Somatic signs and frequent complaints of the patients
- General
  - Reduced somatic condition
  - Reduced appetite, malnutrition, weight loss
  - Bad teeth
  - Frequent inflammatory diseases
  - Actual or past tuberculosis
  - Scars and other signs of frequent accidents (rib fractures, head injuries)
  - Cigarette burns on fingers
  - Dupuytren's disease[11]
  - Loss of libido, erectile impotence
  - Insomnia
  - Excessive sweating
  - "Nervousness"
- Neurologic
  - Reduced sensation in the lower extremities
  - Burning pain in the feet
  - Gait disturbances
  - Dysarthric speech
  - Muscular atrophy (especially in the lower extremities)
  - History of epileptic seizures
- Gastrointestinal
  - Nausea and vomiting, especially in the morning
  - Diarrhea
  - Duodenal and gastric ulcera, history of related internal or surgical treatment
  - Enlargement of the liver
  - Signs of hepatic failure (e.g., hyperbilirubinemia, coagulopathy, edema, ascites)
  - Red nose (acne rosacea), red skin of the face
  - Teleangiektasias, spider angiomas, palmar erythema (as a sign of hepatic failure)
- Diagnostic criteria of abuse or dependence, mainly
  - Signs of intoxication
  - Increased tolerance
  - Loss of control in alcohol consumption
  - Withdrawal signs (tremor, restlessness, sweating)
  - History of abuse of or dependence on other drugs (e.g., benzodiazepines, cannabinoids, stimulants)
- Comorbidity, psychiatric symptoms and complications
  - Depression, present or past suicidal behavior
  - Anxiety disorders (panic disorder, sociophobia, generalized anxiety disorder)
  - Personality disorders (antisocial, borderline)
  - Use of alcohol as self-medication
  - Cognitive deficits (concentration difficulties, impaired short-term memory)
  - Serious neuropsychiatric complications (delirious/psychotic states, amnestic syndrome)
- Laboratory parameters
  - Increased gamma-glutamyl-transpeptidase (GGT)
  - Increased mean corpuscular volume (MCV)
  - Increased carbohydrate-deficient-transferrin (CDT)
  - Anemia
  - Thrombocytopenia
- Social consequences concerning
  - Family life and other relationships
  - Imminent or actual unemployment

TABLE 1.1 (continued)
Summary of Common Alcohol-Specific Clinical Signs

– Legal problems (violence)
– Loss of driver's license
– Imminent or actual homelessness

Elevated levels of GGT, MCV, and CDT as alcohol-specific laboratory markers strongly support the diagnosis.

The social consequences of alcoholism are clearly stronger motivational factors than health problems to get in touch with health or social professionals. Therefore, special attention should be drawn to this complex issue. During initial contact, it is not necessary to ask for all social problems in detail. However, a few direct questions concerning possible problem areas will contribute substantially to the clinician's knowledge of the patient.

Last but not least, questions concerning how the patient got to this first interview can give hints about the psychosocial background of the patient.

Please note that there is also the possibility of overreporting somatic complaints by the patient trying to distract the clinician's attention away from his/her alcohol problem. Chronic intoxication is followed by a serious self-neglect of the patient that may lead to an underreporting of symptoms possibly related to serious disorders as well.

THE UNBEARABLE DIAGNOSIS

The main problem in conducting an interview to get indications of the origin of alcohol-related phenomena is the fact that every question is possibly perceived by the patient as an offense and a condemnation of his/her "bad habits." Thus, as much as alcohol consumption accompanies every conceivable social event, as condemned are those who become dependent on this substance. However, the harshest and most devaluating judges of their illness are the patients themselves. Consequently, your interest in the patient and his/her problems is often misinterpreted by the patient as an inquisitory act that can destroy what little self-esteem he might have left. Patients are not able to accept either the, as they perceive it, incriminating diagnosis of alcoholism or the long-term consequences of such a diagnosis at the moment of first contact. Apart from their low self-esteem, the psychological aspects of the disease itself (i.e., alcohol dependence) make it nearly impossible for the patient to change his/her attitudes. Abstinence can be perceived as a loss that cannot be accepted without feelings of serious despair, anxiety, or aggression. These are the main causes for defense mechanisms and the resulting specific communication problems in the first contact situation. The most common defense mechanisms are *denial, rationalization,* and *projection.* These mechanisms must be understood as protective efforts to keep away feelings of guilt, shame, total submission to significant others (including you as the therapist), or defeat. Nevertheless, it is very difficult for the professional to interpret these phenomena in this way when confronted with an annoyed, angry, and "obviously lying" patient, who rejects all his/her efforts to find a basis of cooperation. If you, for example, find yourself, against your original intentions, in the role of a prosecutor arguing with your patient if the amount of alcohol he reports to have drunk might be plausible or not, you know for sure that you are fighting with the patient's defense mechanisms rather than strengthening his/her motivation toward further treatment. These dynamics are very common in first contact situations, and it can be very frustrating for the professional to be rejected in his/her therapeutic efforts. The clinician is now confronted with his/her own feelings of anger and resignation; as an unintended — and certainly counterproductive — reaction, he might deepen his/her belief that the patient does not want to change anything and the patient's motivation is too low to warrant further therapeutic help.

TABLE 1.2
The Three Goals of Motivational Intervention Strategies

1. Motivate the patient to accept treatment (short-term goal); treatment motivation is proportional to the
   - Extent of suffering
   - Likelihood of success
   - Practicability (amount of subjective costs).
2. Motivate the patient to become and remain abstinent (abstinence motivation; long term).
3. Motivate the patient to change his/her lifestyle (long term).

MOTIVATION AS A DYNAMIC PRINCIPLE

The principle of motivation has been controversial in the past. Nowadays, motivation is defined as a dynamic process that can change over time and can be successfully supported even when it seems to be very low (for detailed information, see Chapter 9). At the time of first contact, being confronted with an "unthinkable" and "unmentionable" fact, your patients simply cannot show sufficient motivation toward long-term abstinence or far-reaching changes in their lifestyles, although many of them know that these consequences may be the only possibility to recover from their bad situation.

Abstinence or dramatic changes in lifestyle are distant or very frightening goals for the patient. Thus, in order to break the overall task into manageable bits, you should seek out, identify, and strengthen the following aspects of the patient's motivation (Table 1.2): motivation to accept treatment in the first place, motivation to become abstinent, and motivation to initiate major changes in his/her lifestyle.[14,15]

From this point of view, it is easy to conclude that the main goal of early intervention is to motivate the patient to undergo further treatment. Clinical experience corroborates that serious suffering from alcohol-related disturbances is often not motivating enough to change addictive attitudes and behavior. There has to be a hope for the patient that the treatment possibilities offered or recommendations made by you can provide a chance for him/her to improve his/her condition. The third factor determining treatment motivation includes the actual subjective costs (material, personal, and social) that arise when the patient accepts further therapy. Thus, it has to be the main therapeutic effort to reach the patient in his/her suffering and to set up an atmosphere of trust and support that gives him/her the opportunity to leave his/her defense behind, at least for a certain period of time.

INTERVIEW TECHNIQUE

Table 1.3 shows the basic principles that should be followed during the initial interview.[14-17]

It is very difficult, even for clinicians trained in this technique for years, to maintain this high level of communication style throughout the interview, especially if an emotionally charged atmosphere develops. In this situation, the challenge for you is to avoid incapacitating the patient by authoritarian impulses on your side on the one hand and to shrink from potential conflicts on the other hand. Be aware that avoiding potential conflicts (e.g., by not confronting the patient with the significance of the clinical signs of chronic harmful alcohol consumption that you just detected on him/her) does not help the patient. Quite the contrary, it is really a disregard of the patient's cry for help. To be a realistic counterpart to the patient and to give him/her the impression of being accepted at the same time is a challenging goal, that will often not be rewarded with instant success. The success of your future first interviews will be variable, and the patient's reaction can range from leaving without any obvious consequences to showing first attempts to reduce alcohol consumption, by getting in contact with specialized treatment facilities for an abstinence-oriented therapy.

TABLE 1.3
Suggested Interview Technique

- Show an empathic, optimistic, and supportive attitude toward the patient (e.g., "From what you have told me and from what the lab tests show, I can understand why you feel pretty badly right now…, but there are a lot of options for you to get better…").
- Let the patient tell his/her story in his/her own words first.
- Summarize with the patient, give neutral feedback (e.g., "So, if I have understood you correctly, you have trouble making it to work on Mondays because of bodily complaints that may have been worsened by your drinking…").
- Check to see if you are avoiding annoying topics (i.e., social problems, amount of alcohol consumed).
- Ask questions in an interested and concerned manner.
- Confront the patient with your perceptions, for example, by giving clear information about the diagnostic indicators you collected (e.g., "I have found several spider naevi on your chest; your liver is enlarged. Very often, these clinical signs indicate liver damage and most often this type of liver damage is due to too much drinking. Do you have problems with your drinking?")
- At the same time, give specific advice on realistic treatment goals and how to reach them (e.g., reduce alcohol consumption, seek hospital admission, join a self-help group, seek admission in a specialized treatment facility, etc.).
- Recommend different treatment strategies and facilities.
- Let the patient make his/her own decision concerning the next steps.

CONCLUSION

Dependence disorders are chronic disorders showing considerable variation with respect to the point in time at which the patient is able to accept treatment. There is evidence, however, that empathic and caring attitudes toward patients with alcohol problems during the initial interview result in better acceptance of treatment and, ultimately, in better outcome results than strict confrontative strategies did in the past. Even if the professional's efforts do not seem to be instantaneously successful in some cases, a first step is taken toward a change in the future. It is never too late to try to find the right moment together with our patients.

REFERENCES

1. Miller, W.R., What motivates people to change? *Motivational Interviewing: Preparing People to Change Addictive Behavior*, Miller, W.R. and Rollnick, S., Eds., Guilford Press, New York, 1991.
2. Kristenson, H., Ohlin, H., Hulten-Nosslin, M. B., Trell, E., and Hood, B., Identification and intervention of heavy drinking in middle-aged men: results and follow-up of 24-60 months of long-term study with randomized controls, *Alcohol Clin. Exp. Res.*, 7(2), 203, 1983.
3. Chick, J., Early intervention for hazardous drinking in the general hospital, *Alcohol Alcohol. (Suppl.)*, 1, 477, 1991.
4. Nilssen, O., The Tromso Study: identification of and a controlled intervention on a population of early-stage risk drinkers, *Prev. Med.*, 20, 518, 1991.
5. Richmond, R., Heather, N., Wodak, A., Kehoe, L., and Webster, I., Controlled evaluation of a general practice-based brief intervention for excessive drinking, *Addiction*, 90, 119, 1995.
6. A cross-national trial of brief interventions with heavy drinkers. WHO Brief Intervention Study Group, *Am. J. Public Health*, 86, 948, 1996.
7. Fleming, M. F., Barry, K. L., Manwell, L. B., Johnson, K., and London, R., Brief physician advice for problem alcohol drinkers. A randomized controlled trial in community-based primary care practices, *JAMA*, 277, 1039, 1997.
8. Senft, R. A., Polen, M. R., Freeborn, D. K., and Hollis, J. F., Brief intervention in a primary care setting for hazardous drinkers, *Am. J. Prev. Med.*, 13, 464, 1997.
9. Welte, J. W., Perry, P., Longabaugh, R., and Clifford, P. R., An outcome evaluation of a hospital-based early intervention program, *Addiction*, 93, 573, 1998.

10. Tomson, Y., Romeslo, A., and Aberg, H., Excessive drinking — brief intervention by a primary health care nurse. A randomized controlled trial, *Scand. J. Health Care*, 16, 188, 1998.

11. Attali, P., Ink, O., Vernier, C., Jean, F., Moulton, L., and Etienne, J. P., Dupuytren's contracture, alcohol consumption, and chronic liver disease, *Arch. Intern. Med.*, 147, 1065, 1987.

12. O'Farrell, T. J., Kleinke, C. L., and Cutter, H. S., Sexual adjustment of male alcoholics: changes from before to after receiving alcoholism counseling with and without marital therapy, *Addict. Behav.,* 23, 419, 1998.

13. Knight, R. G. and Longmore, B. E., *Clinical Neuropsychology of Alcoholism*, Lawrence Erlbaum Associates, Hove Hillsdale, 1994.

14. Schwoon, D. R., Motivierende Interventionen bei Suchtkranken, *Moderne Suchtmedizin. Diagnostik und Therapie der somatischen, psychischen und sozialen Syndrome,* Goelz, J., Ed., Georg Thieme Verlag, New York, 1998.

15. Rosenstock, I.M., The health belief model and preventive health behavior, *Hlth. Educ. Monogr.,* 354, 1974.

16. Mann, K. and Guenthner A., Suchterkrankungen, *Psychiatrie und Psychotherapie*, Berger, M., Ed., Urban & Schwarzenberg, Muenchen, 1999.

17. Senay, E. C., Diagnostic interview and mental status examination, *Substance Abuse. A Comprehensive Textbook*, Lowinson J. H., Ruiz, P., Millman, R. B., and Langrod, J. G., Eds., Williams & Wilkins, Baltimore, 1997.

2 Natural History

Mary E. Larimer and Jason R. Kilmer

OVERVIEW

Conclusions drawn about the natural history of alcohol problems are influenced by the populations studied as well as the research methods used. Early retrospective studies of populations in treatment suggested a chronic, progressive course with average age of onset in the late teens. However, longitudinal studies indicate that the highest incidence of alcohol problems is in early adulthood, with onset in the mid-teen years, and that the majority of these early problems remit over time. Alcohol problems present in middle age are more likely to become chronic, even if onset is recent. Factors that predict both development of and persistence of alcohol problems include comorbid psychiatric conditions (particularly conduct disorder/antisocial personality disorder), early age of onset of drinking, and to some extent family history. The majority of individuals with alcohol problems never seek treatment, and those who do wait more than 10 years on average from onset of symptoms to first attempt at treatment. However, many individuals with alcohol problems recover without formal treatment.

INTRODUCTION

Describing the natural history of alcoholism is a difficult endeavor. The conclusions drawn about time course, progression, chronicity, and remission are heavily influenced by the study sample (age, gender, cohort, treatment or population-based, volunteers or randomly selected representative sample), the design of the research (cross-sectional or longitudinal, retrospective or prospective), and the choice of instruments and diagnostic criteria employed.[1] In part, these difficulties in generalizing from one sample or research strategy to another appear to reflect the fact that alcohol problems, and the people experiencing them, may be more heterogeneous than homogeneous. Thus, it may be easier to answer the question "what is the likely course of problems for this particular patient (or type of patient)?" than it is to answer the question "what is the likely course of alcohol problems for the average patient?" However, limitations specific to certain commonly used research strategies also contribute to the variety of conflicting research findings in this area of study.[1,2]

We begin this chapter with a general overview of the different approaches that have been used to study the natural history of alcohol problems, and discuss the strengths and weaknesses of these approaches. We then review the literature relevant to onset of drinking, adolescent alcohol problems, continuation of alcohol problems into adulthood, progression vs. remission of adult drinking problems, and predictors of treatment seeking or remission without formal treatment. At each stage we discuss findings emerging from different research designs, and highlight areas of agreement as well as areas where additional research is needed to resolve discrepancies. It is hoped that this information will provide a useful guide for clinicians in understanding and predicting the likely course of problems for their patients, and developing appropriate prevention and treatment plans.

RESEARCH DESIGN ISSUES

The earliest studies of the natural history and course of alcohol problems were based on the retrospective accounts of patients with severe alcohol use disorders. Upon entering treatment or during the course of their recovery, these patients were asked to retrospectively recall how their problems with alcohol misuse began. These early studies, although largely descriptive, had a major influence on contemporary conceptualizations of alcohol problems, particularly involving the chronic and progressive nature of alcoholism.[3,4] More recent studies using this approach have investigated the onset, progression, and clustering of various symptoms of alcohol abuse and dependence, the relationship between alcohol abuse and dependence, the temporal relationship between comorbid psychiatric diagnoses and alcohol diagnoses, and a host of other "natural history" phenomena.

There are, of course, considerable advantages to this method of inquiry. Since only subjects who already have the disorder are included, the sample sizes do not have to be as large as a population-based survey. The assessment can often be conducted during a single session using interview or paper and pencil instruments, and yet can yield information about the development of problems over a long period of time prior to the patient entering treatment.

Unfortunately, retrospective studies of treatment populations have several disadvantages for the study of natural history. The first is that patients in treatment for alcohol problems may not be representative of the broader population of individuals with alcohol problems in the community. In fact, as many researchers have demonstrated, a variety of factors in addition to the severity of one's alcohol misuse may contribute to entering treatment.[5,6] A related concern is that retrospective reports by patients in treatment for alcohol problems likely lead to a substantial overestimation of the progressive nature of these disorders; by definition, only those whose alcohol problems progressed to a serious level are included in the sample.[2,7] Finally, retrospective reporting, particularly over a long time period, may be influenced by problems with recall and may also lead to overestimates of the orderly progression of symptoms due to the patient's attempts to understand and describe the development of his or her current problems.[1,8]

One advance in retrospective accounts of patients in treatment is to include a nontreated comparison group drawn from a similar population. Several researchers have used variants of this procedure for assessing the differences in natural history between treated and untreated samples.[2] In addition, several large-scale epidemiological surveys have used representative community samples to retrospectively assess both current and past (lifetime) alcohol use, alcohol abuse or dependence, and often other comorbid psychiatric conditions.[9-13] These studies represent a significant advance over studies of treated samples alone, and yield much better information about prevalence rates and comorbidity in the general population. Unfortunately, these studies are still limited by retrospective recall bias. In addition, the unavoidable confound between age and cohort effects in these samples limits the conclusions that can be made about the course of alcohol problems across the lifespan.[9]

Longitudinal prospective studies of the course of alcohol problems in community-based samples would address many of the limitations of these retrospective approaches. However, due to the prohibitive expense associated with conducting true longitudinal epidemiological studies, few of these have been conducted in the alcohol field. The majority of prospective studies that have been conducted have been of relatively short duration, and there were often sampling limitations. These include a narrowed age range (such as a focus on school-aged or college-aged adolescents, older adults, or other special populations), nonrepresentative samples, and sample sizes too small to analyze higher-order interactions between various predictors of alcohol problems. Many longitudinal studies address some of these concerns,[1,8,14-16] but often at the expense of other design limitations.

Despite limitations, the information gained from these rare long-term longitudinal studies is extremely valuable in understanding the development and course of alcohol problems. When combined with other sources of data from retrospective studies of treatment and community samples, it is possible to draw some conclusions regarding the natural history of alcohol problems, or more appropriately, the variety of "natural histories" that one might encounter. This information is reviewed in the subsequent sections of this chapter.

ONSET OF ALCOHOL USE AND ABUSE

Alcohol use among adults in the U.S. is a common behavior. In the latest Household Survey on Drug Abuse,[17] more than 80% of the adult U.S. population (over age 18) reported lifetime alcohol use, and approximately 60% reported using alcohol in the past year. These results are similar to those obtained in other large-scale epidemiologic studies of U.S. drinking patterns.[9,11-13] Alcohol use by adolescents is also common in the U.S. and other Western societies (see also Chapter 11 on special therapeutic considerations concerning adolescents). Numerous studies report initiation of alcohol use by adolescents as young as 9 or 10 years,[18] and by age 14, 65 to 70% of adolescents in the U.S. have used alcohol at least occasionally.[19] In the most recent wave of data from the Monitoring the Future survey, 70% of 8th grade students (age 14), 84% of 10th grade students (age 16), and 88% of 12th grade students (age 18) reported lifetime use of alcohol. Episodes of heavy drinking (consumption of 5 or more drinks at least once in the past 2 weeks) were also common; 15% of 8th grade students, 25% of 10th grade students, and 31% of 12th grade students reported this drinking pattern.

The experience of at least some alcohol-related negative consequences is also normative among adolescents. Cross-sectional studies indicate the prevalence of alcohol-related negative consequences among adolescents ages 12 to 18 ranges from 25% to more than 50%, depending on the type of consequence. These consequences include social difficulties, academic problems, minor health consequences, such as hangovers and nausea, as well as such risky behavior as driving while intoxicated.[17]

Although the experience of negative consequences and the diagnosis of alcohol abuse are fairly common among drinking adolescents, alcohol dependence is a relatively rare phenomenon. One U.S. study, using a proxy measure of alcohol dependence based on symptoms from the National Household Survey[19] found only 3% of adolescents ages 12 to 17 met DSM-IV criterion for alcohol dependence.[20]

Several demographic, environmental, behavioral, and genetic factors have been investigated as predictors of alcohol abuse and dependence among adolescents. Factors that appear to predict adolescent problem drinking (including abuse and dependence) are earlier age of onset of drinking,[20,28] the co-occurrence of other psychiatric disorders (particularly mood disorders[22,23] and early conduct problems[1,21]), family instability or conflict,[1] and to a lesser extent family history of alcohol problems.[24] Peer norms supporting deviant behavior and heavy drinking are also implicated in predicting adolescent alcohol problems.[25-28] Not surprisingly, many of these risk factors tend to co-occur.[27-29] Research indicates that these risk factors can have both direct effects on problems related to drinking, as well as indirect effects through promoting heavier consumption which then leads to problems.[30] In addition, multiple risk factors can produce interactive effects, increasing the odds of developing alcohol problems.[28,30]

Of all the risk factors for onset of adolescent alcohol problems, early history of problem behaviors (particularly conduct disorder) seems to be the most robust predictor across multiple studies using many different samples and research strategies.[1,8,21,25-28,31] Longitudinal studies, as well as retrospective studies, suggest conduct problems precede the development of alcohol problems among adolescent populations.[1,21,23,25-27] For example, White, Johnson, and Garrison found the relative odds of comorbid substance use with delinquency to be 1.8 for 15-year-old boys and 2.1 for 15-year-old girls.[78] There is a less clear relationship between alcohol problems and other comorbid psychiatric disorders. Retrospective studies tend to suggest that anxiety largely precedes the development of alcohol or other substance use problems in adolescents, and depression often precedes alcohol problems.[22,23] However, longitudinal studies conducted by Vaillant[1,8] suggest depression and anxiety disorders are more the result of, rather than the cause of, alcohol problems, as does the work of Fillmore and colleagues.[15,16]

Age of onset of drinking, and the age at first intoxication, are also strongly correlated with problem drinking during adolescence.[10,24] For example, Fergusson and colleagues[28] found that the best predictor of problem alcohol use at age 16 was the highest amount of alcohol consumed by age 14. However, quantity and frequency of drinking per se are not as strongly linked to the development of abuse or dependence as is age of onset. The correlation between amount of drinking and drinking problems only ranges from 0.30 to 0.60,[32] suggesting other personal or environmental factors play an important role in determining which drinkers will develop problems related to their drinking.

Estimates of the typical age at which the first symptoms of an alcohol use disorder develop vary as a function of the type of research strategy employed. Most retrospective studies indicate that onset is typically during late adolescence or early adulthood. For example, in Shuckit and colleagues'[2] retrospective analysis of 478 alcohol-dependent individuals and 444 drinking but not dependent individuals, they found alcohol-dependent participants typically reported their age at first symptom to be between 19 and 20 years. Buckholz and colleagues,[33] in their retrospective account of symptom progression among clinical, family, and community samples of alcohol-dependent individuals, found first symptoms reported at approximately age 17. Recent surveys of adolescents and young adults, both in treatment and community samples, suggest the average age of onset of first symptoms of an alcohol use disorder is earlier in adolescence, approximately age 14.[20,28,34] As these findings illustrate, the percentage of adolescents experiencing alcohol problems and the average age of onset of drinking in studies of adolescent users reflects earlier and more problematic use than is found in most retrospective studies of the general adult population. This may be the result of a true cohort effect, with younger cohorts somewhat more likely to drink and to progress to alcohol abuse than are older cohorts. This is supported by results of the National Longitudinal Alcohol Epidemiological Survey,[9] a large-scale cross-sectional study of alcohol use in a representative national sample of 42,862 participants, representing age cohorts from 18 to 70 years. Grant found that individuals in the youngest cohort (age 18 to 24) were more likely to drink, drink heavily, and develop alcohol abuse or dependence. He also found more rapid progression from onset of drinking to onset of problems in the younger cohorts. This is somewhat in contrast to the work of Fillmore and colleagues[15,16] who found only limited indication of cohort effects in their earlier longitudinal studies. Observed discrepancies between age cohorts could also reflect the increased mortality rate of individuals with serious alcohol problems, such that members of the older cohorts who experienced early alcohol problems are more likely to die at a younger age, and therefore fewer surviving members of older cohorts report early drinking problems.[8,15] Finally, the increased numbers of adolescents reporting alcohol abuse in concurrent or longitudinal, rather than retrospective, studies may represent a recall or reporting bias, as individuals whose alcohol abuse is far in the past may be less likely to recall or report it than individuals whose drinking problems are more recent.

Despite differences in the age of onset of symptoms based on cohort effects or research methodology employed, the progression of symptoms (among those subjects whose symptoms do worsen) appears from most retrospective studies to be remarkably similar. For example, based on mean age at which symptoms develop, Schuckit and colleagues[2] found alcohol-dependent individuals are most likely to report first experiencing increasingly heavy alcohol use and minor social consequences such as fights or arguments, with typical onset in their late teens to early 20s. Throughout their mid- to late 20s they report progressing to more serious social and occupational disruption, including minor legal difficulties. Finally, during their late 20s to mid-30s on average, these individuals report experiencing more severe health, marital, employment, or legal difficulties. Severe withdrawal symptoms such as delirium tremens appear very late in this progression, and many individuals who meet criteria for alcohol dependence never report experiencing these symptoms. Other researchers report similar findings using retrospective mean-age estimates.[33,35] However, these studies are limited in that the mean age at which symptoms appear is only calculated for those subjects who actually experience a symptom. In a recent survival-hazard analysis of symptom progression among individuals in treatment for alcohol problems,[7] it was found that mean age estimates were good predictors of symptom progression for frequently experienced symptoms, but presented a more linear picture of symptom development than was supported by the study. This discrepancy results in part because some symptoms are rarely experienced (and only very late in the development of the disorder), but those who do experience them have the most severe problems overall, and therefore an earlier age of onset of these rare symptoms.

Although the progression of symptoms appears to be fairly orderly for those individuals who eventually develop alcohol abuse or dependence, the experience of early or mild symptoms cannot be used to predict the onset of adult dependence. Instead, many alcohol-related problems are commonly reported by non-dependent drinking individuals as well as dependent drinking individuals,[2] and appear at a similar age, suggesting the mere presence of these early symptoms does not necessarily indicate a progressive alcohol use disorder.

CONTINUATION OF ALCOHOL PROBLEMS INTO ADULTHOOD

In fact, although alcohol use and negative consequences of drinking are relatively common in adolescence and early adulthood, longitudinal research and population-based studies suggest that only about 20 to 30% of individuals who report early alcohol problems continue to have problems into adulthood.[9,16,36] For example, even in the age group with the highest rate of lifetime dependence (ages 18 to 24), only about 20% of those with a lifetime dependence diagnosis in Grant's[9] sample met DSM-IV criteria for current dependence. This is a much different conclusion than that reached by earlier retrospective studies of treatment populations, and suggests that early problems with alcohol are a relatively poor predictor of long-term drinking patterns, problems, or alcohol dependence.[37] Both cross-sectional and longitudinal studies indicate that alcohol abuse, alcohol dependence, and heavy drinking are most common among younger individuals.[1,9,11,12,15,16,22] Factors predicting the continuation of adolescent alcohol problems into early adulthood are in many ways similar to those that predict the initial development of adolescent alcohol problems. In particular, a history of conduct problems or antisocial personality disorder consistently emerges as a predictor of the continuation of adolescent alcohol problems into adulthood.[1,22,29] Early age of onset of drinking and alcohol problems also predicts continuation of adolescent problems into adulthood.[10,38] For example, using retrospective reports, Grant and Dawson[10] found the risk of developing alcohol dependence at some point in adulthood decreased 8 to 14% per year as age of onset of drinking increased from 12 to 20 years of age, approximately 40% of individuals who began drinking at age 12 or younger met DSM-IV lifetime criteria for dependence. Similarly, Kandel and Logan[39] found the highest risk of developing alcohol dependence at some point in life occurred for those individuals who initiate drinking prior to age 18, and that after age 20, the risk diminishes significantly. Therefore, although adolescent drinking behavior does not necessarily predict later problems, abstinence during adolescence may be a protective factor for reducing risks of problem alcohol use. Other co-occurring psychiatric conditions, such as depression, are somewhat weaker predictors of continuation of problems. Just as quantity and frequency of alcohol use are not good predictors of concurrent alcohol diagnoses, they are also not particularly strong predictors of continuation of alcohol problems into adulthood.

CHRONICITY OF ADULT ALCOHOL PROBLEMS
ACROSS THE LIFESPAN

Early retrospective studies of alcoholics in treatment indicated that adult alcohol problems were both progressive and chronic. These types of studies generally found that symptoms worsened over time as long as the individual continued to drink, and that once a diagnosis of alcohol dependence was made, the disorder would continue until drinking was arrested by treatment, incarceration, occasionally by spiritual conversion, or by death.

This presumption of progression and chronicity of alcohol problems underlies many of the common models of alcoholism and alcohol treatment, particularly the Twelve-Step and disease models.[4] However, epidemiological data, as well as longitudinal data about the natural history of alcohol problems, largely fails to support these presumptions. Arguably, the two best data sources for addressing the question of chronicity are the longitudinal samples followed by Vaillant,[1,8] and the combined longitudinal and cohort studies reported by Fillmore and colleagues.[16,37]

Vaillant and colleagues[1,8,41,42] have followed two longitudinal samples since, for some research participants, 1939 and no later than 1944. The first sample, referred to as the "College sample," was a group of 268 men from a study of healthy college students. The second sample, a group of 456 men referred to as the "Core City sample," was the control group in a study of "juvenile delinquents."

Fillmore and colleagues[16,37,40] have reported on multiple longitudinal samples with follow-up periods ranging from 4 to 20 years, across a variety of age cohorts and national boundaries. These longitudinal studies are supplemented by surveys of nationally representative samples using retrospective assessment of past vs. current alcohol diagnoses.[10,11]

Results of both longitudinal and cross-sectional studies indicate that among adults, whether alcohol abuse or dependence is chronic or not chronic, depend to a large extent on the age of the individual at the time the problem develops, and age at the time of assessment.[10,16,37,40,43] Specifically, although alcohol problems are most common during adolescence and early adulthood, alcohol diagnoses are least stable during this period of time. Young adults, under the age of 30, evidence considerable fluctuation in their experience of alcohol problems, and over time, there is increasing likelihood that their problems will remit.[8,16,37] Problems that are present in middle age (even if onset is relatively recent) are more likely to persist and become chronic, such that alcohol disorder diagnoses are relatively stable during this period of life in longitudinal samples.[8,16,43] Among older adults (over age 50), alcohol diagnoses are again less stable,[40] primarily in the direction of decreases in dependence over time (see also Chapter 12 on special therapeutic considerations concerning geriatric patients). Overall, a meta-analysis of 27 longitudinal studies conducted at different times, in different countries, and with different age groups of subjects supports a decrease in alcohol use quantity and alcohol abuse and dependence over the lifespan, beginning around age 25 to 30.[40] A variety of cultural and environmental factors influence overall rate of drinking and such factors as the age of onset of drinking and the age at which problems develop, peak, and subside.[40,44] Overall, however, Fillmore's work suggests that the tendency for problems to peak early in life and subside as individuals age is relatively universal.

In addition to the age of the individual at the time of the assessment, a variety of other factors have been shown to be related to the chronicity of alcohol problems over time. Once again, comorbid psychiatric conditions are associated with increased severity of and to some extent, chronicity of alcohol dependence (see also Chapter 26 on comorbidity). In addition, several studies indicate family history of alcohol problems as a significant predictor of persistence of adult alcohol abuse and dependence.[24,45,46] Men are also more likely to develop chronic alcohol problems than are women (see also Chapter 13 on special therapeutic considerations concerning women).[47]

TREATMENT SEEKING

Examining research regarding the chronicity of drinking problems over the lifespan inevitably leads to a discussion of the role of treatment in promoting remission. There is conflicting evidence regarding the importance of treatment in the natural history of alcohol problems, arising in part from differences in the research methods and probably in part from differences in the treatment itself. Treatment approaches and treatment outcome are covered elsewhere in this volume, and will not be reviewed here. However, relevant to the discussion of natural history is the question of at what point, and under what circumstances, do individuals seek treatment for their alcohol use disorders, and what happens to those who never seek treatment?

Treatment outcome studies historically indicate that most treatments are better than no treatment, and that individuals who enter and remain in treatment often show considerable improvement in their functioning. It has been less common to find differences between credible treatments with different contents or intensities.[48] The longitudinal work conducted by Vaillant,[8] however, suggested that treatment plays a very minor role in remission of alcohol problems overall, and appeared no more effective than natural healing processes. The discrepancy between treatment outcome trials and natural history studies probably arises from several sources. However, one likely reason for this discrepancy arises out of findings that the vast majority of individuals with clinical levels of alcohol problems never seek treatment. Researchers estimate the rate of untreated to treated individuals may be as high as 13:1.[49-51]

A recent report by the Institute of Medicine[49] estimated 80% of alcohol-dependent individuals in the U.S. never receive treatment. In addition, Shuckit and colleagues[2] found the average length of time between age of first symptoms and age at which the individual sought help or advice was more than 10 years, by which time substantial social, occupational, legal, and health consequences had ensued.

These findings suggest it is important to pay close attention to those pretreatment characteristics and therapeutic techniques that promote entrance into and retention in treatment. Tucker and Gladsjo[6] interviewed current and former problem drinkers regarding their use of treatment resources (including AA) as well as their past drinking patterns and their history of interpersonal, legal, and health consequences of drinking. They found heavier drinking was not related to treatment seeking, but a greater number of interpersonal negative consequences was related to treatment seeking. Although overall severity of problems was not related to treatment seeking in this sample, it was related to successful resolution of problems, with successful abstainers reporting more previous drinking and a higher severity of problems overall. In another study, Sobell and colleagues[49] similarly found individuals who had resolved their drinking problems through treatment reported higher overall severity of drinking problems and a greater overall number of negative consequences than those who had resolved problems without treatment. Similar to the results obtained by Shuckit and colleagues,[2] the Sobell studies indicated participants who sought treatment for their drinking reported problem drinking histories of 13 to 14 years duration.

While it is important to consider what influences individuals to seek alcohol treatment, it is also important to consider what stops the majority from seeking treatment. Pertinent to the topic of natural history, several studies suggest a major reason why many alcohol-abusing or -dependent individuals fail to seek treatment is that they do not believe their problem is serious enough to warrant treatment, and/or they believe they can resolve their problems on their own. These beliefs are often perceived by professionals as an indication of classical denial. However, Sobell and colleagues[53] as well as Sanchez-Craig and colleagues[54] have suggested this reflects the focus of most treatment programs on the severe or chronic alcoholic, rather than those alcohol abusers with less severe patterns of use and problems. Motivational interviewing[55] is one treatment strategy that has been developed to specifically address this problem, through the use of feedback to increase the clients' awareness of their negative consequences and build a discrepancy between their current drinking and their perception of themselves as not having a drinking problem. In addition to this approach, increasing the visibility of services for alcohol abusers and mildly dependent individuals may help shorten the interval between problem development and treatment seeking.

NATURAL RECOVERY

It is apparent from a consideration of the work of Fillmore and colleagues, Vaillant, Grant, and others that rates of alcohol abuse and dependence decline over the lifespan, and that treatment cannot account for this decline. While many persons with problems resulting from alcohol use do improve through participation in alcohol treatment, there appears to be a large percentage of people who become abstainers or moderate drinkers without any formal intervention. This "natural recovery," "spontaneous remission," or "aging-out" phenomenon has received increased attention from researchers investigating effective treatments for alcohol problems, largely because it is suggested that a great deal can be learned from "what works" for these individuals who improve without intervention. Are there commonalities to their experiences that can shed light on ways to improve treatment? What are the pathways out of problematic alcohol use?

Three sources of data about spontaneous remission are longitudinal studies of drinkers, control groups of problem drinkers recruited to measure the effects of a treatment, and studies designed to explore the phenomenon of natural recovery itself that are either cross-sectional, longitudinal, retrospective, or prospective in nature.[14,56] While a great deal of research is dedicated to the development, implementation, and evaluation of alcohol treatment programs and interventions, Sobell and colleagues[5] suggest that most people who recover from alcohol problems do so without professional intervention. Representation in the literature, however, is not accordingly proportionate[57]; note that for every study of natural recovery, there "are literally hundreds of studies of alcoholism treatment outcome." Thus, in many ways, research on natural recovery is in its formative years. As with the study of the natural history of alcohol problems, the study of natural recovery from alcohol problems is hampered by limitations to the research designs, and method-ologies are still being improved upon and refined.

METHODOLOGICAL LIMITATIONS IN THE ASSESSMENT OF NATURAL RECOVERY

Vaillant[1] noted that the natural history of alcoholism depends on the population studied and the methods utilized by researchers. As with the study of natural history, the study of natural or "spontaneous" recovery from alcohol use disorders is limited by methodological flaws and incon-sistencies in the research literature. One concern is whether self-identified remitters are represen-tative of persons who resolve a problematic substance use career without formal or lay interven-tion.[56] Additionally, as previously mentioned, the age of samples at the time of investigation can have a major impact on a study's outcome.[43] A younger sample would be more likely to "mature out" of problematic substance use,[16] while a sample of middle-aged individuals may appear to be more stable. The socioeconomic status of research participants is also important. Tucker and Gladsjo[6] reported that resolved abstinent former drinkers had higher incomes, were more likely to be employed full time, and had greater social stability. Humphreys, Moos, and Finney,[57] however, suggest that because rates of heavy drinking are higher among people with lower income and education, it takes more severe problems for a person to feel "outside of norm" and begin contem-plating change. At that point, they argue, dependence may be severe enough that moderate use is not a workable option.

An additional limitation of existing research is related to measurement. Sobell, Sobell, and Toneatto[49] report that many studies utilize short resolution periods, and Pettinati and colleagues,[58] in their study monitoring a 4-year resolution period, illustrate that variability in problem resolution exists in such a way that sampling only 1 year is potentially quite confounded. Many individuals in early recovery move in and out of abstinent, moderate, and excessive states. Often, data are not separated for those who resolved their problem by achieving abstinence and those who drank in a moderate, non-problem manner.

Similarly, the definition of problem resolution is a limitation of existing research. It is often difficult to distinguish whether persons truly recover naturally based on researchers' definitions of natural recovery. Some researchers include AA attendance in their definition of "no-treatment." Further, definition of abstinence and moderate use is quite variable throughout the literature. For example, Pettinati and colleagues[58] concluded that 29% of a sample of remitters (including persons with and without treatment) were able to maintain abstinence, strictly defined as no alcohol consumption, and showed an overall good adjustment to their lives. Nace[43] observed that if absti-nence is redefined as making room for "slips," that is, "no more than one episode of intoxication in…at least 12 consecutive months," 55% of Pettinati's sample now would have maintained abstinence.* It is important to acknowledge that limitations exist, yet as studies are conducted, researchers are learning new ways to improve the assessment and measurement of natural history and natural recovery.

PREVALENCE OF NATURAL RECOVERY

A look at research over the years highlights that one of the most consistent components of natural recovery is its inconsistency — it exists, it happens, yet studies vary in their report of its prevalence. Studies demonstrate that persons with alcohol problems can improve over time, contrary to the worsening of a progressive disease.[59] Smart concludes that spontaneous remission rates vary from 1 to 33%, depending on the sample studied,[79] while Stall and Biernacki[56] report that spontaneous remission rates range from a low of 4%[8,60] to a high of 59%.[61] Vaillant[8] reported that the rate of stable remission in longitudinal samples is between 2 and 3% a year. However, Sobell and Sobell[62] found that 82% of self-identified former alcohol abusers who resolved their problem for over 1 year did so without treatment, compared to 18% who reported going through treatment of some sort. Similarly Leung, Kinzie, Boehnlein, and Shore[63] reported that 83% of a sample of Native Americans who had previously had problems with alcohol, but were no longer drinking, stopped without ever entering alcohol treatment. In treatment-seeking samples, the rate appears much lower. Armor and colleagues report that 6 months after contacting an alcoholism treatment center without any intervention after the initial contact, 11% of such people achieved abstinence.[64] Emrick[65] reports that 13.6% of persons receiving no or minimal treatment achieve abstinence.

PROCESSES OF NATURAL RECOVERY

Referred to as "autoremission" by Klingemann,[63] coping strategies utilized by people with heroin and alcohol problems who achieved a significant improvement in consumption behavior without any or with minimal treatment were explored. Three phases or stages of remission were described: decision, action, and maintenance.

During the decision stage, where substance-using persons determine that a reduction in their use is necessary, Klingemann found that the experience of "hitting rock bottom" was not the dominant feature of natural recovery.[66] Rather, more important were sudden key experiences or new reference groups. The importance of key experiences is supported by research conducted by Tucker, Vuchinich, and Gladsjo.[67] These researchers found that 65% of individuals becoming abstinent from alcohol without formal intervention acknowledged that physical health problems (e.g., illnesses, injuries, and negative physical effects from drinking) were influential in their decision. Further, 75% of research participants reported long-term influences that evolved over time. Tuchfeld[68] stated that people who resolved drinking problems did so after personal illness or accident, religious experiences, drinking-related financial problems, family interventions, and what was referred to as "extraordinary events." Stall and Biernacki[56] note that important influences on the process of changing one's behavior include health problems, social pressures, religious factors, problems with significant others, and financial difficulties. Leung, Kinzie, Boehnlein, and Shore[63] reported that many remitters realized that drinking was causing many social and financial problems, and reported that "the effort required to acquire and consume alcohol was "not worth it anymore." Vaillant[8] reported that almost one-half of his sample who had achieved abstinence credited willpower. Klingemann's study notes that while many remitters detect social pressures to change, about three-quarters of these people felt they had been left alone and were not able to depend on anyone for help when attempting to change their behavior.

---

* Nace uses Vaillant's[1] "less than rigorous definition of abstinence" to make this point. Abstinence is defined as "at least 12 consecutive months of using alcohol less often than once a month with no more than one episode of intoxication in the abstinent year and that episode less than a week in duration (p. 59)." (Vaillant, G.E., *The Natural History of Alcoholism*, Harvard University Press, Cambridge, MA, 1983.)

Despite research suggesting that specific factors can be identified, others have difficulty identifying precipitating events for natural recovery. Leung, Kinzie, Boehnlein, and Shore[63] found that 45% of remitters from a Native American population could not name a specific reason as to what was influential in achieving abstinence. Additionally, others have reported that a vaguely defined "hitting bottom" is a preliminary event, with studies citing that up to 75% of remitters experience severe problems before changing.[69,70] A review of the literature suggests that hitting "rock bottom" is in the eye of the beholder — much depends on the roles an individual holds and his or her premorbid functioning.

The second stage of spontaneous remission — action — is characterized by a "toolbox" of options. Klingemann reported that most remitters are "conscious strategists" who are motivated to change and rely on a range of strategies and techniques to maintain abstinence or reduced consumption. In fact, many of the approaches utilized by participants in Klingemann's study are similar to components of existing formal treatment. For example, remitters reported that they attempted to create a substance-free environment by removing all alcohol from the home and/or finding a new route home to avoid bars — stimulus control components of Marlatt and Gordon's[71] relapse prevention. Similarly, participants reported attempting to strengthen the personal commitment to change by "symbolic acts," usually involving the performance of a ritual of quitting — also a component of relapse prevention. For some, diversion was important and often reinforcing, since working more and interacting with people strengthens occupational and social contacts and experiences. Behavioral strategies frequently included gradually lengthening drinking intervals while gradually decreasing amounts consumed. Calculating financial and other costs of resuming the habit against the benefits of reduced consumption was also utilized. Finally, ideas about the effects and nature of alcohol, as well as exploring adequate substitute behaviors occurred.

Klingemann suggests that while taking action is important in changing one's substance-use patterns, maintaining these changes is needed. The great American author Mark Twain noted that quitting is easy — he had done it hundreds of times. Multiple quit attempts followed by a return to problematic use can be damaging for a person's self-efficacy and confidence, thus making actions taken during the maintenance stage very important. Klingemann reports that first, persons who have changed their substance-use behavior need to strengthen self-confidence in their ability of self-control by increasing exposure to triggers, testing coping strategies, and staging self-tests. Klingemann found that participants in his study reported that the experience of coping without using drugs or alcohol strengthened self-confidence. Additionally, while not engaging in problematic use, individuals noted that seeing the negative consequences experienced by active substance users supported their decision to change their use. Second, the person increasingly focuses on the gains and rewards made and acquired from their changed consumption. These can include an increase in personal well-being, resumption of hobbies, and rewards based on changes in the surrounding environment (e.g., a person motivated to change because of hurting friends and loved ones now finds renewed trust and opportunities to be with these individuals). Finally, while in the maintenance stage, the individual internalizes new social roles. One problem persons who drastically change their alcohol consumption often find, as opposed to people attempting to remit from other substances, is that it may be difficult to fully remove oneself from their former "alcohol world."[66]

Stall and Biernacki[56] propose a three-stage model of natural recovery as well, in which the central process underlying successful resolution of an alcohol problem is the "successful public renegotiation and acceptance of the user's new, non-stigmatized identity." In the first stage, an individual enhances motivation to quit largely because of the necessity of coping constantly with health problems, social sanctions, problems with significant others, and financial difficulties. The authors suggest that when deciding to quit or to change one's use, individuals are required to redefine important social and economic relationships. In the second stage, a public announcement of behavior change is made, and renegotiation of the user's identity begins. Stall and Biernacki state that at this point, a person may relapse, use substances intermittently, or succeed in achieving abstinence. In the third stage, the individual manages his or her new identity and integrates into a substance-free lifestyle.

MAINTENANCE OF PROBLEM RESOLUTION

While the Klingemann and Stall and Biernacki three-stage models are just two examples of how natural recovery may occur, they illustrate that, regardless of the pathway out of problematic use, maintenance is a key component. Sobell, Sobell, Toneatto, and Leo[5] report that maintenance of successful problem resolution is influenced most commonly by spousal or social support. Another factor important in maintaining problem resolution is changes in one's environment that reinforce the new behavior. Tucker, Vuchinich, and Gladsjo[67] report that in the year prior to problem resolution, heightened health concerns and an uneventful, stable work situation were characteristic of people who went on to achieve abstinence (compared to non-problem-drinking individuals). Those people who achieved abstinence reported that their health events significantly decreased to levels comparable to non-resolved individuals after changing their drinking behavior. A similar decrease in legal events occurred over time for persons who achieved abstinence. The resolved abstinent group experienced a decrease in the total number of negative events over time, while non-resolved persons reported an increase over time. The authors hypothesize that regardless of whether a person is highly motivated or not, and whether a person enters treatment or not, success may depend on stability in important areas of functioning and decreases in negative events after quitting. They found eight factors that appeared to have an impact on resolution maintenance: health changes, role of spouse, role of other family members, changes in friends, hobbies, leisure or recreational activities, social activities, religious involvement, and changes in will power or self-control.

OUTCOMES OF PROBLEM RESOLUTION: IS ABSTINENCE THE ONLY ANSWER?

In a word, no. While abstinence is a valued outcome of attempts to reduce risks and consequences associated with alcohol consumption, moderate drinking is a viable, effective outcome for many who resolve problems on their own. Cahalan and Roizen[72] report that approximately one half of people who were once problem drinkers reduced their drinking 4 years later. Humphreys, Moos, and Finney[57] report that while some untreated individuals do continue drinking in a problematic way, a significant portion either abstain or drink moderately. Sobell, Sobell, and Toneatto[49] reported that 57% of resolved non-abstainers began with a goal of abstinence and later began to use moderately. These researchers suggest that an individual's belief that he or she can achieve control over alcohol plays the largest role in his or her resolution course. Some 58% of Sobell and colleagues' resolved abstainers reported that they selected abstinence as a goal because they *lacked* control over alcohol. Interestingly, half of resolved moderate drinkers selected moderation as a goal because they *wanted* control over alcohol.

Vaillant[1] found that a decrease in alcohol consumption to non-problem drinking without professional help occurred for men who were college-educated, socially stable, and upper-middle-class, while abstinence without formal intervention was the more likely outcome for men who were less educated and of lower socioeconomic status. Armor and Meshkoff's[73] findings support these correlates of different pathways out of problematic drinking for persons who recover with formal treatment. They report that persons with higher socioeconomic status and less severe problems tend to become moderate drinkers, while persons with lower socioeconomic status and more severe problems are more likely to become abstainers if their drinking pattern changes. Rosenberg[74] reports that less severely dependent persons are more likely to become moderate drinkers. Sobell, Sobell, and Toneatto,[49] however, suggest that a range of problem severity, from mid- to severe-dependence, exists across people who moderate problematic use.

Humphreys and colleagues[57] report that past research shows that adopting abstinence over moderate drinking may be associated with age, with older individuals who attempt recovery selecting abstinence as a goal. Additionally, they argue that those with drinking-related health problems may be more likely to select abstinence as a goal rather than moderate drinking. In their study attempting to replicate the pathways out of problem drinking described by Vaillant and Armor and Meshkoff, Humphreys, Moos, and Finney[57] detailed two distinct pathways out of problem drinking that, in their words, "resonate" with Vaillant's findings. Problem drinkers who moderated their alcohol use without problems had higher levels of education, higher levels of occupational status, high self-esteem, and supportive relationships with friends and family. They argue that early problem recognition among these people gives them greater flexibility in their choice of resolution options since severe dependence may not yet be developed. Additionally, these persons had intact social resources that helped to maintain changes in their drinking behavior.

Problem drinkers who resolved problematic use with an outcome of abstinence had lower levels of income and education. These individuals did not perceive their drinking as problematic until severe dependence had developed. The authors report that triggering mechanisms for these individuals may be aging, drinking-related health problems, poor relationships with one's extended family, low self-esteem, and belief that drinking is a very serious problem. Maintenance of changes for these people includes reliance on Alcoholics Anonymous, remission of alcohol-related health problems, rising self-esteem, increased partner support, increased self-efficacy to maintain abstinence, and acknowledgment that they have a significant drinking problem.

FUTURE DIRECTIONS

Moos[75] explains that a better understanding of the process of recovery without formal intervention may help health care providers improve upon professional treatment. As more is understood about the processes that work in those who succeed in resolving problematic use, treatment programs could take advantage of this information.[56] Given that health concerns are often identified as triggers or influences for change, Tucker and colleagues suggest that heavy drinkers identified in general medical settings but who have not presented for assistance with their alcohol use may be a "receptive, at-risk group for cost-effective interventions."[57] While Prugh[70] suggests that a key question involves identifying persons unlikely to remit on their own, Humphreys, Moos, and Finney[57] suggest that steps should be taken to identify those who can remit on their own so that a stepped-care approach to intervention can be utilized and treatment resources could be directed to people less likely to succeed in changing on their own.

The stability of treatment programs and therapies is solid, and the success of persons making changes on their own does not threaten the place of treatment interventions in our health care world. However, given that apparently more people change without professional treatment than with, it may be that society and the public can make changes to avoid threatening spontaneous remission and instead to foster a climate supportive of making healthy changes. Tuchfeld[68] suggests that spontaneous remitters may be reluctant to accept the designation of "alcoholic," which contributes to their decision to attempt change on their own. Research has demonstrated that the negative social consequences of entering treatment appear to be more influential in decisions not to seek professional help than treatment cost and inaccessibility.[66,67,77] If addiction is viewed as a disease that can only get worse without treatment, persons may not acknowledge that they can play a role in their own recovery and improvement.[66] Stall and Biernacki,[56] in fact, even point out that the term "spontaneous remission" maintains the notion that one has remitted from a disease. They observe that if, as their theory suggests, the process of renegotiating a stigmatized identity underlies the process of natural recovery, health policies should promote the idea that problematic substance use can be a temporary phase in a person's life. If the identity of "addict" is incorporated into a person's self-image, perhaps reduced consumption will not be seen as an option.

Stall and Biernacki recommend that health education efforts break down the belief that addiction is permanent, and should publicize the idea that individuals can, in fact, resolve problematic substance use behaviors outside of treatment. Otherwise, it is possible that the belief that substance-use behaviors are permanent and intractable could contribute to a self-fulfilling prophecy. This does not mean that substance use will be encouraged or condoned, only that the public might be taught that addiction "is not a disease that can only get worse without treatment."[66] Mulford[77] suggests that treatment agencies direct effort at accelerating natural recovery in the community by working with problem-drinking individuals to improve connections to families, friends, and self-help groups. Humphreys, Moos, and Finney[57] suggest that education and prevention programs can help to shape community norms so that, if problematic, individuals may perceive their drinking as such before abuse becomes severe dependence. Harm reduction approaches advocate lowering the threshold to entering treatment, and inherent to harm reduction is treating the substance user with respect. In short, a climate where there is less shame involved with seeking the support of friends and family members, an individual who does not see treatment as a viable option may be more likely to make changes him- or herself.

REFERENCES

1. Vaillant, G.E., Natural history of male alcoholism. V. Is alcoholism the cart or the horse to sociopathy? *Br. J. Addict.*, 78, 317, 1983.
2. Schuckit, M.A., Anthenelli, R.M., Bucholz, K.,K., Hesselbrock, V.M., and Tipp, J., The time course of development of alcohol-related problems in men and women, *J. Stud. Alcohol.*, 56, 218, 1995.
3. Jellinek, E.M., *The Disease Concept in Alcoholism*, Hill House Press, New Brunswick, Canada, 1960.
4. Miller, W.R. and Kurtz, E., Models of alcoholism used in treatment: contrasting AA and other perspectives with which it is often confused, *J. Stud. Alcohol.,* 55, 159, 1994.
5. Sobell, L.C., Sobell, M.B., Toneatto, T., and Leo, G.I., What triggers the resolution of alcohol problems without treatment? *Alcohol. Clin. Exp. Res.*, 17, 217, 1993.
6. Tucker, J.A. and Gladsjo, J.A., Help-seeking and recovery by problem drinkers: characteristics of drinkers who attended Alcoholics Anonymous or formal treatment or who recovered with assistance, *Addict Behav.,* 18, 529, 1993.
7. Langenbucher, J.W. and Chung, T., Onset and staging of DSM-IV alcohol dependence using mean age and survival-hazard methods, *J. Abnorm. Psychol.*, 104, 346, 1995.
8. Vaillant, G.E., A long-term follow-up of male alcohol abuse, *Arch. Gen. Psychiatry,* 53, 243, 1996.
9. Grant, B.F., Prevalence and correlates of alcohol use and DSM-IV alcohol dependence in the United States. Results of the National Longitudinal Alcohol Epidemiologic Survey, *J. Stud. Alcohol.*, 58, 464, 1997.
10. Grant, B.F. and Dawson, D.A., Age at onset of alcohol use and its association with DSM-IV alcohol abuse and dependence: results from the National Longitudinal Alcohol Epidemiologic Survey, *J. Subst. Abuse*, 9, 103, 1997.
11. Dawson, D.A., Grant, B.F., Chou, S.P., and Pickering, R.P., Subgroup variation in U.S. drinking patterns: results of the 1992 National Longitudinal Epidemiologic Study, *J. Subst. Abuse*, 7, 331, 1995.
12. Robins, L.N. and Regier, D.A., *Psychiatric Disorders in America: The Epidemiologic Catchment Area Study,* The Free Press, New York, 1991.
13. Kessler, R.C., McGonagle, K.A., Zhao, S., Nelson, C.B., Hughes, M., Eshleman, S., Wittchen, H.U., and Kendler, K.S., Lifetime and 12-month prevalence of DSM-III-R psychiatric disorders in the United States: results from the National Comorbidity Study, *Arch. Gen. Psychiatry,* 51, 8, 1994.
14. Vaillant, G.E. and Hiller-Stuermhofel, S., The natural history of male alcoholism, *Alcohol Health and Research World*, 20, 152, 1996.
15. Fillmore, K.M., Prevalence, incidence and chronicity of drinking patterns and problems among men as a function of age: a longitudinal and cohort analysis, *Br. J. Addict.*, 82, 77, 1987.
16. Fillmore, K.M. and Midanik, L., Chronicity of drinking problems among men: a longitudinal study, *J. Stud. Alcohol.*, 45, 228, 1984.
17. Office of Applied Studies, Substance Abuse and Mental Health Services Administration, National Household Survey on Drug Abuse: Main Findings 1992, DHHS Publication No. (SMA) 94-3012. Rockville, MD, U.S. Department of Health and Human Services, 1995.

18. Oetting, E.R. and Beauvais, F., Adolescent drug use: findings of national and local surveys, *J. Consult. Clin. Psychol.*, 58, 385, 1990.
19. Health and Human Services (June, 1998) (online) http://www.health.org/mtf/hhsfact.htm.
20. Kandel, D., Chen, K., Warner, L.A., Kessler, R.C., and Grant, B., Prevalence and demographic correlates of symptoms of last year dependence on alcohol, nicotine, marijuana and cocaine in the U.S. population, *Drug and Alcohol Dependence*, 44, 11, 1997.
21. Clapper, R.L., Buka, S.L., Goldfield, E.C., Lipsitt, L.P., and Tsuang, M.T., Adolescent problem behaviors as predictors of adult alcohol diagnoses, *Int. J. Addict.*, 30, 507, 1995.
22. Kessler, R.C., Crum, R.M., Warner, L.A., Nelson, C.B., Schulenberg, J., and Anthony, J.C., Lifetime co-occurence of DSM-III-R alcohol abuse and dependence with other psychiatric disorders in the national comorbidity survey, *Arch. Gen. Psychiatry*, 54, 313, 1997.
23. Rohde, P., Lewinson, P.M., and Seeley, J.R., Psychiatric comorbidity with problematic alcohol use in high school students, *J. Am. Acad. Child. Adolesc. Psychiatry,* 35, 101, 1996.
24. Windle, M., On the discriminative validity of a family history of problem drinking index with a national sample of young adults, *J. Stud. Alcohol.*, 57, 378, 1996.
25. Jessor, R., Problem-behavior theory, psychosocial development, and adolescent problem drinking, *Br. J. Addict.,* 82, 331, 1987.
26. Jessor, R. and Jessor, S.L., Adolescence to young adulthood: a twelve-year prospective study of problem behavior and psychosocial development, S. A. Mednick, M. Harway, and K. M. Finello, Eds. *Handbook of Longitudinal Research*, Vol. 2: Teenage and Adult Cohorts, Praeger, New York.
27. Donovan, J. E., Jessor, R., and Jessor, L., Problem drinking in adolescence and young adulthood: a follow-up study, *J. Stud. Alcohol.,* 44, 109, 1983.
28. Fergusson, D.M., Horwood, L.J., and Lynskey, M.T., The prevalence and risk factors associated with abusive or hazardous alcohol consumption in 16-year-olds, *Addiction,* 90, 935, 1995.
29. Yates, W.R., Petty, F., and Brown, K., Alcoholism in males with antisocial personality disorder, *Int. J. Addict.,* 23, 999, 1988.
30. Stice, E., Barrera, M., and Chassin, L., Prospective differential prediction of adolescent alcohol use and problem use: examining the mechanisms of effect, *J. Abnorm. Psychol.*, 107, 616, 1998.
31. Loeber, R. and Keenan, K., Interaction between conduct disorder and its comorbid conditions: effects of age and gender, *Clin. Psychol. Rev.*, 14, 497, 1994.
32. White, H.R. and Labouvie, E.W., Towards the assessment of adolescent drinking, *J. Stud. Alcohol.*, 58, 513, 1989.
33. Buckholz, K. K., Helzer, J.E., Shayka, J.J., and Lewis, C.E., Comparison of alcohol dependence in subjects from clinical, community, and family studies. *Alcohol. Clin. Exp. Res.*, 18, 1091, 1994.
34. Keller, M.B., Lavori, P.W., Beardslee, W., Wunder, J., Drs, D., and Hasin, D., Clinical course and outcome of substance abuse disorders in adolescents, *J. Substance Abuse Treatment*, 9, 9, 1992.
35. Nelson, C. B., Little, R. J., Heath, A.C., and Kessler, R.C., Patterns of DSM-III-R alcohol dependence symptom progression in a general population survey, *Psychol. Med.*, 26, 449, 1996.
36. Kilbey, M.M., Downey, K., and Breslau, N., Predicting the emergence and persistence of alcohol dependence in young adults: The role of expectancy and other risk factors, *Exp. Clin. Psychopharmacol.*, 6, 149, 1998.
37. Temple, M.T. and Fillmore, K.M., The variability of drinking patterns and problems among young men, age 16-31: a longitudinal study, *Int. J. Addict.,* 20, 1595, 1985.
38. Chou, S.P. and Pickering, R.P., Early onset of drinking as a risk factor for lifetime alcohol-related problems, *Br. J. Addict.*, 87, 1199, 1992.
39. Kandel, D.B. and Logan, J.A., Patterns of drug use from adolescence to young adulthood: periods of risk for initiation, continued use, and discontinutation, *Am. J. Public Health,* 74, 660, 1984.
40. Fillmore, K.M., Hartka, E., Johnstone, B.M., Leino, E.V., Motoyoshi, M., and Temple, M.T., A meta-analysis of life course variation in drinking, *Br. J. Addict.*, 86, 1221, 1991.
41. Vaillant, G.E., Natural history of male psychological health: VIII. Antecedents of alcoholism and "orality," *Am. J. Psychiatry*, 137, 181, 1980.
42. Vaillant G.E., Gale, L., and Milofsky, E.S., Natural history of male alcoholism: II. The relationship between different diagnostic dimensions, *J. Stud. Alcohol.,* 43, 216, 1982.
43. Nace, E.P., The natural history of alcoholism versus treatment effectiveness: methodological problems, *Am. J. Drug Alcohol Abuse*, 15, 55, 1989.

44. Bronisch, T. and Wittchen, H.U., Lifetime and 6-month prevalence of abuse and dependence of alcohol in the Munich follow-up study, *Eur. Arch. Psychiatry Clin. Neurosci.*, 241, 273, 1992.

45. Dawson, D.A. and Grant, B.F., Family history of alcoholism and gender: their combined effects on DSM-IV alcohol dependence and major depression, *J. Stud. Alcohol.*, 59, 97, 1998.

46. Turner, W.M., Cutter, H.S., Worobec, T.G., O'Farrell, T.J., Bayog, R.D., and Tsuang, M.T., Family history models of alcoholism: age of onset, consequences and dependence, *J. Stud. Alcohol,* 54, 164, 1993.

47. Fillmore, K.M., Women's drinking across the adult life course as compared to men's, *Br. J. Addict.*, 82, 801, 1987.

48. Project MATCH Research Group, Matching alcoholism treatments to client heterogeneity: Project MATCH posttreatment drinking outcomes, *J. Stud. Alcohol.*, 58, 7, 1997.

49. Sobell, L.C., Sobell, M.B., and Toneatto, T., Recovery from alcohol problems without treatment, Heather, N., Miller, W.R., Greeley, J., Eds., *Self-control and Addictive Behaviors*, Maxwell Macmillan, New York, 1992, 198–242.

50. Nathan, P.E., Treatment outcomes for alcoholism in the U.S.: current research, *Addictive Behaviors: Prevention and Early Intervention*, Lorberg, T., Miller, W.R., and Marlatt, G.A., Eds., Swets & Zeitlinger, Amsterdam, 1989, 87–101.

51. Roizen, R., Calahan, D., and Shanks, P., Spontaneous remission among untreated problem drinkers: in *Longitudinal Research on Drug Use: Empirical Findings and Methodological Issues*, Kandel, D.B., Ed., Hemisphere Publishing, Washington, D.C., 1978, 197–221.

52. Institute of Medicine (IOM), *Broadening the Base of Treatment for Alcohol Problems*. National Academy Press, Washington, D.C., 1990.

53. Sobell, L.C., Cunningham, J.A., Sobell, M.B., Agrawal, S., Gavin, D. R., Leo, G.I., and Singh, K.N., Fostering self-change among problem drinkers: A proactive community intervention. *Addict. Behav.,* 21, 817, 1996.

54. Sanchez-Craig, M., & Lei, H., Disadvantages to imposing the goal of abstinence on problem drinkers: an empirical study, *Br. J. Addict.*, 81, 505, 1986.

55. Miller, W.R. and Rollnick, S. *Motivational Interviewing: Preparing People to Change Addictive Behavior*, Guilford Press, New York, 1991.

56. Stall, R. and Biernacki, P., Spontaneous remission from the problematic use of substances: an inductive model derived from a comparative analysis of the alcohol, opiate, tobacco, and food/obesity literatures, *Int. J. Addict.*, 21, 1, 1986.

57. Humphreys, K., Moos, R.H., and Finney, J.W., Two pathways out of drinking problems without professional treatment, *Addict. Behav.,* 20, 427, 1995.

58. Pettinati, H.M., Sugerman, A.A., DiDonato, N., and Maurer, H.S., The natural history of alcoholism over four years after treatment, *J. Stud. Alcohol.*, 43, 201, 1982.

59. Miller, N.S., The natural history of alcohol abuse: Implications for definitions of alcohol use disorders, *Am. J. Psychiatry*, 148, 1095, 1991.

60. Kissin, B., Rosenblatt, S., and Machover, S., Prognostic factors in alcoholism, *Psychiatr. Res. Rep.*, 23–24, 22–43, February–March, 1968.

61. Edwards, B., Orford, J., Egert, S., Guthrie, S., Hawker, A., Hensman, C., Mitcheson, M., Oppenheimer, E., and Taylor, C., Alcoholism: a controlled trial of "treatment" and "advise," *J. Stud. Alcohol.,* 38, 1004, 1977.

62. Sobell, L.C. and Sobell, M.B., *Cognitive Mediators of Natural Recoveries from Alcohol Problems: Implications for Treatment*, paper presented as part of a symposium on Therapies of Substance Abuse: A View Towards the Future, presented at the *Annu. Meeting of the Assoc. for Advancement of Behavior Therapy,* New York, November, 1991.

63. Leung, P.K., Kinzie, J.D., Boehnlein, J.K., and Shore, J.H., A prospective study of the natural course of alcoholism in a Native American village, *J. Stud. Alcohol.*, 54, 733, 1993.

64. Armor, D.J., Polich, J.M., and Stambul, H.B., Alcoholism and treatment. [Prepared for the U.S. National Institute on Alcohol and Abuse and Alcoholism.] Rand Corp., Santa Monica, CA, 1976.

65. Emrick, C.D., A review of psychologically oriented treatment of alcoholism. II. The relative effectiveness of different treatment approaches and the effectiveness of treatment versus no treatment, *J. Stud. Alcohol.*, 36, 88, 1975.

66. Klingemann, H.K., Coping and maintenance strategies of spontaneous remitters from problem use of alcohol and heroin in Switzerland, *Int. J. Addict.*, 27, 1359, 1992.

67. Tucker, J.A., Vuchinich, R.E., and Gladsjo, J.A., Environmental events surrounding natural recovery from alcohol-related problems, *J. Stud. Alcohol.*, 55, 401, 1994.
68. Tuchfeld, B.S., Spontaneous remission in alcoholics: Empirical observations and theoretical implications, *J. Stud. Alcohol.*, 42, 626, 1981.
69. Ludwig, A.M., Cognitive processes associated with "spontaneous" recovery from alcoholism, *J. Stud. Alcohol.*, 46, 53, 1985.
70. Prugh, T., Recovery without treatment, *Alcohol Health and Res. World*, 11, 71, Fall 1986.
71. Marlatt, G.A. and Gordon, J. R., Eds., *Relapse Prevention: Maintenance Strategies in the Treatment of Addictive Behaviors*, Guilford Press, New York, 1985.
72. Calahan, D. and Roisen, R., Changes in Drinking Problems in a National Sample of Men, presented at the *North American Congress on Alcohol and Drug Problems*, San Francisco, 1975.
73. Armor, D.J. and Meshkoff, J.E., Remission among treated and untreated alcoholics, *Adv. Subst. Abuse*, 3, 239, 1983.
74. Rosenberg, H., Prediction of controlled drinking by alcoholics and problem drinkers, *Psychol. Bull.*, 113, 129, 1993.
75. Moos, R., Treated or untreated, an addiction is not an island unto itself, *Addiction*, 89, 507, 1994.
76. Tucker, J.A. and Sobell, L.C., Influences on help-seeking for drinking problems and on natural recovery without treatment, *The Behavior Therapist*, 15, 12, 1992.
77. Mulford, H.A., Treating alcoholism versus accelerating the natural recovery process. A cost-benefit comparison, *J. Stud. Alcohol.*, 40, 505, 1979.
78. White, H.R., Johnson, V., and Garrison, C.G., The drug-crime nexus among adolescents and their peers, *Deviant Behavior*, 6, 183, 1985.
79. Smart, R.G., Spontaneous recovery in alcoholics: A review and analysis of available research, *Drug Alcohol Depend*, 1, 277, 1976. ·

3   Laboratory Parameters

Alois Saria and Gerald Zernig

OVERVIEW

Alterations in biochemical parameters during alcohol abuse have been the focus of investigations for many years. However, only a very few have been of value as diagnostic markers. The most reliable markers today are carbohydrate-deficient transferrin (CDT) and gamma-glutamyltransferase (GGT). CDT offers the advantage of higher specificity, whereas the sensitivities of GGT and CDT are comparable. A combination of CDT plus GGT may increase diagnostic efficacy. However, as none of the markers exhibit maximum diagnostic efficacy, biochemical markers need to be used with caution and should always be interpreted in connection with other clinical symptoms or diagnostic questionnaires.

INTRODUCTION

Alcohol abuse causes a variety of metabolic changes and organ damage. Therefore, the alterations of biochemical parameters have been the focus of investigations for many years. Many of these parameters have been tested for their value as diagnostic markers or predisposition indicators.[1]

GENERAL PROBLEMS OF LABORATORY TESTS: SPECIFICITY, SENSITIVITY, AND DIAGNOSTIC EFFICACY OF LABORATORY PARAMETERS

Biochemical tests are imperfect by nature. A detailed analysis of the problems associated with testing in general has been published by Brett and Friedman.[2] Here, we will briefly discuss the major issues of this problem. One of them is related to characteristics that are inherent to the biochemical analysis, independent of the clinical context. Some examples are a miscalibrated blood chemistry analyzer, variabilities in measurements of the same parameter in different laboratories, sometimes with apparently the same technique, or by variations in human interpretations of the same data (e.g., different interpretations of the same complex pattern obtained by analysis of a biochemical matrix, comparable to different interpretations of an X-ray film by different radiologists). **Precision** describes the degree to which repeated measurements on one sample give the same result. However, if an apparatus for determining blood alcohol is calibrated defectively, it might produce data with high precision, yet it would not represent the true value. The tendency of a measurement to approximate the true value is expressed with the term **accuracy.** Of course, another source of uncertainty or error arises from the application of a biochemical test to the clinical problem. That is, regardless of the precision or accuracy of the analysis, how well does it assist clinicians in separating diseased from non-diseased persons?

A powerful diagnostic parameter should discriminate the group of patients with the expected diagnosis (e.g., chronic alcoholic patients) from healthy persons or persons with diseases that may affect the diagnostic parameter (e.g., healthy, or liver diseases not resulting from alcohol abuse). To classify a diagnostic parameter for its power, the following definitions are commonly used: specificity, sensitivity, and diagnostic efficacy. **Sensitivity** defines the percentage of individuals from the group of chronic alcoholic patients who are correctly classified, and **specificity** defines the percentage of individuals from the group of healthy or liver-diseased who are correctly classified. In other words, sensitivity is defined as the probability of a positive test result, given the presence of the disease in question, and specificity is the probability of a negative test result given the absence of that disease. Thus, sensitivity is decreased by false-negative and specificity by false-positive laboratory data, respectively. The **false negative rate** (1-sensitivity) is the probability of a negative test result despite the presence of the disease, and the **false positive rate** (1-specificity) is the probability of a false positive test result despite the absence of the disease. **Diagnostic efficacy** is calculated as sensitivity (% sensitivity/100) × specificity (% specificity/100). Thus, maximum possible efficacy is 1. Mohs and Watson[1] defined the term **diagnostic efficiency** as specificity (%) + sensitivity (%), resulting in a maximum (best) value of 200. Values for sensitivity are derived by examining the performance of the test in a population known to have a disease according to an independent standard of reference. The exact figure of sensitivity when a new test is applied depends on the spectrum of the disease in the population under investigation. Similarly, the specificity may vary, depending on parameters such as age, sex, or the incidence of other diseases influencing the test.

The results of most diagnostic tests are not necessarily dichotomous, that is, normal/abnormal or positive/negative, etc. In contrast, diagnostic tests generally yield a range of results. Therefore, it is necessary to define a **cutoff point** that separates positive and negative results. For calculating sensitivity and specificity, it is necessary to define this cutoff point for a positive result. The following example[2] nicely illustrates this problem: "ST" segment depression in exercise electrocardiography indicates possible coronary artery disease. The size of ST depression correlates with the probability of coronary artery disease. If only 1 mm is chosen as the cutoff value, the sensitivity of this method will be very high because the test will give pathological data easily. However, the specificity will be poor because these small abnormalities are often seen in healthy individuals. If the cutoff is increased to 3 mm, the sensitivity decreases because the diseased persons with less dramatic electrocardiographic changes would not be detected. However, the specificity improves because only very few healthy persons will produce such extreme ST depression.

In general, clinical considerations determine the choice of a suitable cutoff point. If clinical arguments speak in favor of identifying as many diseased persons as possible, and harms of a false positive results are minimal, a cutoff point that enhances sensitivity at the expense of specificity is selected. If one wishes to avoid false positive data by maximizing specificity, the cutoff point is set to produce as few false positive results as possible, but the sensitivity will decrease. The tradeoff between sensitivity and specificity at various cutoff points can be plotted graphically for any given diagnostic test. The resulting curve is called the **receiver operating characteristic (ROC)** curve. The area under this curve represents a measure for the performance of the test.

For detecting chronic alcohol abuse in individuals, it is obvious that, in many instances, specificity may be more important than sensitivity, considering the putative negative consequences of a false positive value.

MARKERS FOR POSSIBLE PREDISPOSITION

Human family and twin studies have shown the importance of genetics in alcohol preference and consumption levels (see Chapter 27).[1] Those at increased risk due to familial alcoholism exhibited biochemical changes such as high circulating acetaldehyde levels during alcohol consumption or alcohol-related flushing. In genetic analyses, certain phenotypes with increased incidence in alcoholics could be identified. However, as the diagnostic efficacy is apparently low, genetic markers are not useful in identifying individuals with a predisposition for alcohol abuse with desired accuracy. Moreover, as they cannot serve as indicators of alcoholism, or excessive alcohol consumption, they will not be further discussed in this chapter.

TYPES OF BIOCHEMICAL MARKERS

Alcohol concentrations in blood, breath, sweat, urine, and saliva rapidly decrease due to metabolism. Blood alcohol measurements indicate high alcohol consumption no longer than 24 to 36 h thereafter. Chronic use or abuse cannot be detected. Furthermore, the peak blood alcohol concentrations in different individuals consuming the same amount of alcohol differ considerably. Therefore, measurement of blood alcohol concentration is not useful in determining individual alcohol consumption, even for measurement of immediate drinking. Although serum methanol increases with prolonged use of alcohol, this increase does not persist long enough after cessation of drinking, and methanol is difficult to determine in blood with quantitative chemical methods. Therefore, numerous investigations over the years have concentrated on the large number of adaptive changes of the organism. Table 3.1 summarizes a selected list of biochemical parameters changed by alcohol consumption.

From Table 3.1, it could be argued that a large number of biochemical tests would be applicable for testing excessive alcohol consumption; however, in general, most parameters do not exhibit enough specificity and sensitivity to detect alcohol abusers or avoid non-specific, false positive values. Therefore, only those parameters that have been shown to provide the most reliable data are discussed.

TABLE 3.1
Selected Biochemical Parameters Used
or Tested for Diagnosis of Alcoholism

Alcohol
    Body fluids, breath, blood, urine
Blood constituents
    Proteins in serum
        Albumin
        Total protein
        Carbohydrate-deficient transferrin (CDT)
        Globulins (gamma and alpha)
    Blood cells
        Red blood cell count
        White blood cell count
        Hematocrit
        Mean corpuscular hemoglobin (MCH)
        Mean corpuscular volume (MCV)
    Blood lipids
        Cholesterol
        Triglycerides
        High-density lipoproteins
    Liver enzyme activity in serum
        Aspartate aminotransferase (AST)
        Alanine aminotransferase (ALT)
        AST:ALT ratio
        Creatine kinase
        gamma-glutamyltransferase (GGT)
        Alkaline phosphatase (ALP)
        GGT:ALP ratio
        Glutamate dehydrogenase

Source: Selected and modified from Mohs, M.E. and Watson R.R., Changes in enzymes and other biochemical markers associated with alcohol abuse, *Diagnosis of Alcohol Abuse*, Watson R.R., Ed., CRC Press, Boca Raton, FL, 1989, 69–100.

---

gamma-GLUTAMYLTRANSFERASE (gamma-GT, GGT, EC 2.3.2.2)

Alcohol produces changes in several liver enzyme levels and their relative proportions in mito-chondria vs. cytosol. This is true in some cases even before liver damage is clinically apparent. However, most of the gross enzyme changes are seen with the onset of structural liver damage resulting from chronic alcohol abuse. A large number of studies provide evidence for the clinical importance of GGT. Increased serum levels result from enzyme induction in addition to liver damage. Therefore, a number of isolated reasons for an increase of GGT have been described, such as drug-induced increase (anticonvulsants, barbiturates, benzodiazepines), xenobiotic influences (nicotine, organic solvents), or other non-alcoholic liver diseases.[1]

ASPARTATE AMINOTRANSFERASE, ALANINE AMINOTRANSFERASE, AND MITOCHONDRIAL VS. TOTAL ASPARTATE AMINOTRANSFERASE

Although the serum activity of aspartate aminotransferase (AST or ASAT, sometimes also called glutamic oxaloacetic transaminase, GOT) or alanine aminotransferase (ALT or ALAT, sometimes also called glutamic pyruvic transaminase, GPT) did not prove to exhibit better sensitivity and specificity than GGT, there is some evidence that determination of the ratio between mitochondrial and total AST (mAST:tAST) improves the specificity (i.e., discriminating alcoholic liver disease from liver damage not resulting from alcohol abuse).[1] However, more recent studies have not yet strengthened this view.[3,4] Therefore, it remains unclear at present, whether this ratio provides better test performance than the best markers or combination of markers (see below) in a particular clinical setting or population of individuals.

MEAN CORPUSCULAR VOLUME OF ERYTHROCYTES (MCV)

Macrocytosis as a result of alcohol consumption is assumed to result from toxic lesions of bone marrow by alcohol, but other causes cannot be excluded. In addition, liver damage not caused by alcohol, reticulocytosis, nicotine, or low vitamin B_{12} might cause increases in MCV, thereby reducing the specificity of the method. Although this parameter has been widely used, it has no advantage over GGT, although combination of MCV with other markers could improve specificity and sensitivity (Table 3.2).

TABLE 3.2
Comparison of Specificities and Sensitivities of CDT and GGT in Recent Clinical Studies where CDT and GGT were Compared in the Same Population of Individuals

CDT Specificity	GGT Specificity	CDT Sensitivity	GGT Sensitivity	Population or (Specific Method)	Ref.
>90	>90	44	44	Heavy consumers, female	30
>90	>90	79	65	Heavy consumers, male	30
100	100	60	30	Relapse monitoring	31
92	18	61	85	Alcoholics with liver disease	32
92	75	69	72	Chronic alcohol >50 g per day	33
100	49	83	89	(% CDT with isoelectric focusing)	28
98	83	70	65	General hospital population, rural wine-growing area	34

CARBOHYDRATE-DEFICIENT TRANSFERRIN (CDT)

As outlined in more detail below, the most interesting of the more recently investigated biochemical markers has turned out to be carbohydrate-deficient transferrin. Normal human transferrin contains three or more sialic acid residues, whereas individuals with excessive alcohol consumption are known to present elevated concentrations of transferrin isoforms with a reduced content of sialic acids and other carbohydrate residues.[5] Although the primary mechanism underlying this defect has not been identified, encouraging results have been reported on the use of this phenomenon as a biochemical marker for alcohol abuse.[4,6-18] Several earlier studies have reported sensitivities of 90% or above for carbohydrate-deficient transferrin (CDT), together with a specificity of 90 to 100%, although other investigators have found sensitivities of only 20 to 45% in heavy drinkers. A significant effect of gender on the concentrations of CDT has also been noted, such that both the reference range and the relative diagnostic power of the method differ between males and females.[19,20] Conflicting data have also appeared on the effect of liver disease on CDT concentrations. Recently, it was shown that CDT levels are elevated more often in patients with alcoholic liver disease than in alcoholics consuming similar amounts, yet devoid of apparent liver pathology. In fact, CDT seems to be elevated often in those with the early stages of alcoholic liver disease.[21]

To date, the most widely used methodology for measuring CDT in Europe is based on ion-exchange separation of the desialylated fraction from normal transferrin (CDTect, previously Pharmacia-Upjohn, now Axis). Because of its ease of use and time-saving nature, microanion-exchange chromatography, combined with a radioimmunassay originally developed by Stibler et al.,[6,7,9,10] has also been widely used in routine laboratory work.

CDT isoforms have also been detected and quantitated by an isoelectric focusing/immunoblotting/laser densitometry method developed by Bean and Peter.[22] In a recent study, this method was found to provide similar clinical sensitivity and specificity as the CDTect. Recently, new modifications of CDT test kits have also been introduced. In such modifications, the amount of CDT is expressed as percentage of total transferrin (%CDT).

DESCRIPTION OF COMMERCIAL ASSAYS FOR DETERMINATION OF CDT[23]

CDTect™ Assay (originally from Pharmacia-Upjohn, from 1999 produced by Axis)

With CDTect, transferrin in the serum sample is saturated with Fe^{3+} and the different isoforms are separated on an anion-exchange chromatography microcolumn. Quantitation of CDT is carried out by double antibody radioimmunoassay (RIA). The CDT in the eluate competes with a fixed amount of ^{125}I-labelled transferrin for the binding sites of the antibodies. Bound and free transferrin are separated by addition of a second antibody immunoadsorbent, followed by centrifugation and decanting. The radioactivity in the pellet, which is inversely proportional to the CDT content, is measured by gamma-counting. With this test, the CDT content is expressed as the absolute amount (units/litre; 1U CDT refers to approximately 1 mg transferrin) of transferrin isoforms with a pI of 5.7 or higher (part of di-, mono-, and asialo transferrins). Different cut-off limits between normal and abnormal CDT values are used for males (20U/l) and females (27U/l). The production of an enzyme immunoassay from Pharmacia-Upjohn based on the same analytical principle ceased by end of 1998.

Axis %CDT RIA Assay

In the %CDT RIA test, the serum sample is mixed with Fe^{2+} and ^{125}I-labelled transferrin antibodies. The mixture is applied to an ion-exchange microcolumn, and the antibody–CDT complex is eluted and the radioactivity measured by gamma-counting. The result is expressed as the percentage of a-, mono-, and disialo transferrins to total transferrin. The recommended cutoff level between normal and abnormal values is 2.5% for both females and males.

Axis %CDT Tri TIA Assay

In addition to the a-, mono-, and disialo transferrins, the new %CDTri turbidimetric immunoassay (TIA) test measures the trisialo transferrin isoform as well. The transferrin in the serum is iron-saturated and the sample applied onto an ion-exchange microcolumn. The eluted desialylated isoforms form immune complexes with antitransferrin antibodies and are quantified by turbidimetric measurement at 405 nm. The result is expressed as the relative amount (%) to total transferrin. In this test, the concentration of total transferrins is measured separately, using the same antibodies. The inclusion of the trisialo isoform results in an increased baseline level, and a tentative upper reference limit value of 6% for both females and males has been given by the manufacturer. The intra-assay coefficients of variation (CV) of all three methods were reported to be <10%.

In addition to commercial kits, high-performance liquid chromatography (HPLC) methods have been described, which permit both the quantitation of the individual fractions of sialylated transferrin; asialo-, monosialo-, disialo-, trisialo-, and the normal isoforms, and expression of the results as a percentage.[24-26]

Absolute or Relative Measurements of CDT?

The majority of studies on CDT published to date have used microanion-exchange chromatography to separate the desialylated fraction from normal transferrin, followed by radioimmunoassay or more recently enzyme immunoassay (CDTect, Pharmacia). Results are expressed in absolute units per litre of serum. The development of methods to determine the transferrin fractions and isoforms has started a debate on the merits of absolute vs. relative measurements of CDT, and a recent study has suggested that CDT measured in absolute values may have lower specificity for excess alcohol consumption due to variations in total transferrin concentrations, particularly in patients with chronic liver disease.[27] In any case, the %CDT test certainly has no disadvantages over the CDTect RIA in terms of diagnostic efficacy and accuracy, and may be carried out more easily in many laboratory settings. As both CDTect and %CDT Tri TIA are now manufactured by the same company, it can be expected that the %CDT Tri TIA assay will dominate the market in the near future.

Altogether, CDT currently seems to be the biochemical marker with the best overall performance of all markers. However, it is obvious that the very high sensitivity and specificity (>90% for both) originally thought to be reached even with a cutoff point below 50 g alcohol per day did not prove to be valid after having studied different populations of alcohol abusers, and detecting sex differences, and some false positive values in severe liver disease. However, the data summarized in Table 3.2 provide clear evidence that, using similar set points for cutoff, CDT reaches superior specificity compared with GGT or other markers, the sensitivity being comparable with GGT. The data in Table 3.2 are further supported by recent trials.[28,29]

COMBINATION OF BIOCHEMICAL MARKERS

As none of the biochemical markers reach sensitivity and specificity close to 100% when used alone, it is obvious that a combination of several markers should be considered. In fact, data obtained from an analysis of several markers in a test battery of various biochemical markers, including AST, GGT, and MCV, have been summarized.[1] CDT was not commercially available then. Although this battery resulted in a diagnostic efficacy superior to the single tests, the specificity (90%) and sensitivity (50%) reached values comparable with CDT alone found in a majority of studies (see Table 3.2). Table 3.3 summarizes recent trials in which CDT in combination with GGT was tested.

TABLE 3.3
Comparison of Specificities and Sensitivities of CDT or GGT and Combinations of CDT and GGT in Recent Clinical Studies

Marker	Specificity	Sensitivity	Ref.
CDT	>90	79	
GGT	>90	65	
CDT + GGT	>90	95	30 (males)
CDT	>90	44	
GGT	>90	44	
CDT + GGT	>90	72	30 (females)
CDT	81	69	
CDT + GGT + MCV	88	85	35
CDT		79	
CDT + GGT		95	15
CDT		29	
GGT		40	
MCV		34	
CDT + GGT + MCV		70	36 (female heavy drinkers)

Clearly, the diagnostic efficacy improved when compared with the respective single test in the same population of test persons.

OUTCOME

- None of the biochemical markers reach a maximum diagnostic efficacy.
- If high specificity is desired, CDT appears to be superior to GGT, AST, and MCV.
- A combination of CDT with GGT and/or AST and/or MCV improves sensitivity over GGT or CDT alone. Thus, if sensitivity is a serious matter for the question asked, such test combinations may be recommended.
- Under special circumstances (e.g., obviously false positive values of CDT), analysis of % CDT or CDT/total transferrin ratio or analysis of isoforms might be preferred. However, in mixed heterogeneous populations, the variability of CDT itself seems higher than the differences in test performance of different methods involving CDT measurement.

REFERENCES

1. Mohs, M.E. and Watson R.R., Changes in enzymes and other biochemical markers associated with alcohol abuse, *Diagnosis of Alcohol Abuse*, Watson R.R., Ed., CRC Press, Boca Raton, FL, 1989, 69–100.
2. Brett, A.S. and Friedman, L.S., Principles of diagnostic testing, *Diagnosis of Alcohol Abuse*, Watson R.R., Ed., CRC Press, Boca Raton, FL, 1989, 1–7.
3. Musshoff, F. and Daldrup, T., Determination of biological markers for alcohol abuse, *J. Chromatogr. B. Biomed. Sci. Appl.*, 713, 245, 1998.
4. Sillanaukee, P., Aalto, M., and Seppa, K., Carbohydrate-deficient transferrin and conventional alcohol markers as indicators for brief intervention among heavy drinkers in primary health care, *Alcohol Clin. Exp. Res.*, 22, 892, 1998.
5. Sorvajarvi, K., Blake, J.E., Israel, Y., and Niemela, O., Sensitivity and specificity of carbohydrate-deficient transferrin as a marker of alcohol abuse are significantly influenced by alterations in serum transferrin: comparison of two methods, *Alcohol Clin. Exp. Res.*, 20, 449, 1996.

6. Stibler, H., Carbohydrate-deficient transferrin in serum: a new marker of potentially harmful alcohol consumption reviewed, *Clin. Chem.*, 37, 2029, 1991.
7. Stibler, H. and Borg, S., Glycoprotein glycosyltransferase activities in serum in alcohol-abusing patients and healthy controls, *Scand. J. Clin. Lab. Invest.*, 51, 43, 1991.
8. Carlsson, A.V., Hiltunen, A.J., Beck, O., Stibler, H., and Borg, S., Detection of relapses in alcohol-dependent patients: comparison of carbohydrate-deficient transferrin in serum, 5-hydroxytryptophol in urine, and self-reports, *Alcohol Clin. Exp. Res.*, 17, 703, 1993.
9. Stibler, H., Diagnosis of alcohol-related neurological diseases by analysis of carbohydrate-deficient transferrin in serum, *Acta Neurol. Scand.*, 88, 279, 1993.
10. Stibler, H., Diagnosis of the carbohydrate-deficient glycoprotein syndrome by analysis of transferrin in filter paper blood spots, *Acta Paediatr.*, 82, 55, 1993.
11. Borg, S., Carlsson, A.V., Helander, A., Brandt, A.M., Beck, O., and Stibler, H., Detection of relapses in alcohol dependent patients using serum carbohydrate deficient transferrin: improvement with individualized reference levels, *Alcohol Alcohol. (Suppl.)*, 2, 493, 1994.
12. Sillanaukee, P., Seppa, K., Lof, K., and Koivula, T., CDT by anion-exchange chromatography followed by RIA as a marker of heavy drinking among men, *Alcohol Clin. Exp. Res.*, 17, 230, 1993.
13. Lof, K., Seppa, K., Itala, L., Koivula, T., Turpeinen, U., and Sillanaukee, P., Carbohydrate-deficient transferrin as an alcohol marker among female heavy drinkers: a population-based study, *Alcohol Clin. Exp. Res.*, 18, 889, 1994.
14. Sillanaukee, P., Laboratory markers of alcohol abuse, *Alcohol Alcohol.*, 31, 613, 1996.
15. Behrens, U.J., Worner, T.M., and Lieber, C.S., Changes in carbohydrate-deficient transferrin levels after alcohol withdrawal, *Alcohol Clin. Exp. Res.*, 12, 539, 1988.
16. Behrens, U.J., Worner, T.M., Braly, L.F., Schaffner, F., and Lieber, C.S., Carbohydrate-deficient transferrin, a marker for chronic alcohol consumption in different ethnic populations, *Alcohol Clin. Exp. Res.*, 12, 427, 1988.
17. Lieber, C.S., Xin, Y., Lasker, J.M., and Rosman, A.S., Comparison of new methods for measuring carbohydrate-deficient transferrin (CDT): application to a public health approach for the prevention of alcoholic cirrhosis, *Alcohol Alcohol. (Suppl.)*, 2, 111, 1993.
18. Rosman, A.S., Basu, P., Galvin, K., and Lieber, C.S., Utility of carbohydrate-deficient transferrin as a marker of relapse in alcoholic patients. *Alcohol Clin. Exp. Res.*, 19, 611, 1995.
19. Stauber, R.E., Jauk, B., Fickert, P., and Hausler, M., Increased carbohydrate-deficient transferrin during pregnancy: relation to sex hormones [see comments], *Alcohol Alcohol.*, 31, 389, 1996.
20. Stauber, R.E., Vollmann, H., Pesserl, I., Jauk, B., Lipp, R., Halwachs, G., and Wilders, T.M., Carbo-hydrate-deficient transferrin in healthy women: relation to estrogens and iron status, *Alcohol Clin. Exp. Res.*, 20, 1114, 1996.
21. Sorvajarvi, K., Blake, J.E., Israel, Y., and Niemela, O., Sensitivity and specificity of carbohydrate-deficient transferrin as a marker of alcohol abuse are significantly influenced by alterations in serum transferrin: comparison of two methods, *Alcohol Clin. Exp. Res.*, 20, 449, 1996.
22. Bean, P. and Peter, J.B., A new approach to quantitate carbohydrate-deficient transferrin isoforms in alcohol abusers: partial iron saturation in isoelectric focusing/immunoblotting and laser densitometry, *Alcohol Clin. Exp. Res.*, 17, 1163, 1993.
23. Helander, A., Absolute or relative measurement of carbohydrate-deficient transferrin in serum? Experiences with three immunological assays, *Clin. Chem.*, 45, 131, 1999.
24. Jeppsson, J.O., Kristensson, H., and Fimiani, C., Carbohydrate-deficient transferrin quantified by HPLC to determine heavy consumption of alcohol, *Clin. Chem.*, 39, 2115, 1993.
25. Simonsson, P., Lindberg, S., and Alling, C., Carbohydrate-deficient transferrin measured by high-performance liquid chromatography and CDTect immunoassay, *Alcohol Alcohol.*, 31, 397, 1996.
26. Werle, E., Seitz, G.E., Kohl, B., Fiehn, W., and Seitz, H.K., High-performance liquid chromatography improves diagnostic efficiency of carbohydrate-deficient transferrin, *Alcohol Alcohol.*, 32, 71, 1997.
27. Keating, J., Cheung, C., Peters, T.J., and Sherwood, R.A., Carbohydrate deficient transferrin in the assessment of alcohol misuse: absolute or relative measurements? A comparison of two methods with regard to total transferrin concentration, *Clin. Chim. Acta*, 272, 159, 1998.
28. Cotton, F., Adler, M., Dumon, J., Boeynaems, J.M., and Gulbis, B., A simple method for carbohydrate-deficient transferrin measurements in patients with alcohol abuse and hepato-gastrointestinal diseases [published erratum appears in *Ann. Clin. Biochem.*, 35(3), 445, 1998], *Ann. Clin. Biochem.*, 35, 268, 1998.

29. Reynaud, M., Hourcade, F., Planche, F., Albuisson, E., Meunier, M.N., and Planche, R., Usefulness of carbohydrate-deficient transferrin in alcoholic patients with normal gamma-glutamyltranspeptidase, *Alcohol Clin. Exp. Res.*, 22, 615, 1998.

30. Anton, R.F. and Moak, D.H., Carbohydrate-deficient transferrin and gamma-glutamyltransferase as markers of heavy alcohol consumption: gender differences, *Alcohol Clin. Exp. Res.*, 18, 747, 1994.

31. Anton, R.F., Moak, D.H., and Latham, P., Carbohydrate-deficient transferrin as an indicator of drinking status during a treatment outcome study, *Alcohol Clin. Exp. Res.*, 20, 841, 1996.

32. Bell, H., Tallaksen, C., Sjaheim, T., Weberg, R., Raknerud, N., Orjasaeter, H., Try, K., and Haug, E., Serum carbohydrate-deficient transferrin as a marker of alcohol consumption in patients with chronic liver diseases, *Alcohol Clin. Exp. Res.*, 17, 246, 1993.

33. Bell, H., Tallaksen, C.M., Try, K., and Haug, E., Carbohydrate-deficient transferrin and other markers of high alcohol consumption: a study of 502 patients admitted consecutively to a medical department, *Alcohol Clin. Exp. Res.*, 18, 1103, 1994.

34. Lesch, O.M., Walter, H., Freitag, H., Heggli, D.E., Leitner, A., Mader, R., Neumeister, A., Passweg, V., Pusch, H., Semler, B., Sundrehagen, E., and Kasper, S., Carbohydrate-deficient transferrin as a screening marker for drinking in a general hospital population, *Alcohol Alcohol.*, 31, 249, 1996.

35. Aithal, G.P., Thornes, H., Dwarakanath, A.D., and Tanner, A.R., Measurement of carbohydrate-deficient transferrin (CDT) in a general medical clinic: is this test useful in assessing alcohol consumption? *Alcohol Alcohol.*, 33, 304, 1998.

36. Sillanaukee, P., Aalto, M., and Seppa, K., Carbohydrate-deficient transferrin and conventional alcohol markers as indicators for brief intervention among heavy drinkers in primary health care, *Alcohol Clin. Exp. Res.*, 22, 892, 1998.

4 Psychometric Screening Instruments

Peter A. Vanable, Andrea C. King, and Harriet de Wit

OVERVIEW

Despite the high prevalence of alcohol-related problems in a variety of patient care settings, alcohol problems often go undetected. The routine use of screening tests can dramatically increase the likelihood of identifying patients who are in need of treatment services. This chapter provides an overview of approaches to screening for alcohol-related problems, with a practical emphasis on how psychometric screening tests can improve the clinical management of patients who are at risk for alcohol-related disorders. Issues pertaining to the selection of appropriate screening questionnaires are described, along with a discussion of the relative strengths and weaknesses of the most widely used test instruments. By providing an objective basis for judging the risks associated with a patient's drinking, screening instruments allow clinicians to confidently deliver advice to patients regarding the need for reduced drinking or the need for more intensive, abstinence-based intervention.

INTRODUCTION

This chapter focuses on the use of brief, validated assessment instruments to aid in the screening, diagnosis, and treatment of patients with alcohol-related disorders. Empirically derived assessment questionnaires are widely used in research, but are less often utilized by practicing clinicians and internists. Such underutilization is regrettable: besides providing a standardized, economical means of assessing alcohol-related phenomena, psychometric assessment instruments offer considerable predictive power over simple quantity-frequency and laboratory assessment measures in identifying hazardous drinking and alcohol dependence.[1,2] In this brief primer, we examine several well-validated screening and diagnostic questionnaires, with a practical emphasis on how these paper-and-pencil tools can enhance patient care and improve clinical management of patients who are at risk for alcohol-related disorders. In addition, some of these instruments can be used to monitor patients' progress during the later stages of alcohol treatment. For those interested in a more comprehensive overview of a wide range of alcohol-related measures, we recommend a book recently published by the National Institute on Alcohol Abuse and Alcoholism,[3] as well as several recent review articles.[4-6]

As many as 20% of patients seen in ambulatory care settings meet criteria for "Alcohol Abuse or Dependence."[7-9] Alcohol-related problems are also common to mental health settings, where lifetime estimates of comorbid psychiatric and substance abuse diagnoses range from 20 to 30% among patients with affective disorders, to as high as 55% among those with a severe mental illness such as bipolar disorder or schizophrenia.[10] Yet, despite the high prevalence of alcohol-related problems in a variety of patient care settings, drinking problems often go undetected. Indeed, fewer than half of patients with alcohol-related disorders are known by their physicians to have such problems.[9,11] One source of the under-detection of alcohol problems relates to patient-related variables. For example, many problem drinkers avoid full disclosure of the extent of their drinking.[12] Likewise, few patients who drink in excess seek treatment until serious complications arise from their drinking.[13] However, low detection rates are not simply due to lack of disclosure among patients. Health care workers and clinicians often fail to assess important alcohol-related issues in their patients. Although many physicians are well trained to identify medical complications associated with the advanced stages of heavy, chronic alcohol use (e.g., cirrhosis, hypertension, gastrointestinal difficulties), they often fail to obtain information about heavy social or problematic alcohol consumption during routine clinic visits.[14,15]

Brief and sensitive questionnaires are now available to screen for early signs of alcohol-related problems. They can be readily administered to all patients seen by health care providers and mental health professionals. Unlike earlier screening instruments, which were seen by practitioners to be burdensome and time-consuming, the newer questionnaires can easily be administered by a nurse or administrative staff, or can be included as part of a routine battery of health-screening questionnaires administered in a waiting room. The value of using these questionnaires on a routine basis is further reinforced by the development of highly effective, brief interventions to treat early-phase problem drinking.[16,17] The benefits of administering screening questionnaires as a routine part of medical and mental health practices cannot be overstated: by providing an objective score from which to judge the relative risks associated with a patient's drinking, clinicians can confidently deliver advice to patients regarding the need for reduced drinking, or in the case of the alcohol-dependent patient, the need for referral to a specialist for more intensive, abstinence-based intervention.

GENERAL CONSIDERATIONS

CHOOSING AN APPROPRIATE SCREENING INSTRUMENT

The clinical utility of a particular alcohol screening instrument is determined by its ability to correctly detect an alcohol problem when in fact an alcohol problem is present, while minimizing the degree to which the test produces false positives. These test characteristics are expressed in terms of sensitivity and specificity. Test sensitivity refers to the true positive rate (the proportion of persons with alcohol use disorders who are correctly identified), and specificity refers to the true negative rate of a given test (proportion of patients without an alcohol disorder who are screened as negative).[18] Thus, a test with high sensitivity identifies a minimum number of false negatives, and a test with high specificity provides a minimum of false positives.

Although a detailed discussion of measurement sensitivity and specificity is beyond the scope of this chapter, several issues warrant brief consideration here as they relate to the process of choosing a useful screening instrument. First, it is important for clinicians to consider their particular goals for alcohol screening when evaluating sensitivity and specificity data across different test instruments. As emphasized below, sensitivity and specificity data vary considerably, depending on the definition of problem drinking or alcohol dependence used to validate a particular instrument.[4] For our purposes, the most important distinction concerns whether an instrument is needed for detection of more severe signs of alcohol abuse or dependence, or early-phase problem drinking. Widely used instruments like the CAGE and the Michigan Alcoholism Screening Test (MAST) show strong sensitivity and specificity for identifying alcohol dependence, but they are relatively poor at identifying at-risk patients who could benefit from early intervention to avoid future medical and social complications associated with drinking.[6]

Another important consideration in selecting the best screening instrument concerns its suitability for the particular patient population or setting. In busy outpatient medical settings, very brief screening instruments designed to rapidly identify problematic drinking (e.g., the CAGE) may be preferable to more in-depth screening instruments. In contrast, practitioners working in substance abuse follow-up clinics might prefer more detailed screening instruments like the MAST or the Munich Alcoholism Test (MALT©), which can be used both for screening purposes and as a means of generating descriptive feedback for patients concerning the diversity of problems associated with continued drinking. Finally, clinicians should be aware of the fact that some screening instruments are better suited for use with women. In the past, measurement studies have often neglected to include women, or have failed to present gender-specific analyses (see Chapter 13 of this volume for additional details). As discussed later in this chapter, research that has included separate data on men and women suggest, however, that some screening instruments are preferable for use with women, and that lowered cut-points should be considered when screening women for alcohol disorders.[5]

Thus, clinicians and researchers must be clear in specifying the clinical outcome they are most interested in predicting and be aware of differences in test sensitivity across different patient populations when choosing a screening instrument. Other considerations include the assessment time frame (e.g., lifetime vs. most recent year), ease of administration and scoring, and the availability of staff to assist with test administration. We suggest a flexible approach for choosing appropriate screening instruments, in which clinicians select assessment tools based on the particular needs of their clinic and the patient population being served.

ESTABLISHING A DIAGNOSIS

Screening instruments are designed to rapidly detect individuals who have alcohol-related problems or who are at risk for developing such difficulties. It must be stressed, however, that a positive test result does not establish a definitive diagnosis of alcohol abuse or dependence, nor does it provide a full description of the severity of problems associated with drinking. Following a positive test screen, patients should undergo a more thorough diagnostic evaluation to help establish treatment needs. A number of standardized assessment interviews have been developed to assist in diagnosing alcohol disorders. Popular instruments for use with DSM criteria for *alcohol abuse* and *alcohol dependence* include the substance use sections of the Diagnostic Interview Schedule (DIS)[19] and the Structured Interview Schedule for the DSM-IV (SCID),[20] as well as the Alcohol Use Disorder and Associated Disabilities Schedule.[21] The alcohol use section of the Composite International Diagnostic Interview (CIDI) is the most widely used instrument for establishing a diagnosis of *alcohol dependence* and *harmful drinking* based on ICD-10 criteria.[22]

A chapter elsewhere in this volume deals specifically with differences between the DSM-IV and the ICD-10 in their approaches to diagnoses. For our purposes, it is important to note that most studies designed to validate alcohol screening instruments have relied on DSM-based definitions of alcohol abuse and dependence rather than the ICD system. Because there is a fair degree of concordance between the DSM and ICD definitions of alcohol dependence, it is safe to assume that instruments shown to be effective in detecting alcohol dependence based on DSM criteria are also useful in detecting those with alcohol dependence based on ICD criteria. However, there is relatively poor concordance between ICD-10 criteria for harmful use and the DSM-IV criteria for alcohol abuse, mainly because the ICD-10 criteria do not include any social/legal consequences of drinking. Clinicians and researchers should therefore be mindful of these complexities when evaluating the usefulness of different screening instruments.[4]

OVERVIEW OF SCREENING QUESTIONNAIRES

THE CAGE

The CAGE[23] is perhaps the most widely used screening instrument for the detection of alcohol abuse and dependence. CAGE is an acronym for four easily remembered questions:

Cut down	1. Have you ever felt that you ought to cut down on your drinking?
Annoyed	2. Have people annoyed you by criticizing your drinking?
Guilty	3. Have you ever felt bad or guilty about your drinking? and
Eye opener	4. Have you ever had a drink first thing in the morning to steady your nerves or get rid of a hangover?

Two or more positive responses on the CAGE indicate a strong likelihood that a patient has experienced significant alcohol-related problems or is alcohol dependent. Sensitivity and specificity data for the CAGE range from 73 to 97% and 72 to 96%, respectively, indicating that the CAGE performs well in detecting more severe drinking-related symptoms that warrant a diagnosis of alcohol abuse or dependence using DSM-based criteria.[4] However, the CAGE does not assess frequency of drinking, average consumption per drinking occasion, or episodes of heavy drinking, factors that can help to identify at-risk nondependent patients.[24] Therefore, clinicians should not use the CAGE as a screening tool for detecting hazardous drinking. In addition, recent studies indicate that the CAGE may be less sensitive to detecting alcohol-related problems among women. As a consequence, it has been suggested that a cutoff score of 1 be adopted for use with female patients.[5]

Major advantages of the CAGE include its brevity and ease of administration (it takes approximately 1 minute to administer) and the fact that it can be incorporated into a standard clinical interview as part of a general health screening. Because the CAGE only assesses lifetime usage, patients who score high on this should also be questioned concerning their current alcohol usage. In addition, the CAGE may overestimate alcohol-related problems in general practice settings, where questions about "cutting down" and "feeling guilty" are often answered "yes" by current light drinkers or abstainers.[25] Nonetheless, because of the instrument's brevity and high degree of sensitivity for detecting alcohol problems, the CAGE is a widely used instrument for use in primary care and other medical settings.

THE MICHIGAN ALCOHOLISM SCREENING TEST (MAST)

Much like the CAGE, the MAST[26] was originally developed for use as a screening test for alcohol dependence. In its long form, the MAST consists of 25 face-valid yes/no questions and is typically administered using a self-report questionnaire as opposed to an interview. Questions on the MAST emphasize respondents' perceptions of the social, job-related, and familial problems encountered as a result of excessive drinking, as well as more severe alcohol dependence symptoms such as alcohol-related withdrawal (e.g., alcohol-related delirium tremens), loss of control drinking, and the experience of alcohol-related blackouts. Scoring of the MAST is somewhat cumbersome, involving assignment of weighted values of either 1, 2, or 5 points for "alcohol-dependent" responses. Suggested screening criteria on the MAST are for scores ranging from 0 to 3 to be coded as "non-alcohol dependent," a score of 4 as "probably alcohol dependent," and scores of 5 points or greater as "alcoholic."

The MAST typically takes 5 to 10 minutes to complete. As such, it is not an ideal measure for use in a busy clinical practice setting. However, the MAST is often a good choice for use in more intensive outpatient or inpatient substance abuse settings where time restrictions may be less of a concern. Because the MAST provides a rather detailed list of alcohol-related consequences, patients can benefit both from descriptive feedback concerning the diversity of problems associated with continued drinking, and from the direct feedback regarding the diagnostic implications of their test score. If time is more of a concern, two abbreviated versions of the MAST, the ten-question Brief MAST[27] (BMAST) and the 13-question Short MAST[28] (SMAST), have been developed and are now in wide use as suitable alternative measures.

The accuracy of the MAST and its shorter versions in identifying patients with significant alcohol-related problems appears to be comparable to the CAGE, with sensitivities ranging from 71 to 100% and specificities of 81 to 96% (for a review, see Reference 4). Because the CAGE performs reasonably well in comparison to the MAST, the CAGE is often the preferred choice among family practitioners and general internists. However, as a clinical tool for use in providing patient feedback regarding problem areas associated with heavy drinking, the MAST offers considerable advantages over the CAGE becuase it contains more detailed items to discuss. As with the CAGE, the MAST does not perform well as a tool to identify nondependent patients who are at risk for future alcohol-related problems.[4] Likewise, the MAST only provides information regarding lifetime alcohol-related problems.

THE ALCOHOL USE DISORDER IDENTIFICATION TEST© (AUDIT©)

The AUDIT is a relatively new screening instrument that provides a useful alternative for practitioners who are interested in screening for hazardous or harmful alcohol consumption that may precede development of physical dependence or chronic physical or psychosocial problems. Published in 1989 by the World Health Organization,[29,30] the AUDIT consists of ten items assessing quantity and frequency of alcohol use, dependence symptoms, and personal and social harm related to excessive alcohol use. Responses to individual test items are given a score from 1 to 4, with a total test score of 8 or higher indicating the likely presence of hazardous drinking. As with the CAGE, it is suggested that a lower cut-point of 7 should be used when assessing for hazardous drinking among women.[5] In contrast to the CAGE and the MAST, the AUDIT focuses on the detection of problematic drinking within the last 12 months, and was specifically designed for use within primary care settings.

In an initial six-country sample of 913 primary care patients used to develop the instrument, 92% of patients identified as having hazardous or harmful drinking scored 8 or higher on the AUDIT, and 94% of those without hazardous drinking scored below 8.[30] In this initial validation study, *hazardous drinking* was defined as a hazardous daily level of consumption (average daily consumption of 60 g or more for men and 40 g or more for women), recurrent intoxication (e.g., 120 g per drinking occasion at least weekly), at least one symptom of dependence, at least one alcohol-related problem in the last year, an alcohol-related disease, or a self-perceived drinking problem. More recent studies indicate that the AUDIT is preferable over the CAGE and the MAST for use in detecting problem drinking in its early phases.[31-33]

THE MUNICH ALCOHOLISM TEST© (MALT©)

The MALT is an alcoholism screening instrument initially developed in Germany for use in inpatient and outpatient medical settings.[34] Unlike the other instruments reviewed in this chapter, the MALT includes a seven-item physician rating, along with 24 self-report items completed by the patient. The physician rating section includes items assessing the presence or absence of specific medical complications associated with heavy alcohol use (i.e., liver disease, delirium tremens, and polyneuropathy). The physician section also assesses information supplied by the patient or the patient's family concerning alcohol consumption rates (e.g., consumption of at least 300 ml of pure alcohol on a daily basis) and instances of family members seeking professional help because of the identified patient's alcohol use. The patient self-report section of the MALT assesses a wide range of drinking behaviors and alcohol-related consequences, including the occurrence of withdrawal symptoms, preoccupation with alcohol, loss of control, and social difficulties associated with drinking. For scoring on the MALT, each affirmative response on the seven-item physician-rating section is given a weighted score of 4, whereas each positive response on the self-report section is given a score of 1.

Based on data gathered from the initial MALT validation study of 1335 German patients, the authors of the MALT recommend that patients who score 11 or above be considered alcoholic, and patients scoring between 6 and 10 should be considered as "suspected" alcoholic. The MALT has been found to have a diagnostic specificity of 90% and a diagnostic sensitivity of 98%.[34] However, the independent criterion used for determining a diagnosis of "alcoholic" in this initial study was based on a clinical diagnosis of alcoholism made by a physician or team of physicians. No additional information is provided regarding the criteria used to determine the presence or absence of alcoholism.

Although the MALT is a popular diagnostic screening instrument in Europe, little is known about the comparability of the MALT to other more widely used instruments such as the CAGE or the AUDIT. An advantage of the MALT is that it has been translated into a number of different languages. However, because it requires physicians to complete a portion of the instrument, the MALT is less practical than other brief screening instruments reviewed here. Moreover, because the emphasis for the MALT appears to be on detecting more advanced stages of alcoholism, it is likely to be much less sensitive in identifying patients who could benefit from early intervention for problematic drinking.

THE TWEAK AND THE T-ACE©

As previously noted, validation studies have often neglected to include women or have failed to provide separate analyses by gender to determine the usefulness of screening instruments among women. Indeed, a recent review of the literature on screening instruments in women suggests that the CAGE and the MAST are relatively insensitive to detecting alcohol problems in women.[5] The T-ACE and the TWEAK represent viable alternatives for use as screening instruments for women with alcohol-related problems. Although the T-ACE and the TWEAK were initially developed for use in detecting alcohol-related problems among pregnant women,[35,36] these instruments appear to be suitable for use among women in general. Both the T-ACE and TWEAK are described in greater detail in Chapter 13 this volume on treatment needs among women.

INCORPORATING ALCOHOL SCREENING INTO CLINICAL PRACTICE

Because many patients do not freely volunteer information to their practitioner about drinking-related problems, the routine use of any of the screening instruments reviewed in this chapter can dramatically increase the likelihood of identifying patients who are in need of treatment services. For patients who screen positive for alcohol-related problems, the next step is to provide objective feedback regarding the findings. The goal in providing feedback is to maximize the likelihood that an identified patient will consider taking steps toward reducing or eliminating alcohol use. Toward that end, the assessment and feedback process should be experienced by the patient as a collaboration rather than a confrontation.[3,37] In the end, it is the individual patient who must choose whether to address concerns about his/her alcohol use. Therefore, clinicians should provide patients with as much objective information as possible about potential adverse consequences of drinking, and this information should be incorporated into a larger discussion with the patient of both the positive and negative aspects of continued drinking.

Practitioners who lack experience in working with problem drinkers should take heart in knowing that, even if no additional treatment is pursued, the provision of objective assessment feedback and brief patient advice often leads to increased commitment to change and actual reductions in alcohol use.[3] Beyond providing simple feedback, however, it is also the clinician's responsibility to advise patients about different treatment options. For patients who screen positive for hazardous or early-phase problem drinking (perhaps after completing the AUDIT), an agreed-upon goal of reduced drinking may be acceptable. Under such circumstances, a relatively brief intervention involving education, advice, and goal-setting can lead to reduced drinking and health care utilization.[17] Patients experiencing more severe difficulties associated with drinking should be referred for more intensive treatment through a clinic or inpatient program geared toward abstinence-based interventions.

CONCLUSIONS

Many front-line health care providers and mental health professionals are in an ideal position to screen and identify patients with alcohol-related problems. By incorporating the use of brief screening tools into a routine battery of health-screening questionnaires, clinicians can make informed decisions about treatment for patients with alcohol-related disorders. Although many clinicians are able to recognize the signs associated with the advanced stages of alcoholism, the use of a screening instruments reviewed in this chapter can greatly increase the likelihood that patients in the early stages of at-risk drinking can receive appropriate intervention before major life difficulties or health-related problems arise. It is hoped that this brief overview will serve to motivate practicing clinicians to consider the use of routine alcohol screening as a means of enhancing patient care.

REFERENCES

1. Babor, T. F., Kranzler, H.R., and Lauerman, R.J., Early detection of harmful alcohol consumption: comparison of clinical, laboratory, and self-report screening procedures, *Addict. Behav.,* 14, 139, 1989.
2. Yersin, B., Nicolet, J.F., Decrey, H., Burnier, M., van Melle, G., and Pecoud, A., Screening for excessive alcohol drinking, *Arch. Intern. Med.,* 155, 1907, 1995.
3. Allen, J.P. and Columbus, M., Eds., *Assessing Alcohol Problems: A Guide for Clinicians and Researchers, Treatment Handbook, Series 4.* National Institute on Alcohol Abuse and Alcoholism, Bethesda, MD, 1995.
4. Kitchens, J.M., Does this patient have an alcohol problem? *JAMA,* 272, 1782, 1994.
5. Bradley, K.A., Boyd-Wickizer, J., Powell, S.H., and Burman, M.L., Alcohol screening questionnaires in women: a critical review, *JAMA,* 280, 166, 1998.
6. Nilssen, O. and Cone, H., Screening patients for alcohol problems in primary health care settings, *Alcohol Health Res. World,* 18, 136, 1994.
7. American Psychiatric Association, *Diagnostic and Statistical Manual of Mental Disorders,* fourth edition, American Psychiatric Association, Washington, D.C., 1994.
8. Bradley, K.A. Screening and diagnosis of alcoholism in the primary care setting. *Western J. Med.,* 156, 166, 1992.
9. Rydon, P., Redman, S., Sanson-Fisher, R.W., and Reid, A.L.A., Detection of alcohol-related problems in general practice. *J. Stud. Alcohol.,* 53, 197, 1992.
10. Regier, D.A., Farmer, M.E., Rae, D.S., Locke, B.Z., Keith, S.J., Judd, L.L., and Goodwin, F.K., Comorbidity of mental disorders with alcohol and other drug abuse: results from the Epidemiologic Catchment Area (ECA) Study, *JAMA,* 264, 2511, 1990.
11. Cleary, P. D., Miller, M., Bush, B. T., Warburg. M. M., Delbanco, T. L., and Aronson, M. D. Prevalence and recognition of alcohol abuse in a primary care population, *Am. J. Med.,* 85, 466, 1988.
12. Orrego, H., Blendis, L.M., Blake, J.E., Kapur, B.M. and Israel, Y., Reliability of assessment of alcohol intake based on personal interviews in liver clinic, *Lancet,* 2, 1354, 1979.
13. Bucholz, K.K., Homan, S.M., and Helzer, J.E., When do alcoholics first discuss drinking problems? *J. Stud. Alcohol.,* 53, 582, 1992.
14. Deitz, D, Rohde, F., Bertolucci, D., and Dufour, M. Prevalence of screening for alcohol use by physicians during routine physical examinations, *Alcohol Health Res. World,* 18, 162, 1994.
15. O'Connor, P. G., The general internist, *Alcohol Health Res. World,* 18, 110, 1994.
16. Bien, T.H., Miller, W.R., and Tonigan, J.S., Brief interventions for alcohol problems: a review, *Addiction,* 88, 315, 1993.
17. Fleming, M.F., Barry, K.L., Manwell, L.B., Johnson, K., and London, R., Brief physician advice for problem alcohol drinkers: a randomized controlled trial in community-based primary care practices, *JAMA,* 277, 1039, 1997.
18. Connors, G.J., Screening for alcohol problems, J.P. Allen and M. Columbus, Eds., *Assessing Alcohol Problems: A Guide for Clinicians and Researchers. Treatment Handbook, Series 4,* National Institute on Alcohol Abuse and Alcoholism, Bethesda, MD, 1995, 17–30.
19. Robins, L.N., Helzer, J.E., Croughan, J., and Ratcliff, K.S. National Institute of Mental Health Diagnostic Interview Schedule, *Arch. Gen. Psychiatry,* 38, 381, 1981.
20. Spitzer, R.L., Williams, J.B, Gibbon, M., and First, M.B., The Structured Clinical Interview for DSM-III-R (SCID): I. History, rationale, and description, *Arch. Gen. Psychiatry,* 49, 624, 1992.
21. Grant, B.F., Harford, T.C., Dawson, D.A., Chou, P.S., and Pickering, R.P. The alcohol use disorder and associated disabilities interview schedule (AUDADIS): reliability of alcohol and drug use modules in a general population sample, *Drug Alcohol Depend.,* 38, 37, 1995.

22. Wittchen, H.U., Reliability and validity studies of the WHO Composite International Diagnostic Interview (CIDI): a critical review, *J. Psychiatr. Res.*, 28, 57, 1994.
23. Ewing, J.A., Detecting alcoholism: the CAGE questionnaire, *JAMA*, 252, 1905, 1984.
24. Fleming, M.F., Manwell, L.B. Barry, K.L., and Johnson, K. At-risk drinking in an HMO primary care sample: prevalence and health policy implications, *Am. J. Public Health*, 88, 90, 1998.
25. Chan, A.W.K., Pristach, E.A., Welte, J.W., and Russell, M., Use of the TWEAK test screening for alcoholism/heavy drinking in three populations, *Alcoholism: Clin. Exp. Res.*, 17, 1188, 1993.
26. Selzer, M.L., Michigan Alcoholism Screening Test: the quest for a new diagnostic instrument, *Am. J. Psychiatry*, 127, 1653, 1971.
27. Pokorny, A.D., Miller, B.A., and Kaplan, H.B. Brief MAST: a shortened version of the Michigan Alcoholism Screening Test, *Am. J. Psychiatry*, 129, 342, 1972.
28. Selzer, M.L., Vinokur, A., and VanRooijen, L., Self-administered Short Michigan Alcoholism Screening Test (SMAST), *J. Stud. Alcohol*, 36, 117, 1975.
29. Babor, T.F., Hofman, M., Delboca, F.K, Hesselbrock, V., Meyer, R.E., Dolinsky, Z.S., and Rounsaville, B., The Alcohol Use Disorder Test: Guidelines for Use in Primary Health Care. WHO Publication No. 89.4, World Health Organization, Geneva, 1989.
30. Saunders, J.B., Aasland, O.G., Babor, T.F., de la Fuente, J.R., and Grant, M., Development of the Alcohol Use Disorders Identification Test (AUDIT): WHO collaborative project on early detection of persons with harmful alcohol consumption. II, *Addiction*, 88, 791, 1993.
31. Bohn, M.J., Babor, T.F., and Kranzler, H.R., Alcohol Use Disorders Identification Test (AUDIT): validation of a screening instrument for use in medical settings, *J. Stud. Alcohol.*, 56, 423, 1995.
32. Cherpitel, C.J., Differences in performance of screening instruments for problem drinking among blacks, whites and Hispanics in an emergency room population, *J. Stud. Alcohol.*, 59, 420, 1998.
33. MacKenzie, D.M., Langa, A., and Brown, T.M. Identifying hazardous or harmful alcohol use in medical admissions: a comparison of AUDIT, CAGE and brief MAST, *Alcohol and Alcoholism*, 31, 591, 1996.
34. Feuerlein, W., Ringer, Ch., and Kufner, H., Diagnosis of alcoholism: the Munich Alcoholism Test (MALT), M. Galanter, Ed., *Currents in Alcoholism: Recent Advances in Research and Treatment*, Vol. VII, Grune & Stratton, New York, 1980, 137.
35. Sokol, R.J., Martier, S.S., and Ager, J.W., The T-ACE questions: practical prenatal detection of risk-drinking, *Am. J. Obstet. Gynecol.*, 160, 863, 1989.
36. Russel, M., Martier, S.S., Sokol, R.J., Jacobson, S., Jacobson, J., and Bottoms, S., Screening for pregnancy risk-drinking: tweaking the tests, *Alcohol Clin. Exp. Res.*, 15, 638, 1991.
37. Miller, W.R. and Rollnick, S., Using assessment results, Miller, W.R. and Rollnick, S., Eds. *Motivational Interviewing*, Guilford Press, New York, 1991, 89-99.

Part 2

Acute Treatment

5 Acute Alcohol Intoxication

Christoph Pechlaner, Michael Joannidis, and Christian Wiedermann

OVERVIEW

In this chapter, you will find a comprehensive description of the management of acute ethanol intoxication. The major emphasis will be on the clinical scenario of an emergency presentation. The focus is on adult patients. The concepts and mode of delivery of basic and advanced life support will not be elaborated in detail. In the following presentation, "alcohol" may be substituted by "ethanol" if not explicitly stated otherwise.

MANAGEMENT OF ACUTE ALCOHOL INTOXICATION

- **Clinical presentation: whom to suspect for alcohol intoxication**
- **Assess vital functions**
- **Assess and treat for inadequate circulation**
- **Assess and treat for inadequate breathing**
- **Assess consciousness — sedation and coma**
- **Other general measures**
- **Review differential diagnoses, evaluate for additional complications**
- **Assess and treat for typical complications of alcohol**
- **Observe/monitor the patient until in a safe clinical condition**
- **Comments on blood tests**

SYMPTOMS AND SIGNS: WHOM TO SUSPECT FOR ALCOHOL INTOXICATION

Consider acute alcohol intoxication in any patient presenting with:

- Coma
- Syncope
- Any inappropriate behavior
- Any neurologic abnormality
- Trauma
- Traffic accident
- Hypothermia

In many cases, the patient, friends, or bystanders will be able to give a useful history. But it is not uncommon that patients or relatives will be reluctant to talk about an alcohol excess or a chronic alcoholism background. The drowsy patient may be unable to provide any useful information.

The apparently drunken patient is a frequent visitor to the emergency department. The **typical presentation** is with **incoordination and confusion**. The patient typically has slurred speech and an unsteady gait. He/she may misinterpret perceptions from his or her environment. **Inappropriately aggressive** or **sensitive behavior** is also common.

Intoxicated patients may display a variety of neurologic symptoms; even the neurology consultant may be puzzled because the whole picture resists an easy fit into a single explanation. In any patient with "strange neurology," we therefore are primed to also consider intoxication. With increasing levels of intoxication, CNS depression predominates, and ultimately may result in frank **coma**. Differentiating coma from health-restoring sleep is an ambiguous task, especially in a patient who may have just upset the whole emergency room with his aggressive, combative, or rampant behavior.

Some patients may impress you by **rapid fluctuations of neurologic abnormalities**. For example, you may be puzzled as to whether the Babinski sign is present or not, because it continues to wax and wane within minutes. Patients may abruptly change between sedation and excitation, a feature probably more common with alcohol intoxication as compared to other sedative overdose. The patient may be able to give simple answers, but only a minute later even strong painful stimuli may not elicit any motor response. One of our patients, a 35-year-old male, did not respond at all, even to skillfully applied pain. We decided to intubate his trachea without premedication; but immediately after insertion of the tube past the tongue, he grabbed the tube, threw it away, was on his feet in the next few seconds, and insisted on leaving the emergency room right away — which in effect he did after a half hour discussion with baffled emergency physicians. At this time, he obviously was "drunken," but he left the emergency department walking without aid. His blood alcohol level eventually turned out to be around 500 mg dl^{-1}.

Earlier in the course, the skin is flushed, with increased sweating. Excess alcohol may result in **syncope** — the patient drops "under the table." Such episodes more likely occur in hot air. **Gastrointestinal complaints**, such as nausea, vomiting, and abdominal pain, are early signs of alcohol toxicity. Finally, we have seen patients with acute-onset, severe **vertigo** resolving after a couple of hours as the only symptom of acute alcohol intoxication, or acute-onset **tachycardia-arrhythmia**, especially atrial fibrillation, as the leading complaint prompting the patient to ask for professional help.

Alcohol intoxication is a **frequent risk factor for adverse events** such as traffic accidents, injuries, and hypothermia.

A reliable **history** usually yields the most helpful information. **Physical examination** is less specific, and less sensitive. The breath may smell of alcoholic beverage, but this is neither sensitive, nor specific; in other words, alcohol-induced coma may be present without alcoholic smell, and an alcoholic smell does not prove that alcohol is the main problem. Neurological signs are usually present (e.g., ataxia, nystagmus, divergent bulbi). Respiratory depression, hypotension, bradycardia, and hypothermia indicate more severe intoxication.

ASSESS VITAL FUNCTIONS

- Check responsiveness
- Check breathing
- Check circulation

Assess vital functions, according to the recommendations of your resuscitation council for basic life support (e.g., European Resuscitation Council[1]) in every patient as a first priority.

STEP 1: CHECK RESPONSIVENESS

- Does the patient respond to loud talking, shouting, or shaking?
- If not: do not lose time; immediately proceed to steps 2 and 3. If cough and gag reflexes are likely to be absent, consider tracheal intubation to protect the patient's airways. Put the patient into recovery position while not intubated.

STEP 2: CHECK BREATHING

- Look, listen, feel.
- If inadequate, prepare for intubation; immediately proceed to step 3.

STEP 3: CHECK CIRCULATION

- Palpate the carotid artery.
- If carotid pulse is absent, immediately obtain a ECG rhythm strip — prepare for cardiopulmonary resuscitation.
- Absent breathing or circulation should trigger delivery of advanced life support. Do not hesitate to call immediately for assistance in cardiopulmonary resuscitation.

BLOOD CIRCULATION AND BLOOD PRESSURE

- Palpate carotid artery pulse.
- Pulse absent:
  - Observe ECG rhythm on monitor and
  - Prepare for cardiopulmonary resuscitation
- Pulse weak:
  - Measure blood pressure;
  - If systolic blood pressure below 90, give saline (NaCl 0.9%, 500 ml) by rapid i.v. infusion; repeat as needed.
- In hypotension refractory to saline: give norepinephrine continuous i.v. infusion, starting with 0.5 to 1.0 µg min^{-1}.
- Evaluate for bleeding, aspirate stomach fluid via nasogastric cannula, and consider endoscopy.

Palpate for a carotid artery pulse just lateral to the trachea. Some fear a drop in blood pressure or heart rate by inadvertent carotid sinus stimulation, but available evidence strongly argues for a positive benefit–risk relation of the maneuver. Your palpation should be gentle initially, with slightly increasing pressure if no pulse is palpable; too strong a pressure may even compress the artery and yield a false negative result. A palpable pulse indicates left ventricular ejection and no immediate need for chest compression. The strength of the pulse is a useful indicator for the patient's blood pressure.

If carotid pulses are not palpable, the patient may have asystole, ventricular fibrillation, other arrhythmia incompatible with adequate ventricular ejection, or severe hypotension. Immediately obtain an ECG rhythm strip and be prepared for cardiopulmonary resuscitation.

If carotid pulses are weak, measure blood pressure. A systolic reading of 90 mmHg or more is usually safe; lower readings should arouse concern. A reading of below 80 mmHg should definitely prompt immediate action: give "physiologic" saline (NaCl 0.9%, 500 ml) by rapid infusion; the same volume may be infused repeatedly as dictated by clinical course. Consider continuous i.v. infusion of **vasopressor agents** (starting doses: e.g., norepinephrine, 0.5 to 1.0 µg min^{-1}; or dopamine, 10 µg min^{-1}). Dopamine is the agent preferred by many, but this choice seems to be dictated more by tradition than by scientific data. In the setting of intoxication, our pressor agent of choice is the pure alpha-receptor agonist norepinephrine; in some poisonings, dopamine may cause paradoxical hypotension by virtue of its beta-receptor agonist properties.

Consider gastrointestinal bleeding with hemorrhagic shock, especially in chronic alcoholics, who may have esophageal varices, peptic ulcer, or congestive gastropathy. Another common cause of bleeding in alcohol overdose is mucosal tears after bouts of vomiting (Mallory-Weiss syndrome). Consider insertion of a nasogastric cannula for diagnostic aspiration of gastric fluid. Bloody aspirate

---

TABLE 5.1
Causes of Acute Hypotension

Hypovolemic
   Loss of blood
   Vomiting, diarrhea
   Excessive sweating
   Hyperosmolar states (e.g., ketoacidosis)
   "Third-spacing" (e.g., ascites, pancreatitis)
Cardiogenic
   Dysrhythmia
   Low contractile power (e.g., myocardial infarction)
   Acute valvular dysfunction (e.g., papillary muscle rupture)
Obstructive
   Tension pneumothorax
   Pericardial tamponade
   Massive pulmonary embolism
Distributive
   Sepsis syndrome (systemic inflammatory reaction)
   Anaphylaxis
   Neurogenic (vasodilation by autonomic nervous system dysfunction)
   Vasodilator agents (e.g., other poisons)
   Acute adrenal insufficiency
Most poisons

---

warrants urgent endoscopic treatment, with or without somatostatin iv treatment (e.g., octreotide 50 µg i.v. bolus, followed by 50 µg h^{-1} continuous i.v. infusion for 48 to 72 h).

Causes and contributors to hypotension are listed in Table 5.1.

RESPIRATION

- **Give oxygen to every patient with sedation or respiratory depression.**
- **Observe patient's respiratory movements.**
- **Perform orotracheal intubation if:**
  - **No spontaneous breathing**
  - **Coma**
  - **Airways not protected from aspiration.**
- **If spontaneous breathing is depressed:**
  - **Consider bag-valve-mask while checking for need of intubation;**
  - **Obtain arterial blood gas analysis; if not available, pulse oxymetry.**
- **SaO$_2$ lower than 90 to 92% indicates hypoxia; secure airways, consider intubation.**
- **Acute hypercarbia indicates impending respiratory failure.**

First of all, give oxygen via nasal cannula or face mask in any patient who appears sedated, or who appears to have depressed respiration, at an initial rate of 2 to 4 l min^{-1}.

Observe the patient's respiratory movements — of chest and abdomen. Very shallow respirations may be overlooked. If in doubt:

- Gently place the palm of one hand on the patient's abdomen; feel for any movements.
- Place your ear next to the patient's mouth and nose, and listen and feel for any air movements.
- Place the back of your hand next to the patient's mouth and nose; feel for any air movements.

If spontaneous breathing is absent, check the patient's airways for obstacles, remove dental prostheses and spectacles, and support the patient's breathing by bag-valve-mask or mouth-to-mouth ventilation, while preparing for orotracheal **intubation**.

Spontaneous respiratory movements and absence of cyanosis unfortunately do not exclude inadequate gas exchange.

Obtain an **arterial blood gas analysis**; do not rely solely on pulse oxymetry. Pulse oxymetry is useful for monitoring, but has important limitations: it is applicable only to the patient with pulsatile flow under the probe (which may be absent, e.g., in shock or hypothermia); erratic measurement outputs are not uncommon (e.g., if arrhythmia, shivering, or agitation are present). Pulse oxymetry only measures percent of hemoglobin saturated with oxygen (SpO_2), but gives no information on carbon dioxide (CO_2), which accumulates with inadequate ventilation, and ultimately leads to respiratory depression (carbon dioxide narcosis). And finally, you should know that pulse oxymetry yields false high readings (typically near 100%) in potentially lethal poisoning with carbon monoxide (CO) or cyanide. Thus, pulse oxymetry may inspire a misleading feeling of safety when in reality disaster is impending. Arterial blood gas analysis is a must, at least at initial assessment, in every patient with suspected respiratory depression.

Hypoxia is indicated by low arterial hemoglobin saturation with oxygen ($SaO_2 < 90$ to 92%), or by low arterial partial oxygen pressure ($PaO_2 < 60$–65 mmHg). Further increases in oxygen delivery rate over the initial rate of 2 to 4 $l\,min^{-1}$ are usually followed by only very modest effects on arterial oxygenation. **Hypoxia must be reversed within minutes** to avoid irreversible cerebral damage. Without an immediately reversible cause, intubate the patient. Use of noninvasive ventilation is a respiration aid gaining popularity. Noninvasive ventilation denotes the application of a constant airway pressure via a tight-fitting mask over nose and mouth without tracheal intubation. It allows for more efficient oxygen uptake, because oxygen can be provided to the alveoli at a higher fractional concentration than by conventional face mask, and because the pressure gradient for oxygen between alveoli and pulmonary capillaries can be increased. Unfortunately, **noninvasive ventilation is inadequate for the heavily sedated patient**, and therefore inadequate for the severely alcohol intoxicated because it leaves airways unprotected from aspiration.

Hypercapnia, or hypercarbia denotes elevated carbon dioxide partial pressure (pCO_2), above the normal value of 35 mmHg. For the clinician, pCO_2 is the marker for inadequate ventilation (= gas transport), as opposed to oxygenation (oxygen uptake). Acute hypercapnia is the typical finding in respiratory depression, shallow respirations, or airway obstruction. Acute hypercapnia is a much earlier finding in these settings than is hypoxia.

Acute hypercapnia is characterized by the combination of:

- Hypercapnia ($pCO_2 > 45$ mmHg)
- Acidemia (pH < 7.35)
- (Near)-normal bicarbonate (HCO_3), 22 to 26 mmol l^{-1}

This triad should ring an alarm of impending respiratory disaster. **Acute hypercapnia is a respiratory emergency**. You should be able to recognize it from arterial blood gas analysis, and take appropriate measures: auscultate for abnormal lung sounds, monitor the patient, preferably with pulse oxymetry, and consider tracheal intubation. Do not leave the patient alone; reassess the patient at short intervals.

In contrast, **chronic hypercapnia** is typically seen in severe chronic obstructive pulmonary disease (COPD, lung emphysema). pCO_2 is elevated, usually at 50 to 60 mmHg, but bicarbonate is elevated, typically about 30 mmol l^{-1}, resulting in low-normal or only slightly decreased pH. Elevated bicarbonate is due to renal counterregulation, which requires at least a couple days to come into effect.

Acute hypercapnia is a typical finding in severe alcohol intoxication, as in any other respiratory depressant poisoning. There is no specific antidote for alcohol-induced respiratory depression.

Acute hypercapnia should prompt you to consider possible additional toxins (especially sedatives and opiates) and acute respiratory disease (bronchial obstruction like asthma attack, or exacerbation of preexistent chronic obstructive disease).

HEAVY SEDATION AND COMA

- Speak to the patient in a loud voice.
- If no adequate response, apply a painful stimulus.
- Intubate the trachea if tracheal reflexes are inadequate to prevent aspiration.
- Put the patient in lateral decubitus while not intubated.
- Give oxygen, initial rate 2 to 4 l min^{-1}.
- Thiamine 100 mg i.v.
- Measure blood glucose level by bedside test.
- i.v. glucose 10%, 500 ml, or glucose 30%, 100 ml.
- Search for head trauma.
- Frequently assess pupils.
- Consider additional toxin ingestion.
- Consider cerebral computed tomography.

The patient is breathing spontaneously and has a palpable carotid pulse, but he does not or only inadequately reacts to shouting and to a **painful stimulus**:

- Apply firm pressure with your index fingers just under the ear lobes on both sides, in the easily palpable groove between mandible and mastoid process.
- Or, grab a skin fold over the patient's shoulder and pinch.
- Or, prick the nasal mucosa with a needle.

We prefer the first method: it causes sufficient pain without injury, and may be done from behind the patient. This is a safe place to avoid retaliatory actions of the patient against the offending examiner.

Consider intubation — if in doubt, do it. The patient's airway-protecting reflexes may be inadequate, even if regular breathing is present. Eliciting a gag reflex, or assessing whether it is adequate, is an elusive task. Moreover, it may cause harm by provoking vomiting and tracheal aspiration of gastric fluid. Do not hesistate to obtain advice from a senior colleague, wherever readily available.

As long as the patient is **not intubated**, put the patient into **lateral decubitus** position (= rescue position). In this position, any fluid or material in the oropharynx is expected to more easily exit to the outside through the mouth, instead of going down a potentially unprotected trachea.

Give oxygen via nasal cannula or face mask, at an initial rate of 2 to 4 l min^{-1}.

Ensure **preparation of emergency medication** for reversible causes:

- Thiamine (= vitamin B$_1$) 100 mg i.v. is given to prevent acute Wernicke encephalopathy. Newer preparations pose only minimal risk of anaphylaxis.
- Glucose 25 to 50 g (e.g., glucose 10%, 500 ml = 50 g; glucose 30%, 100 ml = 30 g), which poses no clinically relevant risk even in hyperglycemia, but will correct hypoglycemia if present.

Thoroughly evaluate the patient for possible associated problems, especially head trauma, intracerebral bleeding, and additional sedating agent. Consider cerebral computed tomography (CT), as discussed in the next section. Frequently evaluate the patient's pupils. The most helpful signs are a difference in size between pupils, and an absent reaction to light; in such cases, immediately order a cerebral CT. The absolute size may vary considerably among patients, and therefore is less helpful in our experience.

OTHER GENERAL MEASURES

- **Ensure a functioning intravenous line, except for only trivial symptoms.**
- **Draw blood for emergency laboratory examinations.**
- **The most important laboratory examinations are arterial blood gas analysis, glucose, and potassium.**
- **Carefully search for occult head trauma.**
- **Order a cerebral CT if:**
  - **History of head injury *and* Glasgow coma scale < 15;**
  - **Pupils differ in size;**
  - **Worsening of mental status while under observation;**
  - **No improvement in mental status within 3 h after admission.**

You have now completed the basic evaluation for immediately life-threatening conditions and taken appropriate measures.

Ensure a functioning **intravenous line**. You should have an explicit reason for not doing so; for example, if the patient has only very minor symptoms. Proceed to placement of a central venous catheter if you anticipate large quantities of i.v. infusions. Need for continuous i.v. vasopressor infusion is also a plausible indication for a central venous line, at least if higher doses are needed.

Draw blood for emergency laboratory examinations, as recommended in Table 5.2. Our recommendations are a compromise for practicability, speed, and expected changes in management. The more tests you order, the more time will be required to get them. Omitting tests may lead to potentially dangerous underdiagnosis of conditions that require immediate action. In our emergency room, we are happy to make use of on-site analyzers for arterial blood gas analysis, glucose, and potassium. This allows us to recognize within a minute severe hypoxia, hypercarbia, hypoglycemia, or hyperkalemia; and it is these four derangements, where every single minute counts, where immediate action may be needed to prevent patient death.

You should draw blood for a **bedside glucose assay** as early as possible in any comatose patient. Hypoglycemia is a common cause of coma, may lead to irreversible brain damage, and is one of the few opportunities in internal medicine for doing a "miracle cure" within minutes — without clinically relevant side effects.

You should be paranoid with respect to **occult trauma and intracerebral bleeding** for the following reasons:

- The drunken patient can be anticipated to have a high threshold for pain perception, poor short-term memory, and poor narrative skills — as a consequence of the sedative and analgesic effects of ethanol.
- Incoordination in alcohol intoxication predisposes the patient to falls.
- Chronic liver disease is highly prevalent in chronic alcoholics and predisposes them to bleeding, due to low blood clotting factors and thrombopenia. Typical signs of chronic liver disease are often absent, are easily overlooked, and also are unspecific (e.g., dark complexion, spider nevi, hepatomegaly, splenomegaly).

Carefully inspect the patient, especially his head. **Occult head injury** and intracranial bleeding remain the most easily overlooked and most feared complications. Serious head injuries are easily overlooked; some patients have no history and no external signs of head trauma — which may be difficult to detect, especially on the scalp. The most common serious error in management of alcohol-intoxicated patients is to assume for too long that confusion and sedation are due only to intoxication. It is prudent to perform an emergency **cerebral CT** if you are in any doubt. Order a cerebral CT without further delay if one of the following conditions is met:

TABLE 5.2
Recommended Diagnostic Tests

Do in all patients:

Test:	Normal Range[a]	
Glucose	70–110 mg dl^{-1}	3.9–6.1 mmol l^{-1}
Potassium	3.5–5.2 mmol l^{-1}	
Sodium	135–152 mmol l^{-1}	
Chloride	95–110 mmol l^{-1}	
Arterial blood gas analysis		
pH	7.35–7.45	
pCO_2	35–45 mmHg	
Bicarbonate = HCO_3	22–26 mmol l^{-1}	
SaO_2	Greater than 91%	
Ethanol	0 mg dl^{-1}	
Creatine kinase	14–108 U/l	
Creatinine	0.70–1.40 mg dl^{-1}	62–124 µmol l^{-1}
Urea[b]	10.0–50.0 mg dl^{-1}	
Serum osmolality	280–295 mOsm kg^{-1}	
Peripheral blood cell count		
Hemoglobin		
Leukocytes		
Platelets		

Calculate:

Osmolar gap	<10	
Anion gap	10–14	

Consider:

C-reactive protein	–0.70 mg dl^{-1}	
Toxicology screen (benzodiazepines, opiates)		
Carbon monoxide (carboxy-hemoglobin)		
Electrocardiogram		
Cerebral computed tomography		

[a] Normal values may vary considerably across laboratories, and may depend on age. The values given in this table are those at Innsbruck University Hospital.
[b] Urea (mg dl^{-1}) × 0.46 yields BUN (mg dl^{-1})

- History of head injury and Glasgow coma scale < 15
- Pupils are asymmetric
- Worsening of mental status while under observation
- No improvement in mental status within 3 hours after admission

Complete physical examination, including a thorough evaluation for traumatic skin changes.

REVIEW DIFFERENTIAL DIAGNOSES

Acute ethanol intoxication leads to multiple unspecific symptoms. Acute alcohol intoxication is a frequently encountered condition. The sensory, physiological, and behavioral consequences of alcohol intoxication predispose the patient to an array of complications (Table 5.3). Even if alcohol intoxication is very likely, a thorough evaluation for additional or alternative diseases is warranted.

TABLE 5.3
Complications in Alcohol Intoxication

Coma
Occult head injury
Intracerebral bleeding
Trauma
Hypoglycemia
Coingested poisons, especially cocaine, benzodiazepines, and antidepressants
Hypothermia
Rhabdomyolysis
Wernicke encephalopathy
Methanol poisoning
Hyponatremia
Ketoacidosis
Gastrointestinal bleeding
Hypotension, shock

Relatives, friends, or bystanders, when available, may give useful information. Ask for possible prior diseases, and how the patient felt in prior days.

Syncope may be caused by ethanol intoxication alone (via hypotension or sedation). The most severe differential diagnoses to consider are acute myocardial infarction with arrhythmia, pulmonary embolism, hemorrhagic shock, and cerebral bleeding.

Confusion and coma: the most prominent concern is head trauma and intracerebral bleeding. Other potential causes are listed in Table 5.4.

Hypotension: the most important or most common causes in the setting of alcohol intoxication or alcoholism are bleeding, coingested other poisons, and sepsis syndrome.

TABLE 5.4
Causes of Confusion and Coma

Common:
  Hypoglycemia
  Hypoxia (any cause)
  Focal neurologic disease (cerebrovascular occlusion, hemorrhage in brain)
  Intoxication with sedating agents (benzodiazepines, antidepressants)
  Any other serious intoxication (CO)
  Seizures and postictal state
  Thiamine deficiency (Wernicke-Korsakoff)

Rare:
  Hyperthermia or hypothermia
  Endocrine disease (Addison, myxedema)
  Sepsis or CNS infection
  Psychiatric disease
  Profound electrolyte disturbance
  Uremia, hepatic encephalopathy

TYPICAL COMPLICATIONS AND PROBLEMS IN ACUTE ALCOHOL INTOXICATION

- Ensure dedicated care for every alcohol-intoxicated patient
- Avoid benzodiazepines
- Aggressive patients:
  - Try to listen, and talk
  - Haloperidol 10 mg p.o., i.v., i.m., or s.c.
  - Physical restraints are only a last resort
- Coingested poisons, especially cocaine, benzodiazepines, and antidepressants
- Hypoglycemia
- Hypothermia
- Rhabdomyolysis
- Occult head injury
- Wernicke encephalopathy
- Methanol
- Hyponatremia

A particular problem arises with the old drunkard who is a well-known, frequent guest in the emergency room. In this busy environment, anger and frustration in members of the emergency care team easily develop, which favor a **dangerous tendency for substandard** evaluation and care. We remember one patient who died after weeks of intensive care. He was a hope- and homeless drunkard who had suffered irreversible severe brain damage as a consequence of severe hypoglycemia, unrecognized for many hours. We are aware of another patient whose substandard care led to a delay of 6 hours before it was recognized that he had skull base and orbital fractures with cerebrospinal fluid discharge through the nose.

Aggressive behavior can consume considerable resources, and can compromise the safety of caretakers and other patients (e.g., in the emergency room). Wherever possible, offer the patient a quiet place, sit down, **listen**, limit the number of persons the patient is confronted with, and avoid or remove restraints whenever possible. Reaffirm to the patient that you are on his side; make clear that your only interest is in his well-being and in understanding and alleviating whatever obviously seems to upset him — that you are neither the police (no punishment intended) nor a clergyman (no moral reprimands intended). Try to talk about matters where the patient is competent; for example, how does he feel now; his places or professional history may yield some thread for an empathic conversation. It is often helpful to try to imagine that you are sitting with a buddy in a pub. Almost every team has a member with well-developed skills; he (in many instances, a "she" has advantages) should be assigned the task. In our experience, emotions will smooth in the majority of patients treated this way, and the patient may consent to a "good" medication. The preferred medication is a **neuroleptic** (e.g., haloperidol 10 mg p.o. or i.v./s.c./i.m.) because they do not significantly depress central regulation of respiration. In patients not amenable to such a gentle approach, or with overt physical menace, arrange for immediate restraint. Such patients may develop a terrifying physical power, requiring many physically strong persons to gain control. Inserting a venous line for pharmacologic sedation may be impossible or dangerous; then the i.m. route is an alternative.

DO NOT give benzodiazepines; they are very potent respiratory depressants in combination with alcohol overdose. Be extremely cautious and ensure continuous monitoring if considering benzodiazepine administration in a patient who may be alcohol intoxicated. Recently, readers have been drawn twice to media headlines of a dead patient (and a sued physician); in both, the physician had given diazepam to an alcohol-intoxicated young male with aggressive behavior.

Alcohol intoxication threatens life simply by the sedating and respiratory depressant effects of alcohol, as described above. Further complications are not uncommon, especially in the patient with **chronic alcohol abuse**. Chronic alcohol abuse may have already led to significant organ damage, which predisposes to potentially life-threatening complications. Chronic toxicity may affect nearly every major organ system. Unfortunately, **chronic alcohol abuse is not easily recognizable**. Emergency room physicians — although confronted with alcohol-related adverse health effects virtually every day — fail to recognize 50% of patients with ethanol dependence, a proportion that is similar to that overlooked by specialists caring for inpatients.

Hypoglycemia must not be allowed to go untreated; irreversible brain damage may ensue. This is the reason for recommending an **i.v. glucose drip** as a first priority measure in any comatose patient (i.e., after having checked vital functions as described above). Consider hypoglycemia in **every patient with impaired consciousness**. Perform a bedside glucose test as soon as possible. Reevaluate whenever mental status deteriorates.

Hypothermia is a frequent complication during cold weather, due to the sedating and pain-killing effect of ethanol. Ethanol-induced depression of thermoregulatory central mechanisms may also be involved. Treatment of hypothermia is by physical rewarming, and is the same whether or not ethanol intoxication is present. Hypothermia and rewarming are associated with ECG changes and risk of arrhythmia; monitoring is therefore required.

Rhabdomyolysis is the term for skeletal muscle damage, resulting in release of muscle cell contents into blood. The heme component of myoglobin is a potent renal tubular toxin, and thus a not uncommon cause of acute renal failure. Rhabdomyolysis may result from constant pressure on muscle (e.g., after hours immobilized on a hard underground). The main component of treatment is i.v. infusion of adequate volumes of saline.

Occult head trauma and intracranial bleeding: do not forget — see our detailed discussion above.

Wernicke encephalopathy: the combination of carbohydrate overload and thiamine deficiency may precipitate encephalopathy or even coma. Therefore, thiamine 100 mg i.v. is recommended before infusing glucose, especially in the chronic alcoholic.

Coingestion of other toxins: in alcoholics, cocaine is the most commonly abused second drug. The attraction of taking these two drugs together may relate to the formation of a metabolite, cocaethylene, which has 40 times the affinity for cocaine receptors as cocaine itself. However, the risk of sudden death with both drugs ingested is many times higher as compared to cocaine alone.

Benzodiazepines potentiate the sedating effects of alcohol, and may thus precipitate respiratory depression and suffocation.

Antidepressant drugs may lead to mental depression, seizures, and ventricular tachyarrhythmia. Cardiovascular toxicity is preceded by ECG changes, especially QRS duration ≥ 100 ms and prolonged corrected QT ($QT_c \geq 450$ ms). We recommend NaCl 0.9% 500 ml i.v., followed by NaCl 0.9% 1000 ml overnight. If severe ECG changes are present, sodium bicarbonate 100 mmol is recommended. The preferred agent for ventricular tachycardia or fibrillation is lidocaine 100 mg i.v.; if ineffective after a repeat dose, electrical cardioversion/defibrillation is indicated.

Methanol may be a contaminant of alcoholic beverages, especially homemade liquors. Toxicity is the result of two metabolites: formaldehyde and formic acid. A delay of 12 to 18 h after ingestion is typically seen before symptoms appear: CNS depression similar to ethanol, visual disturbances, abdominal pain, and nausea may ultimately lead to permanent blindness, coma, or death. Laboratory clues to methanol poisoning are an anion gap acidemia and an osmolal gap. Treatment is directed at elimination of the toxic metabolites and inhibition of their generation.

Hyponatremia: excessive ingestion of hypoosmolar, low-sodium content drinks may lead to profound hyponatremia. This is typically the case with large amounts of beer — if approaching 20 liters a day. The sodium content of beer is very low; its main solute contributing to osmolality — ethanol — is metabolized to water. Therefore, beer is equivalent to pure water, and ingestion of extreme amounts is equivalent to water intoxication. Normal kidneys have a huge capacity to reabsorb filtered sodium, and to excrete excessive water by producing low-sodium urine. But, with such extreme volumes, sodium losses may result in profound hyponatremia. Hyponatremia predisposes the patient to cerebral edema. Hyponatremia in alcohol intoxication warrants admission to the intensive care unit (ICU) for close monitoring and appropriate treatment.

OBSERVE THE PATIENT UNTIL REASONABLY SOBER

Any patient with alcohol intoxication can develop a life-threatening condition. As with any other poisoning, never rely on a single evaluation alone. A single assessment rarely allows accurate prognosis of further clinical course. Therefore, an appropriate period of observation is virtually always necessary to recognize or exclude problems other than ethanol toxicity, and to document improvement.

Do not leave the patient alone. You must observe or monitor him, or ensure properly supervised transportation to an appropriate unit.

Unhabituated patients eliminate ethanol from their blood at a rate of 15 to 20 mg dl^{-1} per hour. Chronic alcohol abusers usually are able to a faster rate, at an average 25 to 35 mg dl^{-1} per hour. Therefore, patients who are alcohol intoxicated should be expected to progressively get better. Any deterioration during observation should be considered secondary to causes other than alcohol and managed accordingly.

In most patients, acute alcohol intoxication is moderately severe, as judged by the level of consciousness, blood pressure, respiration, and physical examination. Observation only will be adequate in most cases. Most patients can be safely discharged from the emergency room after documented clinical improvement, which usually takes a couple of hours. Admission for treatment of acute ethanol intoxication as the only problem is only rarely required.

BLOOD TESTS IN SUSPECTED ALCOHOL INTOXICATION: COMMENTS

- Peripheral blood cells
- Ethanol
- Osmolal gap
- Anion gap
- Potassium
- Blood gas analysis: arterial vs. venous sampling

Peripheral blood cell count: the alcohol-intoxicated patient has an elevated risk of bleeding. Anemia may be a clue. With bleeding (e.g., into the gastrointestinal tract), both blood cells and plasma are lost from the vascular space. Therefore, immediately after even massive bleeding, the concentrations of red blood cells and hence hemoglobin are unchanged. Only after shift of fluid from the extravascular interstitial space into the hypovolemic vessels will dilution of blood cells occur, and this will manifest as a drop in hemoglobin and erythrocyte concentrations.

Blood ethanol levels only poorly correlate with degree of intoxication, mainly because of the phenomenon of tolerance. At blood levels of 400 to 500 mg dl^{-1}, unhabituated individuals may die from respiratory depression, whereas some alcoholics may appear unintoxicated at the same blood concentration. One drunkard surviving a blood ethanol concentration of 1510 mg dl^{-1}, with supportive care only, has been reported. Unhabituated individuals may experience significant impairment with levels as low as 5 mg dl^{-1}.

Osmolal gap, anion gap: these simple calculations are useful, although not perfect tools for detecting the presence of larger than normal numbers of unusual substances in plasma. Ethanol is a common cause of a hyperosmolar state, an elevated osmolal gap, and an elevated anion gap. Many other substances may be responsible (see Table 5.4).

Potassium: both hypo- and hyperkalemia predispose to potentially lethal cardiac rhythm disorders, and require immediate action. Hyperkalemia may be precipitated by any tissue damage (e.g., rhabdomyolysis).

Arterial blood gas analysis: arterial punction is a painful procedure. Arterial sampling is required if a reliable measurement of arterial oxygenation is needed.

Venous sampling may substitute for arterial blood sampling only if acid-base analysis is intended; pH and pCO_2 do not differ for clinical purposes, and bicarbonate may be assumed to be 2 mmol l^{-1} higher in venous as compared to arterial sampling. Variable oxygen extraction, depending on the clinical situation, does not allow prediction of arterial oxygenation from venous oxygenation, except that arterial oxygen content must be higher than venous oxygen content. If — rarely — oxygen saturation in a venous sample exceeds 90%, then oxygen saturation in this patient must also be higher than 90%. Thus, only such a safe oxygen saturation in a venous sample makes additional arterial sampling unnecessary.

REFERENCES

1. Bossaert, L., Ed., *European Resuscitation Council Guidelines for Resuscitation*, Elsevier, Amsterdam, 1998.
2. Tintinally, J.E., Ruiz, E., and Krome, R.L., *Emergency Medicine — A Comprehensive Study Guide*, McGraw-Hill, New York, 1996.
3. Rosen, P. and Barkin, R., *Emergency Medicine — Concepts and Clinical Practice*, Mosby, St. Louis, 1998.
4. Aghababian, R.V., *Emergency Medicine — The Core Curriculum*, Lippincott-Raven, Philadelphia, 1998.
5. Wallach, J., *Interpretation of Diagnostic Tests — A Synopsis of Laboratory Medicine*, 5th ed., Little, Brown, Boston, 1992.

TABLE 5A.1
Ethanol measurement units

Conventional units	mg dl^{-1}, ‰^{a}
SI units	mmol l^{-1}
Conversion	
to mmol l^{-1}	mg dl^{-1} × 0.22
	‰ × 23
to mg dl^{-1}	mmol l^{-1} × 4.6
	‰ × 106

^{a}'‰' (Promille) reads "per thousand." This unit is popular in many European countries. 1‰ = 0.1% = 0.1 g per 100 g = 105.5 mg dl^{-1}.

TABLE 5A.2
Causes of osmotic gap > 10
Exogenous:
    Ethanol
    Methanol
    Isopropanol
    Ethylene glycol
    Mannitol
    Acetone
    Ethyl ether
    Paraldehyde
Endogenous:
    Diabetic ketoacidosis
    Alcoholic ketoacidosis
    Starvation ketoacidosis
    Renal failure
Hyperlipidemia[a]
Hyperproteinemia[a]
Laboratory analytical error

[a] If analytical method includes dilution
step. Please inquire at your laboratory.

TABLE 5A.3
Causes of an anion gap ≥ 20

Cause	Examples
Ketoacidosis	Diabetes, ethanol
Toxins	methanol, ethylene glycol, paraldehyde, salicylates
Renal failure	
Lactic acidosis	
Rhabdomyolysis	
Phosphate intoxication	
d-Lactic acidosis	From bowel bacteria (e.g., after bowel surgery)

TABLE 5A.4
Glasgow Coma Scale
(GCS)   **Points**

1. Eye opening
   Spontaneous   4
   To verbal command   3
   To pain   2
   No response   1
2. Best verbal response
   Oriented and converses   5
   Disoriented and converses   4
   Inappropriate words   3
   Incomprehensible sounds   2
   No response   1
3. Best motor response
   Obeys   6
   Localizes pain   5
   Flexion-withdrawal   4
   Abnormal flexion   3
   Extension   2
   No response   1

Determine best response for each of the three categories (eyes, verbal, motor) – sum of points is GCS (3 = worst, 15 = best).

TABLE 5.A5
Useful Conversion Factors

BUN	mg dl^{-1} → mmol l^{-1}	×0.356
BUN	mg dl^{-1} → urea mg dl^{-1}	×2.15
Creatinine	mg dl^{-1} → μmol l^{-1}	×88.4
Ethanol	mg dl^{-1} → mmol l^{-1}	×0.217
Glucose	mg dl^{-1} → mmol l^{-1}	÷18
Mannitol	mg dl^{-1} → mmol l^{-1}	÷18.2
Urea	mg dl^{-1} → mmol l^{-1}	÷6

USEFUL CALCULATIONS

calculation of serum osmolality:
   calculated mOsm l^{-1} = [2 × Na (mmol l^{-1})] + glucose (mmol l^{-1}) + BUN (mmol l^{-1})
osmotic gap
   = measured osmolality – calculated osmolality
estimation of blood alcohol from osmotic gap:
   estimated blood alcohol (mg dl^{-1}) = osmotic gap × (100/22) = osmotic gap × 4.54
anion gap
   = Na – (Cl – bicarbonate)all in mmol l^{-1}

RECOVERY POSITION = LEFT LATERAL DECUBITUS

- Remove patient's spectacles.
- Kneel beside the patient and make sure that both legs are straight.
- Open the airway by tilting the head and lifting the chin.
- Place the arm nearest to you out at right angles to his body, elbow bent with the hand palm uppermost.
- Bring his arm across the chest, and hold the back of the hand against the patient's nearest cheek.
- With your other hand, grasp the far leg just above the knee and pull it up, keeping the foot on the ground.
- Keeping his hand pressed against his cheek, pull on the leg to roll the patient toward you onto his side.
- Adjust the upper leg so that both the hip and knee are bent at right angles.
- Tilt the head back to make sure the airway remains open.
- Adjust the hand under the cheek, if necessary, to keep the head tilted.
- Check breathing regularly.

6 Alcohol Withdrawal Syndrome

Christoph H. Stuppaeck, Alexandra B. Whitworth, and Paul C.C. Stuppaeck

OVERVIEW

Alcohol withdrawal syndrome (AWS) is a common state in patients suffering from chronic alcoholism who stop intake or reduce the amount of alcohol. AWS should be treated with psychopharmacologic agents, if the CIWA-Ar score is higher than 8 (see alphabetical list of psychometric screening instruments in the section on useful data and definitions for the test form). In patients with a history of uncomplicated AWS, high motivation, good social background, and little craving, an outpatient setting may be sufficient. Patients with severe AWS in the past, a history of withdrawal seizures, or relevant concomitant diseases should be treated with inpatient care. Patients with delirium tremens must be treated in an intensive care unit. Benzodiazepines are drugs of first choice in all states of AWS, even delirium tremens. Patients with a history of benzodiazepine abuse and mild to moderate AWS can be treated with the anticonvulsant carbamazepine. Sympatholytics may be of help as concomitant medication in patients with predominately anxiety and autonomic hyperactivity. Thiamine is an essential adjunctive treatment in AWS. Alcohol is absolutely contraindicated in the treatment of AWS. The treatment of AWS should be in the hands of specialists and has to be followed by the offer for a long-term treatment with psychotherapeutic and psychopharmacological strategies (see Chapter 9 on psychotherapy).

INTRODUCTION

Depending on the duration of alcohol abuse and dose of alcohol consumed, about 50% of alcohol-dependent patients show the typical signs of AWS after cessation or reduction of alcohol.[1] The exact dose leading to a physical dependence is still unclear and varies widely. Typical patients with moderate to severe AWS treated in an inpatient setting studied by our group had consumed a mean of approximately 300 g of alcohol a day.[2,3] The mean duration from the beginning of alcohol abuse until the appearance of the first withdrawal symptoms after discontinuation of alcohol is at least 6 years.[4]

SYMPTOMS AND CLASSIFICATIONS OF AWS

The first symptom is usually tremor and appears 6 to 8 hours after the last drink. In some patients, even a marked decrease of the alcohol intake may already lead to the appearance of AWS, although their blood alcohol level has not dropped to 0.0.

DSM-IV[5] tends to see a continuum from mild to severe AWS without diagnosing delirium as a special entity, whereas in ICD-10, the terminus delirium is of importance.[6] ICD-10 differentiates between AWS without complications and AWS with delirium, both with or without withdrawal seizures.

Table 6.1 shows the symptoms of AWS. If the additional symptoms of disorientation, clouding of consciousness, hallucinations, and hyperthermia are present, we suggest the use of the term

---

TABLE 6.1
Symptoms of AWS

Tremor of extended hands, tongue, or eyelids
Hyperhidrosis
Nausea and/or vomiting
Tachycardia and/or hypertonia
Psychomotor agitation
Insomnia
Anxiety
Headache
Decreased attention
Hyperthermia
Disorientation
Clouding of consciousness
Hallucinations
Withdrawal seizures

"delirium" for this most severe form of AWS because it needs a more complex treatment approach in an intensive care unit.

To establish guidelines for the treatment of AWS, as well as for an objective criterion of its severity, the use of a rating instrument such as the CIWA-Ar (Clinical Institute Withdrawal Assessment Scale for Alcohol, revised[7]) is recommended. The scale can be applied once daily to as frequently as hourly in patients suffering from AWS and may be helpful in dosing the drugs accordingly. Especially in clinical trials studying various compounds for the treatment of AWS, the CIWA-Ar proves useful in making results comparable.

Besides clinical symptoms, several other somatic signs and laboratory findings are typical for AWS. On admittance, patients often present with signs of polyneuropathy (such as muscle atrophia or disturbed epicritic sensibility), and various signs of liver diseases (e.g., angiomata). Injuries after accidents due to alcohol intoxication are also a common reason for admission to the emergency room, often preceded or followed by a seizure as a symptom of the beginning withdrawal. Especially for differential diagnostic reasons, laboratory evaluations and toxicological examinations should be done to rule out intoxication with sedatives, hallucinogenics, antidepressants, or neuroleptics, or withdrawal from benzodiazepines or other sedatives. Severe medical (i.e., coma hepaticum, hypoglycemic coma, etc.) or neurological diseases accompanied by clouding of consciousness or hallucinations can be confounded with AWS. Other psychiatric syndromes must be excluded — sometimes by way of interviewing significant others. In particular, hallucinations during alcohol withdrawal delirium are often misinterpreted as symptoms of psychotic disorders such as organic mental disease or even schizophrenia. Important laboratory findings in alcohol withdrawal are shown in Table 6.2.

TABLE 6.2
Abnormal Laboratory Parameters in AWS

Elevated liver enzymes (AST, ALT, GGT)
Elevated alkaline phosphatase
Thrombocytopenia
Hyperchrome anemia (MCV, MCH)
Elevated ammonia and bilirubin
Decreased electrolytes (hypokalimia, hypomagnesemia, hyponatremia)

To diagnose AWS is, in most cases, not too difficult. Typical clinical symptoms and laboratory abnormalities, as well as a history of alcohol abuse, confirm the diagnosis. The most common differential diagnosis is a withdrawal syndrome after prolonged use of sedatives — especially benzodiazepines. Due to the half-life times of the benzodiazepines, withdrawal symptoms may appear as late as several days up to 1 week after cessation of the abused drug. The laboratory findings in this case should be normal; slight elevations in liver enzymes occur very rarely.

PHARMACOLOGICAL TREATMENT OF AWS

The decision to treat AWS with or without a pharmacological agent and in an in- or outpatient setting must take into account the length of abuse, concomitant diseases, and the previous history of AWS.[8] Patients suffering from chronic alcoholism for longer than 6 years, older age, prior seizures, delirium, and/or detoxifications have a higher risk of developing severe withdrawal syndrome, such as delirium.[9] With a CIWA-Ar score over 8, they should be treated pharmacologically, especially with concomitant somatic diseases or a history of withdrawal syndromes or seizures. Patients with CIWA-Ar scores higher than 15 should receive medication in any case, because their risk of developing delirium or seizures is high and medication should be started early to prevent these complications.[8] There are no relevant data showing clear predictors of severity of AWS; so, when in doubt, a pharmacological treatment should be started.

Treatment in an outpatient setting can be sucessful in patients suffering only from mild withdrawal symptoms. No concomitant substance abuse should be present and craving should be low. Patients should be seen daily by their treating physician and if a non-pharmacological approach is chosen, a close monitoring for the worsening of symptoms and development of complications is required.

Patients with severe AWS or those suffering from serious comorbid diseases, with a history of withdrawal seizures or withdrawal delirium, should be treated as inpatients in any case.[8]

BENZODIAZEPINES

Benzodiazepines are drugs of first choice in the treatment of AWS.[10] They are effective in treating withdrawal symptoms, preventing seizures and, in most cases, substantially lowering the risk for developing delirium.[11] There is some evidence that benzodiazepines with longer elimination half-lives are more efficacious than those with a short half-life.[12] On the other hand, the use of long-acting agents may lead to prolonged courses of AWS. It should also be taken into account that some benzodiazepines, e.g., diazepam, have better efficacy against withdrawal seizures than congeners like oxazepam or lorazepam.[13] In severe withdrawal symptoms and delirium, it is necessary to have an intravenously applicable drug available.[14] The following parenteral formulations are available: diazepam, chlordiazepoxid, lorazepam, and midazolam.

The main advantage of benzodiazepines over drugs from other chemical classes is the availability of the antagonist flumazenil. This is of importance — especially in patients with concomitant illnesses — because the serious side effect of respiratory depression can be counteracted immediately. If patients do not wake up, a search for other reasons for the sustained impairment of consciousness (e.g., subdural hemorrhagia, brain edema) should immediately be initiated.

The compound best examined and widely used is diazepam; thus, we will refer to this substance in possible dosing schedules. Three different approaches can be applied.

If a specialized professional team is available, we recommend to treat **symptom-triggered**.[15] Ideally, a rating scale such as CIWA-Ar can be used to dose individually. In case of scores higher than 8, a dose of 10 mg diazepam should be administered. This requires frequent assessments (one to two hourly).

In a **fixed dose regimen**,[11] 10 mg diazepam, four times a day, can be prescribed during the first 3 days; and the dose should be tapered down as soon as possible, which will take a mean period of 3 to 6 days. We do not recommend this strategy because the tolerance to this drug varies widely among patients, and overdosing can lead to dangerous side effects such as breathing difficulties and oversedation. On the other hand, this dose can be too low in cases of severe AWS.

Especially in more severe courses of AWS, a so-called front loading strategy[16] might prove helpful. Single doses of 20 mg diazepam are repeated every 2 hours until AWS subsides.

Delirious states make an intravenous benzodiazepine treatment necessary. Doses required may be much higher than mentioned above and should be given according to the patient's condition and vital parameters; it is therefore difficult to give dose recommendations.[14]

The treatment of alcohol withdrawal delirium must be carried out in an intensive care unit with the possibility of monitoring vital parameters and must be accompanied by certain precautionary steps such as antibiotics to ward off pneumonia.

The drawbacks of benzodiazepines are, first, their cross-tolerance with alcohol, so treatment should not be started until a blood alcohol level of 0.0% is reached; and second, they hold a certain risk of abuse in and of themselves.[17] Due to their long elimination half-life times, the use of chlordiazepoxid and diazepam, in particular, can result in oversedation and prolonged courses of AWS because of accumulation.

Patients with severe liver disease should be treated with oxazepam, because liver metabolism is not affected by this benzodiazepine.[12]

The use of other sedating drugs (such as barbiturates, meprobamate, or clomethiazol) is only of historical value. Since the introduction of benzodiazepines, these substances are superfluous, due to their higher rate of complications, higher toxicity, higher risk of dependency and lack of antagonists.[18]

ANTICONVULSANTS (OTHER THAN BENZODIAZEPINES)

During more recent years, the anticonvulsant *carbamazepine* proved very helpful in AWS with the exception of delirium tremens.[2,19] It is effective in preventing seizures and has no cross-tolerance with alcohol.[20] Carbamazepine can be started very early, even in patients with higher blood levels of alcohol at risk for developing AWS. It seems to have nearly zero abuse potential,[21] and side effects are rare.[2] Its use is compatible with serious liver diseases.[22]

A fixed dose regimen is recommended: during the first 3 days of AWS, 200 mg CBZ, four times a day should be given, a slow down-tapering during the next 3 to 6 days is neccessary because of a possible lowering of the seizure threshold in case of abrupt cessation.[2] CBZ is not efficacious in preventing or treating delirium tremens. If symptoms of delirium appear, treatment should be switched to benzodiazepines without delay.

ANTIPSYCHOTICS

Antipsychotics (e.g., haloperidol) play a role as add-on therapy to benzodiazepines in delirium. Hallucinations can be treated successfully, especially when using butyrophenones.[23] It is even possible to reduce the dose of benzodiazepines by adding antipsychotics.[24] In uncomplicated AWS, their use is not recommended due to their side effect profile, which might even aggravate symptoms (extrapyramidal motor side effects, lowering of the seizure threshold, especially by low-potency antipsychotics).[10]

SYMPATHOLYTICS

Due to the increased sympathetic activity in AWS, sympatholytics are currently under intense research in AWS. So far, the literature shows that only patients with mild AWS may profit from monotherapy with beta-blocking agents. They can play a role as adjunctive therapy in patients with pronounced autonomic signs or if symptoms such as anxiety are prominent.[25] The alpha-adrenergic compound clonidine can be helpful as a comedication in patients with marked hypertension, but

---

TABLE 6.3
Frequent Concomitant Diseases in AWS

Nutritional deficits (e.g., electrolytes, metabolism)
Liver diseases (e.g., cirrhosis)
Gastrointestinal illnesses (e.g., pancreatitis, gastritis, ulcera)
Cardiovascular diseases (alcoholic cardiomyopathia, hypertonia)
Pulmonary diseases (e.g., bronchitis, pneumonia, tuberculosis)
Hematologic diseases (e.g., thrombocytopenia, anemia, leucopenia)
Neurological diseases (e.g., seizures, intracerebral hemorrhagia,
  polyneuropathia, brain atrophia, Wernicke-Korsakow syndrome)

---

its main indication in the field of withdrawal treatment is opiate withdrawal syndrome.[26] Neither beta-blocking agents nor alpha-adrenergic substances are an appropriate monotherapy in moderate to severe AWS, and withdrawal seizures are not effectively prevented.[8]

ADJUNCTIVE PHARMACOTHERAPY

Multivitamin B compounds alone were not effective in the treatment of AWS,[11] although they are necessary as adjunct medication and should be routinely included in the treatment plan. In particular, thiamine is important as prophylaxis for Wernicke encephalopathy,[27] and as a treatment for poly-neuropathy, a very common comorbid state in chronic alcoholics.

Patients with AWS often have to be supplemented with potassium in accordance with the laboratory findings (see also Chapter 19 on kidney and electrolyte disturbances). Some authors even postulated pronounced hypokalemia to be a good predictor for delirium tremens.[28] In general, a careful examination of all patients with withdrawal symptoms must be done, and comorbid states should be treated individually. Table 6.3 shows common concomitant diseases.

The mortality rate of AWS (even today between 1 and 8%)[29] is mostly dependent on successful treatment of concomitant illnesses.

AWS IN PREGNANCY

The prevalence of alcohol abuse in pregnant women is probably underestimated (see Chapter 13 on women). The continued abuse of alcohol during pregnancy very often leads to fetal alcohol syndrome (see Chapter 24 on alcohol embryophathy).[18] The risk of treating severe AWS in pregnancy outweighs the risk of leaving it untreated.[10] No data of controlled trials of the treatment of AWS in pregnant women are available. Several benzodiazepines have been connected with an increased risk of congenital malformations when used in the first trimester. They are not recommended for use during labor and delivery because of neonatal flaccidity and respiratory problems. Children born to women after prolonged use of benzodiazepines are at risk for withdrawal symptoms during the postnatal period. Due to the short application of a benzodiazepine in AWS, this risk should be low.

If the severity of AWS makes pharmacotherapy unavoidable, the use of a shorter-acting benzodiazepine such as oxazepam is recommended; if parenteral application is needed, diazepam should be used cautiously.[10]

Data for carbamazepine from long-term treatment of women suffering from epilepsy show a relatively low risk for congenital malformations, although it should be avoided in the first trimester, as should all other drugs.[30] Carbamazepine also has the advantage of a lack of withdrawal symptoms in both mother and neonate.

CAVEATS AND COMMON MISTAKES IN THE TREATMENT OF AWS

- Late initiation of treatment may increase the risk for the development of delirium tremens.
- Somatic illnesses may be overlooked.
- Missing a substitution of electrolyte deficits may be life threatening.
- Uncontrolled intake (dose and duration) of benzodiazepines and other sedatives (especially barbiturates and chlomethiazol) may cause dependency.
- Lack of vitamine B$_1$ substitution may cause Wernicke's encephalopathy.
- The use of alcohol is not a treatment for AWS.

REFERENCES

1. Grant, B. F., Alcohol consumption, alcohol abuse and alcohol dependence: the United States as an example, *Addiction,* 89, 1357, 1994.
2. Stuppaeck, C.H., Pycha, R., Miller, C., Whitworth, A.B., Oberbauer, H., and Fleischhacker, W.W., Carbamazepine versus oxazepam in the treatment of alcohol withdrawal: a double-blind study, *Alcohol Alcohol.,* 27, 153, 1992.
3. Stuppaeck, C.H., Barnas, C., Hackenberg, K., Miller, C., and Fleischhacker, W.W., Carbamazepine monotherapy in the treatment of alcohol withdrawal, *Int. Clin. Psychopharmacol.,* 5, 273, 1990.
4. Ballenger, J.C. and Post, R.M., Kindling as a model for alcohol withdrawal syndromes, *Br. J. Psychiatry,* 133, 1, 1978.
5. American Psychiatric Association, *Diagnostic and Statistical Manual of Mental Disorders,* 4th ed., Psychiatric Association, Washington, D.C., 1994.
6. World Health Organization, *Tenth Revision of the International Classification of Diseases, (ICD-10),* World Health Organization, Geneva, 1992.
7. Sullivan, J.T., Sykora, K., Schneiderman, J., Naranjo, C.A., and Sellers, E.M., Assessment of alcohol withdrawal: the revised clinical institute withdrawal assessment for alcohol scale (CIWA-Ar), *Br. J. Addict.,* 84, 1353, 1989.
8. Saitz, R. and O'Malley, S.S., Pharmacotherapies for alcohol abuse. Withdrawal and treatment, *Alcohol and Other Substance Abuse,* 81, 881, 1997.
9. Foy, A., March, S., and Drinkwater, V., Use of an objective clinical scale in the assessment and management of alcohol withdrawal in a large general hospital, *Alcohol Clin. Exp. Res.,* 12, 360, 1988.
10. Mayo-Smith, M.F., Pharmacological management of alcohol withdrawal. A meta-analysis and evidence-based practice guide, *JAMA,* 278, 144, 1997.
11. Kaim, S.C., Klett, C.J., and Rothfeld, B., Treatment of the acute withdrawal state: a comparison of four drugs, *Am. J. Psychiatry,* 125, 1640, 1969.
12. Hill, A. and Williams, D., Hazards associated with the use of benzodiazepines in alcohol detoxification, *J. Substance Abuse Treat.,* 10, 449, 1993.
13. Mayo-Smith, M.F. and Bernard, D., Late-onset seizures in alcohol withdrawal, *Alcohol Clin. Exp. Res.,* 19, 656, 1995.
14. Pycha, R., Miller, C., Barnas, C., Hummer, M., Stuppaeck, C., Whitworth, A., and Fleischhacker, W.W., Intravenous flunitrazepam in the treatment of alcohol withdrawal delirium, *Alcohol Clin. Exp. Res.,* 17, 753, 1993.
15. Saitz, R., Mayo-Smith, M.F., Roberts, M.S., Redmond, H.A., Bernard, D.R., and Calkins, D.R., Individualized treatment for alcohol withdrawal: a randomized double-blind controlled trial, *JAMA,* 272, 519, 1994.
16. Sellers, E.M., Naranjo, C.A., Harrison, M., Devenyl P., Roach, C., and Sykora, K., Diazepam loading: simplified treatment with alcohol withdrawal, *Clin. Pharmacol. Ther.,* 34, 822, 1983.
17. Griffiths, R.R. and Wolf, B., Relative abuse potential of different benzodiazepines in drug abusers, *J. Clin. Psychopharmacol.,* 10, 237, 1990.
18. Hobbs, W.R., Rall, T.W., and Verdoorn, T.A., Hypnotics and sedatives; alcohol, Hardman, J.G., Goodman, A.G., and Limbird, L.E., Ed., *Goodman and Gilman's The Pharmacological Basis of Therapeutics,* 9th ed., McGraw-Hill, New York, 1996, 361–398.

19. Malcolm, R., Ballenger, J.C., Sturgis, E.T., and Anton, R., Double-blind controlled trial comparing carbamazepine to oxazepam treatment of alcohol withdrawal, *Am. J. Psychiatry,* 146, 617, 1989.

20. Kuhn, R., The psychotropic effect of carbamazepine in non-epileptic adults with particular reference to the drug mechanism of action, *Epileptic Seizures, Behaviour and Pain,* Birkmayer, W., Ed., University Park Press, Baltimore, 1976.

21. Sillanpaa, M., Carbamazepine: pharmacology and clinical uses, *Acta Neurol. Scand.,* 64 (Suppl. 88), 1–202, 1981.

22. Pynnonen, S., Bjorkqvist, S.E., and Pekkarinen, A., The pharmacokinetics of carbamazepine in alcoholics, *Advances in Epileptology,* Meinardi, H., Rowan, A.J., Eds., Swets and Zeitlinger, Amsterdam, 1978, 285-289.

23. Palestine, M.L. and Alatorre, E., Control of acute alcoholic withdrawal symptoms: a comparative study of haloperidol and chlordiazepoxide, *Curr. Ther. Res.,* 20, 289, 1976.

24. Barnas, C., personal communication, 1997.

25. Kraus, M.L., Gottlieb, L.D., Horwitz, R.I., and Anscher, M., Randomized clinical trial of atenolol in patients with alcohol withdrawal, *N. Engl. J. Med.,* 313, 905, 1985.

26. Gold, M.S., Pottash, A.C., and Sweeney, D.R., Opiate withdrawal using clonidine, *JAMA,* 243, 343, 1980.

27. Wilford, B.B., *Syllabus for the Review Course in Addiction Medicine,* American Society of Addiction Medicine, Washington, D.C., 1990, 178.

28. Wadstein, J. and Skude, G., Does hypokalemia precede delirium tremens?, *Lancet,* ii, 549, 1978.

29. Guthrie, S.K., The treatment of alcohol withdrawal, *Pharmacotherapy,* 9, 131, 1989.

30. Lindhout, D. and Omtzigt, J.G., Teratogenic effects of antiepileptic drugs: implications for the management of epilepsy in women of childbearing age, *Epilepsia,* 35 (Suppl. 4), 519, 1994.

7 Alcohol-Induced Psychotic Disorders

Michael Soyka

OVERVIEW

This chapter focuses on the proper diagnosis, differential diagnosis, and treatment of alcohol-induced psychotic disorders. Pathophysiological mechanisms are discussed.

INTRODUCTION

Although psychotic symptoms are quite frequent in alcoholics (6 to 7%, lifetime prevalence 25%, see below), few studies have addressed their pathophysiology and treatment. Alcohol-induced psychoses are a rather ill-defined group. In ICD-10,[1] the diagnosis of a psychotic disorder in substance abuse can be made if the following criteria are fullfilled:

A. Onset of psychotic symptoms must occur during or within 2 weeks of substance abuse.
B. The psychotic symptoms must persist for more than 48 hours.
C. Duration of the disorder must not exceed 6 months.

   With respect to alcoholism, psychotic disorders usually have a hallucinatory or schizophrenia-like symptomatology. In the older psychiatric literature, the term "alcohol hallucinosis" is used to describe psychotic disorders in alcoholics (DSM-IV Nr. 291.30,[2] ICD-10-Nr. F 10.52[1]). Marcel[3] was the first to describe alcohol hallucinosis in chronic alcoholics. Key symptoms are vivid predominantly acoustic hallucinations that usually develop within 48 hours after cessation of alcohol intake. Symptoms of alcohol delirium such as clouding of sensorium and disorientation are missing.

PREVALENCE

There are no epidemiological studies on the prevalence of alcohol hallucinosis. Tsuang et al.[4] in a cohort of 643 patients reported that one fourth of alcoholics had experienced hallucinations in their lifetime; 48 (7%) of their patients met the DSM-III and ICD-10 diagnosis for alcohol hallucinosis. Victor and Adams,[5] in a consecutive series of 266 patients with complications of alcohol abuse admitted to the Boston City Hospital over a 60-day period, reported that 2% of patients suffered from pure auditory hallucinations, 4% from atypical delirious hallucinatory states, and 5% from typical delirium tremens.

PSYCHOPATHOLOGY

The essential feature is an organic hallucinosis with vivid auditory hallucinations following cessation of or reduction in alcohol ingestion by an individual who apparantly has alcohol dependence.

Onset may accompany a gradual reduction in alcohol intake toward the end of an extended period of intoxication, but the symptoms most often occur soon after cessation of drinking. Alcohol hallucinosis predominantly develops in individuals at about age 40 following long-term episodes of heavy drinking, but may also be seen in people in their 20s.

The psychopathology of alcohol hallucinosis closely resembles paranoid schizophrenia.[6] The prognosis of alcohol hallucinosis in abstinent patients is usually good, but long-term follow-up studies as reviewed by Glass[7] suggest that approximately 10 to 20% of the patients develop chronic alcohol hallucinosis with persisting auditory hallucinations independent of further alcohol intake. Some patients with alcohol hallucinosis are misdiagnosed as schizophrenic and are unnecessarily treated with neuroleptics continuously.

Few studies have addressed clinical features and psychopathology of psychotic disorders in alcoholism.[6-12] The rapid onset of acoustic hallucinations is very typical for alcohol hallucinosis. The hallucinations are predominantly voices and less commonly unformed sounds such as hissing or buzzing or music. The content of the hallucinations is usually unpleasant or frightening. The voices nearly exclusively talk about the patient in the third person and, in contrast to schizophrenia, are localized outside the head or ear in the room or elsewhere. In some cases, the voices may address the individual directly. They can be very frightening and insulting. The voices may call the patient a drinker, liar, or thief, or talk about his execution or his bad health and expected death. The patient may call the police or try to hide from his persecutors. Delusions of persecution (71%) and reference (45%) are more frequent than other delusions such as delusional jealousy (5%).[6] Delusions are poorly systematized. Delusional symptoms without hallucinations are less frequent in alcoholics. Suicidality and aggression or violence are frequent complications of alcohol-induced psychotic disorders. Visual hallucinations are less frequent than acoustic hallucinations. Different from alcohol delirium, visual hallucinations are not scenic; the patient does not experience hallucinations of little animals. Tactile hallucinations are very rare. Other signs of withdrawal such as tremulousness may be present but are not very prominent. The sensorium is usually clear, and symptoms of disorientation are lacking or at least less prominent than in alcohol delirium. Usually there is no amnesia for the psychosis. Different from paranoid schizophrenia, psychotic ego disturbances are very rare. Catatonic symptoms are very rarely ever found in alcohol hallucinosis.

CLINICAL COURSE

Prognosis in patients with alcohol hallucinosis is usually good, but long-term catamnestic studies suggest that in 10 to 20% of patients, a chronic psychosis may emerge.[7] Benedetti,[9] in a long-term catamnestic study, found that after 6 months of persisting psychotic symptomatology, a chronic course was most likely. In these cases of chronic alcohol hallucinosis, a schizophrenia-like psychosis with persisting acoustic hallucinations and delusions of persecution and possibly severe cognitive dysfunction could be found. Clinical experience also suggests that in some cases, a chronic paranoid syndrome with delusions of jealousy may emerge from alcohol hallucinosis.

DIFFERENTIAL DIAGNOSIS

Because the comorbidity between schizophrenia and substance abuse, especially alcoholism, is significant,[13,14] differential diagnosis between psychotic disorders and paranoid schizophrenia can be difficult. Furthermore, a number of other clinical diagnoses must also be excluded (Table 7.1). Surawicz[15] pointed out that patients with alcohol hallucinosis are frequently misdiagnosed as being schizophrenic and unnecessarily treated with neuroleptics continuously.

TABLE 7.1
Important Differential Diagnoses
of Alcohol Hallucinosis

(Paranoid) schizophrenia
Alcohol delirium, other toxic delirium
Alcohol and/or drug intoxication
Affective disorder
Other organic mental disorders

PATHOPHYSIOLOGY

The pathophysiological basis of alcohol hallucinosis is not yet totally understood.[16] Tsuang et al.[4] reported that patients with alcohol hallucinosis start to drink earlier, drink greater amounts of alcohol, and have a greater comorbidity of substance abuse compared to other alcoholics. Alcohol hallucinosis was believed to be part of the schizophrenia spectrum, but family and genetic studies failed to demonstrate a greater prevalence of schizophrenia in relatives of patients with alcohol hallucinosis.[4,7,8,17,18,24,25] Twin studies in patients with both schizophrenia and alcoholism point at a genetic predisposition for both disorders being independent from each other.[25] An interesting finding was reported by Hrubec and Omenn,[26] who studied concordance for alcoholism, alcoholic psychosis, and liver cirrhosis in MZ and DZ twins, each of which was higher in MZ twins. The results of this study might be interpreted as a genetic predisposition for and separate transmission of organ-specific vulnerabilities to alcohol damage.

At the neurotransmitter level, several studies point to an increase in central dopaminergic activity and a dopamine receptor subsensitivity as being involved in the development of hallucinations in alcoholics,[27,28] but an impaired dopaminergic neurotransmission in alcohol hallucinosis has not been shown. Other neurotransmitter systems such as serotonin might also be involved.[16] Other biochemical hypotheses, such as the possible role of elevated beta-carboline levels in patients with alcohol psychoses[29] and variations in the structure of neuronal membranes, have been discussed[29] but warrant replication. Finally, an alcohol-induced impairment of the auditory system and sensory pathways might also contribute to the development of the syndrome.[30,31] However, neurophysiological studies suggest that patients with alcohol hallucinosis or delirium tremens show less impairment of the P300 component (i.e., the positive wave 300 ms after a stimulus as assessed in EEG) compared to healthy controls or other alcoholics with withdrawal symptoms.[31]

TREATMENT

Very few studies have addressed the problem of neuroleptic treatment in alcohol hallucinosis.[32] Most authors feel that neuroleptics such as haloperidol should be given in alcohol hallucinosis, although they often fail to show any significant effect in chronic alcohol hallucinosis. For treatment of alcohol hallucinosis, antipsychotic agents such as haloperidol at 1 to 5 mg up to 20 mg per day are recommended.[33] Neuroleptics are usually necessary because of the vivid psychotic symptomatology with a high degree of aggression and the risk of suicide attempts. High-potency neuroleptics such as the butyrophenones, especially haloperidol, are preferred because of their comparatively low anticholinergenic and alpha-adrenolytic profile with a lower risk of orthostatic hypotension and tachycardia compared to other neuroleptics. The risk of pharmacological interactions with other substances that may also have been consumed is also lower in butyrophenones compared to other antipsychotics. The lowering of the seizure threshold by neuroleptics in alcoholics has repeatedly been stressed as a possible risk of treatment; but in a consecutive series of 104 patients with alcohol hallucinosis being treated with neuroleptics, predominantly haloperidol, not a single case of seizures could be demonstrated.[32]

After stable remission of psychotic symptomatology, neuroleptics can be discontinued. In abstinent alcoholics, the risk of an exacerbation of psychotic symptomatology is very small. In relapsers, alcohol hallucinosis can recur. Some patients with alcohol hallucinosis are misdiagnosed as schizophrenic and unnecessarily treated with neuroleptics continuously.[15] As for other alcoholics, abstinence is essential for further treatment.

As stressed above, the prognosis of chronic alcohol hallucinosis is poor. Little is known about the possible efficacy of new atypical neuroleptics in this field. A recent case report suggested that risperidone, a benzisoxazol derivate with combined dopamine D_2 and serotonin $5HT_2$ receptor-blocking properties, is effective in chronic alcohol hallucinosis.[34] Since dysfunctions in both dopaminergic and serotonergic neurotransmission may play a role in the development of hallucinations in alcoholics,[16] risperidone may be considered a prime candidate for further study in treatment-refractory chronic alcohol hallucinosis.

REFERENCES

1. WHO, *The ICD-10 Classification of Mental and Behavioral Disorders,* The World Health Organization, Geneva, 1993.
2. American Psychiatric Association, *Diagnostic and Statistical Manual of Mental Disorders,* 3rd ed., revised, Washington, D.C., American Psychiatric Association, 1987.
3. Marcel, L.N.S., De la Folie Causée par L'abus des Boissons Alcooliques, Thèsis. Paris, Imprimeur de la Faculté de Médecin. Rignoux, 1847.
4. Tsuang, J.W., Irwin, M.R., Smith, T.L., and Schuckit, M.A., Characteristics of men with alcoholic hallucinosis, *Addiction,* 89, 73, 1994.
5. Victor, M. and Adams, R.D., Effects of alcohol on the nervous systems, *Res. Publ. Assoc. Res. Nerv. Ment. Dis.,* 32, 526, 1953.
6. Soyka, M., Psychopathological characteristics in alcohol hallucinosis and paranoid schizophrenia, *Acta Psychiatr. Scand.,* 81, 255, 1990.
7. Glass, I.B., Alcohol hallucinosis: a psychiatric enigma. 2. Follow-up studies, *Br. J. Addict.,* 84, 151, 1989.
8. Glass, I.B., Alcohol hallucinosis: a psychiatric enigma. 1. The development of an idea, *Br. J. Addict.,* 84, 29, 1989.
9. Benedetti, G., *Die Alkoholhalluzinose,* Thieme, Stuttgart, 1952.
10. Cutting, J., A reappraisal of alcoholic psychoses, *Psychol. Med.,* 8, 285, 1978.
11. Cutting, J., The phenomenology of acute organic psychosis: comparison with acute schizophrenia, *Br. J. Psychiatry,* 151, 324, 1987.
12. Deiker, T. and Chambers, H.E., Structure and content of hallucinations in alcohol withdrawal and functional psychosis, *J. Stud. Alcohol,* 39, 1831, 1978.
13. Mueser, K.T., Yarnold, P.R., Levinson, D.F., Singh, H., Bellack, A.S., Kee, K., Morrison, R.L., and Yadalam, K.G., Prevalence of substance abuse in schizophrenia: demographic and clinical correlates, *Schizophrenia Bull.,* 16, 31, 1990.
14. Soyka, M., Albus, M., Finelli, A., Hofstetter, S., Immler, B., Kathmann, N., Holzbach, R., and Sand, P., Prevalence of alcohol and drug abuse in schizophrenic inpatients, *Eur. Arch. Psychiatry Clin. Neurosci.,* 242, 362, 1993.
15. Surawicz, F.G., Alcoholic hallucinosis: a missed diagnosis, *Can. J. Psychiatry,* 25, 57, 1980.
16. Soyka, M., Pathophysiologic mechanisms possibly involved in the development of alcohol hallucinosis, *Addiction,* 90, 289, 1995.
17. Burton-Bradley, B.G., Aspects of alcoholic hallucinosis, *Med. J. Aust.,* 2, 8, 1958.
18. Cook, B.L. and Winokur, G., Separate heritability of alcoholism and psychotic symptoms, *Am. J. Psychiatry,* 142, 360, 1985.

19. Rommelspacher, H., Schmidt, L.G., and May, T., Plasma norharman (beta-carboline) levels are elevated in chronic alcoholics, *Alcohol Clin. Exp. Res.,* 15, 553, 1991.

20. Johanson, E., Acute hallucinosis, paranoic reactions and schizophrenia as psychosis in alcoholic patients, *Acta Societatis Medicorum Upsaliensis,* 66, 105, 1961.

21. Kendler, K.S., Gruenberg, A.M., and Tsuang, M.T., Psychiatric illness in first-degree relatives of schizophrenic and surgical control patients, *Arch. Gen. Psychiatry,* 42, 770, 1985.

22. Schuckit, M.A., The history of psychotic symptoms in alcoholics, *J. Clin. Psychiatry,* 43, 53, 1982.

23. Schuckit, M.A. and Winokur, G., Alcoholic hallucinosis and schizophrenia: a negative study, *Br. J. Psychiatry,* 119, 549, 1971.

24. Scott, D.F., Alcoholic hallucinosis: an aetiological study, *Br. J. Addict.,* 62, 113, 1967.

25. Kendler, K.S., A twin study of individuals with both schizophrenia and alcoholism, *Br. J. Psychiatry,* 147, 48, 1985.

26. Hrubec, Z. and Omenn, G.S., Evidence of genetic predisposition to alcoholic cirrhosis and pschosis: twin concordances for alcoholism and its biological end points by zygosity among male veterans, *Alcoholism,* 5, 207, 1981.

27. Borg, S., Kvande, H., and Valverius, P., Clinical conditions and central dopamine metabolism in alcoholics during acute withdrawal under treatment with different pharmacological agents, *Psychopharmacology,* 88, 12, 1986.

28. Fadda, F., Mosca, E., Colombo, G., and Gessa, G.L., Effect of spontaneous ingestion of ethanol on brain dopamine metabolism, *Life Science,* 44, 281, 1989.

29. Glen, A.I.M., Glen, E.M.T., Horrobin, D.H., Manku, M.S., Miller, J., Will, S., and MacDonell, L.E.F., *Essential Fatty Acids in Alcoholic Hallucinosis and Schizophrenia,* Amsterdam, Excerpta Medica: 778 (Abs. No 3039), 1989.

30. Spitzer, J.B., Auditory effects of chronic alcoholism, *Drug Alcohol Depend.,* 8, 317, 1981.

31. Kathmann, N., Soyka, M., Bickel, M., and Engel, R., P-300 Latency in patients with alcohol psychosis, *Biol. Psychiatry,* 39, 873, 1996.

32. Soyka, M., Botschev, C., and Voelcker, A., Neuroleptic treatment in alcohol hallucinosis — no evidence for increased seizure risk, *J. Clin. Psychopharmacol.,* 12, 66, 1992.

33. Schuckit, M.A., *Drug and Alcohol Abuse, A Clinical Guide to Diagnosis and Treatment,* 4th ed., Plenum Press, New York, 1995.

34. Soyka, M., Wegner, U., and Moeller, H.-J., Risperidone in treatment-refractory chronic alcohol hallucinosis, *Pharmacopsychiatry,* 30, 135, 1997

Part 3

Treatment of Alcohol Abuse
and Dependence

8 Overview and Outlook

Stephanie S. O'Malley

OVERVIEW

Alcoholism is one of the most prevalent psychiatric disorders, second only to nicotine dependence. However, the majority of individuals with alcohol use disorders never seek treatment. The ratio of untreated to treated individuals with alcohol use disorders in the general population has been estimated to be between 3:1 and 13:1 (see also Chapter 2 on the natural history of alcoholism).[1] Of interest, epidemiological surveys of recovery from alcohol problems suggest that the majority of individuals with alcohol problems who recover do so without treatment.[2] Nonetheless, a substantial number of individuals seek help in addressing their alcohol problems.

TREATMENT

The treatment of alcohol abuse and dependence can occur in a range of settings, including, among others, primary care settings, outpatient specialized programs, inpatient detoxification programs, and inpatient rehabilitation programs. These settings differ in a number of attributes, including level of restriction, cost, and provider characteristics. The patients who present at each of these settings are likely to differ as well. Primary care providers see a spectrum of patients presenting for other complaints, including those who are drinking heavily without major problems to those with severe alcohol dependence that complicates the management of their presenting medical complaints. In this setting, the primary care provider's role is to screen and assess, provide advice, and coordinate care (see Chapter 1 on first contact and early intervention and Chapter 9 on psychotherapy). Brief advice to cut down or quit drinking has been associated with reductions in drinking compared to no intervention among those who are drinking heavily.[3] Less information is available about the effectiveness of primary care interventions for alcohol-dependent individuals. For these patients, the primary care provider is in the unique position to help coordinate care over time because of the provider's continuing relationship with the patient regarding other health concerns apart from drinking. In contrast, specialized alcoholism treatment programs may not have another opportunity to intervene with an individual who discontinues therapy.

Specialized alcoholism treatment programs, however, provide a range of services for patients with alcohol dependence, including individual, family, and group counseling. Some programs provide psychiatric evaluations and employment services. These additional services are potentially important if used appropriately because individuals who seek treatment at alcoholism specialty clinics are more likely to have multiple diagnoses, including other substance use and psychiatric disorders,[4,5] than seen in general population surveys.[6] Specialized programs, primarily inpatient and intensive outpatient programs, can also safely manage detoxification from alcohol for patients at risk of significant withdrawal syndromes. Although the predominant setting for alcoholism treatment in the U.S. had been inpatient rehabilitation programs, research findings demonstrated that outpatient programs were cost-effective.[7,8] In addition, changes in reimbursement occurred and these two factors changed the landscape of treatment to consist primarily of outpatient care. In 1991, for example, 88% of patients receiving care were treated in outpatient programs.[9]

In addition to differences in setting, there are also different theoretical models of treatment. For example, some treatment approaches emphasize participation in the fellowship of Alcoholics Anonymous, others stress cognitive behavioral interventions, and still others the management of comorbid psychiatric problems. The research literature on the treatment of alcohol abuse and dependence has consisted primarily of clinical trials comparing different forms of treatment or treatment in different settings. From this literature, one can conclude that treatment is effective overall in reducing alcohol consumption compared to no treatment, but that there is no one outstanding treatment that is better than all others.[10]

Recognizing the significant morbidity and mortality associated with alcoholism and the fact that not all individuals succeed in treatment, several efforts have been made to optimally match patients to treatments. This has involved matching patients to programs of different intensity, to different theoretical models of behavioral treatment, and to types of services within a program. The potential advantage of combining different treatments to optimize overall outcomes is also under investigation.

PATIENT PROGRAM MATCHING

Ideally, patients are optimally matched to the type and intensity of treatment that would be most effective for them. Criteria for matching patients to intensity of treatment have been proposed, with the most widely used being the criteria established by the American Society of Addiction Medicine (ASAM).[11] This model was established in part in response to changes in the managed care, which required standards for the appropriate placement of patients in treatments that were likely to vary in terms of expense. In this schema, more intensive (and more expensive) treatments are provided to patients with more severe problems, based on an assessment of six dimensions: (1) acute intoxication/withdrawal potential; (2) biomedical conditions or complications; (3) emotional and behavioral conditions or complications; and (4) treatment acceptance/resistance, (5) relapse potential; and (6) recovery environment. These placement criteria are the most widely used in the U.S. currently. However, research is needed to examine whether use of these criteria results in better treatment outcome.[12]

PATIENT TREATMENT MATCHING

Independent of matching to intensity of treatment, other researchers have sought to match patients on the basis of other criteria (e.g., psychological severity, cognitive functioning, personality type) to a particular form of therapy (e.g., motivational enhancement therapy, Twelve-Step facilitation) (see Chapter 33 on patient-to-treatment matching). This approach seemed promising on the basis of a number of single-site studies, leading the National Institute on Alcohol Abuse and Alcoholism (NIAAA) to conduct a large multi-site study of matching patients to alcoholism treatments, called Project MATCH.[13] In this study, nearly 1800 alcohol-dependent subjects were randomized to receive one of three therapies: Twelve-Step facilitation therapy, cognitive behavioral relapse prevention therapy, or motivational enhancement therapy. The ability of several different client attributes to differentially predict response to the different forms of therapy was examined. Although there was strong evidence that patients in all three forms of treatment improved greatly during treatment compared with baseline, there was little evidence for matching effects between patient characteristics and these conceptually distinct active therapies. Instead, the results suggested that carefully implemented alcoholism treatments were effective in improving the percentage of days patients were abstinent and the risk of alcohol-related problems. (For a more in-depth discussion of this study, see Chapter 33 on patient-to-treatment matching and Chapter 9 on psychotherapy.)

PATIENT SERVICE MATCHING

Another form of matching assigns the type of service given to a patient on the basis of the types of problems that the patient is currently experiencing. In a recent study by McLellan and colleagues,[14] subjects from four substance abuse treatment programs were randomized to receive usual care or to receive matched services in addition to usual care. In the matched services condition, patients with significant problems in either employment, family, or psychiatric health were matched to receive at least three individual sessions with a psychologist, psychiatrist, or social worker who would address the target area in addition to usual care. The results indicated that those receiving matched services were more likely to complete treatment, and to show improvements in these problem areas than non-matched subjects. McLellan notes that these data are consistent with earlier studies showing that the addition of specialized services, including professional marital counseling,[15] psychotherapy,[16] employment counseling,[17] and medical care,[18] to substance abuse treatment yields higher improvement rates than drug and alcohol counseling alone.

COMBINED THERAPIES

As described, McLellan's study[14] incorporated matching services to patient problems areas, but it also reflects a study in which additional services were "added" to a base of usual treatment. Until recently, there were few studies involving combined therapies. Indeed, the majority of studies of behavioral therapies have involved clinical trials comparing two or more active treatment strategies that are rarely found to differ in efficacy. Kazdin[19] has argued that the failure to find differences between active treatments may be related to several factors. One important consideration is that these comparisons are of treatments that are theoretically distinct, and potentially incomplete. Taking the area of depression as an example, interpersonal therapy for depression addresses the interpersonal aspects of depression, and cognitive therapy for depression addresses the cognitive distortions associated with depression, when patients may have both problems. In the alcoholism area, the Project MATCH therapies were manualized to be as distinct as possible. Twelve-Step facilitation therapy was designed to encourage the patient's involvement in Alcoholics Anonymous but did not include motivational enhancement techniques or cognitive behavioral (CBT) interventions. Similarly, motivational enhancement and CBT were designed to minimize overlap with each other and with Twelve-Step facilitation therapy. Future research studies may be better served by examining more comprehensive treatments that provide the practitioner with several tools to use with a particular patient, such as motivational interviewing, referral to Alcoholics Anonymous, and the skill acquisition.

Evidence for the value of combined therapy comes from studies examining the effects of the addition of a motivation intervention prior to involvement in substance abuse treatment. Several studies have randomized clients entering treatment for alcohol abuse and dependence to receive or not receive assessment feedback and motivational interviewing prior to beginning standard treatment.[20,21] In these studies, those receiving the motivational intervention showed much greater reductions in drinking that those who did not receive the motivational intervention. One explanation for this finding is that the feedback and motivational interviewing increased the client's motivation for change and, as a result, the client became more receptive to treatment and benefited more from the subsequent treatment that was provided.

Efficacy studies of pharmacotherapies can also be considered studies of combined therapy. For example, all studies of acamprosate and naltrexone have examined the efficacy of these medications when added to a platform of behavioral treatment. Thus, studies that found that the active medication group improved significantly more than the placebo group reflect an additional benefit of the medication above and beyond that obtained from the behavioral treatment (see Chapter 31 on the meta-analysis of pharmacotherapeutic trials and Chapter 10 on pharmacotherapy). To date, there are no studies of alcoholism treatment that test whether the addition of a behavioral therapy increases the percentage of patients who benefit from pharmacotherapy compared to pharmacotherapy without behavioral intervention. However, studies of the addition of behavioral treatment to nicotine replacement strategies in smoking cessation (reviewed in Reference 22), methadone maintenance,[18] and naltrexone for opiate addiction[23] suggest that this should be true.

The potential for additive (and possibly synergistic) effects of combining behavioral and pharmacological treatments could occur through a number of mechanisms. First, the combined use of medications and behavioral interventions may result in additive effects by addressing different aspects of the patient's problems. For example, naltrexone may help prevent a lapse from becoming a relapse to heavy drinking by attenuating the ability of alcohol to "prime" craving and further drinking, while the behavioral treatment may teach the patient how to cope with the cognitive and affective responses to violating abstinence. Another possibility is that the pharmacological agent or behavioral therapy may increase the odds that the patient will benefit from the other treatment by increasing overall retention or compliance. For example, a behavioral intervention may be useful in increasing compliance with the medication and thereby maximize the benefit obtained from the pharmacotherapy. Similarly, a pharmacotherapy that improves treatment retention may increase the likelihood that the patient will remain in a behavioral therapy long enough to learn new skills for coping without the use of alcohol.

As the availability of pharmacological interventions for alcoholism increases, a next step for research will be to study the efficacy of combined pharmacological interventions. One potential combination of interest is the use of naltrexone and acamprosate together because these two medications work through different neurobiological mechanisms and appear to have different effects on outcome. For example, acamprosate is believed to work in part through actions on NMDA receptors and has been shown to increase retention and overall abstinence rates (for a review, see Reference 24). In contrast, naltrexone has its actions through the endogenous opioid system and appears to most strongly reduce the risk of relapse following a lapse in abstinence.[25,26] There is also interest in combining short-term disulfiram to assist in maintaining initial abstinence followed by longer-term treatment with either acamprosate or naltrexone.[27] The answer to whether these combination therapies will be more effective than monotherapy, however, awaits the results of ongoing research. Just as it is conceivable that a combination may be more effective than monotherapy, it is also possible that the combined adverse effects of two individual therapies may not be tolerable to a subset of patients.

SEQUENCING OF THERAPIES

Effective treatment of alcohol abuse and dependence is likely to require a treatment plan that takes into account the needs of the patient based on where the patient is in the recovery process. From a neurobiological perspective, the target of pharmacological interventions is changing over time. During initiation of abstinence, a particular neurobiological system, such as the adrenergic system, may be hyperactive and, after longer periods of abstinence, may be hyporesponsive. Depending on the severity of withdrawal, the patient may benefit from traditional medications used in acute detoxification (i.e., benzodiazepines, see Chapter 6 on alcohol withdrawal syndrome), but these medications are not appropriate for long-term use once acute abstinence has resolved. Among patients without clinically significant withdrawal, however, the effects of a pharmacotherapy during early abstinence may be different than when the medication is administered at a later point. For example, we have found that the risk of naltrexone-induced nausea is greatest among lighter drinkers with shorter periods of abstinence.[28] These differences in tolerability may be influenced by induction of hepatic enzymes from recent drinking or alterations in opioid receptor activity. Future research studies should consider and possibly test the effects of medications under different times in relationship to the onset of abstinence. In practice, clinicians should keep these issues in mind to avoid dismissing the efficacy of a pharmacotherapy when the medication is used in a way inconsistent with the original research literature.

Similarly, the sequencing of behavioral treatments should probably consider where the patient is in terms of the recovery process. In fact, motivational interventions are predicated on the principle that patients are in different stages of readiness for change. Apart from motivational aspects, however, alcohol-dependent patients may need more intensive support during the initiation of treatment, followed by less frequent sessions. Based on the finding that clinical gains are typically associated with time in treatment, McCrady and colleagues (1996) have argued that treatment systems should develop long-term, low-intensity, and intermittent treatment models of care. Low-intensity interventions may be helpful for a subset of individuals as their primary treatment. For other individuals, a low-intensity treatment that is provided intermittently for supportive purposes should be considered as follow-up to more intensive interventions. Here, the primary care provider is in a good position to play this supportive role over time, given the continuing nature of their relationship with the individual. Alcoholics Anonymous and other peer support groups are also a source for continued support for those individuals who have affiliated with these support groups.

WHAT ARE THE GOALS OF TREATMENT REGARDING DRINKING?

There has been a great debate in the U.S. regarding the appropriate goals of treatment, and whether a reduction in drinking rather than sustained abstinence is possible.[30] When one considers the individual with significant dependence, the data suggest that few people are successful in maintaining a reduction in intensity of drinking. Indeed, an emphasis on abstinence during treatment appears to yield better long-term outcomes, particularly for patients with high dependence.[31] However, primary care physicians, compared to alcoholism specialty clinics, are likely to see a broad range of individuals whose drinking ranges from hazardous to severely dependent. In this setting, brief advice to cut down may be more palatable to someone who is drinking heavily but not experiencing significant problems. This may also be a place for a "stepped care" approach in which the patient negotiates a treatment goal with his/her care provider, obtains experience with working on that goal, and this experience is reviewed at a subsequent appointment to determine whether this goal remains feasible or whether another goal should be considered. A review of the literature suggests that success in reducing drinking is more likely among individuals who are younger, socially and psychologically stable, female, have fewer symptoms of dependence, and believe that controlled drinking is possible.[32] A recent epidemiological survey of natural recovery from alcohol problems provides support for these predictors, but also revealed that those who achieved a stable period of nonproblematic drinking were much less likely to be a current smoker than those who achieved recovery through abstinence.[2]

The availability of new pharmacotherapies provides additional input into this discussion. The clinical benefit from acamprosate appears to be in increasing treatment retention and abstinence rates. Pending additional information about whether acamprosate reduces the intensity of drinking, acamprosate appears to be appropriate for patients who would like to abstain from drinking. Naltrexone treatment also improves measures of abstinence, primarily percent days abstinent. However, another effect of naltrexone is to reduce the amount of alcohol consumed on a drinking occasion. These findings suggest that treatment programs should recognize that a reduction in drinking intensity and frequency may be a benefit of naltrexone therapy. However, the patient who achieves abstinence is likely to see better retention of gains once treatment is discontinued[33] because drinking appears to increase once naltrexone is discontinued in a subset of subjects who reduce but do not maintain abstinence. Pending the results of long-term studies of naltrexone's safety and efficacy and other studies specifically testing a harm reduction goal in problem drinkers, alcohol-dependent patients should be encouraged to work toward a goal of abstinence, while acknowledging that one potential effect of naltrexone in some patients is to reduce the risk of continued drinking if they have a lapse in abstinence.

Ultimately, an assessment of the goals of treatment should not focus exclusively on drinking outcomes, but should also focus on overall quality of life and the resolution of other problems that have resulted from drinking (see also Chapter 4 on psychometric instruments to evaluate outcome in alcoholism treatment). From this perspective, a broader view of the desired outcome of therapy is likely to encourage treatment providers to provide treatment interventions that address the full range of problems that motivate individuals to seek help. And in that regard, the primary factor that motivates people to seek treatment is not a view that the substance abuse itself is the problem, but rather their experience of the problematic consequences of their use, such as family and relationship difficulties or health problems.[34]

REFERENCES

1. Roizen, R., *Barriers to Alcoholism Treatment*, Alcohol Research Group, Berkeley, CA, 1977.
2. Sobell, L.C., Cunningham, J.A., and Sobell, L.C., Recovery from alcohol problems with and without treatment: prevalence in two population surveys, *Am. J. Public Health*, 86, 966, 1996.
3. Wilk, A.I., Jensen, N.M., and Havighurst, T.C. Meta-analysis of randomized control trials addressing brief interventions in heavy alcohol drinkers, *J. Gen. Intern. Med.*, 12, 274, 1997.
4. Ross, H.E., Glaser, F.B., and Germanson, T., Psychopathology in hospitalized alcoholics, *Arch. Gen. Psychiatry*, 45, 1023, 1988.
5. Tomasson, K. and Vaglum, P., A nationwide representative sample of treatment-seeking alcoholics: a study of psychiatric comorbidity, *Acta Psychiatr. Scand.*, 92, 378, 1995.
6. Reiger, D.A., Farmer, M.E., Rae, D.S., Locke, B.Z., Keith, S.J., Judd, L.L., and Goodwin, F.K., Comorbidity of mental disorders with alcohol and other drug abuse. Results from the epidemiologic catchment area (ECA) study, *JAMA*, 264, 2511, 1990.
7. Longabaugh, R., McCrady, B.S., Fink, E., Stout, R., McAuley, T., and McNeill, D., Cost-effectiveness of alcoholism treatment in inpatient versus partial hospital settings: six-month outcomes, *J. Stud. Alcohol*, 44, 1049, 1988.
8. Miller, W.R. and Hester, R.K., Inpatient alcoholism treatment: who benefits? *Am. Psychologist*, 41, 794, 1986.
9. U.S. Department of Health and Human Services, Substance Abuse and Mental Health Services Administration, *National Drug and Alcoholism Treatment Unit Survey (NDATUS): 1991 Main Findings Report*, DHHS Pub. No. (SMA)93-2007, Rockville, MD, The Administration, 1993.
10. Miller, W.R. and Hester, R.K., Treatment for alcohol problems: toward an informed eclecticism, R.K. Hester and W.R. Miller, Eds., *Handbook of Alcoholism Treatment Approaches: Effective Alternatives*, 2nd ed., Allyn & Bacon, Boston, MA, 1995, 1–11.
11. Hoffman, N.G., Halikas, J.A, Mee-Lee, D. and Weedman, R.D., *Patient Placement Criteria for the Treatment of Psychoactive Substance Disorders*, American Society of Addiction Medicine, Washington, D.C., 1991.
12. Morey, L.C., Patient placement criteria: linking typologies to managed care, *Alcohol, Health Res. World*, 20, 37, 1996.
13. Project MATCH Research Group, Matching alcoholism treatments to client heterogeneity: Project MATCH posttreatment drinking outcomes, *J. Stud. Alcohol*, 58, 7, 1997.
14. McLellan, A.T., Grissom, G.R., Zanis, D., Randall, M., Brill, P., and O'Brien, C.P., Problem-service "matching" in addiction treatment, *Arch. Gen. Psychiatry*, 54, 730, 1997.
15. McCrady, B.S., Noel, N.E., Abrams D.B., Stout, R.L., Nelson H.F., and Hay, W.M., Comparative effectiveness of three types of spouse involvement in outpatient behavior alcoholism treatment, *J. Stud. Alcohol*, 47, 459, 1986.
16. Carroll, K.M., Rounsaville, B.J., Gordon L.T., Nich, C., Jatlow, P., Bisighini, R.M., and Gawin, F.H., Psychotherapy and pharmacotherapy for ambulatory cocaine abusers, *Arch. Gen. Psychiatry*, 51, 177, 1994.
17. French, M.T., Rachal, J.V., Harwood, H.J., and Hubbard, R.L., Does drug abuse treatment affect employment and earning of clients? *Benefits Q.*, 6, 58, 1983.

18. McLellan, A.T., Arndt, I.O., Woody, G.E., and Metzger, D., Psychosocial services in substance abuse treatment? A dose-ranging study of psychosocial services, *JAMA*, 269, 1953, 1993.

19. Kazdin, A.E., Comparative outcome studies of psychotherapy: methodological issues and strategies, *J. Consult. Clin. Psychol.*, 54, 95, 1986.

20. Bien, T.H., Miller, W.R., and Boroughs, J.M., Motivational interviewing with alcohol outpatients, *Behav. Cognitive Psychother.*, 21, 347, 1993.

21. Brown, J.M. and Miller, W.R., Impact of motivational interviewing on participation in residential alcoholism treatment, *Psychol. Addict. Behav.*, 7, 211, 1993.

22. Fiore, M.C., Jorenby, D.E., Baker, T.B., and Kenford S.L., Tobacco dependence and the nicotine patch: clinical guidelines for effective use, *JAMA*, 19, 2687, 1992.

23. Callahan, E.J., Rawson, R.A., McCleave, B., and Glazer, M.L., The treatment of heroin addiction: naltrexone alone and with behavior therapy, *Int. J. Addict.*, 15, 795, 1980.

24. Wilde, M.I. and Wagstaff, A.J., Acamprosate. A review of its pharmacology and clinical potential in the management of alcohol dependence after detoxification, *Drugs*, 53, 1038, 1997.

25. O'Malley, S.S., Jaffe, A., Chang, G., Schottenfeld, R.S., Meyer, R.E., and Rounsaville, B.J., Naltrexone and coping skills therapy for alcohol dependence: a controlled study, *Arch. Gen. Psychiatry*, 49, 881, 1992.

26. Volpicelli, J., Alterman, A., Hayasguda, M., and O'Brien, C., Naltrexone in the treatment of alcohol dependence, *Arch. Gen. Psychiatry*, 49, 876, 1992.

27. O'Malley, S., Consensus Panel Chair, *Naltrexone and Alcoholism Treatment*. Treatment Improvement Protocol Series 28, U.S. Department of Health and Human Services, Rockville, MD, 1998.

28. O'Malley, S.S., Krishnan-Sarin, S., Farren, C., and O'Connor, P.G., Naltrexone induced nausea in patients treated for alcohol dependence: clinical predictors and evidence of opioid mediated effects, *J. Clin. Psychopharmacol.*, in press.

29. McCrady, B.S. and Langenbucher, J.W., Alcohol treatment and health care system reform, *Arch. Gen. Psychiatry*, 53, 737, 1996.

30. Sobell, M.B. and Sobell L.C., Controlled drinking after 25 years: how important was the great debate? *Addiction*, 90, 1149, 1995.

31. Cooney, N.L., Babor, T.F., and Litt, M.D., Matching clients to alcoholism treatment based on severity of alcohol dependence, *Project MATCH: A Priori Matching Hypotheses, Results, and Mediating Mechanisms*, R.H. Longabaugh and P.W. Wirtz, Eds., NIAAA Project MATCH Monograph Series, U.S. Government Printing Office, Rockville, MD, in press.

32. Rosenberg, H., Prediction of controlled drinking by alcoholics and problem drinkers, *Psychological Bull.*, 113, 129, 1993.

33. O'Malley, S.S., Jaffe, A.J., Chang, G., Rode, S., Schottenfeld, R., Meyer, R.E., and Rounsaville, B., Six month follow-up of naltrexone and psychotherapy for alcohol dependence, *Arch. Gen. Psychiatry*, 53, 217, 1996.

34. Marlatt, G.A.,Tucker, J.A., Donovan, D.M., and Vuchinich, R.E., Help-seeking by substance abusers: the role of harm reduction and behavioral-economic approaches to facilitate treatment entry and retention by substance abusers, *Beyond the therapeutic alliance: Keeping the drug dependent individual in treatment*, National Institute on Drug Abuser Research Monograph, L.S. Onken, J.D. Blaine, and J.J. Boren, Eds., U.S. Department of Health and Human Services, Public Health Service, National Institutes of Health, Rockville, MD, 1996.

9 Psychotherapy

Friedhelm Stetter

OVERVIEW

In order to effectively apply psychotherapy to alcohol-dependent patients, certain therapeutic attitudes are important. Patience is one of the most important. Patience might also be necessary for some when reading this chapter, which tries to explain psychopathological processes and psychotherapy. However, the reader is assured that his/her patience will pay off. In this chapter, you will learn how to interact with alcohol-dependent patients in a positive way and how you can deal with the frustrations your therapeutic interaction with the patient might bring. How to obtain a clear and unequivocal position toward the patient will be covered in the introduction and the section on the therapist; specific examples will be given. The alcohol-dependent patient is your partner in the psychotherapeutic process. This chapter will give you the patient's characteristics as seen from the different viewpoints of the currently prevailing "schools" of psychotherapy: cognitive-behavioral, psychoanalytic, humanistic, systemic, and relaxation-oriented models. Their respective theoretical backgrounds will be illustrated with the help of specific examples. The goals of psychotherapy and effective factors will be identified in another section; you will see that abstinence-oriented psychotherapies do lead to success in most cases. You will be given hints for your behavior upon first contact with the patient and during the early therapeutic stages. Finally, optimal behavior in the different therapeutic settings (e.g., primary care, outpatient clinic, or inpatient setting) will be discussed. This view of alcohol abuse and dependence and the explanation of psychotherapeutic interventions should also remind you that alcohol dependence is nothing mystical, but just a psychiatric disorder of similar prognosis as the other main psychiatric and psychosomatic disorders, such as depression.

BY WAY OF A PREFACE ... HOW TO READ THIS CHAPTER

Maybe you are asking yourself why you should deal with a preface in just a chapter, one chapter among many in this handbook. Maybe you wish for "just the facts, ma'am"; maybe you think that giving the results of the latest randomized controlled studies on psychotherapy with alcohol-dependent patients really are enough to provide clear guidelines. This might be a good way for other therapeutic strategies; however, in the case of psychotherapy, such an approach would not help you to make your interaction with an alcohol-dependent fellow human being a positive experience. So please bear with us and try to follow the reading rhythm of this chapter. The basis of psychotherapy is the interaction between at least two human beings: the patient and you, the therapist. This chapter will help you to free yourself of as much bias as possible when engaging in the therapist–patient exchange. You will be moved by the patient, you will participate in the pathology but also in the strengths and the resources and, finally, in the healing of the dependent patient. You will acquire knowledge that will enable you to do that without being swept away by the patient. The reward for your patience with this chapter will be that you will learn:

- How to interact with alcohol-dependent patients in an empathic manner
- How to deal with your own negative feelings and thoughts that sometimes occur during the therapeutic process

- How to deal with the patient without losing the crucial, clear, and unequivocal position
- How not to risk becoming a — manipulated — player in the dynamic of addiction
- How to retain a realistic hope in the improvement or healing of the patient despite the occurrence of relapses
- How to use relapses in a constructive way to help the patient

The caring, empathic approach to alcohol-dependent patients is one of the basics of psychotherapy that is very often talked about and which all too often is taken for granted. But how can you as a potential therapist gain such an attitude? Maybe you now think of previous, challenging situations: the intoxicated alcoholic in your office or in the emergency room who swore (in face of his having alcohol on his breath) not having touched liquor for weeks; maybe you remember the patient who had just recovered from acute pancreatitis or esophageal bleeding and swore that he had learned his lesson this time — only to reappear intoxicated a few days later. Or you remember that patient whom you could motivate to start rehabilitation — only to see him terminate it abruptly or declare, after having finished the program, that controlled drinking might be a suitable goal for him after all. In the face of all these experiences, how can you approach the next alcoholic patient — or the old one, for that matter — in an empathic manner? Do not look at the alcohol dependence and the way it has changed that patient; maybe it is worth looking at yourself and your motivation for becoming a therapist for a few moments.

Therapists should have a genuine interest in meeting people *on the job*. Their personality should predispose them toward experiencing joy when exchanging with and expressing themselves in presence of other human beings, when being sensitive for and being touched by the other's feelings, thoughts, hopes, and wishes — *on the job*. There is *no* blame in deciding *not* to live all this *on the job* despite being able to do so. None. However, the willingness to live all this during working hours, while on the job, is a prerequisite for the psychotherapist.

Extending this basic attitude in professional training is what makes the psychotherapist. Some interventions, especially those for primary care settings, can be quickly learned and applied. Psychotherapy training, however, requires familiarization with the theoretical basis of a psychotherapeutic "school" as well as continuing structured exchange with similarly trained professionals. This continuing training and exchange helps one to acquire and maintain a different perspective on the problem situations mentioned above: what is incomprehensible, frightening, and repulsive for most people becomes "normal" for the therapist. Pathology may serve as an illustrative example: for most people, the sight or, even more so, the touch of a dead human being is accompanied by strong negative emotions. The pathologist is trained to cope with those emotions and to interact with a dead body in a way that is productive for him and others. The same applies to addiction therapists: certain processes that elicit strong negative emotions in others are simply part of the addiction process. For example, it is "normal" for alcohol-dependent patients not to be able to fully experience their alcohol abuse and/or to repress their realization of their abusive nature of the alcohol consumption, to deny it or to de-emphasize it. They do this to cope with their massive feelings of guilt and shame — which also are part of their dependence. The above-mentioned mechanism help the dependent patient stabilize his self-esteem. The therapist, by combining the repeated experience of such processes with the acquired knowledge about the features of addiction, is now able to "see behind" the — sometimes outright repulsive — behavior and see the person behind it, the human being tormented by a disease. Remember that the alcohol abuse is an *effort* by the patient, albeit an inefficient and misguided one, to cope with his fear and other negative emotions, which might be considerable. This allows the therapist to approach the patient openly. At the same time, it enables the therapist to maintain the "merciless clarity" *toward the disease* and its pathological behavioral expression that is a prerequisite for the unpleasant but bearable interventions that the patient must face in order to overcome his affliction. Despite all training and excercise in professional attitude, the therapist is constantly challenged by the patient. Now it becomes necessary for the therapist to take the specific experience with that specific patient and clarify the therapist's own moods, thought processes, and reactions in a professional setting; this will help the therapist *avoid* succumbing to feelings of being over-taxed, burnt-out, to deflate overblown expectations in his own therapeutic efficacy, and to cope with negative feelings and thoughts. For example, according to the technique developed by Michael Balint of London, about eight therapists meet in group sessions led by a supervisor. One therapist talks about one "problem" patient and his/her therapeutic and emotional reactions to this patient. The group and the supervisor try to develop specific characteristics of this specific therapeutic relationship and the involvement of the therapist in order to help him/her find new perspectives for this very patient. These "Balint groups" have gained wide acceptance in Europe. Another way for the therapist is to seek the help of a supervisor in a one-on-one setting.

The Psychotherapeutic Approach in a Disease with Multifactorial Genesis and Treatment

This chapter focuses on psychotherapy with alcohol-dependent patients. However, it should be recognized that alcohol dependence is caused by a multitude of different factors that efficient treatment must also address. Currently, there are three main approaches:

- Pharmacotherapy of alcoholism itself and the medical treatment of nonpsychiatric ("somatic") sequelae of alcohol abuse (e.g., liver damage, gastrointestinal problems, polyneuropathy) addresses biological factors.
- Contributing social factors are targeted by sociotherapeutic approaches that aim to improve abstinence by stabilizing family life, improving living conditions, and restructuring work and recreational activities.
- Of utmost importance, however, are psychological factors that lead to the development and persistence of alcohol dependence. Changing these pathogenic factors is the main goal of psychotherapy.

Although these psychotherapeutic approaches are central to the treatment of alcohol dependence, one should never forget that they must be integrated into a comprehensive treatment strategy that does justice to the multidimensional genesis and perpetuation of dependent behavior.

The "Therapist" Effect in Psychotherapy

Psychotherapy in its most general sense can be regarded as "treatment of patients by psychological means." These immaterial means aim to change emotional, cognitive, and behavioral processes in the alcohol-dependent patient. Their specific application (i.e., techniques and methods) should be based on a sound theoretical concept, should address a specific disease model, and should have been tested empirically.

As a general rule, there are at least two participants in the therapeutic process: on the one side, the alcohol-dependent patient; on the other side, the addiction therapist, be it a physician, psychologist, social worker, layman, or member of another vocational group. Those two participants (and sometimes, for example, in family therapy, their dependants as well) are the core of the psychotherapeutic exchange, the rapport and interaction between patient and therapist being the most important factor in psychotherapy. Therefore, it is useful to dwell a little longer on these two players and to look more closely at their attitudes and motivations which will, in all likelihood, strongly determine their interaction. In fact, we are talking about you, dear reader, someone who deals with and wants to help addicted patients. Even if your primary interest lies in the biological or social determinants of alcohol dependence, even if you contact the patient only during blood sampling, during an emergency visit, or in an employment agency, your contact allows you — indeed forces you — to interact with the alcohol-dependent patient in a psychotherapeutic manner. Let us concentrate on you, dear reader.

THE ADDICTION THERAPIST

THERAPIST ATTTITUDE AS A NONSPECIFIC BUT CRUCIAL EFFECTIVE FACTOR

Even if we revert to the term "addicition" — mostly for reasons of simplification — we would like to stress that the World Health Organization (WHO) recommended 30 years ago to replace the term "addiction" with the term "dependence" in order to emphasize the disease model of drug dependence and avoid moralistic undertones. This leads us to the essential attitude of the (future) addiction therapist: it is crucial for the therapist to internalize the concept of alcohol abuse and dependence as a disease and to let go of any lingering remains of believing that the alcoholic "just lacks willpower." Furthermore, it is essential for the therapist to be open and empathic toward the patient and not be tempted to morally condemn the patient. Simply changing the terminology from "addiction" to "dependence" might turn out to be only lip service. Alcohol dependence is a disease inflicted on a person of certain character who lives under certain social conditions; try to obtain information on all of these three aspects and apply this information to the patient in front of you. This will help you approach your alcohol-dependent patient in an authentic manner, similar to how you would approach your other "chronic" patients (e.g., diabetics, dialysis patients, hypertensives, etc.). Your patient should experience and feel that you are neither an accuser or controller of his life nor a "savior" or accomplice, but that you are open and prepared to support your patient and accompany him/her on his way out of dependence.[1] This open, empathic, clear, and unequivocal attitude is one of the crucial determinants of successful psychotherapy with alcohol-dependent patients.[2]

WORKING WITH ALCOHOL-DEPENDENT PATIENTS —
STATUS QUO AND NEW PERSPECTIVES

Contacting and working with alcohol-dependent patients is a therapeutic expertise that — despite newer, positive developments — is almost never trained at universities (at least not at German ones), or, for that matter, not intensified and further refined as a part of the usual psychiatric, psychotherapeutic, or other specialized postgraduate training.[3] Thus, it is not surprising that in a 1984 anonymous questionnaire administered to 117 general practitioners from the region of Schleswig-Holstein, Germany, the most frequent response was: "Alcoholics are difficult patients. Their will is weak. They lack insight into their disease and are not cooperative. Their disease is caused by moral weakness or a character fault. Maybe alcoholism is also a social problem; maybe it's simply a bad habit."[4] According to the same physicians, therapeutic work with alcohol-dependent patients in the general practice is jeopardized mainly by limited opportunities to help, but also by time constraints and prejudices formed by previous frustrating experiences with alcoholics. Most likely, the situation is the same for the departments of internal medicine or surgery, which are the "inpatient treatment centers" for many alcohol-dependent patients.[5-8] For example, an estimated 600,000 alcoholics were treated in these nonpsychiatric inpatient facilities in (the former) West Germany each year.[9]

Working with alcohol-dependent patients is difficult indeed. Very often, they present as intoxicated emergency cases in the general practice or in the clinic, and very often they suffer from a multitude of secondary medical problems. Despite their manifest medical problems, these patients — and this is part of the psychopathology of dependence — do not realize the full extent of their impairment, nor do they see the connection between their medical problems and their alcohol abuse. In first-line treatment, alcohol abuse is often de-emphasized or not reported at all. But even if the physician is willing to initiate an extensive treatment of the somatic consequences of alcohol abuse, alcohol-dependent patients often seek discharge from the hospital as soon as their intoxication or their major symptoms abate — only to reappear as an emergency or to obtain medical certificates to apply for social support.

To blame all these difficulties on the alcohol-dependent patient is a nontherapeutic attitude, which may simply be a reflection of the therapist's belief that alcoholism is not a disease but a "bad habit" or a "weakness of character," even when these beliefs are not openly stated. Alcohol-dependent patients often demonstrate to the therapist that psychotherapy indeed has its limits. Putting the blame on the dependent patients might thus also be an — inappropriate — way to deal with the helplessness, impotence, and anger that the frustrated therapist, especially the enthusiastic and engaged therapist, feels. In that case, the therapist should remember that alcohol dependence is one of the severe psychiatric disorders that is most amenable to therapy, long-term abstinence rates being around 50% (at least in Germany[11]). Even pronounced alcohol-related nonpsychiatric medical problems are reversible to a degree at which re-integration into a normal lifestyle is possible.

CLEAR AND UNEQUIVOCAL POSITION — AND HOW TO OBTAIN IT

For all the above reasons, it is imperative that you reflect upon your own therapeutic attitude. Moralistic, punishing, or discriminatory impulses, emotions, attitudes, and behaviors must be openly admitted and worked on in peer groups (e.g., Balint groups), under the supervision of an outside psychotherapist, or in other forms of professional interaction in which one feels comfortable. Recognizing your own counterproductive impulses and discussing them openly with trusted professionals will help you approach your alcohol-dependent patient openly, empathically, and with respect, while maintaining your own, clear, and unequivocal position. This attitude is prerequisite for fostering the willingness of the patient to remain in treatment and remain or become fully abstinent, without becoming manipulative and trying to demand the patient's submission under treatment regimens that serve the therapist's ego more than the patient's well-being.

This continuous reflection of and work on your own therapeutic attitude is one of the most important forms of psychohygiene: do not forget that physicians and other therapists are themselves at an increased risk of suffering from burn-out-syndrome and of developing substance dependence.[12] It is unclear if alcohol dependence is more prevalent among health care professionals than among the general population; abuse of and dependence on psychotropic medications (especially opioids like morphine, or benzodiazepines) are more prevalent among this group, not least due to the fact that health care givers have easier access to these drugs.[13] The following reasons for burn-out-syndrome and substance dependence have been given by afflicted health care professionals: stress on the job, high level of responsibility, large number of patients, time pressure, irregular working hours, lack of a lifestyle that can compensate for the increased stress, such as supportive partnerships or families, social activities, or ability to relax properly.[14] For alcohol dependent physicians and therapists, the same rules as for non-physician alcohol-dependent patients apply: do not de-emphasize or negate the alcohol problem. Of special concern for alcohol-dependent physicians are their role reversal (from therapist to patient) and more severe feelings of guilt and shame resulting from over-emphasizing their role as a moral model ("Of all things, THAT should not have happened to me as a doctor!"). Special treatment and vocational rehabilitation programs for substance-dependent "helpers" have, for example, been developed in the U.S.[15] and Germany.[16]

THE ALCOHOL-DEPENDENT PATIENT

THE ALCOHOLIC PERSONALITY: AN ILLUSION

At the start of this chapter, psychotherapy was defined in general term as a "treatment of patients by psychological means," the process of pychotherapy being determined and formed by the alcohol-dependent patient, the addiction therapist, and their interaction. If we take a closer look at the alcohol-dependent patient, we first have to report that, after decades of intense research, no general "alcoholic personality" could be found. Specific or predisposing personality traits that are relevant for all alcoholics could not be demonstrated beyond reasonable doubt in any of the empirical investigations.[17] In some investigations, a slightly higher frequency of emotional instability, depressive mood changes, or disturbances of the autonomic nervous system were found; these characteristics, however, were of only slight predictive value for substance dependence.[18]

In this regard, one has to distinguish between the concept of a "general alcoholic personality" and the — useful — concept of "typologies" of alcohol-dependent patients. Discussing "typologies" is beyond the scope of this chapter, although sometimes certain personality traits (e.g., "antisocial") contribute to certain "types" of alcoholics.[19]

Although predisposing genetic factors have been found ("alcoholic sons of alcoholic fathers"[20]; see also Chapter 27 on heritability of alcohol dependence), they do not yet play a role in psychotherapeutic strategies. Predisposing psychosocial influences will be discussed below.

As there is no predisposing "alcoholic personality" in general, the psychotherapeutic explanation of alcohol abuse and dependence — and how such behavior might have developed in a specific patient — is heavily influenced by the psychotherapeutic "school" to which the therapist belongs. However, there is agreement between the partisans of the two major psychotherapeutic approaches (i.e., psychoanalyis and cognitive-behavioral therapy) that the DSM-IV- or ICD-10-based, descriptive diagnosis (even when complemented by laboratory diagnosis) must be extended by a more fine-tuned exploration of the patient in order to obtain guidelines for the structuring and implementation of psychotherapy.

Differentiated Diagnosis of Alcohol-Dependent Patients

In order to describe the patient and patient interactions with the therapist in the partnership-based therapeutic process, therapists can choose among the following three major models:

1. Cognitive-behavioral model
2. Psychoanalytic model
3. Stage model of change

Remember that this chapter focuses on how to obtain a productive attitude toward the alcohol-dependent patient and how to explain his or her behavior in a way that opens new therapeutic perspectives for you. Its goal is not to compare the efficacy of the different therapeutic approaches as determined in clinical trials. Evidence from these trials favors the cognitive-behavioral approach for reasons that we do not want to detail in this chapter. Historical differences, transoceanic differences in clinical traditions (i.e., the "CBT in the U.S." vs. the "Psychoanalysis or integrative Psychotherapy in Central Europe"), and differences in health care systems (i.e., the "short-term U.S." vs. the "long-term Central Europe") should not concern you too much. Remain open when trying to help each of your patients — one at a time — each with his/her personal history and special needs. And please remember that the author of this chapter is working with psychotherapeutic approaches that are mainly derived from psychoanalysis but also include aspects of cognitive behavioral as well as relaxation therapy.

Alcohol-Dependent Patients in Cognitive-Behavioral Therapy

Cognitive-behavioral therapy can be regarded as the psychotherapeutic "school" that applies learning theory in practice. In contrast to psychoanalysis, which interprets behavior according to a "sign-(symbol-) approach" (see below), cognitive-behavioral therapy (CBT) regards any behavior as a "representative sample" of overall possible behavior.[21] The symptom (i.e., the expression) is identical to the problem. Modern CBT theory does not restrict itself to observable behavior, but regards affect and emotion, sensation, imagery, cognition, and interpersonal relationships — especially if verbally expressed — as "behavior" and makes all these different behaviors the object of CBT diagnosis and treatment.[22,23]

Concerning alcohol dependence, there are a number of premises in CBT: drinking behavior is seen as a continuum that ranges from complete abstinence to dependent alcohol intake. This entails that there are no "quantum leaps" (i.e., qualitative differences) between an abstinent person, a social drinker, a problem drinker, and a fully dependent alcoholic. Problematic and dependent drinking are, like other ways to deal with alcohol, learned behaviors. Like other behaviors, problematic and dependent drinking can be "unlearned" or modified.[24] In that context, it is useful to differentiate between those factors that have contributed to the *acquisition* of problematic drinking behavior and those that are contributing to the *maintenance* of problematic drinking.

Drinking behavior is part of an individual learning history that, on the other hand, is strongly dependent on cultural and environmental influences. A large proportion of learning processes take place in childhood and adolescence before any alcohol is consumed.[25] This is due to the fact that alcohol consumption is steered predominantly by attitudes and expectations of alcohol's effects. Only later — and with less impact on his learning — does the patient experience actual alcohol effects (operant conditioning). Finally, especially in dependent drinking, classical conditioning (respondent conditioning) takes place. Classical conditioning, however, is more involved in the maintenance than in the acquisition of problematic drinking.

Alcohol-related attitudes and expectations are primarily acquired through model learning, among others from the example of the primary relevant person or from that of peer groups.[25] A cognitive structure (i.e., expectations of alcohol effects) is formed that strongly influences drinking behavior. Frequently encountered expectations that increase the probability of alcohol consumption are, for example, "alcohol relaxes"; "alcohol is a reward"; "everything can be endured better with alcohol"; or "I'm really really attractive only after having drunk a little."

This set of expectations concerning alcohol effects interacts with first experiences of actual alcohol consumption. As we all know, these are not necessarily always positive. Despite possible first negative experiences, and again under the strong influence of the social environment and already-formed expectations, alcohol consumption is continued. Generally, this is when most people have more positive experiences with alcohol, like the disinhibition after lower doses and the sedation after higher doses of alcohol. In the first case, alcohol acts as a positive reinforcer; in the second case, as a negative reinforcer (e.g., diffuse affective tension is escaped from). Because the strength of the reinforcing effect is strongly influenced by situational factors, the alcohol reinforcement is sometimes stronger, sometimes weaker, sometimes absent — intermittent reinforcement takes place. Intermittently reinforced behavior is especially resistant to extinction.[25] If such a development occurs in a person who lacks other reinforcing behaviors (e.g., decreasing stress by efficient relaxation techniques), the probability to develop increasingly regular drinking increases. Thus, lack of social competence is of considerable importance for most alcohol-dependent patients. Because alcohol often induces positive affect (e.g., self-esteem) and/or decreases negative affect, drinking can also be seen as an (inadequate) coping behavior in affect management.[25] At the same time, regular alcohol abuse prevents the development of alternative — and adequate coping strategies. Alcohol consumption thus becomes a sort of "universal coping competence" (so-called "alcohol competence"). With that in mind, it is not surprising that social competence training is a crucial element in almost all CBT programs for alcohol-dependent patients.

The above-mentioned developments illustrate the transition from processes of acquisition to processes of maintenance of problematic drinking behavior. At this stage, dysfunctional beliefs, such as "If I do not drink alcohol, I cannot be happy" or "I have full control over myself only after having drunk a little," become especially important according to CBT theory.[26,27] Continuous alcohol abuse further distorts self-perception and judgment of self in many persons. Now, alcohol consumption itself becomes a problem. However, negative consequences (with respect to psychological, interpersonal, or social problems and their solutions) are sometimes not realized as such — or not attributed to the alcohol consumption. Even if they are recognized as such and even if the alcohol-abusing patient tries to solve his "alcohol problem," these trials often fail, not least because the patient lacks social competence or already suffers from a very limited repertoire of coping behavior (see above). This, in turn, leads to a decrease in self-esteem (e.g., "I am alcohol's prisoner," or "I can't make it through the day without alcohol."[26] A further impairment of self-regulation results.[25] In the end, alcohol tolerance and the appearance of the dread of bodily withdrawal symptoms also maintain dependent behavior, withdrawal serving as a negative reinforcer. At that stage, causal attribution starts to contribute to the maintenance of dependent behavior (e.g., "My body cannot keep on living without alcohol"[26]).

In its beginnings, behavioral therapy focused on treating the symptoms of problematic drinking. A prime example is aversion therapy, which makes use of classical conditioning. Such a treatment consists of administering an emetic (e.g., apomorphine) to the patient. When the drug-induced nausea reaches its peak, the patient has to smell his preferred drink, has to take it into his mouth, or even has to take a sip. This procedure is performed repeatedly. The goal of this therapy is to stably induce aversion in the patient against his preferred drink.[28] Long-term efficacy, however, is rather low. Apart from ethical considerations, short-term decrease in drinking behavior alone does not address any underlying problems that eventually lead to a perpetuation of problematic drinking.[25,29]

In cue exposure (cue reactivity) therapies, abstinent patients are subjected to situations that had previously engendered drinking (e.g., by creating a "social get-together" atmosphere in role play or by inducing negative affect). As in aversion therapy, the preferred drink is available. However, in cue exposure, the patient is prevented from consuming the drink and is trained to develop alternative behavior by model play and instructions. This leads to extinction of drinking behavior and, possibly, even of conditioned withdrawal symptoms.[25,30,31]

Coping deficits in interpersonal relationships are specifically targeted by social competence and assertiveness training.[32,33] Of special importance is the training of specific behaviors that instill in the patient a feeling of security in situations of high relapse risk. There are, for example, special training sessions dedicated to refusing an offered drink (e.g., "I once had an alcohol problem. I've been in therapy and I do not drink any more." See Reference 16). Relaxation techniques (e.g., progressive relaxation) and cognitive training are used to increase the patient's resources. Cognitive approaches try to correct the inappropriate affect and self-damaging drinking by changing the underlying dysfunctional thought patterns (cognitive premises). The patient should be made aware of the connection between his emotional stress and his stress-relieving drinking and/or his pleasure-inducing alcohol consumption. By reframing the patient's dysfunctional cognitive premises, the therapist aims to decrease the patient's craving. At the same time, the patient is trained in techniques that help him control his (drinking) behavior. To that end, the therapist helps the patient become aware how his typical thought patterns lead to emotional tension. The patient is guided in examining these thought patterns more closely and to modify them in a way that allows the patient to access the problems that are really relevant for him. Advantages and disadvantages of alcohol consumption are discussed by the patient in the therapeutic dialogue with the therapist and — outside of therapy sessions and when the actual situation arises — by the patient in the form of a well-reflected inner monologue. The patient learns to recognize self-defeating thoughts and their influence on his frustration tolerance, and he learns to avoid — or at least diminish — these self-defeating thoughts. One of the main techniques is "Socratic dialogue": by asking the patient specific, targeted questions, the therapist helps the patient to view old thought patterns in a new light and experience thoughts that he previously avoided. The goal of this "Socratic dialogue" is to enable the patient to find and consider new solutions.[26]

The creation of a trusting, empathic relationship and the deliberation of pros and cons of alcohol consumption are main features of the *social-cognitive* model as well. In this model, the goal is to strengthen the patient's sense of his own responsibility to change his behavior (e.g., attain abstinence) and thus help him to cope with ambivalence about drinking. Behaviors and environmental conditions are analyzed to identify social, situational, emotional, cognitive, and physiological cues for and consequences of alcohol consumption. After that, the goals of therapy are specifically stated.[24,25]

In practice, cognitive-behavioral therapy rarely relies on a single technique; in most cases, several techniques are applied ("broad-band therapy"). In this broad approach, care is also taken to treat disturbances and deficits that cause or precede problematic drinking or are consequences of it.[25] Emphasis is put on the patient's *self-management*, that is, a sometimes very complex array of techniques and strategies that enable the patient to cope with problem situations without resorting to drinking.

ALCOHOL-DEPENDENT PATIENTS IN THE PSYCHOANALYTIC MODEL

In psychoanalytic diagnostics, a symptom or behavior (drinking in this case) is seen as a sign (symbol) for an underlying, relatively stable disorder (e.g., an unconscious conflict or an ego-deficit).[21] In the diagnostic process — which in fact is already part of the psychoanalytic therapeutical process — the therapist tries to gather information on and create an "image" of the patient and his interactions, diligently putting together the pieces of a puzzle. At this stage, it is expected that the personality of the therapist strongly influences both the diagnostic process and its outcome.[34] It is therefore imperative to recognize that the patient's behavior cannot be interpreted in just one way and that the patient's pathological feeling, thinking, experiencing, and behavior, especially his verbal expression, represents an acceptable — albeit suboptimal–solution for the patient's mental equilibrium. Seen from this perspective, even the dependent consumption of alcohol fulfills a crucial, stabilizing function for the patient at this moment. In psychoanalytic diagnosis, this function of alcohol has be worked through with the patient.[16] Furthermore, it should be made clear that the same function (i.e., acceptable but suboptimal stabilization) determines the way the patient orchestrates his social interactions, including his interaction with the therapist, his co-patients, and his family.[34]

This requires an understanding of transference and countertransference. Briefly, *transference* means that the patient unconsciously and inappropriately re-enacts attitudes, feelings, thoughts, and wishes that originated with important figures in the past — and that in all probability were at that time the best solution for interactions with these important past figures. This triggers a similar process in the therapist — *countertransference*. It is the task of the therapist to recognize and control these attitudes, feelings, and behaviors. The following three levels can be distinguished: manifest actions, latent actions, and unconscious fantasies.

Manifest actions are the conscious feelings, experiences, and behaviors that refer to social norms, intentions, and regulations, and that may be openly declared by the patients. For example, a patient who had rarely voiced his thoughts and emotions, and very rarely had voiced them in an "unfiltered" way, might say, if specifically asked about it, that "Silence is golden. I always think twice before saying anything."

Latent actions signify habitual positions and roles that serve as defenses and stabilizers for the patient and help him to cope with drives, instincts, narcissistic needs, or infantile fears and, thus, deal with concrete situations. In the above example, one might wonder if the patient has difficulties allowing himself emotionally more intense relationships. This might be, for example, because the patient had experienced important figures of reference (e.g., his parents, his siblings) as unreliable. This (infantile) fear of always being disappointed in intense relationships might be contributing to the habitual defensive position observed in therapy. The therapist should respect the protective and stabilizing function of this habitual position for the patient.

Unconscious fantasies relate to regressive transference, that is, a reactivation of (early) childhood experiences and behaviors. They indicate an (imagined) basic conflict.[34] In the above example, this basic conflict might be an autonomy-dependence-conflict ("I do not need anybody to confide in; confiding in anyone might make me need him too much").

If psychoanalytic diagnosis emphasizes dysfunctions of emotional regulation as major causes for mental disorders, alcohol abuse can be regarded as a self-medication effort, because alcohol is known to blunt unpleasant emotions and is euphorigenic, at least initially. Self-medication efforts are especially alluring for patients with a type of developmental impairment that entails disturbed perception of emotions and diffuse emotional states (of either positive or negative nature). Such diffuse emotional states do not lead to concrete behavioral instructions. Initially, alcohol is in fact able to terminate diffuse emotions of tension and dysphoria.[35] Even when strong emotions of, for example, anxiety or dysphoria exist in alcohol-dependent patients, these emotions may not induce the patient to do something about them, because their origin remains unclear to the patient. In that case, alcohol helps the patient to distance himself from an unbearable reality. Because, initially, alcohol is such an effective means for the termination of diffuse unpleasant emotions and thus helps to keep the patient in equilibrium (functionality of the drug of abuse), it is difficult for alcohol-dependent patients to renounce alcohol.[35] For effective therapy planning, it is important to determine if the ego dysfunction (e.g., the patient's differentiated perception of his own emotions) is a *result* of the alcohol dependence or if structural ego deficits have existed before the onset of the alcohol dependence. Many comorbid alcohol-dependent patients who suffer from depression or anxiety do possess differentiated psychic structures, in particular relatively mature ego functions (e.g., the ability to separate inner processes and outward reality; differentiation of affect) and a differentiated superego structure (simplified, "conscience"; value-based censorship of urges and drives). Under abstinence, alcohol-induced impairment of structures is reversed, and the therapist is able to make use of the patient's developmental stage that had existed before the onset of dependence. These patients, who were termed "neurotic" by previous nomenclatures, will benefit from clarifications (e.g., "Did you often experience your father as unreliable?"), confrontations (e.g., "Why did you miss work the last three Mondays?"), and interpretations (e.g., "If you say that silence is golden, might this also mean that you do not want to be hurt by others after exposing yourself to them?").[35] In interpretations, favored explanations by the patient are put under question and new, more adequate explanations are offered. An example: a patient with a predominantly depressive structure had an alcohol excess after his wife told him that she wanted to go on vacation with her girlfriend instead of with him. After clarification and working through defenses, the following interpretation might be offered: "Maybe you felt like a child who needs his mother but is left alone by her. For a child, this is indeed threatening and frightening. And a child cannot handle this enormous and diffuse fear. Maybe you felt such a childlike, enormous fright, at that moment, as an adult. And like a child, at that moment, you didn't know how to handle this situation. At that moment, it may have seemed sensible to you to drink a lot of alcohol to make that negative feeling go away."

In interpretation, conflict-laden scenarios (in the above example, a dependence-autonomy-conflict) are uncovered and effect–cause relationships that have been disrupted by defense mechanisms are identified and restrengthened.[34] Interpretations can often change the perception of present, real situations that have become distorted by previous experiences;[35] at the same time, these previous experiences can be remembered by the patient but are not brought into the context of the present situation, because he does not realize how important they, indeed, have become for his perception of present situations. Interpretations that make use of conscious material (i.e., memories of previous experiences) are especially useful in the initial stages of psychotherapy. The therapist can take over auxiliary ego functions (i.e., perform ego functions that the patient is unable to perform at the moment, e.g., reality testing) and report his own feelings (i.e., report on countertransference phenomena) to the patient. Supportive psychotherapy[36,37] is especially helpful as an initial therapy: direct support of the ego is accomplished through direct measures (e.g., fostering of reality testing by the patient, utilization of the patient's resources, strengthening of self-esteem and reduction of anxiety, direct guidance) as well as indirect measures (relief from feelings of guilt and shame).[38]

In the further course of psychoanalytic therapy, emphasis is put on the patient's description of his feelings and experiences in recent situations and his description of his relationship to currently important relevant persons. It is important that the patient also actively experiences and reflects upon his relationship with the therapist and that the patient corrects distortions in his perceptions. The therapist (of the psychoanalytic-interactional school) can encourage the patient by serving as a role model who openly talks about emotions, perceptions, and experiences.[4, 35]

If, however, structural ego defects can be identified that were present before the onset of alcohol use, and have not been caused by the alcohol abuse — and thus will not be reversible under abstinence — the therapeutic strategy will change considerably. These patients lack the stable inner structures and the tensions that are necessary for accepting interpretations by the therapist.[34] This group of alcoholics can be further separated into "alcohol-dependent patients with weak ego" and patients in whom a disturbance in primary identity formation has led to self-hatred, self-destructiveness, and to frequent change of symptoms (change of drug of abuse, too).[39] The DSM-IV term for this disturbance is "borderline personality disorder."[40]

Both groups suffer from impaired interpersonal relationships. Structurally disturbed patients, for example, try to instrumentalize the therapist without seeing him as a whole and independent person. This may induce a feeling of being manipulated or used by the therapist (and/or other relevant persons), who, in turn, become reluctant to help, become upset, or even try to punish the patient. The therapist must learn to register these feelings and make use of them without behaving according to the feelings and fantasies that the patient induces in him. For a nontraditional psychoanalyst who is working according to the interactional method, this means that the therapeutic process can be advanced by giving the patient those "authentic and affective responses" that the patient has induced in the therapist.[34]

An example: a patient had trouble taking his own position because his perception of himself and others was impaired. When asked if he wanted a co-therapist to be present in future sessions, he did not respond. The request to decide was transformed by the patient in the following way: he told the prospective co-therapist that the therapist was not sure if the co-therapist's presence was useful or not. After clarifying the situation and possible explanations for the patient's behavior in a therapist–co-therapist discussion, an authentic affective response might be for the co-therapist to express her confusion to the patient while telling the patient that the same confusion might be something that the patient himself is currently experiencing. By putting herself into his situation, she can easily imagine that his (i.e., the patient's) inability to find a position in the therapeutic setting might be a reflection of his tension and maybe even of his being afraid of what the planned therapy has in stock for him.

In order to be able to give these "authentic affective responses," the therapist must have realized which specific form of transference and countertransference has taken place in that specific situation and he must be aware what his authentic affective reponse will most likely induce in the patient. Authentic affective responses can only be given when taking the therapeutic attitude of presence, of acceptance, and of respect.

By giving authentic affective responses, "information-processing affects" like a startling response or surprise can be induced. These emotions can help the patient to loosen preformed attitudes and to reach new self-reflective experiences. Take into account the patient's ability to regulate his affects,[34] as, according to psychoanalytic theory, the inability to control overwhelming affects is crucial for the development and maintenance of addictive behavior.[41]

ALCOHOL-DEPENDENT PATIENTS IN THE STAGE MODEL OF CHANGE

Prochaska and DiClemente[42] described five discrete stages in the process of changing a habit pattern:

1. Precontemplation
2. Contemplation
3. Preparation
4. Action
5. Maintenance

At the *precontemplation* stage, there is no intention to change yet; most patients are not even aware of their alcohol problem. If the patient has an inkling that his alcohol consumption pattern is problematic, continuing to drink alcohol is still much stronger than his willingness to address the alcohol-related problems. Accordingly, the patient has not even started to really become ambivalent about his drinking yet. The patient is still caught in his "alcohol competence" and sees neither the necessity nor the possibility to let go of the apparent security that alcohol gives him and seek out alternative coping strategies. Hints by significant others that he may be consuming too much alcohol are not taken seriously. The patient de-emphasizes his alcohol consumption. Some patients start to drink secretly at this stage.

The *contemplation* stage is a phase in which the patient's awareness of his alcohol problem increases while he still does not contemplate any action. The patient acknowledges that he cannot continue drinking the way he has. However, similar hints by significant others or by the therapist are still met with resistance. In contrast to the precontemplation stage, the patient is now strongly ambivalent about his drinking. Balancing the pros and cons of drinking still gives varying results. If the patient takes any decisions regarding his drinking, these decisions are not very stable. The instability of the patient is experienced by the social environment as fickleness and unreliability of the patient; significant others are disappointed and upset. At this stage, psychotherapy should focus on motivation enhancement; persuasion usually does not lead to stable decisions and change yet.[25]

In the *preparation* stage, the patient plans concrete actions. He commits himself to change (e.g., abstinence). Very often, the patient tries to quit drinking on his own — either permanently or for specified periods — or to control his drinking and drink only at special occasions. Failure to do so may result either in the patient seeking help from others or in the patient falling back into the precontemplation phase. If the patient seeks help at this stage, it is essential that the therapist creates a trusting atmosphere and give specific help. This, in turn, enables the patient to build a commitment that is stable and can withstand problematic situations. For this reason, the late contemplation stage is also termed the *decision* stage or the *commitment* stage.[25]

The *action* stage is characterized by the first obvious changes in behavior (e.g., abstinence). Many patients first accept low-threshold treatment offers; for example, they seek advice from their family physician or attend self-help groups "out of curiosity." Often, however, they do not quite succeed in continuously living according to their commitment (e.g., stay abstinent). The experienced "failures" decrease their feeling of self-reliance, self-control, and self-esteem. These sometimes unbearable emotions often lead to defense scenarios and problematic alcohol use. Often, patients relapse into earlier stages. On the other hand, the experience of a "failure" can lead to a more intense search for outside help and can render the patient ready for a more intense abstinence program.

At the *maintenance* stage, the new behaviors (e.g., abstinence) are perpetuated. New attitudes, thought patterns, and behavioral changes that were acquired in therapy are tried out and anchored in everyday life. This stage is characterized by changes that involve significant others and the patient's social environment as well. Often, alcohol-dependent patients have relinquished responsibilities within the family and/or their job. Spouses, children, and co-workers have adapted to this situation and taken over responsibilities. Now, the abstinent patient returns and demands to be given back his old responsibilities. This often leads to considerable tensions and even disappointments with significant others and the social environment.

As indicated above, all these stages can be lived through repeatedly. Relapses into previous stages — but also a very rapid progession through them — are always possible and require flexibility on the part of the therapist. Relapse to drinking might occur at any time. A multitude of intrapersonal and extrapersonal factors determine how far the patient is thrown back and how quickly he recovers.

Knowledge of the five stages of change will enable the physician working in a primary care or outpatient setting to establish a *motivational therapy* with the goal of patient self-management and willingness to change. According to Miller and Rollnick,[43] motivational therapy starts by building encouragement to change. The therapist encourages verbalization of self-motivational thoughts, listens empathically, asks open questions, gives personal feedback, confirms the patient in his first positive steps of change, works with (not against) the patient's defenses, strengthens the patient, and summarizes again and again what has been discussed so far. In the second phase, the patient's commitment is supported by strengthening the patient's willingness to change and by helping the patient to plan a strategy that can be broken down into small, concrete steps (intermediate goals). The focus is on the patient's ability to choose, his willingness to change, and on the consequences of continuing the old drinking behavior. The advantages of abstinence are emphasized and specific advice for steps of change is given. The patient's commitment is reinforced. If the patient agrees to do so, then significant others are included in the therapeutic process. At the last stage, relapse preventation and maintenance of new, beneficial behaviors are the main goals of psychotherapy. Again, strengthening the patient's commitment, increasing his motivation are most important. If a relapse has occurred, it has to be discussed as specifically as possible: perhaps more intensive treatment strategies have to be described to the patient and, the patient willing, he has to be referred to the respective treatment facilities.

OTHER PSYCHOTHERAPEUTIC APPROACHES

CLIENT-CENTERED THERAPY (NON-DIRECTIVE THERAPY)

One of the main premises of this approach is that the existence of a positive, empathic relationship between therapist and patient is in itself enough to enable the patient (client) to change. Therefore, this approach focuses on the therapeutic interaction itself.[44,45] The therapist has to create an atmosphere that is coninducive for patient-initiated positive changes. Three main therapist characteristics have been identified:

1. Authenticity (the therapist should always express his true feelings toward the patient)
2. Unconditional respect (change can be induced if the patient feels himself accepted as he is)
3. Empathy (the therapist has to "walk in the patient's shoes," i.e., should approach the patient in a warm-hearted and open way and try to see things from the patient's perspective)

These three features are of utmost importance — not only for client-centered therapy, but also for the creation of patient–therapist relationships in general. The patient should be willing to embark on an intensive self-exploration in order to facilitate the intended changes.

Elements of client-centered therapy can often be found in *addiction counseling*, be it in screening for abstinence therapies, in aftercare, or when counseling significant others (e.g., relatives). Client-centered therapy is considered a *humanistic* form of psychotherapy.[46] Another form of humanistic psychotherapy is *psychodrama*,[47] which focuses on role play: conflicts, imageries, and crucial situations are acted out by patients in a group therapy setting. This may result in loosening the encrusted behavioral patterns and in viewing emotionally demanding situations from a new perspective. Role play is an important technique for other psychotherapies in the addiction field as well, especially when training how to cope with high-risk situations.

SYSTEMIC THERAPY

The term "systemic" describes an approach that explains the behavior of elements (e.g., the alcohol-dependent patient, his spouse, etc.) of a system (e.g., all persons suffering — or profiting — from the patient's alcohol dependence), primarily on the basis of the interactions of the elements with each other and does not focus on the individual element.[48-50] Thus, all systemic approaches are inter*personally (as opposed to intra*personally) oriented. In systemic therapy, often the entire family (or several members of the family) is invited to therapy sessions. If therapy sessions are conducted with the patient alone, the focus is still on the entire family (or larger system) and on personal interactions, role designations, role-taking, etc. Systemic therapy posits that the symptoms that appear in the patient (and lead him to therapy) are caused and maintained by the entire system (e.g., a couple, a family). Several members of a system can be "symptom carriers." Thus, the patient presenting with the symptom is an "index patient," that is, his symptoms indicate a dysfunction of the entire system. The goal of systemic therapy is to make this dysfunction visible to all concerned members of the system, to induce changes (e.g., abolish fixed roles within the system) so that the symptom no longer becomes necessary for the stability of the system — the patient can get rid of his "load," the symptom disappears. In recent years, systemic therapy has developed a number of solution-oriented interventions. Systemic theory is validated by the fact that working with significant others has become a fixed part of essentially all broad-band addiction therapies.

When working with significant others of alcohol-dependent patients, the following goals should be attained: acquistion of knowledge about alcohol dependence; demystification; specific planning of coping strategies in high-risk situations, in relapse, or in marital crises. For the latter, it is important to have both spouses attend therapy sessions. Help the patient and his spouse to look at their respective roles. During the course of the disease, other family members have very often taken over roles previously filled by the dependent patient, while the patient has become dependent on their care. These family members might not necessarily be willing to relinquish these ego-strengthening roles when the patient becomes abstinent and demands his old roles back. Interventions like role designation or close observation of self and others all aim at making the automatic perserverance in old roles as difficult as possible and enhancing the probability of change. Dysfunctional communication patterns are made visible and both partners are enabled to consciously steer through such situations. Taboos can be identified and made accessible in therapy sessions.[51]

RELAXATION TECHNIQUES

Relaxation is one of the most frequent expectations in alcohol consumption, both by social and problem drinkers. This expectancy is also reflected in the development of the *tension reduction hypothesis*:[52] alcohol is thought to diminish tension, which acts as a negative reinforcer for further alcohol consumption. Results from empirical research into this hypothesis remain equivocal.[25] However, on the strength of the patients' expectancies themselves, efficient psychotherapy has to offer alternative methods for relaxation to the alcohol-dependent patient. Accordingly, relaxation techniques are an integral part of most treatment regimens. Please note that the exercise of these techniques and the experience of their success by the patient feed back into his feeling of self-reliance and self-esteem and, thus, become effective coping strategies.[53]

Autogenic training, progressive relaxation, relaxing hypnosis, and biofeedback are techniques that are backed by a sound empirical basis. They are used as adjuncts in other psychotherapeutic regimens. Closely related techniques are employed in *body therapy* (which enjoys increasing popularity and certainly has its place in the treatment of alcohol dependence); here, relaxation is not the final goal but serves (or is a result of) other, more far-reaching aims.[54] Feldenkrais therapy, concentrative motion therapy, and functional relaxation can all be subsumed under body therapy. The relaxation techniques mentioned above can be distinguished from meditation in that they do not stem from religious traditions. Common to all is their ability to create conditions that are inducive for psycho-physiological processes leading to relaxation. Focusing, imagery, and re-attribution of bodily sensation (which had been perceived as life-threatening before; e.g., "My heart beats so fast, I think I'll have a stroke.") as features of life, and relaxation (e.g., "My heart beats steadily like a machine; that's wonderful.") are major components of these techniques. It should be stressed again that the regular autonomous exercise of these techniques enhances the patient's self-esteem and feeling of self-efficacy.[53]

Autogenic Training

Autogenic training (self-hypnosis) is a well-structured technique for "concentrative self-relaxation." It was developed by the neurologist and psychotherapist I. H. Schultz[55,56] on the basis of his observation of hypnotized patients. In contrast to hypnosis, however, autogenic training relies exclusively on self- (i.e., auto-) suggestion. This means that — contrary to general lore — the session supervisor remains silent during the training and does not issue "orders" (i.e., suggestions) to the trainees. At the basal level (i.e., after a few weeks of training), autosuggestions of heaviness and warmth enable an autonomic (organismic) switch to a relaxed state. Bodily self-perception is increased by focusing on individual organs. Brief resolution-type auto-suggestions are used as well for personal enrichment. A similar approach, *graduated active hypnosis*, can be used to intensify the training experience.[57] At the advanced level, the trainee uses imagery during self-induced trance; at this level, autogenic training becomes more than a simple relaxation technique.[53] As a general rule, abstinent alcohol-dependent patients acquire basic competence in autogenic training rather quickly. The crucial point here is that they exercise daily in their everyday environment.[58] Diaries and protocol sheets — which they are instructed to keep to record their experiences — can help the patients to maintain the necessary discipline.

Progressive Relaxation

At the beginning of this century, E. Jacobson[59] observed that muscle tension is usually accompanied by restlessness, anxiety, and mental tension. He used this interrelationship for a systematic training that focuses on the perception of the contrast between willfully contracted and relaxed muscle groups. Progressive relaxation was established in the U.S. at about the same time as autogenic training was in Germany. "Progressive" means that the trainee is increasingly able to specifically relax the targeted muscle group. Step by step, he learns to perceive, contract, and relax all important muscle groups of the body. Well-trained individuals are able to reach and maintain a state of relaxation *automatically.*

Hypnosis

Hypnosis, equivocally, signifies both a certain state of consciousness and the technique by which this state is attained. It is suggested to use the term "trance" for this certain state of consciousness and the term "hypnosis" for the suggestive method to reach this state.[61-63] Beyond comprising all features of relaxation, trance can be characterized by a changed perception of time, trance logic, greater emotionality, facilitation of dissociative processes, and increased suggestibility. Suggestibility itself is a personality trait that is normally distributed in the general population. Hypnosis makes therapeutic use of the characteristics of trance; similar to systemic therapy, hypnosis aims to give the patient new perspectives on old situations in order to help him find positive solutions and change his behavior.[124] Physiological changes in hypnosis-induced trance are similar to those obtained with relaxation techniques.[61] Despite extensive and highly differentiated theoretical approaches, there is as yet no generally accepted theory of hypnosis therapy.

Biofeedback

In biofeedback,[64,65] physiological responses — which otherwise are accessible to the patient only after the patient has been trained to focus attention inward — are brought to the patient's attention by instruments and are fed back via optical or acoustic signals. The patient is instructed to reach a certain set point (e.g., increase his surface temperature to a certain level), which is signaled to the patient (e.g., by a lower-frequency tone). As biofeedback can be viewed as operant conditioning, some investigators count it among the behavioral techniques,[46] although others point out that biofeedback contains suggestive, cognitive,[66] motivational, nonspecific, or placebo effects as well.[67]

GOALS, EFFECTS, AND EFFECT FACTORS

GOALS OF PSYCHOTHERAPY OF ALCOHOL-DEPENDENT PATIENTS: A CREDO FOR ABSTINENCE

We think that the overriding goal of psychotherapy (and the entire treatment, for that matter) of alcohol-dependent patients still should be lifelong "contented abstinence," although others (e.g., Sobell and Sobell's group after its first outcome study in the 1970s[68]) have demanded a paradigm change to "controlled drinking" in the treatment of alcohol dependence.[69] There is evidence that controlled drinking is feasible, especially for problem drinkers, who, on the other hand, might be classified as "abusers" rather than "alcohol dependent."[70,71] For alcohol-dependent patients, results from controlled drinking trials are not satisfactory.[72-74] In addiction, there is evidence that patients whose goal was abstinence relapsed less frequently than patients whose goal was controlled drinking.[75,76]

Apart from trial outcomes, there are further reasons for abstinence as a goal of therapy,[77,78] including

1. Self-help groups, which are of demonstrated efficacy in the treatment of alcohol dependence,[79-80] very often make abstinence a prerequisite for admission of a prospective member or declare abstinence as the common goal for the group.
2. Building the contrasting image of the "non-drinker" is easier for an alcoholic than building that of an "average drinker."
3. Controlled drinking requires a considerable amount of discrimination with respect to the level of intoxication; such a discriminatory ability might not be available to the patient.
4. It is true that abstinent patients are subjected to considerable peer pressure in a variety of social contexts. However, abstinence is still possible under those conditions.
5. Long-term longitudinal studies have shown that most of those problem drinkers and alcohol-dependent patients who have sought treatment either remain abstinent or relapse to abusive drinking; only a few patients actually managed to control their drinking.[81-83]

All of these considerations suggest that complete abstinence — and *not* controlled drinking — should be the main goal of therapy for alcohol-dependent patients. Other goals include: better social adaptation, psychic and somatic well-being, improved coping and problem-solving strategies. Again and again, it has been shown that the latter goals are decisively influenced by alcohol consumption.[84] Thus, if abstinence is terminated during treatment, these goals cannot be efficiently worked toward until abstinence resumes.

EFFECTS AND EFFECT FACTORS OF PSYCHOTHERAPY

As an introduction to this section, we again remind the reader of the abilities of an effective therapist. Formal training and supervision can accomplish a great deal, including correct grandiose expectations of therapeutic efficacy and spare the future therapist the "cyclothymic" mood swings that in fact might be due to the respective therapy phase of his patient.[29]

Along with the supposed or empirically demonstrated effect factors of the various psychotherapies (see above), one must not forget *nonspecific effect factors*, which play a role in all kinds of medical treatment, and thus in psychotherapy as well. The fact alone that there is a therapist who cares about the patient's well-being can strengthen the patient's self-esteem and activate the patient's resources. Psychotherapy of alcohol-dependent patients is based on techniques and methods that have proved successful in the treatment of other psychiatric disorders as well. Therefore, we would like to discuss those general effect factors that have been distilled by Grawe and co-workers[46,85] from their meta-analysis of psychotherapy trials and which are of relevance in the psychotherapy of dependence:

- Actualization of the problem (e.g., the relevant problem, such as drinking alcohol to overcome inhibitions to approach other people, must surface in the therapeutic setting and must be talked about)
- Activation of resources (available strengths of the patient are evaluated for their usefulness in coping with the alcohol problem)
- Active help in problem solution (the therapist develops problem solution strategies together with the patient and makes suggestions)
- Clarification (therapist and patient together try to explain developments and try to find alternative explanations for cause–effect relationships)

Psychoanalytically oriented researchers have obtained similar general effect factors, and identified two more factors:[86]

- Mobilization of hope
- Offering a theory that explains the path to healing

Beyond common effect factors between the psychotherapy of alcohol dependence and other psychiatric disorders, there are features particular to alcohol dependence:[87]

- Abstinence is not only the overall goal of psychotherapy but, in most cases, also one of its prerequisites. As a general rule, psychotherapy with intoxicated patients is useless.
- Self-help groups have an impact on the treatment of alcohol dependence that has not (yet) been attained to the same extent by self-help groups for patients with other psychiatric disorders.

Clinical trials with emphasis on psychotherapy have been evaluated for their efficacy; the outcome criteria most often referred to drinking behavior. A meta-analysis of such studies by Emrick[88] led to two conclusions: (1) there seems to be a "rule of thirds," i.e., 34% of the patients were abstinent, 33% improved, and 33% worsened; (2) there is considerable intertrial variability, which renders the above rule-of-thumb essentially useless. A 4-year follow-up study on 44 treatment centers in the U.S. (the so-called RAND report)[89] yielded an average abstinence rate of only 9%, whereas a similar study on 21 German treatment centers yielded an average abstinence rate of 46%.[90] A meta-analysis of 36 trials in both English- and German-speaking countries showed an abstinence rate of 34% at an average of 1.5 years;[91] 23% of the patients had not improved. Trials with longer follow-up times had abstinence rates of 26 to 28%. Abstinence rates dropped considerably between 6 to 12 months after termination of treatment. After that, abstinence rates remained rather stable. We found a similarly pronounced risk of relapse in the first months after discharge.[92]

When comparing various psychotherapies, behavioral therapy (i.e., multimodal broad-band therapy; see below) proved superior to other psychotherapies. Eclectic standard addiction therapies (see below for definition) fared better than treatments focusing almost exclusively on pharmacotherapy (e.g., disulfiram) or minimal therapies (placebo, or short counseling).[91] We found a similar pronounced difference in efficacy between minimal therapy and inpatient abstinence-oriented treatment.[93]

In the meta-analysis by Suess,[91] the most striking result is the fact that German-speaking countries — in which the duration of inpatient treatment is much longer than that in English-speaking countries — had higher abstinence rates (45 vs. 31%). Similar results were obtained in a meta-analysis by Feuerlein and Kuefner.[11] When comparing trials in the German-speaking countries, there was a significant positive correlation between duration of inpatient treatment and outcome. When treatments lasted only 2 to 6 weeks, no such correlation could be found.

The question if inpatient treatment settings are more efficacious than outpatient treatment settings is not yet fully resolved. However, if one focuses on abstinence rates (as opposed to less stringent outcome criteria), inpatient settings still seem to be superior to outpatient settings.[94] This finding is corroborated by the results of Project MATCH[95,96] (see Chapter 33 on patient-to-treatment matching): patients who received short inpatient treatment before being routed to the different outpatient treatments (the comparison of which was the main focus of the study) had an abstinence rate almost 20% higher than that of patients who were routed directly to outpatient treatment.[95] Although patients were not randomly assigned to one of these two arms of the study — which limits the methodological relevance of this result — the higher abstinence rate of patients who received inpatient care is of great clinical and practical importance and should encourage further research.

In summary, cognitive-behavioral therapies and so-called eclectic therapies (i.e., psychotherapies that combine psychodynamic, systemic, and addiction-specific elements, e.g., Twelve-Step programs fashioned after the Alcoholics Anonymous program) proved effective in the treatment of alcohol-dependent patients. The considerable and specific effects of motivation enhancement are discussed below. The overall goal of psychotherapy should be abstinence. Inpatient settings seem superior to outpatient settings. Optimal treatment combines early diagnosis and motivation of the patient in an outpatient setting with inpatient detoxification and addiction therapy and intensive outpatient aftercare.

PSYCHOTHERAPEUTIC INTERVENTIONS IN DIFFERENT SETTINGS AND IN DIFFERENT PHASES OF READINESS TO CHANGE

When comparing the different institutionalized approaches to treating alcohol-dependent patients, the following questions must be asked:

1. In which setting (family physician or primary care provider, outpatient clinic, inpatient facility, intensive care unit, psychiatric department, etc.) is the patient contacted?
2. In which phase of readiness to change is the patient currently?
3. Which psychotherapeutic approach is used? (e.g., cognitive-behavioral therapy or psychoanalysis) Is this psychotherapeutic approach of proven efficacy?
4. What are the attitudes and abilities of the therapist, his/her training, his/her demonstrated expertise in treating alcohol-dependent patients?
5. Does the therapist see the patient alone or in group therapy?
6. How much time is available for therapy? (e.g., brief motivational therapy lasting one to four sessions; inpatient treatment of several months' duration) How intensive will the treatment be? (4 hours a day? 8 hours? Will treatment last 6 weeks? 12 weeks?)

The referring physician — who wants the best possible treatment for his patient, i.e., an optimal patient-to-treatment matching — must consider the *specific requirements* of the patient. For example, how could an inpatient treatment center deal with a patient who just had a relapse and, thus, was thrown back from the maintenance phase to the early contemplation phase, while the inpatient treatment center can offer a maximum treatment duration of 3 weeks? In all probability, the patient would not be able to resolve the problems associated with the early contemplation phase to make full use of the inpatient treatment facility. In that case, keeping the patient under primary care or referring him to an outpatient treatment center would be preferable. Another example: should a patient who has just begun his abstinence be taken into psychoanalytic treatment by a nearby psychotherapist who is well trained in psychoanalysis? Has the patient recovered enough from the alcohol-induced damage to profit from psychoanalytic treatment? How are his ego functions? Does he have the necessary psychological structures to profit from it? Such decisions would require a degree of knowledge that cannot be imparted within the scope of this review. The relevant expertise, however, can be obtained by practice-oriented postgraduate training.

On the other hand, there is as yet not enough evidence that such a differentiated patient-to-treatment matching is really possible after all. Project MATCH tried to match patient characteristics with several different psychotherapeutic approaches in order to obtain optimal patient-to-treatment matching (see Chapter 33 on patient-to-treatment matching).[95,96] The major finding was that patients who had received at least a 7-day inpatient treatment before being randomized to receive one of three low-frequency outpatient treatments (which really were focus of the trial) showed a 1-year abstinence rate that was almost twice as high as that of patients who were directly routed into the outpatient treatments. In the aftercare arm, approximately 35% of the patients reported continuous abstinence, while in the outpatient arm, only 19% of the patients did.[95,96] There were, for us, no strong predictors for optimal patient-to-treatment matching of relevance *in practice*. However, it should be noted that in this study, baseline intervention (i.e., intake interviews, follow-up interviews, testing, etc.) was quite intensive, while the tested psychotherapies were of rather low intensity; they consisted of 12 sessions (in one case, only of 4 sessions spread over a period of 3 months). On average, patients attended only two thirds of these sessions. Thus, the time invested in study-related interviews and tests (at least eight hours!) was, in all likelihood, longer than that invested in the actual treatments. The psychotherapy durations might have been too short to detect any beneficial effects, while the high-intensity evaluation of the trial — which certainly can be considered a nonspecific effect factor (see above) — might have masked any smaller differences between the tested psychotherapies.

As patient-to-treatment matching is not yet sufficiently evidence-based, we will concentrate in the following on a short (and incomplete) description of various psychotherapeutic interventions that are most appropriate for selection of typical therapeutic settings.

OUTPATIENT SETTING IN PRIMARY CARE

About 75% of alcohol-dependent patients in Germany contact their family physician at least once a year.[9] This situation should be similar in other countries. The primary care physician is not expected to dedicate his time to specialized treatment of addictions. His most important function is to take alcohol dependence into account when patients — or their significant others — present with complaints and symptoms. Every patient should be examined for increased alcohol consumption. Simple clinical signs (e.g., red face or red palms; but see Chapter 23 on dermatological problems of alcohol-dependent patients; spider naevi), simple laboratory parameters (GGT or MCV; see Chapter 3 on laboratory markers for alcoholism), observation during house visits, and social abnormalities (i.e., requesting a certificate for calling in sick every Monday; complaints or remarks by significant others) are all that is necessary to quickly decide whether an alcohol problem may be present. Careful, empathic, sober, and open discussions help to dispel the first suspicion or yield a first diagnosis. If the diagnosis is confirmed, the patient should be informed about the consequences of alcohol abuse in a non-threatening way. Awareness of alcohol-induced problems should be furthered, and inconsistencies in the patient's responses should be identified and pointed at, again in a non-threatening manner. The primary care physician should then refer the patient to a specialized treatment facility, to a self-help group (e.g., Alcoholics Anonymous), or may start psychotherapy himself, provided he has the necessary training.

How does the primary care physician choose the best psychotherapist for his patient? The psychotherapeutic "school" to which the therapist belongs is by far less important than his experience in treating dependent patients and his ability to tailor his psychotherapeutic approach to the special needs of dependent patients. The psychotherapist demonstrates this ability by continuously raising dependence-relevant topics (e.g., ambivalence about drinking) during all stages of therapy. The primary care physician can see this if, for example, the psychotherapist seeks his cooperation, for example, to obtain laboratory parameters to corroborate the patient's claim to be abstinent or to obtain medical help in the treatment of alcohol-related nonpsychiatric problems (e.g., ulcer).

According to the stage model of Prochaska and DiClemente (see above), most patients are still in the first stage (i.e., the precontemplation stage) when they see their primary care physician. Remain calm, clear, and empathic. Point out the problematic consequences of drinking. Do not use threatening reports of alcohol-induced damage; they are counterproductive. Point out that abstinence is possible and that abstinence can offer presently unimagined possibilities — in spousal and family relations, on the job, etc. Be patient.

Codependent behavior by any therapist, the primary care physician included, must be recognized, reflected upon, and diminished. Co-dependent behavior is a result of the wish to handle the dependent patient and avoid problems and harm as much as possible. Paradoxically, this can worsen the patient's dependence.[51] For example, co-dependent behavior could consist of meeting the patient's demand for hypnotics (seemingly to treat his insomnia) or antidepressants (to treat the patient's alcohol-induced depression). Codependent behavior is writing a medical certificate of absence, repeatedly, on a Monday, after the patient has only called your office and requested one. Co-dependent behavior occurs when a primary care physician trained in psychotherapy does *not* corroborate the patient's claim to be abstinent during a motivational discussion or a supportive psychotherapeutic intervention. Only an empathic, clear, reflective attitude by the primary care physician enables further therapeutic interventions.

Fortunately, primary care physicians increasingly obtain basic competence in addiction psychotherapy. On the basis of such a training, *supportive psychotherapeutic interventions*[38] become possible, even in the primary care setting. Following the approach by Luborsky,[36,37] the very first session can be used to create an atmosphere that enables the patient to talk openly about himself, to describe his psychological and bodily complaints, and to describe his social situation. The primary care physician uses direct ego-support by, for example, helping the patient to perform a reality check ("Is it true that your wife ALWAYS/ONLY criticizes you? … that you are ALWAYS depressed?"). The patient is encouraged to identify strengths, resources, and coping strategies that have remained ("In which situations could you remain abstinent?"). The physician tries to reduce the often-present anxiety ("If you want, I will be there and accompany you on your discovery of yourself and the reasons for your alcohol problem. You will call the shots and tell me how far you want to go and how often you want me here by your side.") and tries to strengthen the patient's self-esteem ("It takes a lot of courage to confront one's alcohol problem and seek help. You have shown that you have the guts to do that. You are here. You did it. For the moment, that is the most important thing."). The physician can also use indirect means of ego-support, which in alcohol-dependent patients consists mainly of verbalizing and relieving feelings of guilt and shame which can be agonizing for the patient ("Could it be that you are sad, that you feel guilty, that you are ashamed that you cannot stop drinking although you want to stop so much? For me, what you suffer from is a disease like any other disease. It is not your fault that you are hit by it. And still you managed to come here and do something about it.").

In later sessions, focus shifts to experience and reflects upon feelings that are present at the moment ("How do you feel if I talk about the changes in your liver? What sort of emotion does that trigger?"). Here, the physician often has to be active as a model ("I would be scared. Maybe I would feel hopeless."). In such a supportive therapy sequence, which may be completed within a few sessions, even intrapersonal conflicts, for example, as pertaining to the functionality of alcohol, may be accessed ("I have the impression that you demand a lot from yourself, and that you are rarely really satisfied with what you have done. But still you seem to expect a lot of approval and recognition from others, secretly. And if this does not happen, you are disappointed and your inner tension increases. And that's when you take alcohol, to fight that inner tension.").

One of the big advantages for the primary care physician is his knowledge of the family setting. Very often, it is the spouse or other significant others who first approach the family physician for advice. Now, it becomes important to find out what the dynamics in the family or problem system is. Well-intentioned behavior by significant others may, paradoxically, bind the dependent patient even tighter to his drug of abuse. This behavior and their underlying interpersonal relationships are termed "codependent." Codependent spouses, for example, take over control functions (e.g., lock away alcohol or pour it down the sink) in the — always disappointed — hope that the dependent patient will thus be able to control his alcohol problem. Codependent spouses cover up for the dependent patient, if he is (again) unable to meet his social or occupational obligations because he is intoxicated or hung over. Codependent spouses threaten to leave the patient if he does not drink without acting on that threat. That way, they induce intensive feelings of shame and guilt which, however, increase the dependent behavior even more, because feelings of shame and guilt are often responsible for maintaining dependent alcohol consumption. The main task for the physician in this situation is to recommend simple actions (e.g., "Do not use empty threats. If you decide to give your husband a choice between yourself and his drink, follow through. If you decide to use other sanctions, follow through."), and to point out the possibility of professional help or self-help groups for significant others of alcohol-dependent patients (e.g., AL-ANON groups).

The patient might be motivated to keep a drinking diary that he has to write in every evening. Instructions for keeping the diary (i.e., structural help) should be given: What was my goal today? When and how much alcohol did I drink today? Or, in the case of intended abstinence: Was I abstinent today? Did I experience craving? In which situations did I experience craving? Which feelings were dominant today? How did others react to me? Did I make use of the techniques that I've learned? (e.g., practiced progressive relaxation or autogenic training; called AA friends).

If the patient is already able to maintain abstinence — at least for certain periods of time — relaxation techniques (e.g., progressive relaxation, autogenic training) can already be taught in primary care. Under appropriate coaching and regular practice, the patient does not only benefit from the relaxation and relief from diffuse tension, but also from the experience of self-efficacy ("I am able to do something about my tensions. I hadn't thought I could do anything about them. Now I myself am working this problem out."); the experience of self-reliance strengthens the expectancy of further self-reliant behavior.[53]

It is not sufficient only to recommend a self-help group to the patient. You should be able to answer the patient's questions about the structures and methods of the self-help groups available in your area. Encourage the patient to try out several different groups to find the one that best fits his personality and in which, in turn, he best fits. If the patient chooses to attend meetings of such a self-help group, support attendance by asking the patient how his/her integration into the group is proceeding.

These primary care psychotherapeutic interventions will, in many cases, help the problem drinker (i.e., the patient suffering from alcohol abuse) to abstain from drinking and perhaps become able to control his drinking. However, for alcohol-dependent patients, the psychotherapeutic help that can be given in the average primary care setting is, most likely, not enough. Accordingly, the decision to yield to the patient's wish for outpatient withdrawal in the primary care setting is a difficult one. Positive results have been obtained if the primary care physician is available the entire week (including weekends) and if the course of the withdrawal is uncomplicated.[97] You must decide if you are able and willing to commit yourself to that level of intensity. Do not simply prescribe a benzodiazepine (or any drug), send the patient home, and tell him to come back only if problems occur. Withdrawal is a potentially life-threatening procedure and should not be treated as a banal cough. If the patient is willing to be withdrawn in more intensive therapeutic settings, the primary care physician should actively maintain contact with these specialized treatment facilities.

WITHDRAWAL AND MOTIVATIONAL THERAPY

Medically Supervised Withdrawal Is the Start of a Qualified Treatment

The main goal in withdrawal is to minimize harm to the patient. This entails proper pharmacotherapy (see Chapter 6 on the treatment of withdrawal). Thorough diagnostics should be followed by medical therapy of alcohol-induced organ damage; this can be done perfectly well in non-psychiatric hospitals as well. However, *detoxification* should be more than simple relief from withdrawal symptoms; it has to include appropriate psychotherapy. After the initial medical care, the therapist should listen very carefully if the patient is indeed willing to continue abstinence or is not yet really ready for this step. The process of deciding for abstinence should be supported by the therapist using motivational interventions.

Deciding to withdraw or being persuaded by a significant other to withdraw as an "emergency case" in an inpatient setting constitutes a crisis for many patients. In such a crisis, most patients are more open to a psychotherapeutic approach. This applies to alcohol-dependent patients as well. Actualization of a problem is one of the documented effect factors in successful psychotherapy.[46] A crisis facilitates problem actualization considerably. In order to make proper use of the favorable situation, the therapist should take great care to take the patient seriously and make the patient feel accepted with his specific problems. This first psychotherapeutic intervention changes "simple" detoxification into professional detoxification and motivational therapy. Creating a warm and trusting atmosphere is not enough; as soon as withdrawal symptoms abate, a larger number of patients recommence the use of old and often used defenses: denial, dismissal of the alcohol problem, projection, etc. Stay empathic, be patient, be clear, and use confrontation if necessary.

Features of Specific Interventions

Contents and techniques of psychotherapy must be tailored to the patient's needs as much as possible. In addition, there are some general features of successful psychotherapy in withdrawal:

- Establish personal contact as soon as possible.[98,99]
- It is not necessary to let the patient experience his withdrawal symptoms to the fullest. Do not let the patient "hit the bottom." Always use pharmacotherapy to alleviate the patient's symptoms (see Chapter 6 on the pharmacotherapy of withdrawal).
- Split the entire recovery process into intermediate goals that are realistic; beware of grandiose plans.
- The steps necessary to reach these intermediate goals should be discussed again and again between the therapist and the patient — maybe also in group therapy. That way, the therapist does what self-help groups such as AA do: give active help to the patient.[46]
- The patient and the therapist should openly discuss that the goal of "contented abstinence" is worthwhile pursuing, but that the processes necessary to maintain that goal usually take months and, thus, that they probably will not be completed within the time frame of the withdrawal treatment. Therefore, the patient will, in all likelihood, need psychotherapy after the withdrawal phase as well.
- Thus, the main goal of motivational psychotherapy is to motivate the patient to accept further psychotherapy. The patient should be told that the quality of life of dependent patients improves through continuing psychotherapy.[100] Motivational therapy also consists of imparting information about alcohol-induced organ damage on the basis of a patient's laboratory data or nonpsychiatric medical diagnoses and making use of the patient's concern about these findings: acceptance of the existence of the alcohol problems and willingness to change are the rewards for such an endeavor. Specific active help is given by informing the patient about available therapy settings, about their contents and structure (e.g., what constitutes the daily routine in an inpatient facility) and to help to commit to specific steps to contact these treatment facilities.[92]
- Help the patient to contact former dependent patients who "have made it" (e.g., in self-help groups). This might help the patient to gain new perspectives and accept advice (from such a person) that is not as easily accepted when it comes from the therapist's mouth.

TABLE 9.1
Evidence for the Effectiveness of Motivational Therapy in Different Treatment Settings

Type of Intervention	Controlled Trials (Reference)	Evaluation Studies (Reference)
Motivational therapy during withdrawal in nonpsychiatric inpatient setting (e.g., departments of internal medicine)	98, 100, 101	5, 102
Motivational therapy as part of a more comprehensive approach during withdrawal in psychiatric inpatient setting	103, 104	92, 97, 105–109
Two-phase treatment in psychiatric inpatient setting: after short detoxification, motivational therapy was offered only to informed patients who specifically asked for it	110, 111	112
Outpatient psychotherapy after inpatient withdrawal	113	114, 115

All of these interventions can be be made in nonpsychiatric hospitals. Table 9.1 lists evidence for the efficacy and for the effectiveness of the above-mentioned interventions in various settings.

Examples of Therapy Settings 1:
Inpatient Detoxification and Motivational Therapy

In order to give the reader of this chapter an idea of what the daily routine in a specialized inpatient treatment facility might look like, we will briefly describe typical therapeutic settings with which we are very familiar (i.e., Department of Psychiatry, University of Tuebingen and Oberbergklinik at Extertal, both located in Germany). Similar therapy settings can, of course, be found in other countries as well.

At the Department of Psychiatry in Tuebingen, patients are treated by "broad-band therapy," with special emphasis on motivational therapy.[92] Admitted patients are welcomed by two *personal therapists* — one physician and one nurse. One to two single patient sessions per week are offered by each of the two personal therapists. In addition, the following treatment is offered as group therapy:[116]

- Information (general information on alcohol dependence as a disease and specific encouragement of willingness to be treated)
- Clinical round 1: group (the remission of alcohol-induced impairment under inpatient detoxification conditions is used for motivational therapy; discussion of intermediate goals and concrete steps to reach them)
- Clinical round 2: visit of the single patient in his room (contents of therapy as in clinical round 1)
- Relaxation technique (autogenic training; creates alternative for alcohol as a relaxant)[58]
- Body training (enhancement of bodily self-perception)
- Significant others group (relevant persons are informed about the disease and about available treatments and are also encouraged to express their feelings)
- Self-help groups introduce themselves

This program lasts 2 to 3 weeks and is generally very well accepted.[117] Eight months after the end of this inpatient treatment, 469 (89%) of the initial 529 patients were followed up; 242 patients (46% of the original sample) achieved the treatment goal and started further addiction treatment, mainly as inpatients. At the follow-up after 8 months, 187 patients were discharged from further treatment; 127 of these patients reported continuous abstinence after that treatment. Another 55 of these patients were abstinent. However, they were still under treatment (24% and 10.5%, respectively [summed up: 34.5%] of the original sample; 75% of the subsample with further treatment). Some 60 patients relapsed after that further treatment (11.5% of the original sample; 25% of the subsample with further treatment); and 227 patients did not start further addiction therapy (43% of the original sample). At the follow-up after 8 months, 113 of these patients without further treatment had relapsed (21.5% of the original sample; 50% of the subsample without further treatment), while 114 reported continuous abstinence without further therapy (21.5% of the original sample; 50% of the subsample without further treatment). This beneficial effect of further abstinence-oriented addiction treatment after inpatient detoxification and motivation therapy was even more pronounced at a 2.5-year follow-up in a smaller subsample.[92]

Inpatient Addiction Psychotherapy

Psychotherapy seems to be more efficient when offered as an inpatient (as opposed to an outpatient) regimen (see above). Inpatient abstinence-oriented treatments last, on average, 4 to 16 weeks. The following are further examples of such treatment settings.

Examples of Therapy Settings 2:
Combined Inpatient–Outpatient Psychotherapy

At the Department of Psychiatry in Tuebingen, a 6-week inpatient treatment is followed by 1-year outpatient treatment. Patients are examined by members of the department and admitted if they fulfill the following criteria: dependence on alcohol only, no severe psychiatric (e.g., psychosis) or neurological comorbidity, and residence not more than 30 miles from the hospital. Ten to twelve patients are taken in every 6 weeks. They are detoxified if necessary and then start their 6-week inpatient treatment. In the last 3 weeks, they must spend weekends at home. After discharge, the same group of patients meets weekly for 1 year and is supervised by the same two therapists who had accompanied the patients through their inpatient phase. If a crisis occurs or if relapse threatens, patients can be admitted again for a few days to the inpatient facility. If the crisis is resolved, the patient is allowed to return to the outpatient group. Abstinence is checked regularly by breathalyzers and laboratory samples.

The offered psychotherapy is multimodal with psychoanalytic as well as addiction-specific elements. Again, the following therapy features are more or less typical of state-of-the-art treatment facilities worldwide:[118]

- Well-structured daily routines obligatory for all (wake-up at the same time each day, meals taken together, kitchen duty, obligatory attendance at group therapies, regular field trips)
- Two personal therapists for each patient (one physician, one nurse), each of whom offers to the patient one to two single therapy sessions per week
- Group therapy (three times a week; basic psychoanalysis, subject-centered interactions)
- Information group (two times a week; information on alcohol dependence as a disease)
- Role play (two times a week; pedagogic and psychodramatic elements; enacting of critical situations). An example: the group plays a "self-help group." Members draw lots; two of them are marked as "relapsers." The group does not know who the two "relapsers" are. The task of the two "relapsers" is to out themselves and then to talk about their feelings when they drew the "relapser" lot and in the role as "relapser" when confronting the "self-help group." The task of the group is to adequately react to such expression of emotions or to the silence of the two "relapsers" and later to reflect on the group's reaction.

- Autogenic training (two times a week; learn relaxation without alcohol)
- Body therapy as a group (daily; develop bodily self-perception; experience group play; experience self and others in interaction)
- Occupational therapy (crafts or creative art)
- Ward group (learn to organize recreational activites and to arrive at group decisions)
- Evening events and field trips (transform group decisions into action; learn how to enjoy leisure time without alcohol)
- Significant others group and seminar (relevant persons are invited to attend a group separate from that of the patients, receive information on the disease and the therapy in the course of a weekend seminar, and then are given ample time to work on coping strategies for positively reacting to the patient's return, and are encouraged to express their feelings)

Between 1982 and 1990, 790 patients were treated according to this program.[125] At a 10-year follow-up on a 96-patient representative sample, 24% of the patients had remained continuously abstinent, and 27% had relapsed but had resumed abstinence and were continuously abstinent in the 12 months before the 10-year follow-up.[82] At the 15-year follow-up, 22% of the patients had remained continuously abstinent, and 11% had been abstinent for the last 10 years.[119]

Examples of Therapy Settings 3: Intensive Inpatient Therapy

At the Oberbergklinik in Extertal, Germany, patients at all stages of alcohol abuse and dependence, even severely intoxicated ones (exception: patients requiring intensive care), are admitted to an internistic-psychiatric ward. During the first few days, an extensive somatic and pychiatric examination is performed (e.g., sonography of the abdomen, 24-h ECG, 24-h blood pressure measurements, etc.) The internists at Oberbergklinik are trained in psychotherapy. Single-patient sessions with the internist and the psychotherapist are held to ensure that the patient becomes aware of both his psychiatric and nonpsychiatric alcohol-induced medical problems. The patient is checked for possible comorbid psychiatric disorders initially and then at 2 to 4 weeks' abstinence.

Psychotherapy begins right at patient intake, first emphasizing motivational therapy. The patient is offered daily, single-patient sessions with his personal therapist. In addition, group therapy (group size: eight patients) is performed 100 minutes each day. Patients are encouraged to express their problems nonverbally (body therapy, psychoanalytic forms of expressive therapy) and verbally. Relapse prevention training (see below), information about alcohol dependence as a disease, relaxation training, and abstinence competence training (CBT; see below) — either in the group or in single-patient sessions — complement the therapeutic program. Pair therapy with the significant other is done whenever possible, and patients are encouraged to briefly return to their family and job to apply their acquired coping skills. Self-help groups are visited during the inpatient treatment, and specific steps are planned for the patient's joining self-help groups and attending a local outpatient facility after discharge. Overall, the patient is offered 35 hours of therapy per week. For the 50–60 patients that can be admitted to the Oberbergklinik, 25 psychotherapists (10 to 12 physicians and 8 psychologists and special addiction therapists) are available. This extremely high-intensity care allows shortening of therapy duration.[16]

Aftercare and Relapse Prevention

Substance dependence disorders are chronic diseases; their underlying processes may stretch over several years. Often, it also takes the dependent patient years to start serious attempts to break out of the deadly cycle of addiction. Therefore, it is not surprising that such an endeavor is often not successful at the first trial. Even during qualified psychotherapy in inpatient settings, a number of patients relapse. However, this does not mean that these patients are "lost cases." Relapses can be used to better cope with problem situations the next time; relapses can help the patient overcome ambivalence about wanting to stop drinking. Relapsing patients may very well attain "contented abstinence" at the next trial, or the one after that.

A considerable proportion of patients do remain abstinent after a detoxification and abstinence-oriented therapy (see above). Do not forget this.

Aftercare

In our view, the most important effect factor of successful aftercare is the involvement of the withdrawn and abstinent patient in self-help groups (at least one meeting per week of the patient's "home group"), preferably in the patient's home town. In addition, addiction-oriented outpatient facilities should continue to train social competence and work through unconscious conflicts and other intrapersonal problems of the patient. Psychotherapists or addiction counselors in practice or in outpatient clinics are available for such a treatment. Pair or family therapy (systemic therapy) can address interpersonal problems (e.g., between spouses, within the family) that tend to exacerbate once the abstinent patient returns home from inpatient treatment. Comorbid psychiatric disorders must be properly treated, that is, covered by psychotherapy and proper pharmacotherapy. However, drugs that can cause a dependence should not be prescribed! Social workers can help the patient cope with debts, or with finding a new job. The primary care physician should coordinate these efforts and monitor and, if necessary, treat the alcohol-induced organ damage.

Relapse Prevention

Previously, and according to an "all-or-nothing" dogma, every single drink that terminated a period of abstinence was seen by the therapist as a catastrophe. This counterproductive therapeutic attitude has, fortunately, given way to a more differentiated view. Accordingly, many therapists call the first drink after abstinence (the alcohol content of which, in most cases, can be limited by the patient) a "slip" or a "lapse." Still, any slip constitutes a crisis that must be taken very seriously. The proper approach to this crisis decides if the slip helps the alcohol-dependent patient to resume abstinence or if the slip escalates to full-blown alcohol relapse. To emphasize, these considerations do not mean that a slip is a necessary part of the treatment of alcohol-dependent patients. However, should a slip occur, it can be used in a positive way by the experienced therapist and the patient. Thus, a slip is no cause for giving up hope for the eventual full recovery of the alcohol-dependent patient.

For the effective prevention and treatment of relapse, the model developed by Marlatt and Gordon[70] is considered the most influential.

Triggers of relapse and high-risk situations can be sorted according to general principles; however, they have to be identified and targeted for each patient individually.

Intrapersonal triggers include:

• Negative emotions: diffuse tension, annoyance, dysphoria, lonesomeness
• Positive emotions (less frequent): the dependent patient may be tempted to "top off" his euphoria with alcohol (e.g., after a personal success or in a romantic situation)
• Craving (which might be induced by external stimuli, i.e., "cues", e.g., the sight and smell of beer)
• Wishes to see if the patient can change to "controlled drinking"

We have found that alcohol-dependent patients may develop association patterns that are resistant to forgetting and that stably transform formerly neutral external stimuli into cues for craving, even after prolonged abstinence.[120-122]

Interpersonal triggers of relapse include:

- Conflicts (e.g., with spouse, family members, friends, or colleagues at work)
- Social situations with high drinking pressure (e.g., weddings, holidays, etc.)
- Stressful life events (e.g., prolonged sickness, divorce, death of a significant other, loss of job, debts, etc.)

Marlatt and Gordon[70] have stressed that it is extremely important how the abstinent patient meets these challenging situations. Predisposing to relapse is an unbalanced lifestyle (e.g., too many duties in the face of too few rewards or pleasant life events; living-out of extremes; being a workaholic; boredom; lack of a structured daily routine). Cognitive distortions (e.g., denial, rationalization) can also play a role in relapse.

As a result, a chain of seemingly minor decisions leads to a full-blown risk situation. For example, an abstinent patient might decide to invite a social drinker to his house. The patient knows that his guest will expect to be served alcohol. So the patient breaks his resolve to never keep alcohol in his house, seemingly just to please the expected guest, shops for alcohol, and stores the alcohol in his house. The visit itself can escalate into a high-risk situation. But even if the guest decides not to consume any alcohol, the next seemingly trivial decision might be cooking a sauce for his significant other that contains a little alcohol. Step by step, seemingly rational or irrelevant conditions can lead to relapse.

Additional relapse risk factors are an experienced and expected low degree of self-control and self-efficacy.

If the abstinent patient has acquired effective coping strategies, even high-risk situations do not lead to relapse. On the negative side, this might tempt the patient to overestimate his abilities in the next risk situation. On the positive side, emerging from a high-risk situation without relapse might considerably strengthen the patient's feelings of self-control and self-reliance — which in turn are beneficial for maintaining abstinence.

Relapse may trigger an *abstinence violation effect*:[70] the patient experiences a conflict between his commitment to abstinence and the actual behavior (cognitive dissonance). For the further course of the lapse, it is decisive if the patient attributes his behavior (i.e., the slip) to himself in a global and inflexible manner ("once an alcoholic, always an alcoholic"; "all my efforts were in vain; I have always been a loser"; "my alcoholism is inherited from my father, and I cannot do anything about it anyway"), or if the patient is able to analyze his relapse in a differentiated manner that considers internal as well as external factors ("This wasn't my day today. I really felt shitty. And on top of that, my buddy offered me this cold beer. But, no more drinks. I'll feel better tomorrow."). Pervasive feelings of guilt, shame, hopelessness, and personal defects, as well as sadness, often also contribute to a full-blown relapse in this situation.[25] In dependent patients, a full-blown relapse often leads to loss of control.

Permanent awareness, a feeling of being responsible for oneself, and a feeling of being able to do things on one's own, negative expectations with regard to resumption of alcohol abuse (e.g., loss of spouse or job, progression of ulcer), coping strategies for unavoidable risk situations, and support by a functioning social network are all important factors for the prevention of relapse.[123]

ACKNOWLEDGMENTS

The author thanks G. Zernig for his very helpful support throughout all phases of writing this chapter. Dr. Zernig not only helped by providing outstanding editorial care and support and by translating this chapter, but also by his continuous constructive advice, which was based on his profound knowledge of psychotherapeutic approaches. Without Dr. Zernig's suggestions and help, this chapter would not exist in its present form.

REFERENCES

1. Schmidt, L., *Alkoholkrankheit und Alkoholmissbrauch*, Kohlhammer, Stuttgart, 1993.
2. Glatt, M.M., Psychologische Grundlagen der Alkoholikerbehandlung, *Muench. Med. Wochenschr.*, 107, 2477, 1966.
3. Mann, K. and Kapp, B., Zur Lehre in der Suchtmedizin. Eine Befragung von Studenten und Professoren, *Suchtforschung und Suchttherapie in Deutschland*, K. Mann and G. Buchkremer, Eds., Neuland, Geesthacht, 1995, 38-40.
4. Reimer, C. and Freisfeld, A., Einstellungen und emotionale Reaktionen von Aerzten gegenueber Alkoholikern, *Therapiewoche*, 34, 3514, 1984.
5. Katz, A., Morgan, M.Y., and Sherlock, S., Alcoholism treatment in a medical setting, *J. Stud. Alcohol*, 42, 136, 1981.
6. Schneider, J., Die Behandlung Alkoholabhaengiger im Allgemeinkrankenhaus: Ein Blick in die Dunkelzone, *Die vergessene Mehrheit. Zur Realitaet der Versorgung alkohol- und medikamentenabhaengiger Menschen*, G. Wienberg, Ed., Psychiatrie-Verlag, Berlin, 1992, 114-119.
7. Moeller, H.J., Angermund, A., and Muehlen, B., Praevalenzraten von Alkoholismus an einem chirurgischen Krankenhaus: Empirische Untersuchungen mit dem Muenchner Alkoholismus-Test, *Suchtgefahren*, 33, 199, 1987.
8. Moore, R.D., Bone, L.R., Geller, G., Mamon, J.A., Stokes, E.J., and Levine, D.M., Prevalence, detection, and treatment of alcoholism in hospitalized patients, *JAMA*, 261, 403, 1989.
9. Wienberg, G., Struktur und Dynamik der Suchtkrankenversorgung in der Bundesrepublik — ein Versuch, die Realitaet vollstaendig wahrzunehmen, *Die vergessene Mehrheit. Zur Realitaet der Versorgung alkohol- und medikamentenabhaengiger Menschen*, G. Wienberg, Ed., Psychiatrie-Verlag, Berlin, 1992, 12-60.
10. Schwoon, D.R., Motivation — ein kritischer Begriff in der Behandlung Suchtkranker, *Die vergessene Mehrheit. Zur Realitaet der Versorgung alkohol- und medikamentenabhaengiger Menschen*, G. Wienberg, Ed., Psychiatrie-Verlag, Berlin, 1992, 170-182.
11. Feuerlein, W. and Kuefner, H., Langzeitverlaeufe des Alkoholismus, *Suchtkranke. Die ungeliebten Kinder der Psychiatrie*, D.R. Schwoon and M. Krausz, Eds., Enke, Stuttgart, 1990, 69-80.
12. Maeulen, B., Gottschaldt, M., and Damm, K., Unterstuetzung durch die Aerztekammern: Hilfsmoeglichkeiten fuer abhaengige Aerzte, *Dtsch Aerzteblatt*, 92, C2083, 1995.
13. Soyka, M., *Die Alkoholkrankheit — Diagnose und Therapie*, Chapman & Hall, Weinheim, 1995.
14. Fengler, J., *Helfen macht muede*, Pfeiffer, Munich, 1998.
15. Talbott, G.D., Gallegos, K.V., Wilson, P.O., and Porter, T.L., The Medical Association of Georgia's Impaired Physicians Program. Review of the first 1000 physicians: analysis of specialty, *JAMA*, 257, 2927, 1987.
16. Gottschaldt, M., *Alkohol und Medikamente — Wege aus der Abhaengigkeit. Was uns im Leben praegt — Sucht als emotionales Problem*, Trias, Stuttgart, 1997.
17. Rist, F. and Watzl, H., Clusteranalysen von Persoenlichkeitsmerkmalen — ein Weg zur differentiellen Zuweisung von Alkoholkranken?, *Z. Klin. Psychol.*, 18, 166, 1989.
18. Ellgring, H. and Vollmer, H.C., Veraenderungen von Persoenlichkeitsfaktoren in der Therapie, *Suchttherapie — psychoanalytisch, verhaltenstherapeutisch*, A. Heigl-Evers and H.C. Vollmer, Eds., Vandenhoeck & Ruprecht, Goettingen, 1991, 140-151.
19. Cloninger, C.R., Sigvardsson, S., and Bohman, M., Childhood personality predicts alcohol abuse in young adults, *Alcohol Clin. Exp. Res.*, 12, 494, 1988.
20. Schuckit, M.A., Genetic and clinical implications of alcoholism and affective disorder, *Am. J. Psychiatry*, 143, 140, 1986.
21. Kraemer, S., Differentialdiagnostik und Indikation zur Verhaltenstherapie bei Alkoholabhaengigkeit, *Suchttherapie — psychoanalytisch, verhaltenstherapeutisch*, A. Heigl-Evers and H.C. Vollmer, Eds., Vandenhoeck & Ruprecht, Goettingen, 1991, 57-72.
22. Lazarus, A.A., *Brief but Comprehensive Psychotherapy: The Multimodal Way*, Springer, New York, 1997.
23. Lazarus, A.A., *Multimodale Verhaltenstherapie*, Klotz, Frankfurt, 1977.

24. Jung, M., Abhaengigkeit als gelerntes Verhalten — die Sicht der Verhaltenstherapie, *Sucht — die Lebenswelten Abhaengiger*, G. Laengle, K. Mann, and G. Buchkremer, Eds., Attempto, Tuebingen, 1996, 99–108.

25. Arend, H., *Alkoholismus — Ambulante Therapie und Rueckfallprophylaxe*, Beltz, Weinheim, 1994.

26. Beck, A.T., Wright, F.D., Newman, C.F., and Liese, B.S., *Cognitive Therapy of Substance Abuse*, Guilford Press, New York, 1993.

27. Beck, A.T., Wright, F.D., Newman, C.F., and Liese, B.S., *Kognitive Therapie der Sucht*, Beltz, Weinheim, 1997.

28. Wolpe, J., *The Practice of Behavior Therapy*, Pergamon Press, New York, 1969.

29. Watzl, H., Verhaltenstherapie des Alkoholismus, *Drogen und Alkohol*, D. Ladewig, Ed., Ispa-press, Lausanne, 1986, 86–104.

30. Rist, F. and Davies-Osterkamp, S., An alcohol contact program: training for increased security of alcoholics in trial situations, *Drug Alcohol Depend.*, 2, 163, 1977.

31. Rist, F., Watzl, H., and Cohen, R., Versuche zur Erfassung von Rueckfallbedingungen bei Alkoholkranken, *Rueckfall und Rueckfallprophylaxe*, H. Watzl and R. Cohen, Eds., Springer, Heidelberg, 1989, 126-138.

32. Monti, P.M., Abrams, D.B., Kadden, R.M., and Cooney, N.L., *Treating Alcohol Dependence: A Coping Skills Training Guide*, Guilford Press, New York, 1989.

33. Monti, P.M., Gulliver, S.B., and Myers, M.G., Social skills training for alcoholics: assessment and treatment, *Alcohol Alcohol*, 29, 627, 1994.

34. Heigl-Evers, A. and Standke, G., Die Beziehungsdynamik Patient-Therapeut in der psychoanalytisch-orientierten Diagnostik, *Suchttherapie — psychoanalytisch, verhaltenstherapeutisch*, A. Heigl-Evers and H.C. Vollmer, Eds., Vandenhoeck & Ruprecht, Goettingen, 1991, 43-56.

35. Koenig, K., Vorbereitung und Einleitung der Therapie, *Suchttherapie — psychoanalytisch, verhaltenstherapeutisch*, A. Heigl-Evers and H.C. Vollmer, Eds., Vandenhoeck & Ruprecht, Goettingen, 1991, 73–84.

36. Luborsky, L., *Einfuehrung in die psychoanalytische Therapie. Ein Lehrbuch*, Vandenhoeck & Ruprecht, Goettingen, 1998.

37. Luborsky, L., *Principles of Psychoanalytic Psychotherapy*, Basic Books, New York, 1984.

38. Woeller, W., Kruse, J., and Alberti, L., Was ist supportive Psychotherapie? Supportive psychotherapy, *Der. Nervenarzt.*, 67, 249, 1996.

39. Rost, W.D., Konzeption einer psychodynamischen Diagnose und Therapie der Alkoholabhaengigkeit, *Suchtgefahren*, 32, 221, 1986.

40. American Psychiatric Association, *Diagnostic and Statistical Manual of Mental Disorders*, 4th ed., (DSM-IV), American Psychiatric Association, Washington, D.C., 1994.

41. Wurmser, L., Flucht vor dem Gewissen. Zur Dynamik der Toxikomanie bei jungen Erwachsenen, *Wr. Z. Suchtforsch.*, 10, 29, 1987.

42. Prochaska, J.O. and DiClemente, C.C., In search of how people change. Applications to addictive behavior, *Am. Psychol.*, 47, 1102, 1992.

43. Miller, W.R. and Rollnick, S., *Motivational Interviewing*, Guilford Press, New York, 1991.

44. Rogers, C.R., *Client-Centered Psychotherapy*, Houghton Mifflin, Boston, 1951.

45. Tausch, R., *Gespraechstherapie*, Hogrefe, Goettingen, 1975.

46. Grawe, K., Donati, R., and Bernauer, F., *Psychotherapie im Wandel. Von der Konfession zur Profession*, Hogrefe, Goettingen, 1995.

47. Fox, J., *The Essential Moreno: Writings on Psychodrama, Group Therapy, and Spontaneity*, Springer, New York, 1988.

48. vonSchlippe, A. and Schweitzer, J., *Lehrbuch der systemischen Therapie und Beratung*, Vandenhoeck und Ruprecht, Goettingen, 1996.

49. Schweitzer, J. and Weber, G., Stoere meine Kreise. Zur Theorie, Praxis und kritischen Einschaetzung der Systemischen Therapie, *Psychtherapeut.*, 42, 197, 1997.

50. Becvar, D.S. and Becvar, R.J., *Family Therapy: A Systemic Integration*, Allyn and Bacon, New York, 1996.

51. Czisch, P., Der Abhaengige in der Familie, *Sucht — die Lebenswelten Abhaengiger*, G. Laengle, K. Mann, and G. Buchkremer, Eds., Tuebingen, 1996, 172-181.

52. Conger, J.J., Alcoholism: theory, problem, and challenge. II. Reinforcement theory, *Q. J. Stud. Alcohol,* 17, 296, 1956.

53. Stetter, F., Was geschieht, ist gut. Entspannungsverfahren in der Psychotherapie, *Psychotherapeut,* 43, 209, 1998.

54. Mueller-Braunschweig, H., Zur gegenwaertigen Situation der koerperbezogenen Psychotherapie, *Psychotherapeut,* 42, 132, 1997.

55. Schultz, I.H., *Das autogene Training,* Thieme, Stuttgart, 1987.

56. Langen, D., Autogenic training and psychosomatic medicine, *Handbook of Hypnosis and Psychosomatic Medicine,* G.D. Burrows and L. Dennerstein, Eds., Elsevier, Amsterdam, 1980, 497–507.

57. Stetter, F., Gestufte Aktivhypnose, autogenes Training und zweigleisige Psychotherapie. Historischer Hintergrund und aktuelle Bedeutung der Therapieansaetze von Ernst Kretschmer, *Fundam. Psychiatr.,* 8, 14, 1994.

58. Stetter, F. and Mann, K., Der Wunsch nach Entspannung — eine autonome Entscheidung. Das autogene Training als Komponente in der Behandlung Alkoholabhaengiger, *Psycho,* 17, 305, 1991.

59. Jacobson, E., *Progressive Relaxation,* University of Chicago Press, Chicago, 1928.

60. Wahl, R. and Kohl, F., Entspannungsverfahren bei Angsterkrankungen, *Angst- und Panikerkrankungen,* S. Kasper and H.J. Moeller, Eds., Fischer, Stuttgart, 1995, 448-468.

61. Bongartz, W. and Bongartz, B., *Hypnosetherapie,* Hogrefe, Goettingen, 1998.

62. Havens, R.A., *The Wisdom of Milton H. Erickson: Hypnosis and Hypnotherapy,* Vol. 1, Irvington, New York, 1996.

63. Hunter, R.C., *The Art of Hypnosis: Mastering Basic Techniques,* Kendall Hunt, New York, 1996.

64. Futterman, A.D. and Shapiro, D., A review of biofeedback for mental disorders, *Hosp. Community Psychiatry,* 37, 27, 1986.

65. Childress, A.R., McLellan, A.T., and O'Brien, C.P., Behavioral therapies for substance abuse, *Int. J. Addict.,* 20, 947, 1985.

66. Krampen, G., *Einfuehrungskurse zum autogenen Training,* Verlag fuer angewandte Psychologie, Goettingen, 1929.

67. Haag, G., Biofeedback, *Muench. Med. Wochenschr.,* 138, 50, 1996.

68. Sobell, M.B. and Sobell, L.C., Individualized behavior therapy for alcoholics, *Behav. Ther.,* 4, 49, 1973.

69. Klepsch, R., Paradigmenwechsel in der Behandlung von Alkoholabhaengigkeit — ein Interview mit Prof. Dr. Mark Sobell und Prof. Dr. Linda Sobell. *Sucht,* 35, 394, 1989.

70. Marlatt, G.A. and Gordon, J.R., *Relapse prevention: Maintenance Strategies in the Treatment of Addictive Behaviors,* Marlatt, G. A. and Gordon, J. R., Eds., Guilford Press, New York, 1985.

71. Rosenberg, H., Prediction of controlled drinking by alcoholics and problem drinkers, *Psychol. Bull.,* 113, 129, 1993.

72. Pendery, M.L., Maltzman, I.M., and West, L.J., Controlled drinking by alcoholics? New findings and a reevaluation of a major affirmative study, *Science,* 217, 169, 1982.

73. Miller, W.R. and Hester, R.K., *The Effectiveness of Alcoholism Treatment Methods: What Research Reveals,* Miller, W. R. and Heather, N., Eds., Plenum Press, New York, 1986, 121-174.

74. Kunkel, E., Kontrolliertes Trinken und Abstinenz — Therapieziele bei Alkoholikern, *Suchtgefahren,* 33, 389, 1987.

75. Hall, S.M., Havassy, B.E., and Wasserman, D.A., Commitment to abstinence and acute stress in relapse to alcohol, opiates, and nicotine, *J. Consult. Clin. Psychol.,* 58, 175, 1990.

76. Gallant, D.M., Prognosis and relapse in alcoholism, *Alcohol Clin. Exp. Res.,* 13, 465, 1989.

77. Watzl, H., Kontrolliertes Trinken als Alternative fuer Alkoholabhaengige?, *Suchtgefahren in unserer Zeit,* V. Faust, Ed., Hippokrates, Stuttgart, 1983, 99-110.

78. Feuerlein, W. and Kuefner, H., Therapieziele bei der Behandlung von Alkoholikern und Medikamentenabhaengigen, *Methoden der Behandlung von Alkohol-, Drogen- und Medikamentenabhaengigen,* O. Schrappe, Ed., Schattauer, Stuttgart, 1983, 3-10.

79. Baekeland, F., Evaluation of treatment methods in chronic alcoholism, *The Biology of Addiction. Vol. V. Treatment and Rehabilitation of the Chronic Alcoholic,* B. Kissin and H. Begleiter, Eds., Plenum Press, New York, 1977, 385-440.

80. John, U., Alkoholiker nach Therapien: Teilnahme an Selbsthilfegruppen, *Oeffentl Gesundheitswesen,* 46, 309, 1984.

81. Edwards, G., As the years go rolling by. Drinking problems in the time dimension, *Br. J. Psychiatry*, 154, 18, 1989.
82. Laengle, G., Mann, K., Mundle, G., and Schied, X., Ten years after — The posttreatment course of alcoholism, *Eur. Psychiatry*, 8, 95, 1993.
83. Miller, W.R., Leckman, L., Delaney, H.D., and Tinkcom, M., Long-term follow-up of behavioral self-control training, *J. Stud. Alcohol*, 53, 249, 1992.
84. National Institute on Alcohol Abuse and Alcoholism, *Seventh Special Report to the U.S. Congress on Alcohol and Health*, National Institute on Alcohol Abuse and Alcoholism, Rockville, MD, 1990.
85. Grawe, K., Research-informed psychotherapy, *Psychotherapy Res.*, 7, -1, 1997.
86. Meyer, A.E., Kommunale Faktoren in der Psychotherapie als Erklaerung fuer nicht grob unterschiedliche Ergebnisse — Ein Mythos mehr in der Psychotherapieforschung?, *Psychother. Psychosom. Med. Psychol.*, 40, 152, 1990.
87. Mann, K., Czisch, P., and Mundle, G., Psychotherapie der Alkoholabhaengigkeit, *Alkoholismus als psychische Stoerung*, M. Soyka and H.J. Moeller, Eds., 1997, 119-132.
88. Emrick, C.D., A review of psychologically oriented treatment of alcoholism. II. The relative effectiveness of different treatment approaches and the effectiveness of treatment versus no treatment, *J. Stud. Alcohol*, 36, 88, 1975.
89. Polich, J.M., Armor, D.J., and Braiker, H.B., *The Course of Alcoholism: Four Years after Treatment*, Wiley, New York, 1981.
90. Kuefner, H., Feuerlein, W., and Huber, M., Die stationaere Behandlung von Alkoholabhaengigen: Ergebnisse der 4-Jahres Katamnesen, moegliche Konsequenzen fuer Indikationsstellungen und Behandlungen, *Sucht*, 34, 157, 1988.
91. Suess, H.M., Zur Wirksamkeit der Therapie bei Alkoholabhaengigen: Ergebnisse einer Meta-Analyse, *Psychol. Rundschau.*, 46, 248, 1995.
92. Stetter, F. and Mann, K., The course of alcohol dependency after inpatient detoxification and motivation treatment [Zum Krankheitsverlauf Alkoholabhaengiger nach einer stationaeren Entgiftungs- und Motivationsbehandlung], *Der Nervenarzt*, 68, 574, 1997.
93. Schwaerzler, F., Stetter, F., Kuehnel, P., and Mann, K., Zum Stellenwert einer niederfrequenten ambulanten Therapie fuer Alkoholabhaengige in der Post-Entzugs-Phase, *Nervenheilkunde*, 16, 397, 1997.
94. Feuerlein, W., Kuefner, H., and Soyka, M., *Alkoholismus — Missbrauch und Abhaengigkeit*, Thieme, Stuttgart, 1998.
95. Project MATCH Research Group, Matching alcoholism treatments to client heterogeneity: Project MATCH posttreatment drinking outcomes, *J. Stud. Alcohol*, 58, 7, 1997.
96. Project MATCH Research Group, Project MATCH secondary *a priori* hypotheses. Project MATCH Research Group, *Addiction*, 92, 1671, 1997.
97. Hayashida, M., Alterman, A.I., McLellan, A.T., O'Brien, C.P., Purtill, J.J., Volpicelli, J.R., Raphaelson, A.H., and Hall, C.P., Comparative effectiveness and costs of inpatient and outpatient detoxification of patients with mild-to-moderate alcohol withdrawal syndrome, *N. Engl. J. Med.*, 320, 358, 1989.
98. Chafetz, M.E., Blane, H.T., Abram, H.S., Golner, J., Lacy, E., McCourt, W.F., Clark, E., and Meyers, W., Establishing treatment relations with alcoholics, *J. Nerv. Ment. Dis.*, 134, 395, 1962.
99. Haigh, R. and Hibbert, G., Where and when to detoxify single homeless drinkers, *Br. Med. J.*, 301, 848, 1990.
100. Fishbein, M., Ajzen, I., and McArdle, J., Changing the behavior of alcoholics. Effects of persuasive communication, *Understanding Attitudes and Predicting Social Behavior*, I. Ajzen and M. Fishbein, Eds., Prentice-Hall, Englewood Cliffs, NJ, 1980, 215-247.
101. Kuchipudi, V., Hobein, K., Flickinger, A., and Iber, F.L., Failure of a 2-hour motivational intervention to alter recurrent drinking behavior in alcoholics with gastrointestinal disease, *J. Stud. Alcohol*, 51, 356, 1990.
102. Castaneda, R., Lifshutz, H., Galanter, M., Medalia, A., and Franco, H., Treatment compliance after detoxification among highly disadvantaged alcoholics, *Am. J. Drug Alcohol Abuse*, 18, 223, 1992.
103. Koumans, A. and Muller, J.J., Use of letters to increase motivation for treatment in alcoholics, *Psychol. Rep.*, 16, 1152, 1965.
104. Koumans, A., Muller, J.J., and Miller, C.F., Use of telephone calls to increase motivation, *Psychol. Rep.*, 21, 327, 1967.

105. Gordis, E., Dorph, D., Sepe, V., and Smith, H., Outcome of alcoholism treatment among 5578 patients in an urban comprehensive hospital-based program: application of a computerized data system, *Alcohol Clin. Exp. Res.,* 5, 509, 1981.

106. McGovern, M.P., Comparative evaluation of medical versus social treatment of alcohol withdrawal syndrome, *J. Clin. Psychol.,* 39, 791, 1983.

107. Vaitl, B., Bender, W., Metzler, F., and Wernitz, W., Motivation zur Entwoehnungsbehandlung: Gibt es Prognosekriterien bei Alkoholikern in der Entgiftungsphase fuer eine Teilnahme an einer weiter-fuehrenden stationaeren Entgiftungstherapie?, *Neuropsychiatrie,* 1, 75, 1987.

108. Schwoon, D.R., Veltrup, C., and Gehlen, A., Ein mehrstufiges Behandlungsangebot fuer Alkohol-kranke: Inanspruchnahme und Behandlungsergebnisse, *Psychiatr. Praxis,* 16, 161, 1989.

109. Vinson, D.C. and Menezes, M., Admission alcohol level: a predictor of the course of alcohol with-drawal, *J. Fam. Pract.,* 33, 161, 1991.

110. Krampen, G. and Petry, J., Klinische Evaluation eines Gruppenprogramms zur Motivation und Infor-mation von Alkoholabhaengigen, *Z. Klin. Psychol.,* 16, 58, 1987.

111. Veltrup, C. and Driessen, M., Erweiterte Entzugsbehandlung fuer alkoholabhaengige Patienten in einer psychiatrischen Klinik, *Sucht,* 39, 168, 1993.

112. Talmon-Gros, S., Dilling, H., Jost, A., and Kok, H.G., Katamnestische Ergebnisse der stationaeren Motivationsgruppen-Behandlung von Alkoholabhaengigen, *Suchtgefahren,* 35, 110, 1989.

113. Pfeiffer, W., Feuerlein, W., and Brenk-Schulte, E., The motivation of alcohol-dependent patients to undergo treatment, *Drug Alcohol Depend.,* 29, 87, 1991.

114. Blasius, J., Alkoholismus und Therapieteilnahme, *Sucht,* 37, 215, 1991.

115. Timko, C., Finney, J.W., Moos, R.H., Moos, B.S., and Steinbaum, D.P., The process of treatment selection among previously untreated help-seeking problem drinkers, *J. Subst. Abuse,* 5, 203, 1993.

116. Stetter, F. and Axmann-Krczmar, D., Psychotherapeutische Motivationsarbeit bei Alkoholkranken in der Entgiftungsphase, *Sucht: Grundlagen, Diagnostik, Therapie,* K. Mann and G. Buchkremer, Eds., Fischer, Stuttgart, 1996, 255-264.

117. Zaehres, S., Stetter, F., and Mann, K., Behandlungskomponenten einer Entgiftungs- und Motivation-stherapie aus der Sicht der Alkoholkranken, *Sucht,* 39, 332, 1993.

118. Schied, H.W., Konzepte der Alkoholismus-Behandlung, *Der chronische Alkoholismus,* N.N, Ed., Fischer, Stuttgart, 1989, 253-266.

119. Schaefer, D., Langzeitverlaeufe bei Alkoholabhaengigen, *Sucht — Die Lebenswelten Abhaengiger,* G. Laengle, K. Mann, and G. Buchkremer, Eds., Attempto, Tuebingen, 1996, 154-164.

120. Stetter, F., Ackermann, K., Bizer, A., Straube, E.R., and Mann, K., Effects of disease-related cues in alcoholic inpatients: results of a controlled "Alcohol Stroop" study, *Alcohol Clin. Exp. Res.,* 19, 593, 1995.

121. Stetter, F., Ackermann, K., Scherer, E., Schmid, H., Straube, E.R., and Mann, K., Distraction resulting from disease related words in alcohol-dependent inpatients: a controlled dichotic listening study, *Eur. Arch. Psychiatry Clin. Neurosci.,* 244, 223, 1994.

122. Stetter, F., Ackermann, K., Chaluppa, C., Straube, E.R., and Mann, K., Experimentelle Hinweise auf ein alkoholbezogenes semantisches Netzwerk. Eine kontrollierte Verlaufsuntersuchung mit dem Stroop und "Alkohol-Stroop" Test bei Alkoholpatienten, *Sucht,* 40, 171, 1994.

123. Koerkel, J. and Lauer, G., Rueckfaelle Alkoholabhaengiger, *Sucht und Rueckfall,* J. Koerkel, G. Lauer, and R. Scheller, Eds., Enke, Stuttgart, 1995, 1-2.

124. Revenstorf, D., Klinische Hypnose, Gegenwaertiger Stand der Theorie und Empirie, *Psychother., Psychosom. med. Psychol.,* 49, 5, 1999.

125. Mann, K. and Bantra, A., Die gemeindenahe Versorgung von Alkoholabhaengigen, *Psychiatr. Praxis,* 20, 102, 1993.

10 Pharmacotherapy

*Gerald Zernig, Alois Saria, W. Wolfgang Fleischhacker,
Martin Kurz, and Hartmann Hinterhuber*

OVERVIEW

Double-blind controlled clinical trials of drugs promising for the treatment of alcohol abuse and dependence were mostly performed with men in their 40s who presented with at least a 10-year history of harmful drinking. In these patients, and applying the most stringent and psychopathologically most important criterion of *continuous abstinence*, only two compounds — acamprosate (main adverse effect: diarrhea) and naltrexone (main adverse effect: nausea) — proved effective; the effectiveness of acamprosate is currently far better documented than that of naltrexone. When "*relapse*" was defined not as the consumption of a single drink but as a return to more severe drinking, naltrexone's efficacy improved. The effects of these two compounds and other drugs on other outcome criteria (percent abstinent days, amount of alcohol consumed, etc.) are discussed in detail below.

The following drugs may be considered promising lead compounds in that they all have been shown to be efficacious with respect to one or more outcome criteria: nalmefene, gamma-hydroxybutyrate (GHB), and tiapride. Similarly, disulfiram still must be considered an efficacious drug. However, before any of these compounds can be fully recommended for the pharmacotherapy of alcohol dependence, a number of issues (e.g., amount of supporting clinical evidence, harmful or prohibitive adverse effects) must be resolved. In comorbid depressive alcohol-dependent patients, the SSRI fluoxetine increased percent abstinent days; lithium's efficacy depended on compliance and on plasma lithium levels >0.4 mmol l^{-1}. Buspirone may prove its efficacy in comorbid anxious patients if tested in a larger sample. The pharmacotherapy of alcoholism should always be part of a comprehensive therapeutic approach, comprising psychotherapeutic, sociopsychiatric, and non-psychiatric medical support as well.

INTRODUCTION

A plethora of drugs from vastly different pharmacological classes have been proposed to be effective in the treatment of alcohol abuse and dependence on the basis of widely differing molecular mechanisms. In order to provide the reader with an orientation in a complex field, this review risks oversimplification for the sake of clarity. Thus, we will not thoroughly cover the alleged mechanisms of action in this review. Consult Chapter 34 on the molecular pharmacology and neuroanatomy for a comprehensive review. Very briefly, the tested compounds are thought to decrease alcohol consumption by modulating the following receptor systems: naltrexone and nalmefene, mu- and delta-opioid (but see Chapter 35 on behavioral pharmacology); acamprosate, gamma-aminobutyric acid (GABA$_A$), and glutamate (i.e., *N*-methyl-*D*-aspartate; NMDA); tiapride and bromocriptine, dopamine (DA; but see Chapter 36 on controversial research issues); selective serotonin reuptake inhibitors (SSRIs) fluoxetine and citalopram, serotonin (5HT); buspirone, 5HT$_{1A}$, DA D$_2$, and alpha$_2$-adrenergic; gamma-hydroxybutyrate (GHB), a distinct GHB receptor and the GABAergic system.

We evaluated all double-blind controlled clinical trials that were available to us through Medline® searches, information from other reviews on the pharmacotherapies of alcoholism, meta-analyses, information from drug companies, and word-of-mouth. Trials that did not require abstinence at the start or lasted less than 3 months were not included. Details of our evaluation are available in the form of a list upon request (gerald.zernig@uibk.ac.at). Please direct our attention to trials that we might have overlooked.

Most controlled clinical trials were performed with subjects, mostly men in their 40s, who presented with at least a 10-year history of harmful drinking and considerable socioeconomic deterioration. Thus, the currently available clinical trials focus on severely impaired alcohol-dependent patients and are therefore not necessarily generalizable to a less severely ill patient population. Trials that evaluate promising compounds in primary care settings have only just begun.[1]

Outcome criteria varied across trials. The most stringent and arguably the most psychopathologically relevant outcome criterion was *continuous abstinence*. Interestingly, in clinical trials of naltrexone and nalmefene, additional use was made of a definition of "relapse" or "full" relapse that was less stringent than simple termination of abstinence by a single drink (sometimes called "lapse" in these studies). Thus, a "relapse" was defined as a return to (1) drinking five or more drinks per occasion, or (2) five or more drinking days per week, or (3) coming to treatment with a blood alcohol level of 100 mg dl^{-1} or more.

Most trials also used the outcome criterion of *percent abstinent days*. The criterion most useful for those health care providers who focus on overall harm reduction (i.e., the amount of alcohol consumed) was sometimes expressed as *average amount consumed per day, amount consumed overall,* or as *amount consumed per drinking event*. Sometimes, craving scores from visual analog scales or discrete scales were given as well, as were laboratory values (GGT, AST=GOT, ALT=GPT, MCV, and CDT; please consult the final chapter for a list of abbreviations).

Clinical trials varied significantly with respect to the type and intensity of psychotherapy and sociopsychiatric interventions that were offered in addition to the tested pharmacotherapy. We believe that this confounding variable may be reason for the considerable intertrial variability (see below).

EVALUATION OF COMPOUNDS

Applying the most stringent and most psychopathologically important criterion of *continuous abstinence*, only two compounds (i.e., acamprosate and naltrexone), proved to be effective. Table 10.1 gives dosage, adverse effects, and comments. Effect sizes (i.e., measures of the efficacy of a compound) seem to be comparable among the two drugs (see Chapter 31 on the meta-analysis of pharmacotherapeutic trials). However, the effect of acamprosate[2-8] is far better documented than that of naltrexone.[9-11] The total number of patients evaluated in clinical trials that are in the public domain currently is 2195 (nine double-blind controlled trials) for acamprosate, and 211 (three double-blind controlled trials) for naltrexone. A meta-analysis is available for two of the three naltrexone trials.[12] Unfortunately, an analysis of the pooled acamprosate data (claiming to comprise 3338 patients in 11 clinical trials) is only available in abstract form.[13] For a meta-analysis of either drug, see Chapter 31. If you would like to perform meta-analyses on your own, consult Chapter 32 for step-by-step instructions.

Table 10.1 shows that both naltrexone and acamprosate are both efficacious drugs and, in contrast to the "classic" disulfiram, do not result in a potentially harmful situation if the patient ingests alcohol. Neither drug has serious adverse effects. Thus, both drugs can be fully recommended for the pharmacotherapy of alcohol abuse and dependence even in primary care settings,[1] provided they are part of a multimodal therapeutic approach comprising psychotherapeutic, sociopsychiatric, and nonpsychiatric medical support as well. In that respect, please consider that the nonpharmacotherapeutic aspects of comprehensive therapy — especially any well-structured psychotherapeutic interventions — might be more difficult to implement in the primary care setting.

Table 10.2 lists those drugs that can be considered promising lead compounds in that they all have been shown to be efficacious with respect to one or more outcome criteria: nalmefene, gamma-hydroxybutyrate (GHB), and tiapride. Similarly, disulfiram must still be considered an efficacious drug. However, before any of these compounds can be fully recommended for the pharmacotherapy

TABLE 10.1
Currently Recommended Pharmacotherapies

Drug (total number of patients, references for double blind clinical trials)	Dosage	Adverse effects (frequency significantly higher than for placebo) Contraindications	Comments
Acamprosate (n = 2195)[2-8,24,25]	3 tablets 2 times a day (= 999 mg × 2) for patients > 60kg 2 tablets 2 times a day (= 666 mg × 2) for patients up to 60 kg	Adverse effect: • Diarrhea Contraindications:[26] • Known hypersensitivity to the drug • Pregnancy • Breast-feeding • Renal impairment (serum creatinine > 0.12 mmol l^{-1}, i.e., ≥ 1.4 mg dl^{-1}) • Severe hepatic failure (Pugh grade C, i.e., liver transplant candidates)	• Best-documented effect for the most stringent outcome criterion, i.e., continuous abstinence • Increases % abstinent days • No data available on amount of alcohol consumed • No adverse effect after alcohol intake
Naltrexone (n = 211)[9-11]	1 tablet a day (= 50 mg × 1)	Adverse effects: • Nausea • Dizziness • Weight loss Contraindications:[27] • Known hypersensitivity to the drug • Acute hepatitis • Severe hepatic failure • Patients receiving opioid analgesics • Opioid-positive urine • Known opioid withdrawal syndrome • Pregnancy • Breast-feeding	• Much smaller database than acamprosate • Significantly reduces risk of heavy drinking after relapse • Increases % abstinent days • Decreases amount of alcohol consumed • Effect disappears after stopping drug[28] • No adverse effect after alcohol intake

of alcohol dependence, a number of issues (e.g., amount of supporting clinical evidence, harmful or prohibitive adverse effects) must be resolved.

A look at the different compounds from the perspective of the outcome criterion reveals the following: for the outcome criterion of *percent abstinent days*, acamprosate, naltrexone, disulfiram, gamma-hydroxybutyrate (GHB), and tiapride were effective. Naltrexone, disulfiram, fluoxetine, and tiapride decreased *alcohol consumption*. Statistics are not available for gamma-hydroxybutyrate, which is claimed to decrease alcohol consumption. Unfortunately, no data on alcohol consumption is available for acamprosate and nalmefene.

All other drugs tested in abstinence-oriented trials (i.e., atenolol,[14] bromocriptine,[15] desipra-mine,[16] and the SSRI citalopram[17,18]) were ineffective with respect to *continuous abstinence, percent abstinent days*, or *amount of alcohol consumed*. Some trials on buspirone[19] or carbamazepine did not report on

TABLE 10.2
Promising Drugs with Unresolved Issues (compounds are listed in alphabetical order)

Drug (total number of patients investigated, references for double blind clinical trials)	Comments
Buspirone (n = 61)[20]	• May be effective in comorbid anxious patients (HAM-A score 15) • Small study: no statistical significance at $p < 0.05$ level despite differences in % continuous abstinent subjects, % abstinent days ($p < 0.1$), and amount of alcohol consumed
Disulfiram (n = 648)[29,30]	• Increases % abstinent days and decreases amount of alcohol consumed • Potentially fatal disulfiram-alcohol reaction after alcohol intake: fall in blood pressure, raised pulse rate, hyperventilation, nausea, headache, and flushing[31]
Gamma hydroxybutyrate (GHB) (n = 71)[32]	• Increases % abstinent days and may decrease amount of alcohol consumed • U.S. FDA re-issued warning against GHB because of its abuse liability and potentially fatal adverse effects (vomiting, dizziness, tremors, seizures)[33] • Use outside of approved clinical trials currently prohibited in the U.S.[34]
Lithium (n = 579)[35,36]	• Effective only in alcohol-dependent patients with comorbid depression: increases continuous abstinence • Efficacy[35] dependent on compliance and lithium levels >0.4 mmol l^{-1}
Nalmefene (n = 21)[23]	• Reduces relapse rates significantly ONLY if "relapse" is defined as >5 drinks per day or >5 drinking days per week • Currently, only one clinical trial with a total of 21 patients divided into 3 groups of 7 each
SSRI fluoxetine (n = 180)[37-39]	• Effective only in alcohol-dependent patients with comorbid depression: increases % abstinent days and decreases amount of alcohol consumed[39]
Tiapride (n = 100)[40]	• Increases % abstinent days and amount of alcohol consumed only in study completers • Risk of neuroleptic malignant syndrome and tardive dyskinesia at dose employed (i.e., 100 mg t.i.d.)[41]

any of the above-mentioned outcome criteria (i.e., *percent continuously abstinent subjects*, *percent abstinent days*, or *amount of alcohol consumed*). In the one trial on buspirone (alcohol-dependent patients suffering from comorbid anxiety) that reported on these measures, buspirone's effects failed to reach the $p < 0.05$ level of significance (percent abstinent days reached the $p < 0.1$ level).[20]

DISCUSSION AND OUTLOOK

Acamprosate and naltrexone are drugs of proven efficacy and safety in the treatment of alcohol dependence. As acamprosate is thought to modulate the glutamate (NMDA) and GABA$_A$ system and naltrexone supposedly decreases alcohol intake via the opioid system (see Chapters 34, 35, and 36 for detailed discussions and references), one can expect that the combined administration of acamprosate and naltrexone should yield at least an additive (if not synergistic, i.e., supra-additive) beneficial effect in alcohol dependence. Indeed, the National Institute on Alcohol Abuse and Alcoholism (NIAAA) is sponsoring COMBINE, a multicenter trial that will study, among other therapeutic interventions, the combination of naltrexone and acamprosate (Stephanie O'Malley and Barbara Mason, personal communications). This study, unfortunately, is not yet completed. Preliminary results from other studies suggest that the combination of acamprosate and naltrexone can be safely administered (Barbara Mason, personal communication). Alas, the only currently available trial in the public domain is an open study that directly compares acamprosate, naltrexone, and disulfiram.[21,22] There were no significant differences with respect to percent continuously abstinent subjects and percent abstinent days. Upon relapse, however, disulfiram patients drank significantly more alcohol (165 g d^{-1}) than acamprosate (86g d^{-1}) or naltrexone (59g d^{-1}) patients.

The currently available trials differ considerably with respect to the success rate of the placebo group, most likely due to different psychotherapeutic and sociopsychiatric approaches used in combination with the tested pharmacotherapy, as well as to different intensities of trial-related interaction with the patient. Patient characteristics did not differ dramatically across trials: the typical study subject was a 40-year-old male, with at least a 10-year history of problem drinking, who was not homeless, and had significant others who could be relied upon for collateral reports of his drinking behavior. Specific inclusion and exclusion criteria as well as run-in periods, however, did differ across trials, as did the type and intensity of the concomitant psychotherapy and socia-psychiatric interventions. Thus, in future pharmacotherapy trials, more effort must be put into standardizing concomitant psychotherapy, social therapy, and study-related interaction with the patient (see Friedhelm Stetter's critique of the project MATCH design in Chapter 9 on psychotherapy).

Some of the compounds listed above are touted as "anti-craving" drugs. However, despite the attractiveness of the concept, the evidence for such an effect is highly controversial. "Craving" itself is a poorly defined concept (see Chapter 36 on controversial research issues) which, in its currently tested form, is most likely irrelevant for the prediction of dependent alcohol consumption. Accordingly, changes in amount of alcohol consumed or percent abstinent days did not correlate well with changes in craving scores in most of the studies. Specifically, in the naltrexone study by O'Malley and coworkers, craving scores in the supportive therapy groups did not differ significantly between naltrexone and placebo, while naltrexone significantly increased the percentage of continuously abstinent subjects as well as significantly increased the percentage of abstinent days; in other words, naltrexone significantly decreased alcohol intake in the face of unchanged craving scores.[10] The same effect (i.e., effect on drinking despite a lack of effect on craving) was found for acamprosate[5] and nalmefene.[23]

The overall effect of the compounds mentioned above is modest. However, patients suffering from a disease with such a serious prognosis as alcohol dependence most certainly need — and deserve — all the help their physician can give them. The clinical efficacy and safety of acamprostate and naltrexone have definitely been proven, and they should indeed become a fixed part of a multimodal therapeutic approach comprising psychotherapeutic, sociopsychiatric, nonpsychiatric medical, and pharmacotherapeutic interventions.

Unfortunately, the interest of pharmaceutical companies in developing drugs for the treatment of alcohol dependence has, in general, not been great. Considering that alcohol dependence is a disease affecting 5% of the adult population (see Chapter 25 on epidemiology) — indeed, a huge prospective market offering long-term customers, similar to the market for antidepressants — one should encourage pharmaceutical companies to take a second look and (at least partially) shift the burden of drug development from the public sector.

REFERENCES

1. O'Connor, P.G., Farren, C.K., Rounsaville, B.J., and O'Malley, S.S., A preliminary investigation of the management of alcohol dependence with naltrexone by primary care providers, *Am. J. Med.*, 103, 477, 1997.

2. Lhuintre, J.P., Moore, N.D., Saligaut, C., Boismare, F., Daoust, M., Chretien, P., Tran, G., and Hillemand, B., Ability of calcium bis-acetyl homotaurine, a GABA antagonist, to prevent relapse in weaned alcoholics, *Lancet*, 4, 1014, 1985.

3. Ladewig, D., Knecht, T., Leher, P., and Fendl, A., Acamprosat — ein Stabilisierungsfaktor in der Langzeitentwoehnung von Alkoholabhaengigen, *Ther. Umsch.*, 50, 182, 1993.

4. Paille, F.M., Guelfi, J.D., Perkins, A.C., Royer, R.J., Steru, L., and Parot, P., Double-blind randomized multicentre trial of acamprosate in maintaining abstinence from alcohol, *Alcohol Alcohol.*, 30, 239, 1995.

5. Sass, H., Soyka, M., Mann, K., and Zieglgaensberger, W., Relapse prevention by acamprosate. Results from a placebo-controlled study on alcohol dependence, *Arch. Gen. Psychiatry*, 53, 673, 1996.

6. Whitworth, A.B., Fischer, F., Lesch, O.M., Nimmerrichter, A., Oberbauer, H., Platz, T., Potgieter, A., Walter, H., and Fleischhacker, W.W., Comparison of acamprosate and placebo in long-term treatment of alcohol dependence, *Lancet*, 347, 1438, 1996.

7. Geerlings, P.J., Ansoms, C., and vandenBrink, W., Acamprosate and prevention of relapse in alcoholics. Results of a randomized, placebo-controlled, double-blind study in out-patient alcoholics in the Netherlands, Belgium and Luxembourg, *Eur. Addiction Res.*, 3, 129, 1997.

8. Besson, J., Aeby, F., Kasas, A., Lehert, P., and Potgieter, A., Combined efficacy of acamprosate and disulfiram in the treatment of alcoholism: a controlled study, *Alcohol Clin. Exp. Res.*, 22, 573, 1998.

9. Volpicelli, J.R., Alterman, A.I., Hayashida, M., and O'Brien, C.P., Naltrexone in the treatment of alcohol dependence, *Arch. Gen. Psychiatry*, 49, 876, 1992.

10. O'Malley, S.S., Jaffe, A.J., Chang, G., Schottenfeld, R.S., Meyer, R.E., and Rounsaville, B., Naltrexone and coping skills therapy for alcohol dependence. A controlled study, *Arch. Gen. Psychiatry*, 49, 881, 1992.

11. Oslin, D., Liberto, J.G., O'Brien, J., Krois, S., and Norbeck, J., Naltrexone as an adjunctive treatment for older patients with alcohol dependence, *Am. J. Geriatr. Psychiatry*, 5, 324, 1997.

12. O'Malley, S.S., Croop, R.S., Wroblewski, J.M., Labriola, D.F., and Volpicelli, J.R., Naltrexone in the treatment of alcohol dependence: a combined analysis of two trials, *Psychiatr. Ann.*, 25, 681, 1995.

13. Sass, H., Results from a pooled analysis of 11 European trials comparing acamprosate and placebo in the treatment of alcohol dependence, *Alcohol Alcohol.*, 30, 484, 1995.

14. Gottlieb, L.D., Horwitz, R.I., Kraus, M.L., Segal, S.R., and Viscoli, C.M., Randomized controlled trial in alcohol relapse prevention: role of atenolol, alcohol craving, and treatment adherence, *J. Subst. Abuse Treatm.*, 11, 253, 1994.

15. Naranjo, C.A., Dongier, M., and Bremner, K.E., Long-acting injectable bromocriptine does not reduce relapse in alcoholics, *Addiction*, 92, 969, 1997.

16. Mason, B., Kocsis, J.H., Ritvo, E.C., and Cutler, R.B., A double-blind, placebo-controlled trial of desipramine for primary alcohol dependence stratified on the presence or absence of major depression, *JAMA*, 275, 761, 1996.

17. Naranjo, C.A., Bremner, K.E., and Lanctot, K.L., Effects of citalopram and a brief psycho-social intervention on alcohol intake, dependence and problems, *Addiction*, 90, 87, 1995.

18. Tiihonen, J., Ryynaenen, O.P., Kauhanen, J., Hakola, H.P., and Salaspuro, M., Citalopram in the treatment of alcoholism: a double-blind placebo-controlled study, *Pharmacopsychiatry*, 29, 27, 1996.

19. Malcolm, R., Anton, R.F., Randall, C.L., Johnston, A., Brady, K., and Thevos, A., A placebo-controlled trial of buspirone in anxious inpatient alcoholics, *Alcohol Clin. Exp. Res.*, 16, 1007, 1992.

20. Kranzler, H.R., Burleson, J.A., DelBoca, F.K., Babor, T.F., Korner, P., Brown, J., and Bohn, M.J., Buspirone treatment of anxious alcoholics. A placebo-controlled trial. *Arch. Gen. Psychiatry*, 51, 720, 1994.

21. Knoch, H., Biedert, E., Bardeleben, U.v., Ihde, T., and Ladewig, D., Naltrexone, acamprosate and disulfiram combined with cognitive-behavioral therapy in relapse prevention, *Alcohol Clin. Exp. Res.*, 22, 37A, 1998.

22. Bardeleben, U.v., Knoch, H., Biedert, E., Ihde, T., and Ladewig, D., Naltrexone and acamprosate compared to disulfiram — preliminary results, *Alcohol Clin. Exp. Res.,* in press, 2000.

23. Mason, B.J., Ritvo, E.C., Morgan, R.O., Salvato, F.R., Goldberg, G., Welch, B., and Mantero-Atienza, E., A double-blind, placebo-controlled pilot study to evaluate the efficacy and safety of oral nalmefene HCl for alcohol dependence, *Alcohol Clin. Exp. Res.,* 18, 1162, 1994.

24. Pelc, I., Verbanck, P., Le, B.O., Gavrilovic, M., Lion, K., and Lehert, P., Efficacy and safety of acamprosate in the treatment of detoxified alcohol-dependent patients. A 90-day placebo-controlled dose-finding study, *Br. J. Psychiatry,* 171, 73, 1997.

25. Poldrugo, F., Acamprosate treatment in a long-term community-based alcohol rehabilitation programme, *Addiction,* 92, 1537, 1997.

26. Wilde, M.J. and Wagstaff, A.J., Acamprosate: a review of its pharmacology and clinical potential in the management of alcohol dependence after detoxification, *Drugs,* 53, 1038, 1997.

27. Jentzsch, A. and Jasek, W., *Austria-Codex Fachinformation 1997/98,* Oesterreichische Apotheker-Verlagsgesellschaft, Vienna, 1997.

28. O'Malley, S.S., Jaffe, A.J., Chang, G., Rode, S., Schottenfeld, R., Meyer, R.E., and Rounsaville, B., Six-month follow-up of naltrexone and psychotherapy for alcohol dependence, *Arch. Gen. Psychiatry,* 53, 217, 1996.

29. Azrin, N.H., Sisson, R., Myers, R., and Godley, M., Alcoholism treatment by disulfiram and community reinforcement therapy, *J. Behav. Ther. Exp. Psychol.,* 13, 105, 1982.

30. Fuller, R.K., Branchey, L., Brightwell, D.R., Derman, R.M., Emrick, C.D., Iber, F.L., James, K.E., Lacoursiere, R.B., Lee, K.K., Lowenstam, I., Maany, I., Neiderhiser, D., Nockes, J.J., and Shaw, S., Disulfiram treatment of alcoholism: a Veterans Administration cooperative study, *JAMA,* 256, 1449, 1986.

31. Christensen, J.K., Moller, I.W., Ronsted, P., Angelo, H.R., and Johansson, B., Dose-effect relationship of disulfiram in human volunteers. I. Clinical studies, *Pharmacol. Toxicol.,* 68, 163, 1991.

32. Gallimberti, L., Ferri, M., Ferrara, S.D., Fadda, F., and Gessa, G.L., Gamma-hydroxybutyric acid in the treatment of alcohol dependence: a double-blind study, *Alcohol Clin. Exp. Res.,* 16, 673, 1992.

33. Food and Drug Administration, FDA re-issues warning on GHB, *FDA Talk Paper* (www.fda.gov), 1997-02-17, 1-2, 1997.

34. Food and Drug Administration, GHB warning, FDA Communication, 1998-02-17, 1-2, 1998.

35. Clark, D.C. and Fawcett, J., Does lithium carbonate therapy for alcoholism deter relapse drinking?, *Rec. Dev. Alcohol.,* 7, 315, 1989.

36. Dorus, W., Ostrow, D.G., Anton, R., Cushman, P., Collins, J.F., Schaefer, M., Charles, H.L., Desai, P., Hayashida, M., Malkerneker, U., Willenbring, M., Fiscella, R., and Sather, M.R., Lithium treatment of depressed and nondepressed alcoholics, *JAMA,* 262, 1646, 1989.

37. Kranzler, H.R., Burleson, J.A., Korner, P., DelBoca, F.K., Bohn, M.J., Brown, J., and Liebowitz, N., Placebo-controlled trial of fluoxetine as an adjunct to relapse prevention in alcoholics, *Am. J. Psychiatry,* 152, 391, 1995.

38. Kabel, D.I. and Petty, F., A placebo-controlled, double-blind study of fluoxetine in severe alcohol dependence: adjunctive pharmacotherapy during and after inpatient treatment, *Alcohol Clin. Exp. Res.,* 20, 780, 1996.

39. Cornelius, J.R., Salloum, I.M., Ehler, J.G., Jarrett, P.J., Cornelius, M.D., Perel, J.M., Thase, M.E., and Black, A., Fluoxetine in depressed alcoholics. A double-blind, placebo-controlled trial, *Arch. Gen. Psychiatry,* 54, 700, 1997.

40. Shaw, G.K., Waller, S., Majumdar, S.K., Alberts, J.L., Latham, C.J., and Dunn, G., Tiapride in the prevention of relapse in recently detoxified alcoholics, *Br. J. Psychiatry,* 165, 515, 1994.

41. Peters, D.H. and Faulds, D., Tiapride. A review of its pharmacology and therapeutic potential in the management of alcohol dependence syndrome, *Drugs,* 47, 1010, 1994.

11 Adolescent Patients

Norbert Kriechbaum and Gerald Zernig

OVERVIEW

In the treatment of alcohol abuse and dependence in adolescent (i.e., 14- to 18-year old) patients, the therapist has to consider special features that distinguish the adolescent from the adult patient with respect to therapeutic setting, specific drug abuse behavior, and prognosis. This chapter describes how to create the optimum therapeutic setting and how to make use of the special psychopathological and somatic situation that the adolescent finds her/himself in.

SPECIAL FEATURES OF ADOLESCENTS

The following details nine special features that distinguish alcohol abuse and dependence in adolescents (i.e., 14- to 18-year old) from those of adults. These features characteristic for adolescent alcohol abuse and dependence can be explained by the rapid physiological and psychological changes in adolescents as well as their social roles in the family and in peer groups.

At the beginning of puberty, feelings of (sexual) desire increase. The intensity of these feelings is new for the adolescent and destabilizes the adolescent's psychological equilibrium. Coping strategies for expression of desire in a socially accepted form that have been successful in the past now fail. The body of the adolescent changes into its adult form under the strong impact of hormones. The task of adapting his/her sexual urges to social conventions requires a considerable amount of sensibility and flexibility on the part of the adolescent. Adolescents reach limits; they become victims and perpetrators; crises might occur; the adolescent may fail in this difficult task.

Here, the familial social environment usually provides a position to which adolescents can retreat. Intrafamily relations familiar to the adolescent are less threatening, but not free of conflict. The adolescent must distance her/himself from the infantile demands on her/his parents and develop a new form of relationship with them.

On the basis of these considerations, the following features of adolescent abuse and dependence can be identified:

1. Prognosis of alcohol abuse and dependence in adolescents is better compared to the prognosis in adults due to the developmental potential of adolescents.
2. On the other hand, manifest alcohol abuse and dependence in a developing person lead to developmental arrest and, thus, to immature personality.[1]
3. Because of the shorter duration of possible abusive and dependent alcohol consumption, organ damage and psychosocial impairment are less pronounced than in the adult (e.g., less liver damage, less neurological impairment, less social isolation).
4. Dependence on alcohol develops faster than in the adult. Thus, a recent study found that 40% of patients who had started to drink at age 15 developed alcohol dependence during their lifetime, whereas only 10% of those who had started to drink at age 21 to 22 developed alcohol dependence.[2]
5. Adolescents are still strongly attached to and dependent upon their family. Thus, conflict situations, traumatization, abuse, and a locus of control that resides predominantly with

the parents, as well as the indirect influence of alcohol-dependent parents are all factors that impact more on the development of alcohol abuse and dependence in the adolescent.

Sexual development heightens conflicts between the adolescent and her/his parents; "the drama of separation" takes place.[3] The incest taboo makes it impossible for the adolescent to satisfy her/his awakening sexual urges within the family. Thus, the adolescent is forced to open up new "worlds" outside the family. This process of separation leads to a sometimes quite intensive psychological tug-of-war between the adolescent and the parents.

Maturation of motor coordination, strength, social skills, and genital sexuality enable the adolescent — for the first time — to imagine an independent life (i.e., a life independent of her/his parents). The omnipotence that the adolescent has imbued the parents now shrinks. The adolescent discovers parental mistakes and flaws and responds to them with disappointment. This disappointment leads to anger directed toward the parents, because they do not fulfill the wishful expectations of childhood. Parents and other adult significant others (e.g., grandparents, a close and frequently contacted neighbor) have to expect reproaches and devaluation. At the same time, the adolescent wistfully mourns for past love relationships. Rapidly changing back and forth between painful longing for this past and abrupt flight from it causes the difficulties adolescents and adults experience in interaction with each other. Adolescents abruptly switch between loving trust and uncompromising rejection.

In urban industrialized society, there is no defined time point at which separation from parents should take place. Thus, it becomes the task of the adolescent to choose this time point. Adolescents question their parents' authority. At the same time, critical reflection of her/his parents' values serves as an essential point of reference, as an anchor, for the adolescent. Lack of parental authority leaves the adolescent without orientation. Similar to their rapid switching between loving trust and uncompromising rejection of their parents, the adolescents' attitude toward their parents' authority rapidly changes back and forth: a yearning for guidance and for persons whom the adolescent can entrust with anything exists side by side with a vehement rejection of any curtailing of adolescent autonomy.

6. The risk of alcohol-induced organ damage and other negative consequences of alcohol abuse is almost always underestimated by adolescents.
7. Each therapeutic measure also has a strong preventive character, because abstinent adolescents have a long life expectancy and thus contribute significantly in epidemiological evaluations. Conversely, 40% of alcohol-dependent patients started to drink at age 15.[2] Adolescents who started to drink early have a higher risk to develop dependence on other psychotropic drugs later in life.[4]
8. Substance-abusing adolescents are, as a general rule, polytoxicomanic. Only 20 to 40% of alcohol-abusing adolescents stick to alcohol as their only drug of abuse; the remainder abuse drugs from a variety of chemical classes, either sequentially — often rapidly changing drugs of abuse — or simultaneously.[5]
9. Adolescents are in general truthful about their alcohol consumption pattern and the amount of alcohol consumed.

GRADING OF THE ALCOHOL PROBLEM AND THERAPEUTIC APPROACHES

There is general agreement among epidemiological studies that 80 to 90% of 18-year-olds had tried alcohol at least once (see also Chapter 2 on the natural history of alcoholism).[6] The grading of the severity of the adolescent's alcohol problem is difficult, remains controversial, and lacks specific guidelines. When trying to grade the adolescent's alcohol problem, take into account the age, the maturational stage, the frequency and then intensity of the adolescent's alcohol consumption, and the social context.

1. **Severe intoxication** is usually a result of regional customs that have replaced the initiation rites of pre-industrialized societies. The final step of adolescence is the entry into the adult world. Initiation rites of various cultures set a fixed time point at which adolescents become adults, found a family, and support themselves. The right to vote, the acquisition of a driver's license, or the draft constitute modern society's attempts to replace the initiation rites of pre-industrialized societies. In industrialized urban society, sexual maturation takes place at an increasingly younger age (biological acceleration). Authority to enter into contracts is long withheld from today's adolescents. Vocational training takes increasingly longer; thus, adolescents have to wait longer and longer until they can support themselves (social retardation).

   As a result, the biological and social maturation processes separate further and further. This leads to tensions that must be endured by the adolescent and the family, sometimes over years, while the adolescent has to relinquish the realization of her/his physical and sexual drives. In this conflict, some adolescents try to use alcohol consumption, especially alcohol intoxication, as an initiation rite.

   A productive way to cope with the stress of separation from one's parents consists of seeking out a reference group of same-age persons (peer group) in which a certain degree of acceptance and security can be experienced. The conflict-laden family relationships are avoided; at the same time, positive, trusting relationships (including libidinous ones) can be formed with members of the peer group. As supportive as these peer groups can be, they still contain the danger of becoming cult centers of substance abuse, inducing members to abuse alcohol.

   Although there is increasing awareness of the necessity of rituals (including initiation rites) and although there are first efforts to establish explicit rituals in psychotherapy, theoretical models are still missing. Religious rites of initiation (e.g., bar mitzvah, confirmation) are of diminishing importance in industrialized urban society. Thus, a stimulating approach for the therapist lies in developing family-specific rites of initiation and encouraging the family and the adolescent to enact it; for example, a family feast, a journey, the giving of a special present, or some other creative solution for the adolescent's need for an intiation rite.

2. A **problem drinker** is someone who, in the face of an overwhelming conflict situation (e.g., divorce of the parents, unfulfilled expectations of performance), hopes to diminish his feelings of tension with the help of alcohol.

3. **Alcohol abuse**: 25 to 50% of the 12- to 18-year-olds in the U.S. fulfill the criteria for alcohol abuse as defined in the Diagnostic and Statistical Manual of Mental Disorders (DSM-IV)[7] of the American Psychiatric Association (see the section on DSM-IV definitions on how to obtain the DSM; and see Chapter 2 on the natural history of alcoholism for more epidemiological data). Additional symptoms in adolescents are high frequency of intoxication and the failure to fulfill the expected social roles in school, on the job, or at home. Alcohol consumption in adolescents often presents a high risk of bodily harm. Alcohol-abusing adolescents often have legal problems and often continue their alcohol abuse despite social and interpersonal problems.

4. **Alcohol dependence**: 3% of 12- to 17-year-olds in the U.S. fulfill DSM-IV criteria for alcohol dependence (see Chapter 2 on the natural history of alcoholism for more epidemiological data).

Of special importance in adolescence are the following symptoms:

a. Development of tolerance
b. Drinking occurs more often than intended
c. Repeated unsuccessful attempts to quit drinking
d. A lot of time is spent drinking
e. Social activities are given up because of drinking

Criteria which are less applicable to adolescents are:

a. Continuing use despite awareness of alcohol-induced bodily and psychological problems
b. Drinking despite existing medical problems

Reports on withdrawal symptoms in adolescents vary. The highest reported prevalence in a hospital sample was 8%,[5] although most authors estimate the withdrawal prevalence to be considerably lower.[8] Still, the occurrence of withdrawal symptoms is the best diagnostic criterion for adolescent alcohol dependence.

As mentioned above, if questioned in an empathic manner, adolescents are usually truthful in their reporting of the quantity of alcohol consumed and the frequency of alcohol consumption. The following questions will help you identify the alcohol consumption pattern more precisely:[1]

1. How often do you drink?
2. What is your favorite alcoholic beverage?
3. How much do you drink when you drink?
4. Could you estimate how much your best friends drink when you go out? Do you drink more or less than they do when you go out?
5. How many days each month do you drink any alcohol?
6. Have you ever been drunk?
7. Where do you usually drink?
8. When do you usually drink?

The parents should be asked the following questions:

1. What patterns of alcohol use has your child seen in your family?
2. Does your child associate with other adolescents who drink?
3. Are your child's grades and socializing patterns changing?
4. Has your child become more secretive about destinations and companions?
5. Have you found drug paraphernalia or alcohol hidden in your child's room?
6. Has your child had problems with the law?

RISK FACTORS

The following factors aggravate alcohol abuse and dependence in adolescents:

1. Positive family history of alcohol abuse, compulsive behavior, depression (i.e., major depression according to DSM-IV or the International Classification of Diseases, ICD-10), or personality disorders
2. Early onset of drinking
3. Dysfunctional family, especially conflicts, divorce of parents, physical and/or verbal abuse, traumata, neglect
4. Lack of role model for moderate alcohol consumption
5. Previous or present learning disorder and attention deficit disorder

6. Pre-existing depression
7. Anxiety disorder or obsessive-compulsive disorder with frequent social withdrawal
8. Easy access to alcohol
9. Sociocultural background favoring alcohol consumption (e.g., wine-growing area)
10. Alcohol-abusing peer groups

CONSEQUENCES OF ADOLESCENT ALCOHOL ABUSE

Alcohol consumption is a major contributor to adolescent morbidity and mortality: 40 to 50% of adolescents who died as a result of violent events (i.e., traffic accidents and homicide) were found in postmortem investigations to have drunk alcohol; 30% of adolescents who committed suicide had significantly increased blood alcohol levels. Alcohol consumption is also associated with accidents (e.g., burns or falls from great heights).[9,10]

Children and adolescents who frequently use alcohol often also show high-risk behavior. They have a record of violence and other deviant behavior, use contraceptives inadequately, often suffer unwanted pregnancies, and have difficulties at school or have prematurely terminated their education. These adolescents have trouble holding down a job and have to deal with the ensuing long-term consequences and instabilities within the family. Alcohol abuse also leads to developmental regression, because alcohol interferes with steps in normal development. Finally, heavy alcohol consumption can mask other severe psychological problems (e.g., abuse by parents).

DIFFERENTIAL DIAGNOSIS

When alcohol use, abuse, and dependence are present, the following underlying causes should be considered:

1. Self-medication in major depression (but see Chapter 26 on comorbidity)
2. Tension reduction in schizophrenic disorders
3. Self-medication by obsessive-compulsive patients
4. Self-destruction by adolescents with adjustment disorder
5. Alcohol intoxication as part of a suicidal attempt
6. Bulimia

However, as the processes leading to alcohol dependence in most of these cases have not had enough time to develop, unmasking of the above underlying psychiatric disorders should not be too difficult.

THERAPY

The following six items summarize elements of efficient therapy in adolescent alcohol abusers and alcohol-dependent patients:

1. CONSIDER THE CONTEXT

If the physician is contacted, she/he can safely assume that there have been a number of conflicts between the adolescent and her/his parents. Very often, a request for drug screening is the actual reason for contacting the physician. You have to realize that you are entering a highly charged situation. Overblown and unrealistic expectations of you and your therapeutic abilities must be corrected. Thus, your first step should be to clarify who expects what from you. Often, the parents have much more precise — and more precisely verbalized — expectations than the adolescent. However, even if adolescents often cannot express their expectations well, they certainly do have them. Be aware of this situation throughout your therapeutic interactions!

2. MAKE CONTACT

In order to adequately approach the patient — and to avoid unrealistic expectations on your part — you should explore the motivation of the adolescent with respect to her/his alcohol consumption. At the time of first contact, many adolescents are in a stage that almost excludes any change. Here, the therapist can only provide information and maintain contact with the adolescent. At this stage, it is important not to provoke or increase resistance, defenses, and spite. You can assume that the adolescent is ambivalent about her/his alcohol consumption. Even when she/he presents her/himself as very alcohol-oriented to the therapist, we know that her/his other side rejects alcohol. If the therapist emphasizes this alcohol-rejecting side within the adolescent, she/he risks a compensatory increase of the alcohol-affirming side within the adolescent. You have to find out how prepared the adolescent is to accept help.

Try to build a contract, maybe even a written one, with the adolescent. This contract should affirm the adolescent's willingness to change, but also your commitment to help and take over responsibilities. If the contract is broken, work through your disappointment and view the breach of contract as a (failed) effort of the adolescent to commit her/himself.

3. PROCEED ACCORDING TO THE SEVERITY OF THE ALCOHOL PROBLEM

If alcohol is used only once or twice a year, the physician has only to provide information. If pathological intoxication (i.e., consumption and loss of control, "blackouts") and if alcohol consumption has occurred more often than once a month, there should be regular visits and therapeutic interventions. This degree of alcohol consumption might already possess symptom character, that is, it might indicate an underlying problem. Problem drinkers show similar symptoms; however, underlying problems are clearly visible at this stage. Problems should be solved as quickly as possible (e.g., complete divorce of parents). Find out how much impact the peer group has with respect to the patient's drinking. Do the parents serve as drinking role models? Discuss these influences with the adolescent and work with her/him to establish alternatives to drinking.

If alcohol dependence is diagnosed, the adolescent should be admitted to a specialized treatment facility at which the level of treatment intensity (outpatient, day clinic, inpatient) will be agreed upon with the adolescent. For the adolescent, admittance to an inpatient treatment facility brings considerable anxiety and stress; be careful when discussing and planning such an intervention with the adolescent. If, however, suicide threatens, you have to act quickly and have the patient committed — if necessary, against her/his will and, of course, in compliance with the local laws. Special treatment centers for adolescents yield the same treatment results as in treatment centers for adults.[11,12]

4. INDIVIDUALIZE THERAPY

Look for comorbid psychiatric disorders; 89% of alcohol-abusing adolescents present with a second major psychiatric disorder (i.e., axis I diagnosis according to DSM-IV),[13,14] the most frequent being affective disorders and obsessive-compulsive disorders, followed by those listed in this chapter under "Differential Diagnosis" (see above). Comorbid psychiatric disorders should be treated comprehensively (including pharmacotherapy, e.g., selective serotonin reuptake inhibitors (SSRIs) for comorbid major depression). Deficits in social skills should be amended by social skills training and communication training. Dependent alcohol consumption should be pharmacologically treated as well (naltrexone 50 mg once a day).[15,16]

5. INVOLVE THE FAMILY

An important principle during formation of contact is "symmetry": For example, if a concerned mother wants the therapist to talk to her 16-year-old son, the therapist should take care to dedicate the same amount of time to each of them, preferably by talking to each separately. Even in highly charged situations, the therapist should not accept the role of arbitrator.

Instead, strive to obtain and maintain comparable levels of interaction quality and intensity with all family members. This is a goal that is difficult to reach — and more easily attainable if two therapists care for the family. Often, parents approach you because they cannot "handle" their kid anymore. Despite this expectation, take the side of the adolescent, implicitly (i.e., nonverbally), even against her/his parents. Try to take the adolescent seriously, to perceive her/him fully, and to signal her/him support and protection. Try to find out what the adolescent's problems are — and mostly they concern her/his parents. In the second step, approach the parents. This might be difficult because you have already taken the adolescent's side. Regardless, try to maintain empathy. Remind yourself that you can assume that the parents in front of you, like all parents, try to do the best for their kid. You can only help the child if you can help the parents. Armed with these attitudes, you should now translate your impression of the adolescent's behavior in a careful and acceptable form to the parents. Your role is now that of a mediator, perhaps that of a buffer. Your task is to encourage the defusion of the "drama of separation," its transformation into a constructive dialogue and, possibly, a reconciliation between adolescent and parents.

6. INITIATE SOCIAL THERAPY

In extremely high-tension familial situations, it is sometimes wise to take the adolescent out of that situation for a while. It might even be necessary to let the adolescent complete her/his separation at a safe distance from her/his parents. There are therapeutic communities (either fully or partially supervised, e.g., halfway houses) for adolescents of almost all stages of development. When referring the adolescent to such a therapeutic community, do not jeopardize the adolescent's school attendance. Actively seek cooperation with the adolescent's teachers.

Some consider the social therapeutic measures to be the most important effect factor in the treatment of adolescent patients. It is crucial to help the adolescent find fulfilling vocational training or occupation by offering her/him specialized career counseling. If your patient has legal problems, decrease the stress that this might hold for her/him by helping her/him to contact a legal adviser.

To conclude, avoid any fixed treatment scheme when trying to help your adolescent patients, but respond flexibly to their needs, deficits, and difficulties. That way, you will be able to help them effectively.

REFERENCES

1. Beth, A., Alcohol abuse in adolescents, *AFP*, 43, 527, 1991.
2. Grant, B.F. and Dawson, D.A., Age at onset of alcohol use and its association with DSM-IV alcohol abuse and dependence: results from the National Longitudinal Alcohol Epidemiologic Survey, *J. Subst. Abuse*, 9, 103, 1997.
3. Stierlin, H., *Eltern und Kinder. Das Drama von Trennung und Versoehnung im Jugendalter*, Suhrkamp, Frankfurt, 1996.
4. Clark, D.B., Kirisci, L., and Tarter, R.E., Adolescent versus adult onset and the development of substance use disorders in males, *Drug Alcohol Depend.*, 49, 115, 1998.
5. Stewart, D.G. and Brown, S.A., Withdrawal and dependency symptoms among adolescent alcohol and drug abusers, *Addiction*, 90, 627, 1995.
6. Johnston, L., Bachman, J.G., and O'Malley, P.M., *National Trends in Drug Use and Related Factor among American High-School Students and Young Adults 1975–1986*, National Institute on Drug Abuse, Rockville, MD, 1987.
7. American Psychiatric Association, *Diagnostic and Statistical Manual of Mental Disorders,* 4th ed., (DSM-IV), American Psychiatric Association, Washington, D.C., 1994.

8. Brown, S.A., Myers, M.G., Lippke, L., Tapert, S.F., Stewart, D.G., and Vik, P.W., Psychometric evaluation of the Customary Drinking and Drug Use Record (CDDR): a measure of adolescent alcohol and drug involvement, *J. Stud. Alcohol,* 59, 427, 1998.

9. Windle, M., Substance use, risky behaviors, and victimization among a U.S. national adolescent sample, *Addiction,* 89, 175, 1994.

10. Bass, J., Gallagher, S., and Menta, K., Unintentional injuries among adolescents and young adults, *Ped. Clin. N. Am.,* 32, 231, 1985.

11. Marshall, M.J. and Marshall, S., Homogeneous versus heterogeneous age group treatment of adolescent substance abusers, *Am. J. Drug Alcohol Abuse,* 19, 199, 1993.

12. Marshall, M.J. and Marshall, S., Treatment paternalism in chemical dependency counselors, *Int. J. Addict.,* 28, 91, 1993.

13. Keller, M.B. and Baker, L.A., The clinical course of panic disorder and depression, *J. Clin. Psychiatry,* 53 (Suppl.), 5, 1992.

14. Keller, M.B., Lavori, P.W., Beardslee, W.R., Wunder, J., Schwartz, C.E., Roth, J., and Biederman, J., The disruptive behavioral disorder in children and adolescents: comorbidity and clinical course, *J. Am. Acad. Child Adolesc. Psychiatry,* 31, 204, 1992.

15. Wold, M. and Kaminer, Y., Naltrexone for alcohol abuse [letter], *J. Am. Acad. Child Adolesc. Psychiatry,* 36, 6, 1997.

16. Lifrak, P.D., Alterman, A.I., O'Brien, C.P., and Volpicelli, J.R., Naltrexone for alcoholic adolescents [letter], *Am. J. Psychiatry,* 154, 439, 1997.

12 Geriatric Patients

Goetz Mundle

OVERVIEW

Until a few years ago, drinking problems among the elderly were neglected. The accepted view was that the elderly do not drink alcohol. However, alcohol consumption at risk level can be assumed in 10 to 20% of men over the age of 60 years and in 5 to 10% of women. Alcohol abuse and alcohol dependence is known in 2 to 3% of males and 0.5 to 1% of women over the age of 60 years. This chapter focuses on those special diagnostic and therapeutic problems that might occur when treating alcohol abuse and dependence in patients of more advanced age.

INTRODUCTION

For a long time, drinking problems among the elderly were neglected. This can be attributed to Magnus Huss' 1849 hypothesis that "it is the exception to meet an alcoholic over the age of 60." In addition, it was presumed that alcohol dependence is a "self-limiting disease" and alcoholics do not reach old age. This chapter describes how we are now faced with a different situation, due mainly to developments in the population pyramid, and that we are confronted with an increasing number of elderly people with alcohol problems. Also, it will be made clear that alcohol dependence in elderly people is usually easy to diagnose and that adequate treatment has a good prognosis.

EPIDEMIOLOGY

Elderly people regularly consume alcohol.[1,2] The high rate of abstinence in the elderly reported in the past is no longer valid. The over-60s show only irrelevantly lower consumption levels than the younger generation; indeed, a higher consumption of certain types of alcohol can be seen.[3] An alcohol consumption at risk level can be assumed in 10 to 20% of men over the age of 60 years and in 5 to 10% of women.[4] Alcohol abuse and alcohol dependence is known in 2 to 3% of males and 0.5 to 1.0% of women over the age of 60 years.[5-7]

The proportion of older patients with alcohol problems in hospitals and old people's homes can be demonstrated to be up to 50%.[8-10] A German study showed in a general hospital, the prevalence of alcohol abuse and dependence in 65- to 69-year-old patients was over 20%.[11] In an American study, the proportion of residents in a senior citizen home with alcohol problems was around 50%.[12] A questionnaire to 24 geriatric home directors in Germany showed an alcohol abuse rate among residents of 11%.[13] In the Mannheim geriatric care study, 4% of the home residents were diagnosed as alcohol abusive or dependent.[14]

DIAGNOSIS

The guidelines used to diagnose alcohol abuse or dependence in elderly people are the same as those for young patients according to DSM-IV[15] or ICD-10.[16] These operational criteria are also reliable when diagnosing elderly people (Table 12.1).

TABLE 12.1
Diagnostic Criteria of Alcohol Dependence in the Elderly (ICD-10)

Compulsion to drink (craving)
Impaired control
Withdrawal syndrome
Increased tolerance
Progressive neglect of alternative pleasures and interests
Persistent alcohol use despite negative consequenses (social, physical, psychological)

Note: Three of the six criteria must be met at any time during the last year or continually during the last 4 weeks.

It is noticeable that despite these diagnostic guidelines, alcohol abuse or dependence is rarely diagnosed in elderly people. Whereas general practitioners identify most cases in young patients, this only occurs for 40% of elderly patients with alcohol problems. In hospitals, a correct diagnosis is even rarer. Alcohol dependence or abuse is correctly diagnosed in less than 20% of elderly patients.[17,18]

Inadequate diagnostics is only partly the result of the specific problems in differential diagnosis of the elderly. More likely is that the deficiency in diagnostics reflects a serious lack in teaching and training in the sphere of dependence, and that it shows a fatalistic attitude toward the success of therapy, especially for older patients.[19] Most doctors do not realize that even a rudimentary intervention, in the sense of a correct diagnosis, and consultation with the patient can lead to evident modifications in behavior.[20]

An additional background for diagnostic difficulties could be the slightly changed clinical symptoms. Typical negative consequences of younger patients, such as loss of work or driver's license or difficulties with colleagues or the family, are rare in elderly people. Increased tolerance can occur due to physiological developments by relatively low quantities of alcohol and inconspicuous drinking behavior. A progressive neglect of other interests and social isolation are often difficult to differentiate from the inclination of the elderly to retreat. Denial and the tendency to play down problems are not so immediately recognized in a reduced social sphere, and sooner accepted by the family and welfare workers.[21]

COMORBIDITY

An important part of the diagnostic process for elderly patients is an in-depth medical history of psychiatric and physical illness.[22] Depending on the time of examination, up to 50% of all patients show additional psychiatric diagnoses. In addition to the common psychiatric concomitant diagnoses of depression and anxiety[23-25] in old age, cognitive deficits and dementia are frequent.[26,27] The differential diagnosis of these comorbid diseases at the beginning of treatment is difficult. The development of cognitive impairment and dementia can have ethyltoxic reasons or be caused by vascular dementia or Alzheimer's disease.[28] The same applies for the development of depressive or paranoid symptoms, which can be caused by chronic intoxication, protracted detoxification, or develop independent of alcohol dependence. Interaction of alcohol with internal or psychiatric medication can result in serious psychiatric symptoms due to a lowered metabolic rate and a lower detoxification capacity. A conclusive differential diagnostic classification is often only possible after weeks or months of consistent abstinence.

Also, all concomitant physical illness (e.g., liver, pancreas, heart diseases, etc.) should be taken into consideration. A detailed summary of limitations in flexibility and mobility due to physical illness is essential for planning treatment strategies.

TABLE 12.2
Biological Markers for Alcoholism

Marker	Sensitivity (%)	Specificity (%)
GGT		
Alcohol abuse	20–50	55–100
Alcohol dependence	60–90	
MCV		
Alcohol abuse	20-30	65–100
Alcohol dependence	40–50	
CDT		
Alcohol abuse	25–60	>90
Alcohol dependence	65–95	

LABORATORY PARAMETERS AND QUESTIONNAIRES

Biological markers are important supports in the diagnosis of alcoholic patients. Typical changes in biological markers due to increased alcohol consumption also occur in older patients.

The most common biological marker and the easiest to identify, is gamma-glutamyl-transferase (GGT). The sensitivity for alcohol dependence is 60 to 80%, the specificity varies between 50 and 90%, according to population. Carbohydrate-deficient transferrin (CDT) is a new marker for alcoholism.[29] The advantage of CDT is its high specificity of over 90%. Because both markers increase independently, it is useful to combine them. The sensitivity for a diagnosis of alcoholism can be increased to 80 to 90% without a significant loss in specificity. Another marker for alcoholism that has been used for many years is the Mean Corpuscular Volume (MCV). The advantage of MCV is its high specificity of around 90%; the disadvantage of MCV is its low sensitivity, particularly in males, of sometimes less than 50%. For females, initial studies suggest that MCV has good sensitivity rates comparable to those of GGT or CDT.[30,31] An important factor in the analysis of laboratory parameters is the time between the last alcohol consumption and taking of the blood sample. Even short periods of abstinence of a few days can lead to a significant drop in test results and a decrease in sensitivity due to the short half-life of CDT (15 days) and GGT (28 days).[32,33] If a longer period of abstinence is suspected, MCV should also be included in laboratory tests due to its long half-life of 120 days (Table 12.2).

Questionnaires are also an important supplement in the diagnostic process of alcohol-dependent patients. In German-speaking countries, the most commonly used questionnaire is the Munich Alcoholism Test (MALT).[34] Internationally, the questionnaires more often used are the Alcohol Use Disorders Identification Test (AUDIT) and the Michigan Alcohol Screening Test (MAST), of which a special version (MAST G) has been developed for screening geriatric patients.[35] The easiest questionnaire, with only four questions, is the CAGE. With few limitations, all tests can be used for older patients.[36-38]

TYPOLOGY

Contrary to the previous school of thought and in particular contrary to DSM-III, which asserted that onset of alcohol dependence after age 45 is extremely rare, several studies have demonstrated that onset after age 60 occurs often. In around a third of older patients, alcohol dependence began after the 60th year. Accordingly, a distinction is made between "early onset" before age 60 and "late onset" of dependence after age 60.[39-41]

TABLE 12.3
Characteristics of Early and Late Onset

Characteristic	Early Onset	Late Onset
Age	<60 years	≥60 years
Number	2/3	1/3
Personality	Unstable	Stable
Social and family status	Maladjusted	Adjusted
Family history of alcoholism	Positive	Negative
Days of intoxication	Frequent	Less frequent
Treatment outcome	Poor	Favorable

Patients with early onset often have more severe symptoms due to higher drinking amounts and a longer drinking history. The social and family situation is often more unstable, and negative physical consequences are seen more frequently.[42] Also, family history is more often positive. Patients with late onset usually have a more stable social and family status.[43] The personality structure and the physical health are usually due to the short drinking history in a better condition. Changes in drinking habits are usually caused by the changes accompanying becoming elderly, such as loss of workplace, friends, or physical health. Due to the short drinking history and the stable psychosocial status, prognosis for patients with late onset is more favorable, and treatment is agreed to and completed more often[44,45] (Table 12.3).

Apart from the onset of dependence, many other factors are of prognostic relevance. For therapy planning, onset should be only one factor among many others. All clinical criteria should be considered, such as motivation, comorbid disorders, especially cognitive impairment, limited mobility and flexibility and psychosocial support by significant others.

CLINICAL SYMPTOMS

GENERAL FINDINGS

Geriatric alcohol-dependent patients show the same clinical symptoms as younger patients. General findings include reduced physical health with nutritional deficits,[46] inadequate hygiene and vegetative symptoms. Typical abdominal symptoms are dysfunction of the liver, stomach, and intestines.[47,48] Peripheral neuropathia, hypertension, and cardiac arrhythmia are also common. Depression and anxiety are the most frequent psychological symptoms. Compared to younger patients, cognitive impairments and dementia are observed more often in the elderly[49] (Table 12.4).

Due to physiological changes in the elderly, symptoms occur with lower amounts of alcohol consumption.[50] With the same quantity of alcohol, older patients show higher blood alcohol levels. This is most probably due to a reduced activity of alcohol dehydrogenase (ADH) in the stomach and a lower water distribution volume in the body. Because of these physiological processes and an increased ZNS sensitivity for alcohol in older people, severe intoxication symptoms can appear after a low alcohol consumption. Older patients feel drunk more quickly.[51]

Also, the interactions of general medications and alcohol in elderly people are more pronounced. Side effects and toxicity are more common. One reason is a generally lowered enzyme metabolism and especially a lower liver detoxification capacity. A detailed history of medication in elderly alcoholic patients is absolutely necessary.[52,53]

WITHDRAWAL SYMPTOMS

Withdrawal symptoms are more intense and persist longer in the elderly; cognitive deficits are observed more often. An increase in the occurrence of delirium is under discussion. The intensification of

TABLE 12.4
Clinical Symptoms of Alcoholism in the Elderly

General	Vegetativum	Neurological	Psychological
Reduced health status	Sweats, headaches, weakness	Epileptic seizures (grand mal)	Psychomotoric agitation, irritability, nervousness
Malnutrition, inadequate hygiene	Sleep disorder	Peripheral neuropathia	Mood disturbance, depression, anxiety
Abdominal pain, nausea, vomiting, gastritis, ulcera	Sexual dysfunction	Cerebellar dysfunction tremors, dysarthria, ataxia	Cognitive impairment, dementia, blackouts
Liver and pancreas dysfunction			
Hypertension, cardiac arrhythmia			
Red cheeks, spider nevi muscleatrophia (cave muscles)			

withdrawal symptoms has been attributed to life-long alcohol consumption, increased sensitivity of the nervous system in old age, and recurrent episodes of withdrawal treatment in the sense of a kindling mechanism. If medication is necessary, doses should be adapted individually to around half of the usual quantity. The risk of an accumulation or overdose due to lowered enzymatic activities must be taken into consideration.[54,55]

TREATMENT

At first, one must consider whether the usual alcoholism treatment can be used for elderly patients. This greatly depends on cognitive abilities, psychosocial status, and any comorbid diseases that may limit the patient's flexibility and mobility. If there are no major cognitive or physical deficits ("young elderly"), treatment as usual with only few modifications can be carried out without age limits. If a patient is limited in cognitive and physical flexibility, caused by comorbid health problems ("older elderly"), individualized treatment should be planned in cooperation with geriatric and socialpsychiatric services.[56]

With sufficient vitality and mobility ("young elderly"), the usual methods and phases for the treatment of alcohol-dependent patients are valid for all age groups. Depending on motivation, early intervention, detoxification, or long-term in- or outpatient treatment should be carried out. Relapses into previous addictive behaviors are common and a part of the treatment. Even with frequent relapses, therapeutic nihilism should be avoided. The primary goal of treatment is abstinence[57] (Table 12.5).

EARLY INTERVENTION

Important components of early intervention include a discussion with the patient of all symptoms and medical findings related to alcoholism. The basis of the discussion is an emphatic attitude free of prejudice; confrontational and extensively affective interventions are not helpful.[58] Small and reasonable therapeutic steps should be agreed to with patients and their families. Short-term, repeated appointments and laboratory tests or regular home visits are necessary for change. Positive improvements made by the patient should be elaborated and emphasized. If necessary, agreement should be reached with the patient for inpatient detoxification or long-term treatment in an appropriate addiction center.[59]

Age-specific factors, such as changes caused by retirement or loss of a partner, should be part of early intervention or motivational treatment. Integration of family members in the therapeutic process is particularly important in the case of elderly patients because, then, any tendency to

TABLE 12.5
Treatment Modalities for Elderly Patients

Young Patients (<60) (standard treatment)	"Young Elderly" (>60) (standard treatment with age-specific aspects)	"Older Elderly" (>60) (modified treatment)
Detoxification:		
Withdrawal up to 10 days	Withdrawal slightly extended	Protracted withdrawal
Standard medication	Adapted medication doses	Adapted medication doses
Comorbidity without persistent deficits	Comorbidity without persistent deficits	Multimorbidity with limitations of mobility (physical, psychological, cognitive)
Rehabilitation:		
Abstinence	Abstinence	Harm reduction (reduction of drinking amounts, drinking days, alcohol-free environment)
Autonomy	Autonomy	Acknowledgment of existing limitations and deficits (physical, cognitive, affective)
	Discussion of possible future restrictions	
Social and professional reintegration	Social reintegration	Establishing social network
		Cooperation of different professional and non-professional help systems

minimize or ignore the problem become obvious. "Alcohol ought to be allowed in old age after a life of working," and "treatment at this age is not acceptable" are common defensive strategies.[60]

"QUALIFIED" DETOXIFICATION

The goals of "qualified" detoxification are, besides the physical detoxification, the detailed diagnosis of physical or mental comorbidity and the motivation for further abstinence-oriented treatment.[61] At the end of a "qualified" detoxification program, a treatment plan must be completed. The following steps in the treatment process should be discussed with the patient. The patient and his family must be informed about his disease and possible treatments. For elderly patients, it is important to decide if the patient is capable of completing the treatment intended for younger and middle-aged patients ("young elderly") or if, because of cognitive and physical deficits, an individual treatment plan in cooperation with geriatric and socialpsychiatric services is necessary ("older elderly") (Table 5).

Rehabilitation

"Young elderly": Older patients who are capable of attending and completing usual rehabilitation programs ("young elderly") should begin rehabilitation as soon as possible after detoxification. Along with the standard themes, a central part of the treatment should be the recognition of age-specific features and requirements. Anxiety about loss of independence and autonomy, or fears of possible loss of physical and mental performance are common in the elderly. In contrast to middle-aged people, elderly people do not usually aim for renewed autonomy, but wish to preserve existing abilities and resources. The decisive changes in the new period of life caused by retirement, physical changes, or any loss of attachment figures should be made subjects of discussion.[62]

It is still not clear whether rehabilitation of elderly people should be completely separate from that of younger people, or whether integration in standard rehabilitation settings with specific adaptations is beneficial. The real situation now is that elderly people are often treated together with younger patients and usually age-specific modifications in therapy are carried out. The advantage of combined treatment is that younger patients are often motivated and stimulated by the the elderly patients' experiences. Also, in mixed-age groups, typical everyday relationships and inter-relational difficulties between elderly and young occur and can be part of the therapeutic process. However, in special groups for elderly people, specific problems can be dealt with more intensively.[63,64]

Because it is sometimes difficult to motivate elderly people in their last phase of life to leave their familiar environment for treatment, a much more individual form of therapy planning is required. Community-based treatment options would be desirable. Combined inpatient/outpatient or primarily outpatient treatment programs are necessary[65-67] (Table 12.5).

"Older elderly": Individual treatment settings are needed for "older elderly" patients, who due to typical age-specific deficits (multi- and comorbidity) are not able to visit usual rehabilitation centers. According to the possibilities and needs of the patient individualized treatment programs should be compiled in cooperation with home doctors, family members, local welfare services, and specific geriatric therapy centers.[68,69] Long periods of therapy should be expected. It is often necessary to deviate from the standard methods of treatment. Due to physical or mental illness with restrictions in mobility, accompanying social therapy measures are needed for patients who are no longer able to care for themselves and go to an addiction service center. The rule of abstinence can be temporarily adjusted in favor of other therapeutic priorities. A reduction of consumption of substances (alcohol and medicaments), with the corresponding positive effects on general health, can become the primary goal of therapy ("harm reduction"). If, due to impaired cognitive abilities, patients cannot be relied upon to take their medication and keep their appointments with the therapist, an appropriate social welfare service should be arranged, or long-term medical care in an institution such as a home for the elderly.[70]

ANTICRAVING SUBSTANCES

Rehabilitation program studies have been completed in recent years using pharmacological treatment possibilities that included "anticraving" medications.[71,72] As in the treatment of depression or psychosis, psychopharmacological treatment can support — but not replace — classical addiction treatment.[73,74] Double-blind, random, and placebo-controlled studies have demonstrated that a combination of psychotherapeutic and pharmacological treatment is more successful than a single form of treatment alone.[75] The future will reveal the extent to which these results can also be used in the treatment of geriatric patients.

PROGNOSIS

Elderly patients with alcohol problems usually have a good prognosis if their mobility and physical health is retained ("young elderly").[76-78] Elderly patients sometimes show even better success of rehabilitation compared to younger patients. In the MEAT study, older patients, when compared with the very young patients, demonstrated higher rates of abstinence. In males under 24 years of age, the rates of abstinence were 37%; in the over-55 age group, 69%. In females, the rates increased from 23 to 47%.[79]

Therefore, nihilism in the diagnostic and therapeutic process of elderly alcohol-dependent patients does not have any objective basis. Instead, efforts must be made to establish and extend treatment services for older patients. Community-based outpatient, daycare, or combined in-/outpatient facilities should be developed and offered. Also, additional training curricula for personnel working in addiction services should be established to establish unified standards for diagnosis and treatment, particularly for elderly patients.[80,81]

REFERENCES

1. Adams, W.L. and Cox, N.S., Epidemiology of problem drinking among elderly people, *Int. J. Addict.,* 30, 1693, 1995.
2. Beresford, T.P., Alcoholism in the elderly, *Int. Rev. Psychiatry,* 5, 477, 1993.
3. Junge, B. and Stolzenberg, H., Alkoholkonsum, *Die Gesundheit der Deutschen — Ein Ost-West-Vergleich,* Soz.Ep-Hefte 4/1994, Institut fuer Sozialmedizin und Epidemiologie des Bundesgesundheitsamtes, Berlin, 1994.
4. Adams, W.L., Barry, K.L., and Fleming, M.F., Screening for problem drinking in older primary care patients, *JAMA,* 276, 1964, 1996.
5. Holzer, C.E., Robins, L.N., Myers, J.K., Weißmann, M.M., Tischler, G.L., Leaf, P.J., Anthony, J., and Bednarski, P.B., Antecedents and correlates of alcohol abuse and dependence in the elderly, *Nature and Extent of Alcohol Problems among the Elderly,* Eds. Maddox, G., Robins, L.N., Rosenberg, N., Research Monograph 14, National Institute on Drug Abuse, DHHS U.S. Governement Printing Office, Rockville, MD, 1984.
6. Fichter, M.M., *Verlauf psychischer Erkrankungen in der Bevoelkerung,* Springer, Heidelberg, 1990.
7. Atkinson, R.M., Aging and alcohol use disorders: diagnostic issues in the elderly, *Int. Psychoger.,* 2, 55, 1990.
8. Adams, W.L., Yuan, Z., Barboriak, J.J., and Rimm, A.A., Alcohol-related hospitalizations of elderly people. Prevalence and geographic variation in the United States, *JAMA,* 270, 1222, 1993.
9. Bristow, M.F. and Clare, A.W., Prevalence and characteristics of at-risk drinkers among elderly acute medical in-patients, *Br. J. Addict.,* 87, 291, 1992.
10. Schmitz-Moormann, *Alkoholgebrauch und Alkoholismusgefaehrdung bei alten Menschen,* Neuland Geesthacht, 1992.
11. John, U., Hapke, U., Rumpf, H. J., Hill, A., and Dilling, H., *Praevalenz und Sekundaerpraevention von Alkoholmißbrauch und -abhaengigkeit in der medizinischen Versorgung,* Schriftenreihe des Bundesministeriums fuer Gesundheit, Band 71, Nomos, Baden-Baden, 1996.
12. Joseph, C.L., Ganzini, L., and Atkinson, R.M., Screening for alcohol use disorders in the nursing home, *J. Am. Geriatr. Soc.,* 43, 368, 1995.
13. Luderer, H. J. and Rechlin, T., Alkohol- und Medikamentenmißbrauch in Altenheimen, *Psychische Krankheit im Alter,* Eds., Meyer-Lindenberg, J., Moeller, J., Rohde, H., Springer, Berlin, 1993.
14. Weyerer, S. and Zimber, A., Abhaengigkeit und Mißbrauch von Alkohol und Medikamenten in Alten- und Pflegeheimen, *Abhaengigkeit und Mißbrauch von Alkohol und Drogen,* Eds., Watzl, H., Rockstroh, B., Hogrefe, Goettingen, 1997.
15. American Psychiatric Association, *Diagnostic and Statistical Manual of Mental Disorders,* 3rd ed., revised, American Psychiatric Association, Washington, D.C., 1987.
16. Dilling, H., Mombour, W., and Schmidt, M.H., *Internationale Klassifikation psychischer Stoerungen,* Huber, Bern, 1991.
17. Curtis, J.R., Geller, G., Stokes, E.J., Levine D.M.M., and Moore, R.D., Characteristics, diagnosis and treatment of alcoholism in elderly patients, *J. Am. Geriatr. Soc.,* 37, 310, 1989.
18. DeHart, S.S. and Hoffmann, N.G., Screening and diagnosis of "alcohol abuse and dependence" in older adults, *Int. J. Addict.,* 30, 1717, 1995.
19. Mann, K. and Kapp, B., Zur Lehre in Suchtmedizin. Eine Befragung von Studenten und Professoren, *Suchtforschung und Suchttherapie in Deutschland,* Eds., Mann, K., Buchkremer, G., Neuland, Geesthacht S. 38–40, 1995.
20. Wilk, A.I., Jensen, N.M., and Havighurst, T.C., Meta-analysis of randomized control trials addressing brief interventions in heavy alcohol drinkers, *J. Gen. Intern. Med.,* 12, 274, 1997.
21. Miller, N.S., Belkin, B.M., and Gold, M.S., Alcohol and drug dependence among the elderly: epidemiology, diagnosis, and treatment, *Compr. Psychiatry,* 32, 153, 1991.
22. Gurnack, A. M., Ed., *Older Adults Misuse of Alcohol, Medicines, and Other Drugs: Research and Practice Issues,* Springer, New York, 1997.
23. Cook, B.L., Winokur, G., Garvey, M.J., and Beach, V., Depression and previous alcoholism in the elderly, *Br. J. Psychiatry,* 158, 72, 1991.
24. Merikangas, K.R. and Gelertner, C.S., Comorbidity for alcoholism and depression, *Psychiatr. Clin. N. Am.,* 13, 613, 1990.

25. Saunders, P.A., Copeland, J.R., Dewey, M.E., et al., Heavy drinking as a risk factor for depression and dementia in elderly men. Findings from the Liverpool longitudinal community study, *Br. J. Psychiatry,* 159, 213, 1991.

26. Cutting, J.C., Alcohol cognitive impairment and aging: still an uncertain relationship, *Br. J. Addict.,* 83, 995, 1988.

27. Tivis, R., Beatty, W.W., Nixon, S.J., and Parsons, O.A., Patterns of cognitive impairment among alcoholics: are there subtypes? *Alcohol Clin. Exp. Res.,* 19, 496, 1995.

28. Smith, D.M. and Atkinson, R.M., Alcoholism and dementia, *Older Adults' Misuse of Alcohol, Medicines, and Other Drugs: Research and Practice Issues*, Ed., Gurnack, A.M., Springer Publishing, New York, 1997, 132.

29. Stibler, H., Carbohydrate-deficient transferrin in serum: a new marker of potentially harmful alcohol consumption reviewed, *Clin. Chem.,* 37, 2029, 1991.

30. Mundle, G., Ackermann, K., Guenthner, A., and Mann, K., Biological markers in alcoholism treatment: gender differences, *Alcohol Clin. Exp. Res.,* 21, 30A, 1997.

31. Yeastedt, J., LaGrange, L., and Anton, R.F., Female alcoholic outpatients and female college students: a correlation study of self-reported alcohol consumption and carbohydrate-deficient transferrin levels, *J. Stud. Alcohol,* 59, 555, 1998.

32. Agelink, M.W., Kirkes-Kerstin, A., Zeit, T., Bertling, R., Malessa, R., and Klieser, E., Sensitivity of carbohydrate-deficient transferrin (CDT) in relation to age and duration of abstinence, *Alcohol Alcohol.,* 33, 164, 1998.

33. Mundle, G., Ackermann, K., Steinle, D., and Mann, K., Influence of age, alcohol consumption and abstinence on the sensitivity of CDT, GGT and MCV, *Alcohol Alcohol.,* 34, 760, 1999.

34. Speckens, A.E., Heeren, T.J., and Rooijmans, H.G., Alcohol abuse among elderly patients in a general hospital as identified by the Munich Alcoholism Test, *Acta Psychiatr. Scand.,* 83, 460, 1991.

35. Blow, F.C., Brower K.J., Schulenberg, J.E., Demor-Dananberg, L.M., Joung, J.S., and Beresford, T.P., The Michigan Alcoholism Screening Test — Geriatric Version (MAST-G): a new elderly specific screening instrument, *Alcohol Clin. Exp. Res.,* 16, 372, 1992.

36. Jones, T.V., Lindsey, B.A., Yount, P., Soltys, R., and Farani Enayat, B., Alcoholism screening questionnaires: are they valid in elderly medical outpatients?, *J. Gen. Intern. Med.,* 8, 674, 1993.

37. Morton, J.L., Jones, T.V., and Manganaro, M.A., Performance of alcoholism screening questionnaires in elderly veterans, *Am. J. Med.,* 101, 153, 1996.

38. Clay, S.W., Comparison of AUDIT and CAGE questionnaires in screening for alcohol use disorders in elderly primary care outpatients, *J. Am. Osteopath. Assoc.,* 97, 588, 1997.

39. Zimberg S., Two types of problem drinkers: both can be managed, *Geriatrics,* 14, 221, 1974.

40. Liberto, J.G. and Oslin, D.W., Early versus late onset of alcoholism in the elderly, *Int. J. Addict.,* 30, 1799, 1995.

41. Beechem, M., Beechem Risk Inventory for late-onset alcoholism, *J. Drug Educ.,* 27, 397, 1997.

42. Welte, J.W. and Mirand, A.L., Drinking, problem drinking and life stressors in the elderly general population, *J. Stud. Alcohol,* 56, 67, 1995.

43. Epstein, E.E., McCrady, B.S., and Hirsch, L.S., Marital functioning in early versus late-onset alcoholic couples, *Alcohol Clin. Exp. Res.,* 21, 547, 1997.

44. Fitzgerald, J.L. and Mulford, H.A., Elderly vs. younger problem drinker 'treatment' and recovery experiences, *Br. J. Addict.,* 87, 1281, 1992.

45. Schonfeld, L. and Dupree, L.W., Antecedents of drinking for early- and late-onset elderly alcohol abusers, *J. Stud. Alcohol,* 52, 587, 1991.

46. Klein, S. and Iber, F.L., Alcoholism and associated malnutrition in the elderly, *Nutrition,* 7, 75, 1991.

47. Fink, A., Hays, R.D., Moore, A.A., and Beck, J.C., Alcohol-related problems in older persons. Determinants, consequences, and screening, *Arch. Intern. Med.,* 156, 1150, 1996.

48. Smith, J.W., Medical manifestations of alcoholism in the elderly, *Int. J. Addict.,* 30, 1749, 1995.

49. Carlen, P.L., McAndrews, M.P., Weiss, R.T., et al., Alcohol-related dementia in the institutionalized elderly, *Alcohol Clin. Exp. Res.,* 18, 1330, 1994.

50. Ozdemir, V., Fourie, J., Busto, U., and Naranjo, C.A., Pharmacokinetic changes in the elderly. Do they contribute to drug abuse and dependence? *Clin. Pharmacokinet.,* 31, 372, 1996.

51. Dufour, M. and Fuller, R.K., Alcohol in the elderly, *Annu. Rev. Med.,* 46, 123, 1995.

52. Solomon, K., Manepalli, J., Ireland, G.A., and Mahon, G.M., Alcoholism and prescription drug abuse in the elderly: St. Louis University grand rounds [clinical conference], *J. Am. Geriatr. Soc.,* 41, 57, 1993.

53. Seitz, H., Lieber, S., and Simanowski, U., *Handbuch Alkohol-Alkoholismus-alkoholbedingte Organschaeden,* Bart. Leipzig-Heidelberg, 1995.

54. Brower, K.J., Mudd, S., Blow, F.C., Young, J.P., and Hill, E.M., Severity and treatment of alcohol withdrawal in elderly versus younger patients, *Alcohol Clin. Exp. Res.,* 18, 196, 1994.

55. Mundle, G., Die Alkoholabhaengigkeit im Alter, *Sucht. Grundlagen, Diagnostik, Therapie,* Mann, K., Buchkremer, G., Eds., Gustav Fischer, Stuttgart, 1996.

56. Oslin, D.W., Streim, J.E., Parmelee, P., Boyce, A.A., and Katz, I.R., Alcohol abuse: a source of reversible functional disability among residents of a VA nursing home, *Int. J. Geriatr. Psychiatry,* 12, 825, 1997.

57. Mundle, G., Wormstall, H., and Mann, K., [Die Alkoholabhaengigkeit im Alter] Alcoholism in the elderly, *Sucht,* 43, 201, 1997.

58. Miller, W.R. and Rollnick, S., *Motivational Interviewing. Preparing People to Change Addictive Behavior,* Guilford Press, New York, 1991.

59. Mann, K. and Mundle, G., Alkoholismus und Alkoholfolgekrankheiten in der Gerontopsychiatrie, *Lehrbuch der Gerontopsychiatrie,* Ed. Foerstl, H., Enke Verlag Stuttgart, 1996.

60. Feuerlein, W., Abhaengigkeit im Alter, *Zeitschrift fuer Gerontopsychologie und -psychiatrie,* 8, 153, 1995.

61. Mundle, G. and Mann, K., Stationaerer Entzug, *Der Abhaengige Patient.* Ed. Goelz J., Georg Thieme, Stuttgart, 1998.

62. Scholz, H., *Syndrombezogene Alkoholismustherapie,* Hogrefe, Goettingen, 1996.

63. Mulford, H.A. and Fitzgerald, J.L., Elderly versus younger problem drinker profiles: do they indicate a need for special programs for the elderly? *J. Stud. Alcohol,* 53, 601, 1992.

64. Stoddard, C.E. and Thompson, D.L., Alcohol and the elderly: Special concerns for counseling professionals, *Alcohol. Treatm. Q.,* 14, 59, 1996.

65. Fortney, J.C., Booth, B.M., Blow, F.C., and Bunn, J.Y., The effects of travel barriers and age on the utilization of alcoholism treatment aftercare, *Am. J. Drug Alcohol Abuse,* 21, 391, 1995.

66. Mundle, G. and Mann, K., Ein Modell zur Integration stationaerer und ambulanter Therapie von Alkoholabhaengigen, *Psycho,* 22, 444, 1996.

67. Pratt, C.C., Schmall, V.L., Wilson, W., and Benthin, A., Alcohol problems in later life: evaluation of a model community education program, *Community Ment. Health J.,* 28, 327, 1992.

68. Evans, D.J., Street, S.D., and Lynch, D.J., Alcohol withdrawal at home. Pilot project for frail elderly people, *Can. Fam. Physician,* 42, 937, 1996.

69. Hanson, B.S., Social network, social support and heavy drinking in elderly men — a population study of men born in 1914, Malmo, Sweden, *Addiction,* 89, 725, 1994.

70. Fleischmann, H., Suchtprobleme im Alter, *Lehrbuch der Suchterkrankungen,* Eds., Gastpar, Mann, Rommelspacher, Georg Thieme, Stuttgart, 170–178, 1999.

71. Mann, K. and Mundle, G., Die pharmakologische Rueckfallprophylaxe bei Alkoholabhaengigen — Bedarf und Moeglichkeiten, *Sucht. Grundlagen, Diagnostik, Therapie,* Eds., Mann, K., Buchkremer, G., Gustav Fischer, Stuttgart, 1996.

72. Volpicelli, J.R., Altermann, A.I., Hayashida, M., and O'Bien, C.P., Naltrexone in the treatement of alcohol dependence, *Arch. Gen. Psychiatry,* 49, 876, 1992.

73. Sass, H., Soyka, M., Mann, K., and Zieglgaensberger, W., Relapse prevention by acamprosate: results from a placebo controlled study in alcohol dependence, *Arch. Gen. Psychiatry,* 53, 673, 1996.

74. Mundle, G., Acamprosat — Paradigmenwechsel in der Alkoholismustherapie, *Arzneimitteltherapie,* 9, 273, 1999.

75. O'Malley, S.S., Jaffe, A.J., Chang, G., Schottenfeld, R.S., Meyer, R.E., and Rounsaville, B., Naltrexone and coping skills therapy for alcohol dependence. A controlled study, *Arch. Gen. Psychiatry,* 49, 881, 1992.

76. Schuckit, M.A., Assessment and treatment strategies with the late life alcoholic, Introduction, *J. Geriatr. Psychiatry,* 23, 83, 1990.

77. Bercsi, S.J., Brickner, P.W., and Saha, D.C., Alcohol use and abuse in the frail, homebound elderly: a clinical analysis of 103 persons, *Drug Alcohol Depend.,* 33, 139, 1993.

78. Schutte, K.K., Brennan, P.L., and Moos, R.H., Remission of late-life drinking problems: A 4-year follow-up, *Alcohol Clin. Exp. Res.,* 18, 835, 1994.

79. Kuefner, H., and Feuerlein, W., *In-patient-Treatment for Alcoholism. A Multi-centre Evaluation Study,* Springer, Berlin, 1989.

80. Lakhani, N., Alcohol use amongst community-dwelling elderly people: a review of the literature, *J. Adv. Nurs.,* 25, 1227, 1997.

81. Mundle, G., Aktuelle Entwicklungen in der Suchttherapie, *Sucht,* 43, 283, 1997.

Part 4

Treatment of Non-Psychiatric Alcohol-Related Disorders

13 Women

Rajita Sinha

OVERVIEW

Alcohol affects men and women's bodies differently, leading to differing patterns of drinking, amount, frequency, and years of alcohol consumption and differences in rates of alcoholism. These differences have been linked to biological, psychological, and social factors that contribute to the causes and consequences of problem drinking. This chapter first reviews the biological, psychological, and social factors that contribute to the gender differences in alcohol consumption, rates of alcoholism, treatment seeking, and recovery from alcoholism. As a result of these differences, there is growing consensus that alcoholism treatment for women may differ from the treatment offered to men. The special therapeutic needs of alcoholic women are identified, and a clinical model of treatment to address these needs is presented.

INTRODUCTION

There is increasing awareness that women may require alcoholism treatment that differs from the treatment offered to men. This idea is based on the evidence that some of the causes and consequences of alcohol dependence differ between men and women, thus necessitating gender-specific treatment approaches. This chapter will first summarize the major gender differences in the causes and consequences of alcohol dependence, as well as the differences among men and women in treatment response and recovery from alcoholism. This will be followed by an outline of the specific therapeutic needs of women and how best to address these needs in designing women-oriented treatment programs.

Studies in the general population indicate that fewer women than men drink. Epidemiological studies have found about 14 million U.S. adults (i.e., 7.5% of the adult population) meet criteria for alcohol abuse or dependence at any given time, and approximately one-third are women.[1,2] This gender gap in problem drinking is getting smaller, especially for the younger age group, with recent surveys indicating that the ratio of problem drinking women as compared to men for the 18 to 29 age group is 2:1.[3] An examination of drinking patterns indicates that women tend to begin drinking heavily later in life than men, consume smaller quantities of alcohol, and abuse alcohol for fewer years before seeking treatment.[4] Although they tend to report fewer alcohol-related problems and dependence symptoms than men, among the heaviest drinkers, women equal or surpass men in the number of problems resulting from their drinking.[1] These gender differences in rates of alcoholism, age of onset, drinking patterns, amounts of alcohol consumption, and years of drinking before treatment may be linked to the biological, psychological, and social differences between the sexes in the causes and consequences of problem drinking.

GENDER DIFFERENCES IN THE BIOLOGY OF ALCOHOL CONSUMPTION

Alcohol affects women's bodies differently than men. Women become intoxicated after drinking smaller quantities of alcohol as compared to men. After consuming the same amount of alcohol, women achieve higher blood alcohol levels than men (see Chapter 39 on the basic pharmacokinetics of ethanol). These physiological differences are related to several factors. First, women have lower total body water than men of comparable size. As alcohol diffuses uniformly in all body water after consumption, and women have less body water than men, they achieve higher concentrations of alcohol in their blood than men after drinking equivalent amounts of alcohol.[1] Second, there is evidence to suggest that women have reduced activity of alcohol dehydrogenase, the primary enzyme involved in alcohol metabolism in the stomach where a substantial amount of alcohol is metabolized before it enters systemic circulation.[5] This diminished activity leads to less metabolism of alcohol in the stomach for women and higher amounts entering the bloodstream and available for its effects on various organ systems. In fact, alcoholic women have virtually non-existent amounts of gastric alcohol dehydrogenase, making them more vulnerable to alcohol's negative effects.[6] Finally, there is some evidence that fluctuation in gonadal hormonal levels during the menstrual cycle may affect the rate of alcohol metabolism and contribute to the increased blood alcohol concentrations among women.[7,8] These physiological differences in response to alcohol may be partially responsible for the increased vulnerability to alcohol-related consequences among alcoholic women.

HEALTH CONSEQUENCES OF HEAVY DRINKING IN WOMEN

Studies of women alcoholics in treatment suggest that they often experience greater physiological impairment earlier in their drinking careers, despite having consumed less alcohol than men.[9] Due to the biological differences among men and women, the negative consequences of heavy drinking appear accelerated or "telescoped" in women. Table 13.1 lists the alcohol-related health consequences

---

TABLE 13.1
Health Consequences of Alcoholism in Women

Physiologic effects of alcohol consumption
    Intoxication at lower doses
    Toxic effects of alcohol occur at lower doses
Death rates are 50 to 100% higher in women than men
Deaths are related to suicides, alcohol-related accidents,
    circulatory disorders, and liver cirrhosis
Alcohol-induced liver disease
    Greater incidence in women
    More rapid progression of disease in women
Neurological and cognitive impairment
    Greater cerebral atrophy in women
    Greater susceptibility to alcohol-related cognitive impairment has been implicated
Breast cancer
    Increased risk for breast cancer has been suggested
Menstrual cycle disorders and gynecologic problems
    Painful menstruation, heavy flow, and greater premenstrual discomfort
    Irregular and absent cycles
    Early menopause
    Infertility
    Ovarian dysfunction
Pregnancy-related problems
    Fetal alcohol syndrome
    Miscarriage
    Stillbirth
    Preterm birth

---

that occur at a greater frequency among women alcoholics and the health consequences unique to women alcoholics. Female alcoholics have death rates 50 to 100% higher than those of male alcoholics. A greater percentage of alcoholic women die from suicides, alcohol-related accidents, circulatory disorders, and cirrhosis of the liver.[1] Alcohol-induced liver damage is a well-known consequence of heavy drinking; however, it is less well known that women have a heightened vulnerability to alcohol-induced liver damage, possibly due to the above-mentioned physiological differences and the differences in body weight and fluid content in women as compared to men. Heavy drinking has also been linked to an increased risk for breast cancer (see also Chapter 20 on immunological disorders).[10,11] Menstrual disorders such as painful menstruation, heavy flow, pre-menstrual discomfort and irregular and absent cycles, and early menopause are common consequences of heavy drinking. Fertility can be adversely affected by the above-mentioned problems.[1] There is also some evidence that women may be more susceptible to the neuropsychological consequences of heavy drinking.[12] Finally, heavy drinking among pregnant women can result in fetal alcohol effects or fetal alcohol syndrome in their offspring — the leading preventable cause of mental retardation.[1] Thus, the increased vulnerability to health-related consequences of alcohol consumption among women identifies them as a group that could benefit from early and special interventions.

PSYCHOLOGICAL AND SOCIAL INFLUENCES ON HEAVY DRINKING IN WOMEN

VIOLENT VICTIMIZATION

Several studies have found a significant association between childhood sexual abuse and heavy drinking in women. The prevalence of incest and childhood sexual abuse is significantly elevated among alcoholic women in treatment.[13,14] In a general population survey, twice as many women with a history of problem drinking reported childhood sexual abuse as compared to those without the history of problem drinking.[14] In an extensive study, Miller and Downs[13] examined a broad range of childhood victimization of women, ranging from sexual abuse, moderate to severe verbal aggression by father and mother, and moderate to severe physical violence. Their findings indicated the alcoholic women in treatment were significantly more likely to report histories of violent victimization, including childhood sexual abuse histories and father-to-daughter verbal aggression (67 to 70%) as compared to women in treatment without alcohol problems (49 to 52%) and a community-matched sample of women with no alcohol problems (31 to 35%).

Several studies have also found an association between partner violence toward adult women and their drinking behavior.[13,15] In a 1992 U.S. survey of alcohol and family violence, a wife's drinking, whether alone or with her husband, led to more severe violence both by and toward the wife.[16] The above-mentioned studies underscore the need to pay close attention to childhood and adult victimization issues among alcoholic women seeking treatment.

CO-OCCURRING PSYCHOPATHOLOGY

A link between depression and problem drinking among women has been consistently reported in the literature.[16-19] Women report more psychiatric problems and are more likely to drink to relieve negative affect as compared to men.[20-22] Women with alcohol problems are often reported to have higher overall comorbid psychiatric disorders, especially affective disorders, borderline personality disorder, and post-traumatic stress disorder. On the other hand, men are more likely to be diagnosed with antisocial personality disorder.[23-26] There is also recent evidence that alcoholics with major depression at the time of detoxification relapse significantly more quickly than those without depression.[27]

Alcoholic women entering treatment also have lower self-esteem as compared to alcoholic men, which may be related to high rates of physical and sexual abuse among alcoholic women.[16] These

---

TABLE 13.2
Psychological and Social Influences on Problem Drinking in Women

Psychological Factors
　　High rates of childhood sexual abuse, verbal aggression, and partner violence
　　Significantly greater prevalence of anxiety and depressive disorders, eating disorders,
　　　borderline personality disorder and posttraumatic stress disorder in alcoholic women
　　Low self-esteem
Social factors
　　Peer and spouse pressure
　　　Adolescent girls are more susceptible to peer pressure
　　　Alcoholic women are more likely to have alcoholic men as spouses
　　Role-related issues
Lack of social role or loss of social roles
　　Involuntary social roles relating to work/career, marriage, childcare, and education
　　　Marital and employment status predicts heavy drinking in women
　　　Unemployment and financial problems are associated with heavy drinking
　　Societal stigma and negative stereotyping of alcohol use in women
　　Social isolation and poor support network predicts heavy alcohol consumption

---

higher rates of comorbid psychopathology are the reason why women are more likely to seek treatment due to psychological problems, while men seek treatment for social–environmental reasons.[28] Clearly, co-occurring psychological problems are significant for women and warrant special attention in women-oriented treatment programs (Table 13.2).

Peer/Spouse Pressure

The social context appears to affect women's drinking more significantly than men. Adolescent girls are more strongly influenced by peer drinking than boys,[29] and group pressure contributes significantly to alcohol misuse among female adolescents.[30] Both clinical and epidemiological data have consistently revealed strong relationships between women's drinking and their partners' drinking across the world.[14,31] Essentially, the data indicate that women with problem drinking are more likely than their male counterparts to have spouses or significant others who are problem drinkers.[16,25,32] Such relationships may contribute to the evidence of greater marital disruption and relationship difficulties among problem drinking women.[33] Thus, the social context factors are more salient for women and need to be taken into account in treating and managing an alcoholic woman in recovery.

Social Role-related Issues

Women in their 20s and 30s often take on multiple social roles, involving education, work/career, marriage, and childbearing. Women are more likely to become caretakers for family members with chronic illnesses, in addition to being responsible for children as single parents.[28] Fulfilling these roles in socially acceptable ways places multiple demands on women, and women with less internal coping resources and fewer social supports may become more vulnerable to using alcohol as a way of coping with the multiple obligations in their lives.[16] There is also a significant amount of social stigma and stereotyping in society regarding alcohol use among women. The stigma serves to victimize and place pejorative labels on substance-abusing women, which in turn contributes to denial of heavy drinking among women and serves as a barrier to seeking treatment for alcohol problems.[16,28]

　　Upon examination of the data on how women's roles impact their alcohol consumption, several interesting patterns emerge. Marital status plays a significant role in drinking patterns among women. Young women who are single, divorced, or separated are more likely to drink frequently and in larger quantities than married women. This finding may be related to the fact that women with drinking problems seem to have less social support available to them.[34,35] Findings on the association between career, employment, and drinking appear more complex. In general, risk for problem drinking among women in the workplace is associated with nontraditional occupations, low-status jobs, part-time employment, and recent lay-off or unemployment.[14] Among women in their 40s, one study found that 70% of nonalcoholic control women were employed, compared with 40% of problem drinking women. The authors suggest that this demographic difference may be because homemakers not working outside the home are more likely to drink because of boredom or because they are less likely to seek employment.[16] Coping with the demands of raising children adds to the stresses in the lives of women, and yet concern about their children often brings women to treatment.[2] Data suggest that when treatment focuses on relationship and family issues, outcomes for families and the women themselves are enhanced.[36,37] These findings indicate that the social role-related issues play an important part in the development and maintenance of their problem drinking.

GENDER DIFFERENCES IN TREATMENT SEEKING, OUTCOME, AND RECOVERY PATTERNS

Alcoholic men are more likely to receive treatment than women.[38] Although one in three alcoholics is a woman, the sex ratio of those treated is 4 or 5 men to 1 woman. This discrepancy in treatment seeking has been explained by the multiple barriers that women face in accessing treatment.[2] External social factors such as stigmatization of women with alcohol problems, childcare responsibilities, or financial problems have been noted as significant, and internal barriers such as fear of losing their children, multiple roles and demands that interfere with women making treatment a priority, and denial of a drinking problem are also common. Grant[39] recently identified that individual predisposing factors such as lack of confidence in alcohol treatment effectiveness, stigmatization, and denial were more significant barriers to treatment than lack of financial resources or facilities for childcare. Based on the above findings, it is no surprise that women tend to enter treatment with more severe alcohol and psychiatric problems than men.[2,40]

As women experience greater physical problems and psychological difficulties associated with their drinking, they are more likely to seek help from a personal physician, primary care settings, or psychiatric facilities rather than substance abuse agencies.[2] It is essential that primary care settings and psychiatric facilities evaluate alcohol consumption among women seeking their services, and provide a continuum of services or adequate linkages to substance abuse services to address the alcohol problems among women. A greater discussion of such services follows in the "Treatment Components" section below.

Although gender differences in treatment outcomes have not been well studied, some evidence showing differences in treatment variables does exist. For example, group therapy appears to work better for men, while individual therapy and education programs are more helpful to women.[32] Matching the gender of the client and the therapist has also shown positive effects.[41] Sanchez-Craig and colleagues found that when the treatment goal was moderation of drinking, women who were not severely dependent on alcohol were more successful than men.[41] Women achieved better results than men through a self-monitoring program that emphasizes behavioral self-control. Jarvis[42] reported that women had slightly improved treatment outcomes compared with men in the first 12 months after treatment, whereas men showed greater improvement than women in long-term follow-up. While some evidence with regard to AA and self-help groups indicates that women may have better outcomes with participation in self-help groups,[28,41] others have reported that AA involvement was less beneficial to women as compared to men.[43] There are mixed findings with regard to aftercare as well, with some evidence that women are more likely to benefit from aftercare than men,[44] and another study showing that men had a better success rate in aftercare than women.[32]

Several alcohol treatment outcome studies have been conducted to examine the efficacy of various treatment approaches on drinking outcomes, and the general consensus is that there are few differences in effectiveness of current treatments for alcoholism among men and women.[45,46] However, women have been underrepresented in most treatment studies. Studies examining the efficacy of new medications such as naltrexone for alcohol dependence reported that women comprised only 20% of the sample.[47,48] Given that women represent 20% of the treatment population in substance abuse treatment facilities, the lower representation of women in treatment studies is understandable. On the other hand, gender differences will be difficult to identify without adequate sample sizes. This argues for either oversampling of women in treatment studies or conducting studies on alcoholic women alone, to examine whether specific treatment approaches are efficacious.

RECOVERY PATTERNS

There is some evidence that men and women differ in their post-treatment experiences and their efforts toward recovery. Relationship with family, role performance, psychological impairment, effort toward recovery, and drinking patterns were assessed in male and female alcoholics 3 and 15 months after discharge from inpatient treatment.[49] Findings indicated that at 3 months after discharge, being married for men is protective for relapse, while for women, being married is a risk factor for relapse. This suggests that as spouses, women are perhaps more supportive than men, and with evidence indicating that alcoholic women are often married to alcoholic men,[32] obtaining spouse support may be more of a challenge for women. The study also found that for women, fewer years of problem drinking was protective of relapse and that the earlier the women entered treatment, the better the outcomes. Finally, consistent with other findings in the literature,[50-52] psychological problems were associated with heavier drinking among women and were predictive of relapse over the course of 15 months after discharge. These findings suggest that women appear to have a different course of recovery from men, and the physiological, psychological, and social factors that impact heavy drinking among women continue to affect women's lives during recovery.

WOMEN-SPECIFIC TREATMENT NEEDS

The above sections highlight the key differences among men and women in the development and maintenance of alcoholism, and emphasize the need to specifically address the unique needs of alcoholic women in treatment. To summarize, the findings outline that women metabolize alcohol differently, such that the impact of drinking less amounts for fewer years as compared to men can often have worsened health consequences for women. Data also suggest that women do not come to treatment unless their alcohol and psychiatric problems are more severe as compared to men. When they do come to treatment, they are more likely to have verbal, physical, and sexual abuse histories, and concurrent psychopathology that would need specific attention. Further, they often have social problems such as unemployment, financial difficulties, problems with childcare, denial, stigmatization, social isolation, and other factors that contribute to their participation in treatment and would need to be targeted to enhance success in treatment. Finally, social isolation — along with the continued dependence on old problem relationships — are difficult to overcome for women, and interfere significantly with the recovery process.

To address the above key gender differences, there is growing consensus that women-specific programs better serve women's needs.[53] The development of such programs and the research in the area is still in its infancy and yet significant strides have been made. The next section outlines the key developments in addressing women's treatment needs and the research that supports it.

IDENTIFICATION, SCREENING, AND TREATMENT ACCESS

As described earlier, women are more likely to seek treatment initially from their medical doctors or from psychiatric facilities for alcohol-related physical problems or psychological difficulties associated with heavy drinking. These health care facilities can be seen as excellent entry points to engage women in treatment. However, there is evidence that physicians are less effective in identifying alcohol abuse in women than in men.[54] Thus, there is a need to train health care providers to competently diagnose, refer, and treat women with alcohol problems. Brief, easy-to-read, and specific information about heavy drinking and its consequences can be routinely distributed to women accessing primary care and psychiatric services. Social workers or health professionals at these facilities should be trained to further discuss the relevance of the information with women individually. Patient-oriented handouts such as *Alcohol and You*, developed by Miller et al.,[55] can be useful in providing information in a non-judgmental manner. An adaptation of such handouts to address women-specific issues such as stigma, social support, health consequences, and alcohol treatment effectiveness can be designed to address some of the barriers to treatment.

Identification and screening of alcohol problems are becoming part of the standard assessment in primary care and psychiatric facilities. Excellent tools such as the CAGE[56] (see the alphabetical list of psychometric instruments in Chapter 42) have been developed for screening of alcohol problems. Identification of risk drinking among non-abstaining pregnant women has been shown to be further enhanced when the CAGE questionnaire was modified to include a tolerance question on how many drinks it takes to make the person feel high. This modified questionnaire called the T-ACE[57] (see the alphabetical list of psychometric instruments in Chapter 42) takes 1 minute to administer and represents a valid and sensitive screen for identifying risk-drinking among women. The TWEAK[58] (see the alphabetical list of psychometric instruments in Chapter 42) is a similar modification that includes a question on relatives and friends being worried or complaining about the individual's drinking. In a recent assessment of the leading alcohol screening questionnaires, the TWEAK was found to perform the best in detecting heavy drinking among both Caucasian and African-American women.[59] These self-reported assessment tools are quick and superior to laboratory tests for detecting heavy and problem drinking in unselected populations.[59]

Screening is only the first step in the identification of problem drinking among women. A positive result on the screening questionnaires should lead to an assessment of current drinking patterns, adverse consequences of drinking, dependence symptoms, and motivation to change drinking behavior. Time and staffing constraints at primary care facilities may prevent more thorough assessment from occurring. However, it is important that a thorough assessment take place, and linkages with local substance abuse evaluation units or even an ambulatory evaluation unit that provides liaison and case management services could help in conducting the evaluation and making the appropriate referrals. Depending on the severity of problem drinking, a level of care must be determined. A step-down model of care that assesses the need for detoxification (whether it is inpatient or ambulatory), intensive/day program, or outpatient services should be followed.[60] Women may often be reluctant to accept the recommendation to more intensive modalities such as inpatient, residential, or detoxification services because of their multiple demands. Again, case managers can be effective in problem-solving with the patient on management of her social responsibilities such as childcare, etc., so that she is served at the appropriate level of care. Failure to address detoxification or the need for structured treatment programming can seriously impact outcomes.

It is critical that the clinical approach in this initial process of assessment and engagement be empathic, non-judgmental, and nonconfrontational. Brief motivational approaches that provide information, feedback, advice, and support are known to be effective in addressing alcohol problems,[46,55,61] and should be used at entry point to engage women in the treatment system. Case managers can be involved in bridging the link between the entry point and the specific treatment provider and in addressing specific external barriers to accessing care. Finally, there is a need to

TABLE 13.3
Strategies to Improve Treatment Access For Women

Providing information and education in a non-pejorative manner
   Inform women about alcohol-related consequences and risk factors for heavy drinking
   Provide information on types of treatments available and their effectiveness
   Educate public, and increase awareness on societal stigmatization of alcohol use in women
   Educate social service agencies regarding drinking in women
Educating health professionals and case managers at social service agencies on screening and detection of alcohol problems
  in women and referral options
Increase routine screening for alcohol problems in clinics/social agencies addressing women's needs
Screening and referral information should be provided in women's health clinics, pregnancy and family planning clinics,
  and obstetrics and gynecology doctors' offices
Screening and referral information should be provided in psychiatric facilities and social services agencies such as legal
  assistance programs, rape, trauma and domestic violence support services, and state general assistance programs
Improve the availability of services for children
   Availability of childcare services while women participate in treatment
   Provide assessment, referral, and treatment of behavioral problems in children
   Educate children about mother's alcoholism
Improve case management services for alcoholic women
Linkages through case management services between social service agencies, primary care and psychiatric facilities, and
  alcohol treatment agencies
Expand the role of case management to link alcoholic women to treatment and help in removing barriers to treatment
Outreach services to women at-risk for drinking should be improved, with outreach workers educated on screening and
  treatment referrals for alcohol problems

provide better access to treatment for women. Table 13.3 lists some of the measures that can be taken to improve access for alcoholic women.

COMPONENTS OF WOMEN-SPECIFIC TREATMENTS

It has been suggested that because a large proportion of alcoholic women face multiple problems, there is a need to provide broad and comprehensive services for women.[28,53] The services identified range from health services, treatment of other problems such as incest, sexual assault, and violence, multiple substance abuse, co-occurring mental health problems, family services, services for children, parenting skills, development of positive relationships and social support, development of adaptive coping and building self-esteem, along with employment/vocational counseling, legal assistance, and women's support groups. While this is a comprehensive list targeting the range of needs that women seeking alcohol treatment may have, it may be useful to also provide a treatment model that helps organize these services in a clinical framework (Table 13.4). The model presented emphasizes building treatment to match the service needs of the patient. There is some evidence that when patients are matched to services that address their specific needs, they have better outcomes relating to treatment completion and substance use.[62] The treatment framework focuses on a team approach where a primary therapist coordinates the care of the patient by including the necessary components required to address the multiple needs of the patient, and the team provides support and consultation to the primary therapist. The various components of this treatment model are described below.

ENVIRONMENT OF CARE

Several setting characteristics have been identified as necessary for a women-oriented alcoholism treatment program.[53,63] These are (1) a physical and social setting that is compatible with women's

TABLE 13.4
Components of Women-Specific Alcohol Treatment

Environment of care:
    Setting should be compatible with women's interpersonal styles and their various social roles
    Setting that does not allow exploitation or sexual harassment and does not support passive, dependent roles
    Clinical and administrative capability to provide the various components of services needed for women
Primary therapist model:
    Establish a collaborative treatment alliance targeting specific problem areas identified by a primary therapist and the patient and develop a comprehensive treatment plan
    Therapist is responsible for coordinating the range of services needs in collaboration with the team of professionals such as the psychiatrist, case manager, skills trainer, and other team therapists/supervisors available
    Therapist targets alcohol use, treatment engagement and commitment, and treatment for other problems such as multiple substance abuse and psychiatric issues (other treatment resources are activated when necessary)
Case management component:
    Case managers or primary therapists coordinate and provide the following:
        Links to specialized alcohol treatment centers
        Remove barriers to accessing treatment
        Health services
        Family services
        Services for children
        Coordinate employment and vocational counseling
        Coordination of financial and legal assistance
        Accessing crisis services in collaboration with the primary therapist
Pharmacotherapy component:
    For problem drinking
    For psychiatric symptoms
Skill building component:
    To develop adaptive coping strategies which cover the following when and as needed by the patient:
        Coping with drinking triggers and high-risk situations
        Assertiveness and interpersonal effectiveness training
        Stress management skills
        Regulating emotions
        Parenting skills
        Development of self-mastery and self-esteem building
Social support component:
    Building positive relationships and support networks in the community
    Accessing women's support groups and self-help groups

interactional styles and personal orientations; (2) an environment that is considerate of and accounts for gender roles, female socialization, and women's status in society; (3) an environment that is not exploitative of women and does not allow sexual harassment of female patients or support passive, dependent roles for women; and (4) an environment that addresses women-specific treatment issues. Such an environment can be incorporated in a mixed-gender program that still provides women-only groups and female therapists to match with women patients, or in women-only programs.

In recognizing the different patterns of alcohol-related problems and the different treatment needs of women, women-only treatment programs are being implemented with increasing frequency.[53] Women-only treatment programs are thought to be more advantageous as they may attract women to treatment earlier, and may attract women who are otherwise more hesitant to seek treatment at mixed-gender programs.[53] While more research on the effectiveness of women-only programs is needed, there is some evidence indicating that patients who received treatment in a women-only program did better with alcohol consumption and social adjustment over a 2-year follow-up period as compared to a traditional mixed-gender program.[64] There is also some support that women-only programs attracted more women with dependent children, lesbian women, and women with histories of childhood sexual abuse.[65] While this evidence supports developing women-only programs, if women-only programs are not an option, it is still important to address the setting issues listed earlier within a mixed-gender program, or else such programs may risk being less attractive to women.[63]

PRIMARY THERAPIST MODEL

A good therapeutic alliance is a non-specific factor that consistently predicts good outcome.[66] For women, evidence suggests that individual therapy leads to better outcomes, which may be related to their greater need for an interpersonal connection and the lack of social support that women experience in their environments.[41] Selection of a primary therapist is critical and should be determined by the needs of the individual patient. If the patient has alcohol problems as well as other psychiatric issues such as depression, anxiety, and trauma, a therapist who can provide both substance abuse and psychiatric services should be selected. This is often a challenge, as most service delivery systems provide substance abuse and mental health services in separate facilities. However, dual diagnosis units that employ professionals with expertise in both areas are gaining popularity in behavioral health service systems and a therapist with a good understanding of the interplay between substance abuse and mental health problems would be more suitable.

The assigned primary therapist may provide individual therapy or be the primary therapist for a woman in a women-only group. This individual would be responsible for developing a relationship with the patient and working collaboratively with the patient to identify her treatment needs. She would then be responsible to coordinate her care, based on the range of services needed for the patient. The primary therapist would need to address (1) alcohol use and (2) treatment engagement and retention, as these are key in mobilizing the patient toward recovery. Treatment retention is an important target because motivation is a dynamic state and patients often fluctuate in their determination to address alcohol use. If the patient is not ready to address her alcohol use, treatment engagement and retention needs to target motivation to address alcohol use by using established motivational approaches to alcoholism treatment.[55] Once the person begins to engage in treatment and starts making changes in alcohol use behaviors, the primary therapist would pay attention to issues such as other drug use, psychological difficulties, trauma, and other social problems that may relate to the patient's drinking.

CASE MANAGEMENT COMPONENT

This component may function best as an ambulatory case management team that initially, at the point of entry, assigns a case manager (CM) who links the patient to appropriate treatment services and works to eliminate barriers to treatment. In the next phase, the CM collaborates with the primary therapist to help the patient obtain other services in the system. When the primary therapist targets a particular service need in collaboration with the patient, the case manager continues to help the client access these services. The services range from health/medical services, services for children and families, vocational and educational services, and legal assistance. During this early treatment phase, the CM provides support and continuity across service delivery systems and becomes an important person in the woman's treatment network. There is evidence from studies on substance abusing pregnant women who often need multiple services that a case management component can greatly enhance treatment outcomes.[67-69] It is important to note that when a well-defined case management component is unavailable, such as in a general private practice setting, the case management functions can certainly be performed by the primary therapist.

PHARMACOTHERAPY COMPONENT

As there is evidence that women enter treatment with more severe alcohol and psychiatric symptoms,[2,40] availability of psychiatric services to address both alcohol use and psychiatric problems are needed. Informing the patient early in treatment that her psychiatric needs will be addressed can be reassuring to the patient and promote early treatment engagement. The primary therapist can determine the need for a psychiatric evaluation and coordinate this need with the psychiatrists. Depression, anxiety, and sleep difficulties are common complaints among alcoholic women. While these are often secondary to protracted withdrawal from alcohol, it may be difficult to assess if the patient is not completely abstinent. A more aggressive approach to treating the co-occurring psychiatric symptoms has gained support, especially as treating these symptoms may enhance treatment retention and efforts toward recovery from alcoholism.[70,71]

SKILL-BUILDING COMPONENT

The notion that heavy drinking is the primary form of coping with stressful events and the emotional pain of previous trauma is especially applicable to alcoholic women.[13,28] An avoidant coping style that involves denial and minimization of problems is characteristic of women problem drinkers.[28] A skill-building component that focuses on teaching alternate adaptive coping strategies to cope with life's problems is a core aspect of effective alcohol treatment approaches.[72,73] Skills can be taught as part of the individual therapy by the primary therapist, or the patient can attend separate skills groups that focus on helping the patient acquire and practice the new skills in real-life situations. The primary therapist functions as a coach, helping the patient remember and apply her newly learned skills to promote skills generalization to new day-to-day problems of living. This component increases self-efficacy and builds self-esteem, both of which are important issues to address in alcoholic women.

Women may come to treatment because of their children, and improving their relationship with their children is often an important target for them. Improved family functioning and relationships with children can sustain recovery after treatment has ended.[49] Promising, new parenting skills modules have been developed as add-on components to substance abuse treatment[74] and these can be used when appropriate.

BUILDING THE SOCIAL SUPPORT NETWORK

As social support is an important predictor of treatment outcome for women,[75] it is crucial to identify key relationships that are supporting or obstructing the patient's recovery. Including supportive individuals from the patient's network into treatment may help to further strengthen those alliances. Difficulties in marital relationships can be identified and, if willing, the couple can be referred to couples/family treatment. Ethnic and cultural differences may exist in terms of social support, and the therapist would need to understand the cultural issues of her patient in addressing this problem area. Finally, involvement in women self-help groups can help in building an alcohol-free support network. An on-site Alcoholics Anonymous group for women can initiate participation in self-help groups while the patient is still in treatment. The patient is more likely to participate in aftercare self-help groups if she begins to use it effectively while in treatment.[43]

The above components highlight the specific types of services that should be available to address the broad range of service needs of alcoholic women. While not all alcoholic women will require every component, treatment programs can benefit by having the capability in each of the above areas so that the specific services can be matched with patient needs. The treatment model is presented as a clinical framework for use by professionals in formulating the special therapeutic needs of alcoholic women.

REFERENCES

1. *Ninth Special Report to the U.S. Congress on Alcohol and Health,* U.S. Department of Health and Human Services, NIH Publ. No. 97-4017, 1997.
2. Weisner, C. and Schmidt, L. Gender disparities in treatment for alcohol problems. *JAMA,* 268, 1872, 1992.
3. Wilsnack, S., Patterns and trends in women's drinking: findings and some implications for prevention, *N.I.A.A.A. Research Monogr.* 32, NIH Publ. No. 96-3817, 19-63, 1996.
4. Wilsnack, R. and Wilsnack, S. Women, work, and alcohol: failures of simple theories, *Alcohol Clin. Exp. Res.,* 16, 172, 1992.
5. Julkunen, R., Tannenbaum, L., Barona, E., and Lieber, C., First pass metabolism of ethanol: an important determinant of blood levels after alcohol consumption, *Alcohol,* 2, 437, 1985.
6. Frezza, M., DiPadova, C., Pozzato, G., Terpin, M., Baraona, E., and Lieber, C., High blood alcohol levels in women: the role of decreased gastric alcohol dehydrogenase and first-pass metabolism, *N. Engl. J. Med.,* 322, 95, 1990.
7. Zeiner, A. and Kegg, P., Menstrual cycle and oral contraceptive effects on alcohol pharmacokinetics in Caucasian females, M. Galanter, Ed., *Currents in Alcoholism* Vol. 8, Grune & Stratton, New York, 1981, 47.
8. Sutker, P., Goist, K., and King, A., Acute alcohol intoxication in women: relationship to dose and menstrual cycle phase, *Alcoholism: Clin. Exp. Res.,* 11, 74, 1987.
9. Hill, S., Vulnerability to the biomedical consequences of alcoholism and alcohol-related problems among women, S. Wilsnack and L. Beckman, Eds., *Alcohol Problems in Women: Antecedents, Consequences, and Intervention,* Guilford Press, New York, 1984, 121.
10. Longnecker, M., Berlin, J., Orza, M., and Chalmers, T., A meta-analysis of alcohol consumption in relation to risk of breast cancer, *JAMA,* 260, 652, 1988.
11. Katsouyanni, K., Trichopoulou, A., Stuver, S., Vassilaros, S., Papadiamantis, Y., Bournas, N., Skarpou, N., Mueller, N., and Trichopoulos, D. Ethanol and breast cancer: An association that may be both confounded and casual, *Int. J. Cancer,* 58, 356, 1994.
12. Glenn, S., Sex differences in alcohol-induced brain damage, *N.I.A.A.A. Res. Monogr. 22,* NIH Pub. No. 93-3549, 195-212, 1993.
13. Miller, B., Downs, W., and Testa, M. Inter-relationships between victimization experiences and women's alcohol use, *J. Stud. Alcohol,* 11 (Suppl.), 109, 1993.
14. Wilsnack, S. and Wilsnack, R. Epidemiology of women's drinking, *J. Subst. Abuse,* 3, 133, 1991.
15. Kaufman Kantor, G. and Straus, M. Substance abuse as a precipitant of wife abuse victimizations, *Am. J. Drug Alcohol Abuse,* 15, 173, 1989.
16. Gomberg, E., Women's drinking practices and problems from a lifespan perspective, *N.I.A.A.A. Res. Monogr. 32.,* NIH Pub. No. 96-3817, 185-214, 1996.
17. Schuckit, M. and Morrisey, E., Alcoholism in women: some clinical and social perspectives with an emphasis on possible subtypes, M. Greenblatt and M. Schuckit, Eds., *Alcoholism Problems in Women and Children,* Grune and Stratton, New York, 1976, 5.
18. Corrigan, E., *Alcoholic Women in Treatment,* Oxford University Press, New York, 1980.
19. Hesselbrock, M., Meyer, R., and Keener, J., Psychopathology in hospitalized alcoholics, *Arch. Gen. Psychiatry,* 42, 1050, 1985.
20. Ross, H., Glaser, F., and Stiasny, S., Sex differences in the prevalence of psychiatric disorders in patients with alcohol and drug problems. *Br. J. Addiction,* 83, 1179, 1988.
21. Gomberg, E. and Nierenberg, T., Eds., *Women and Substance Abuse,* Ablex Publishing, Norwood, NJ, 1993.
22. Hesselbrock, M. and Hesselbrock, V., Depression and antisocial personality disorder in depression: gender comparison, E. Gomberg and T. Nirenberg, Eds., *Women and Substance Abuse,* Ablex Publishing, Norwood, NJ, 1993.
23. Helzer, J. and Pryzbeck, T., The co-occurrence of alcoholism with other psychiatric disorders in the general population and its impact on treatment, *J. Stud. Alcohol,* 49, 219, 1988.
24. Regier, D., Farmer, M., Rae, D., Locke, B., Keith, S., Judd, L., and Goodwin, F., Comorbidity of mental disorders with alcohol and other drug abuse: results from the Epidemiologic Catchment Area (ECA) study, *JAMA,* 264, 2511, 1990.

25. Windle, M., Windle, R., Scheidt, D., and Miller, G., Physical and sexual abuse and associated mental disorders among alcoholic inpatients, *Am. J. Psychiatry,* 152, 1322, 1995.

26. Kessler, R., Crum, R., Warner, L., Nelson, C., Schulenberg, J., and Anthony, J., Lifetime co-occurrence of DSM-III-R alcohol abuse and dependence with other psychiatric disorders in the National Comorbidity Study, *Arch. Gen. Psychiatry,* 54, 313, 1997.

27. Greenfield, S., Weiss, R., Muenz, L., Vagge, L., Kelly, J., Bello, L., and Michael, J., The effect of depression on return to drinking, *Arch. Gen. Psychiatry,* 55, 259, 1998.

28. Gomberg, E., Women and alcohol: use and abuse, *J. Nerv. Ment. Dis.,* 181, 211, 1993.

29. Margulies, R., Kessler, R., and Kandel, D., A longitudinal study of onset of drinking among high school students, *J. Stud. Alcohol.,* 38, 897, 1977.

30. Schulenberg, J., Dielman, T., and Leech, S., Individual versus social causes of alcohol misuse during early adolescence: a three-wave prospective study, Paper presented at the *Research Society on Alcoholism,* San Antonio, TX, June, 1993.

31. Hammer, T. and Vaglum, P., The increase in alcohol consumption among women: a phenomenon related to accessibility or stress? A general population study, *Br. J. Addiction,* 84, 767, 1989.

32. Moos, R., Finney, J., and Cronkite, R., *Alcoholism Treatment, Context, Process, and Outcome,* Oxford University Press, New York, 1990.

33. Robbins, C. Sex differences in psychosocial consequences of alcohol and drug abuse, *J. Health Soc. Behav.,* 30, 117, 1989.

34. Wilsnack, R., Wilsnack, S., and Klassen, A., Women's drinking and drinking problems: patterns from a 1981 national survey, *Am. J. Pub. Health,* 74, 1231, 1984.

35. Schilit, R. and Gomberg, E., Social support structures of women in treatment for alcoholism, *Health Soc. Work,* 12, 187, 1987.

36. Finkelstein, N., Treatment programming for alcohol and drug-dependent pregnant women, *Health Soc. Work,* 19, 7, 1994.

37. Ravndal, E. and Vaglum, P., Treatment of female addicts: the importance of relationships to parents, partners, and peers for the outcome, *Int. J. Addictions,* 29, 115, 1994.

38. Blume, S., Chemical dependency in women: important issues, *Am. J. Drug Alcohol Abuse,* 16, 297, 1990.

39. Grant, B., Barriers to alcoholism treatment: reasons for not seeking treatment in a general population sample, *J. Stud. Alcohol.,* 58, 365, 1997.

40. Farid, B. and Clarke, M., Characteristics of attenders to community based alcohol treatment centre with special reference to sex difference, *Drug Alcohol Depend.,* 30, 33, 1992.

41. Sanchez-Craig, M., Leigh, G., and Davila, R., Superior outcomes of females over males after brief treatment for the reduction of heavy drinking: replication and report of therapist effects, *Br. J. Addiction,* 86, 867, 1989.

42. Jarvis, T., Implications of gender for alcohol treatment research: a quantitative and qualitative review, *Br. J. Addiction,* 87, 1249, 1992.

43. Tonigan, J. and Hiller-Sturmhofel, Alcoholics Anonymous: who benefits? *Alcohol Health Res. World,* 18, 308, 1994.

44. Annis, H. and Liban, C., Alcoholism in women: treatment modalities and outcomes, O. Kalant, Ed., *Alcohol and Drug Problems in Women: Research Advances in Alcohol and Drug Problems,* Vol. 5, Plenum, New York, 1980, 385.

45. Vannicelli, M., Treatment outcomes of alcoholic women: the state of the art in relation to sex bias and expectancy effects, S. Wilsnack and L. Beckman, Eds., *Alcohol Problems in Women,* Guilford Press, New York, 1984, 369.

46. Project Match Research Group, Matching alcoholism treatments to client heterogeneity: Project MATCH posttreatment drinking outcomes, *J. Stud. Alcohol,* 58, 7, 1997.

47. Volpicelli, J., Alterman, A., Hayashida, M., and O'Brien, C., Naltrexone in the treatment of alcohol dependence, *Arch. Gen. Psychiatry,* 49, 876, 1992.

48. O'Malley, S., Jaffe, A., Chang, G., Schottenfeld, R., Meyer, R., and Rounsaville, B., Naltrexone and coping skills therapy for alcohol dependence: a controlled study, *Arch. Gen. Psychiatry,* 49, 881, 1992.

49. Schneider, K., Kviz, F., Isola, M., and Filstead, W., Evaluating multiple outcomes and gender differences in alcoholism treatment, *Addictive Behav.,* 20, 1, 1995.

50. Boothroyd, W., Nature and development of alcoholism in women, O. Kalant, Ed., *Alcohol and Drug Problems in Women: Research Advances in Alcohol and Drug Problems,* Vol. 5, Plenum, New York, 1980, 299.

51. Finney, J. and Moos, R., The long-term course of treated alcoholism. 1. Mortality, relapse and remission rates and comparisons with community controls, *J. Stud. Alcohol,* 52, 44, 1991.

52. Rounsaville, B., Dolinsky, Z., Barbor, T., and Meyer, R., Psychopathology as a predictor of treatment outcome in alcoholics, *Arch. Gen. Psychiatry,* 44, 505, 1987.

53. Beckman, L., Treatment needs of women with alcohol problems, *Alcohol Health Res. World,* 18, 206, 1994.

54. Moore, R., Bone, L., Geller, G., Mamon, J., Stokes, E., and Levine, D., Prevalence, detection, and treatment of alcoholism in hospitalized patients, *JAMA,* 261, 403, 1989.

55. Miller, W., Zweben, A., DiClemente, C., and Rychtarik, R., *Motivational Enhancement Therapy Manual,* Vol. 2, National Institute on Alcohol Abuse and Alcoholism, Rockville, MD, 1994.

56. Ewing, J., Detecting alcoholism: the CAGE questionnaire, *JAMA,* 252, 1905, 1984.

57. Sokol, R., Martier, S., and Ager, J., The T-ACE questions: practical prenatal detection of risk-drinking, *Am. J. Obstetr. Gynecol.,* 160, 863, 1989.

58. Russell, M., Martier, S.S., Sokol, R.J., et al., Screening for pregnancy risk-drinking, *Alcohol Clin. Exp. Res.,* 18, 1156, 1994.

59. Bradley, K., Boyd-Wickizer, J., Powell, S., and Burman, M., Alcohol screening questionnaires in women, *JAMA,* 280, 166, 1998.

60. American Psychiatric Association, *Practice Guidelines for Treatment of Patients with Substance Use Disorders. Alcohol, Cocaine, Opioids,* American Psychiatric Association, Washington D.C., 1995, 15.

61. Miller, W.R. and Rollnick, S., *Motivational Interviewing,* Guilford Press, New York, 1991.

62. McLellan, A., Grissom, G., Zanis, D., Randall, M., Brill, P., and O'Brien, C., Problem-service 'matching' in addiction treatment, *Arch. Gen. Psychiatry,* 54, 730, 1997.

63. Reed, B., Developing women-sensitive drug dependence treatment services: why so difficult? *J. Psychoactive Drugs,* 19, 151, 1987.

64. Dahlgren, L. and Willander, A., Are special treatment facilities for female alcoholics needed? A controlled 2-year follow-up study from a specialized female unit (EWA) versus a mixed male/female treatment facility, *Alcohol. Clin. Exp. Res.,* 13, 499, 1989.

65. Copeland, J. and Hall, W., Comparison of women seeking drug and alcohol treatment in a specialist women's and two traditional mixed-sex treatment services, *Br. J. Addiction,* 87, 1293, 1992.

66. Hartley, D., Research on the therapeutic alliance in psychotherapy, *Psychiatry Update: American Psychiatric Association Annual Review,* Vol. 4, American Psychiatric Association, Washington, D.C., 1985, 532.

67. Laken, M. and Ager, J., Effects of case management on retention in prenatal substance abuse treatment, *Am. J. Drug Alcohol Abuse,* 22, 439, 1996.

68. Klein, D. and Zahand, E., Perspectives of pregnant substance using women: findings from the California perinatal needs assessment, *J. Psychoactive Drugs,* 29, 55, 1997.

69. Haller, D., Knisely, J., Elswick, R., Dawson, K., and Schnoll, S., Perinatal substance abusers: factors influencing treatment retention, *J. Subst. Abuse Treatment,* 14, 513, 1997.

70. Anton, R., Medications for treating alcoholism, *Alcohol Health Res. World,* 18, 265, 1994.

71. Litten, R. and Allen, J., Pharmacotherapy for alcoholics with collateral depression or anxiety: an update of research findings, *Exp. Clin. Psychopharmacol.,* 3, 87, 1995.

72. Marlatt, G. and Gordon, J., Eds., *Relapse Prevention,* Guilford Press, New York, 1985.

73. Monti, P., Abrams, D., Kadden, R., and Cooney, N., *Treating Alcohol Dependence: A Coping Skills Training Guide,* Guilford Press, New York, 1989.

74. Luthar, S. and Walsh, K., Treatment needs of drug-addicted mothers: integrated parenting psychotherapy interventions, *J. Subst. Abuse Treatment,* 12, 341, 1995.

75. Macdonald, J., Predictors of treatment outcome for alcoholic women, *Int. J. Addictions,* 22, 235, 1987.

14   Primary Care Setting

Patrick G. O'Connor

OVERVIEW

Primary care physicians should assume ongoing responsibility for patients with alcohol problems and provide comprehensive and coordinated care. All patients should be educated about "at-risk" drinking and screened for alcohol problems. At-risk patients should be assessed for alcohol-related medical, psychiatric, and behavioral problems and advised to decrease their alcohol consumption to a level below "at-risk" levels using brief intervention techniques. Alcohol-dependent patients should be advised to abstain from alcohol and referred for appropriate alcohol treatment. They should also be examined and treated for alcohol-related medical, psychiatric, and behavioral problems. Primary care physicians should monitor patients in recovery over time and promote abstinence.

INTRODUCTION

Because alcohol use is associated with a wide range of medical and behavioral disorders,[1-3] patients with alcohol-related problems are likely to present to primary care physicians for care.[4] Studies of medical patients have demonstrated that up to 40% may experience problems related to alcohol.[5] Thus, the "yield" of screening for alcohol problems can be expected to be quite high in medical settings. As with other chronic diseases commonly cared for by primary care physicians such as cardiac disease or diabetes, alcohol use disorders can range in clinical severity from relatively asymptomatic to severe, and require intervention at a variety of levels and from a variety of providers. Primary care physicians should be equipped to identify all stages of alcohol abuse and be able to participate in the management of patients along the entire spectrum of the "disease" process.

In this chapter, the roles of primary care physicians will be delineated as they pertain to three sets of patients: all patients in their practice, nondependent problem drinkers, and alcohol-dependent patients. With each of these sets of patients, the overall approach should to be to provide comprehensive and longitudinal treatment, in conjunction with professionals from other disciplines when necessary.

ALL PATIENTS: SCREENING FOR ALCOHOL PROBLEMS

Despite the prevalence of alcohol problems in medical practice, physicians do not regularly screen for or detect alcohol problems in their patients.[6,7] A variety of explanations have been proposed for this phenomenon, including poor physician education about substance abuse and negative attitudes about substance-using patients. Although physicians are more likely to identify patients experiencing severe medical complications such as cirrhosis,[8] early intervention and prevention strategies depend on the detection of patients who have few or no obvious medical complications due to their alcohol use. Epidemiologic data demonstrating high rates of alcohol problems and the availability of brief and simple screening instruments strongly support the need to screen all medical patients for alcohol problems.[9]

Patients with alcohol problems are likely to be sensitive about their drinking and may be apprehensive when questioned about their alcohol use. Thus, a matter-of-fact and nonjudgmental approach is very important. In addition, discomfort or denial may interfere with the accuracy of patients' responses. Thus, questions may need to be asked on multiple occasions to get a clear picture of the patient's alcohol use history. A four-step process may facilitate screening and diagnosis of alcohol problems.[4,10-12]

1. ASK ABOUT CURRENT AND PAST ALCOHOL USE IN ALL PATIENTS

It is important to ask about current *and* past use, given that many patients with a history of alcohol dependence may be currently abstinent and in recovery. Thus, asking patients, "Have you ever used alcohol?" and then providing specificity as to the time frame of their alcohol use is critical. When taking a family history, it is also important to ask about relatives who may have had alcohol problems. This may indicate increased risk in the patient being interviewed.[13]

2. OBTAIN A MORE DETAILED HISTORY REGARDING QUANTITY AND FREQUENCY OF ALCOHOL USE IN PATIENTS WHO HAVE USED ALCOHOL

Distinguishing past and current alcohol use and the change in the pattern over time is a major goal of the physician when examining patients. Initial questions such as, "How often do you drink?" and "How much do you usually drink on a typical drinking day?" will help to establish a baseline of self-reported alcohol use. Once a baseline is established, it is important to screen for "binge" drinking by asking, "Do you ever drink more than your 'usual' amount?" and to determine what that amount is. In addition, asking "What type of alcohol do you use?" is important to determine the variety of alcohol-containing beverages (beer, wine, spirits) consumed. These quantity and frequency questions may help distinguish "moderate" (not harmful) from "at risk" (e.g., >2 drinks/day and >4 drinks/occasion in men ≤65, or >1 drink/day in women and men >65)[12] and "problem" drinking.

3. USE A STANDARDIZED SCREENING QUESTIONNAIRE TO DETECT POSSIBLE ALCOHOL PROBLEMS

The CAGE questionnaire is the most commonly studied screening instrument in medical settings (Table 14.1). The CAGE is scored from 0 to 4, depending on the number of "yes" responses to the four questions; a score of 2 or more is generally considered to be a "positive" result. It is designed to screen for lifetime alcohol abuse and dependence.[14-16] In one study of patients seen in a general medical outpatient setting, the positive predictive value of the CAGE was demonstrated to be 32% for one positive response, 59% for two positive responses, 81% for three positive responses, and 97% for four positive responses.[17] Although it has been generally accepted as the "standard" screening instrument for primary care settings,[18] the CAGE may perform less well in specific sociodemographic subgroups such older patients[19] and women.[20]

The Alcohol Use Disorder Identification Test (AUDIT) is another approach to screening in primary care which may provide additional information (Table 14.1).[21] Developed by the World Health Organization (WHO), the AUDIT was designed to identify "hazardous" and "harmful" drinking and provides information about current as well as past alcohol problems. The three "quantity/frequency" questions regarding current drinking provide information similar to that discussed earlier in step 2. The additional seven questions about past drinking help to complete the picture. The individual questions are scored on a scale of 0 to 4, and a total score ≥8 is a positive result. Studies of medical patients have demonstrated the AUDIT to have a sensitivity and specificity of 92 and 96%, respectively.[22,23]

TABLE 14.1
Screening Instruments for the Identification of Alcohol Problems

CAGE

Have you felt you should **C**utdown on your drinking?

Have people **A**nnoyed you by criticizing your drinking?

Have you ever felt bad or **G**uilty about your drinking?

Have you ever had a drink first thing in the morning to steady your nerves or get rid of a hangover (**E**ye opener)?

AUDIT

How often do you have a drink containing alcohol?

    (0) Never

    (1) Monthly or less

    (2) Two to four times a month

    (3) Two to three times a week

    (4) Four or more times a week

How many drinks containing alcohol do you have on a typical day when you are drinking?

    (0) 1 or 2

    (1) 3 or 4

    (2) 5 or 6

    (3) 7 to 9

    (4) 10 or more

How often do you have six or more drinks on one occasion?

    (0) Never

    (1) Less than monthly

    (2) Monthly

    (3) Weekly

    (4) Daily or almost daily

How often during the last year have you found that you were not able to stop drinking once you had started?

    (0) Never

    (1) Less than monthly

    (2) Monthly

    (3) Weekly

    (4) Daily or almost daily

How often during the last year have you failed to do what was normally expected from you because of drinking?

    (0) Never

    (1) Less than monthly

    (2) Monthly

    (3) Weekly

    (4) Daily or almost daily

How often during the last year have you needed a first drink in the morning to get yourself going after a heavy drinking session?

    (0) Never

    (1) Less than monthly

    (2) Monthly

    (3) Weekly

    (4) Daily or almost daily

How often during the last year have you had a feeling of guilt or remorse after drinking?

    (0) Never

    (1) Less than monthly

    (2) Monthly

    (3) Weekly

    (4) Daily or almost daily

TABLE 14.1 (continued)
Screening Instruments for the Identification of Alcohol Problems

How often during the last year have you been unable to remember what happened the night before because you had been drinking?

    (0) Never

    (1) Less than monthly

    (2) Monthly

    (3) Weekly

    (4) Daily or almost daily

Have you or someone else been injured as a result of your drinking?

    (0) No

    (2) Yes, but not in the last year

    (4) Yes, during the last year

Has a relative or a friend, or a doctor or other health worker, been concerned about your drinking or suggested you cut down?

    (1) Now

    (2) Yes, but not in the last year

    (4) Yes, during the last year

---

4. PERFORM A DETAILED ASSESSMENT ON PATIENTS WHO SCREEN POSITIVE FOR ALCOHOL PROBLEMS

Patients identified as having potential alcohol problems during screening should undergo a detailed assessment concerning specific alcohol-related problems. This includes a thorough review of all medical problems associated with alcohol, as discussed elsewhere in this handbook, alcohol-related psychiatric problems, especially anxiety and depression, and other behavior-related and social problems (e.g., family, legal, and employment problems). The use of other substances, including tobacco and illicit drugs, should also be examined. In addition, besides identifying "at-risk" drinking, criteria for alcohol abuse and alcohol dependence should be evaluated (see also Chapters 42 and 43).[24] Prior alcohol-related diagnoses and treatment for alcohol problems should also be determined.

"AT-RISK" AND NON-DEPENDENT PROBLEM DRINKERS

Much of the research on intervening with non-dependent, at-risk, or problem drinking has focused on the role of primary care physicians in the management of these patients. The use of "brief intervention" techniques is well suited to primary care practice in that they involve counseling strategies familiar to primary care physicians and can be within the time frame of an office visit. These include giving feedback and advice, along with patient education. In addition, brief intervention techniques can be provided within the longitudinal pattern of care that is typical of primary care practice. The overall treatment goal with "at-risk" drinkers is to have them reduce their alcohol consumption to levels considered medically safe (e.g., below the level of "at-risk" drinking).

Two meta-analyses have examined the efficacy brief intervention therapies.[25,26] In a review of over 30 controlled studies of brief interventions enrolling over 6000 problem drinkers, Bien et al. concluded that, overall, "these studies indicate that brief interventions are more effective than no counseling, and often as effective as more extensive treatment."[25] A subsequent meta-analysis of randomized control trials, focused on methodologic quality, examined studies with sample sizes greater than 30.[26] Methodological quality was assessed using an established scoring, and outcome data were combined so that a pooled odds ratio could be calculated. Twelve studies were included, and the outcome data were combined with resulting pooled odds of 1.91 (95% confidence interval, 1.61–2.27) in favor of brief interventions over no intervention. In subgroup analyses, the authors found that this treatment effect was present regardless of gender, intervention intensity, and type of clinical setting.[26]

Three recent randomized trials illustrate the techniques and effectiveness of brief intervention strategies. In the WHO international study, over 1500 "heavy" drinkers recruited from primary care, hospital, and other settings were randomized to no intervention, 5 minutes of simple advice, or 20 minutes of brief counseling.[27] In this study, the 5-minute intervention was as effective as the 20-minute intervention, and both were more effective than no intervention in males who decreased their daily alcohol consumption by 17% in comparison to controls.[27] Another study of "problem drinkers" identified in 46 physicians' private practices compared "simple advice" to 3 hours of nurse-administered behavioral counseling; it was found that 46% in the "advice" group and 70% in the "counseling" group reduced their drinking, and that behavioral counseling was superior to "simple advice" in reducing alcohol consumption, serum GGT, and physician visits.[28]

In a study by Fleming et al., a sample of 723 subjects (problem drinkers) were recruited from 17 primary care practices.[29] The brief intervention was provided during two physician visits, which were followed by a "reinforcement" phone call from a nurse. For the brief intervention group, the mean number of drinks in the previous 7 days, the number of binge drinking episodes over a 30-day period, and episodes of excessive drinking decreased significantly compared to the control group. In addition, the treatment group had a significantly shorter number of hospital days during the study.[29]

Thus, data from several studies suggest that physicians can play an important role in decreasing at-risk drinking behaviors in their patients and that health benefits may result.

ALCOHOL-DEPENDENT PATIENTS

When patients with alcohol dependence are identified in their practices, primary care physicians will generally need to provide more intensive services, including management of more severe medical morbidity, management of the alcohol withdrawal syndrome, and referral to an alcohol treatment program. In addition, referral to self-help groups such as Alcoholics Anonymous is a step that well-informed primary care physicians can use effectively with their patients. While the management of comorbid medical problems is discussed in other chapters, this chapter discusses the primary care physician's role in the initiation of treatment and follow-up for patients who are alcohol dependent.

MANAGEMENT OF ALCOHOL WITHDRAWAL SYNDROME

Alcohol withdrawal can be associated with a wide range of symptoms, from minimal to severe (see also Chapter 6 on the alcohol withdrawal syndrome). A major role for the primary care physician is to evaluate the patient's level of potential withdrawal severity and provide the appropriate level of medical management. Signs and symptoms of alcohol withdrawal include abnormalities in vital signs (e.g., tachycardia, hypertension), tremor, diaphoresis, insomnia, gastrointestinal symptoms (e.g., nausea, vomiting, diarrhea), and central nervous system manifestations (e.g., anxiety, agitation, hallucinations, seizures, and delirium).[30] Withdrawal severity and response to treatment may be assessed using the revised Clinical Institute Withdrawal Assessment (CIWA-Ar), which describes ten clinical features of withdrawal that are rated by patient observation.[31] Patients presenting with mild withdrawal can be managed as outpatients,[32] oftentimes by primary care physicians. More severe withdrawal or patients with significant comorbid medical or psychiatric problems may require inpatient care.[33] The treatment of alcohol withdrawal should be viewed as a first step in the treatment process. It is critical to refer all patients who are treated for alcohol withdrawal to ongoing treatment to prevent relapse.

Pharmacological therapy for the alcohol withdrawal syndrome primarily involves the use of the benzodiazepines (e.g., chlordiazepoxide, diazepam, lorazepam, and oxazepam) as these drugs have been established as the safest and most effective treatment.[33] Besides providing effective symptom control, benzodiazepines also decrease the incidence of seizures and possibly delirium tremens.[33,34] The American Society of Addiction Medicine published an evidence-based guideline for the management of alcohol withdrawal, and suggested that the longer-acting benzodiazepines provided a smoother withdrawal and may be more effective in preventing seizures than short-acting preparations.[33] Short-acting agents may be more appropriate for the elderly and for patients with severe liver disease.

REFERRING PATIENTS TO TREATMENT

Recent research has demonstrated that Alcoholics Anonymous (AA) attendance may be associated with more successful drinking outcomes in alcohol-dependent patients.[35] Alcoholics Anonymous has major advantages, including its widespread availability and the fact that it is free of charge. In order to "prescribe" AA meetings for their patients, physicians should obtain a meeting schedule from their local AA organization. A critical first step is for patients to find a group that is convenient and suitable. Thus, many patients will only be comfortable in groups with sociodemographic characteristics similar to their own. For example, sending a 60-year-old patient to a meeting dominated by persons in their late teens or early 20s may be counterproductive. Often, trial and error is necessary before appropriate meeting sites are identified. It is often recommended that physicians attend at least one "open" AA meeting themselves to help prepare them to counsel their patients on how AA works.[36]

Patients who meet criteria for alcohol abuse and dependence generally require referral to specialists and formal alcohol treatment programs. Physicians should familiarize themselves with the structure and services available within their local treatment programs so that the most appropriate referrals can be made. It is critical to communicate effectively with alcohol treatment programs and reinforce their treatment strategies when patients present for follow-up medical care.

Criteria have been developed by The American Psychiatric Association[37] and the American Society of Addiction Medicine[38] that are designed to match patients to an appropriate treatment level. Most patients can be managed safely in an outpatient setting, although patients with a high level of medical or psychiatric comorbidity, a low level of social support, or multiple prior outpatient treatment failures may require inpatient treatment. While the psychotherapeutic approaches used in alcohol treatment programs may vary from one program to another, the basic goals motivating patients to change their behavior and lifestyles, teaching them coping skills to avoid alcohol use, encouraging them to develop activities that do not reinforce drinking and reward abstinence, and helping patients to improve interpersonal interactions are common features of all programs.[39]

Pharmacotherapy using disulfiram, naltrexone, and acamprosate has been demonstrated to be a useful adjunct to psychotherapy for alcohol dependence.[40] To date, only naltrexone has been evaluated in detail in the hands of primary care providers.[41] Naltrexone, an opioid antagonist, has been demonstrated to decrease the pleasurable effects and craving associated with alcohol use and was approved by the FDA in 1994.[42-44] In the initial studies of naltrexone, alcohol-dependent subjects were given 50 mg day^{-1} while enrolled in outpatient or day hospital alcohol treatment programs and followed for 12 weeks. These subjects demonstrated a 54% rate of abstinence over 12 weeks.[45] In a more recent study of 29 alcohol-dependent subjects, the investigators demonstrated that naltrexone may also be effective in the hands of primary care providers.[41] In this study, patients received a primary care model of psychotherapy referred to as "Advice and Clinical Management," which incorporated many of the simple counseling techniques used in brief interventions. In this study, the majority of patients (72%) completed treatment and a minority (35%) relapsed to heavy drinking. When compared to baseline, all drinking behaviors improved significantly in these subjects, including percent of days abstinent (increased from 36.6 to 88.8%) and mean number of drinks per occasion (decreased from 9.5 to 2.5).[41] Subjects in this study also reported high levels of satisfaction with primary care-based treatment, suggesting that this approach may be suitable for many patients. Ongoing research will compare the effectiveness of this primary care-based approach to a more traditional coping skills therapy model. Acamprosate has been studied extensively in Europe and may also be suitable in the hands of primary care physicians in selected patients.

REFERENCES

1. Eckardt, M.J., Harford, T.C., Kaelber, C.T., Parker, E.S., Rosenthal, L.S., Ryback, R.S., Salmioraghi, G.C., Vanderveen, E., and Warren, K.R., Health hazards associated with alcohol consumption, *JAMA*, 246, 648, 1981.
2. *Ninth Special Report to the United States Congress on Alcohol and Health*, U.S. Department of Health and Human Services, 1997.
3. Lieber, C.S., Medical disorders of alcoholism, *N. Engl. J. Med.*, 333, 1058, 1995.
4. O'Connor, P.G. and Schottenfeld, R.S., Patients with alcohol problems, *N. Engl. J. Med.*, 338, pp. 592-602, 1998.
5. Magruder-Habib, K., Durand, A.M., and Frey, K.A. Alcohol abuse and alcoholism in primary health care settings, *J. Fam. Pract.*, 32, 406-13, 1991.
6. Cleary, P.D., Miller, M., Bush, B.T., Warburg, M.M., Delbanco, T.L., and Aronson, M.D. Prevalence and recognition of alcohol abuse in a primary care population, *Am. J. Med.*, 85, 466-71, 1988.
7. Coulehan, J.L., Zettier-Segal, M., Block, M., et al., Recognition of alcoholism and substance abuse in primary care patients, *Arch. Intern. Med.*, 147, 349, 1987.
8. Moore, R.D., Bone, L.R., Geller, G., Mamon, J.A., Stokes, E.J., and Levine, D.M., Prevalence, detection, and treatment of alcoholism in hospitalized patients, *JAMA*, 261, 403, 1989.
9. United States Preventive Services Task Force, *Guide to Clinical Preventive Services*, 2nd ed., Williams & Wilkins, Baltimore, MD, 1996.
10. Institute for Health Policy, Brandeis University and The Robert Wood Johnson Foundation, *Substance Abuse: The Nation's Number One Health Problem*, 1993.
11. Kitchens, J.M. Does this patient have an alcohol problem?, *JAMA*, 272, 1782-7, 1994.
12. National Institute on Alcohol Abuse and Alcoholism, *The National Institutes of Health, The Physicians' Guide to Helping Patients With Alcohol Problems*, 1995.
13. Light, J.M., Irvine, K.M., and Kjerulf, L., Estimating genetic and environmental effects of alcohol use and dependence from a national survey: a "quasi-adoption" study, *J. Stud. Alcohol*, 57, 507, 1996.
14. Fleming, M.F. and Barry, K.L., The effectiveness of alcoholism screening in an ambulatory care setting, *J. Stud. Alcohol*, 52, 33, 1991.
15. Liskow, B., Campbell, J., Nickel, E.J., and Powell, B.J., Validity of the CAGE questionnaire in screening for alcohol dependence in a walk-in (triage) clinic, *J. Stud. Alcohol*, 56, 277, 1995.
16. Beresford, T.P., Blow, F.C., Hill, E., Singer, K., and Lucey, M.R., Comparison of CAGE questionnaire and computer-assisted laboratory profiles in screening for covert alcoholism, *Lancet*, 336, 482, 1990.
17. Buchsbaum, D.G., Buchanan, R.G., Centor, R.M., Schnoll, S.H., and Lawton, M.J., Screening for alcohol abuse using CAGE scores and likelihood ratios, *Ann. Intern. Med.*, 115, 774, 1991.
18. Samet, J.H., Rollnick, S., and Barnes, H., Beyond CAGE. A brief clinical approach after detection of substance abuse, *Arch. Intern. Med.*, 156, 2287, 1996.
19. Adams, W.L., Barry, K.L., and Fleming, M.F., Screening for problem drinking in older primary care patients, *JAMA*, 276, 1964, 1996.
20. Steinbauer, J.R., Cantor, S.B., Holzer, C.E., and Volk, R.J., Ethnic and sex bias in primary care screening tests for alcohol use disorders, *Ann. Intern. Med.*, 129, 353, 1998.
21. Allen, J.P., Maisto, S.A., and Connors, G.J., Self-report screening tests for alcohol problems in primary care, *Arch. Intern. Med.*, 155, 1726, 1995.
22. Saunders, J.B., Aasland, O.G., Babor, T.F., de la Fuente, J.R., and Grant, M., Development of the Alcohol Use Disorders Identification Test (AUDIT): WHO Collaborative Project on Early Detection of Persons with Harmful Alcohol Consumption — II, *Addiction*, 88, 791, 1993.
23. Isaacson, J.H., Butler, R., Zacharek, M., and Tzelepis, A., Screening with the Alcohol Use Disorders Identification Test (AUDIT) in an inner city population, *J. Gen. Intern. Med.*, 9, 550, 1994.
24. American Psychiatric Association, *Diagnostic and Statistical Manual of Mental Disorders, Fourth Edition (DSM-IV)*, The American Psychiatric Association, Washington, D.C., 1994.

25. Bien, T.H., Miller, W.R., and Tonigan, J.S., Brief interventions for alcohol problems: a review, *Addiction*, 88, 315, 1993.

26. Wilk, A.I., Jensen, N.M., and Havighurst, T.C., Meta-analysis of randomized control trials addressing brief interventions in heavy alcohol drinkers, *J. Gen. Intern. Med.*, 12, 274, 1997.

27. WHO Brief Intervention Study Group, A cross-national trial of brief interventions with heavy drinkers, *Am. j. Public Health*, 86, 949, 1996.

28. Israel, Y., Hollander, O., Sanchez-Craig, M., Booker, S., Miller, V., Gingrich, R., and Rankin, J.G., Screening for problem drinking and counseling by the primary care physician-nurse team, *Alcohol. Clin. Exp. Res.*, 20, 1443, 1996.

29. Fleming, M.F., Barry, K.L., Manwell, L.B., Johnson, K., and London, R., Brief physician advice for problem alcohol drinkers. A randomized controlled trial in community-based primary care practices, *JAMA*, 277, 1039, 1997.

30. Turner, R.C., Lichstein, P.R., Peden, J.G., Busher, J.T., and Waivers, L.E., Alcohol withdrawal syndromes: a review of pathophysiology, clinical presentation, and treatment, *J. Gen. Intern. Med.*, 4, 432, 1989.

31. Sullivan, J.T., Sykora, K., Schneiderman, J., Naranjo, C.A., and Sellers, E.M., Assessment of alcohol withdrawal: the revised clinical institute withdrawal assessment for alcohol scale (CIWA-Ar), *Br. J. Addict.*, 84, 1353, 1989.

32. Horwitz, R.I., Gottlieb, L.D., and Kraus, M.L., The efficacy of atenolol in the outpatient management of the alcohol withdrawal syndrome. Results of a randomized clinical trial, *Arch. Intern. Med.*, 149, 1089, 1989.

33. Mayo-Smith, M.F., Pharmacological management of alcohol withdrawal. A meta-analysis and evidence-based practice guideline. American Society of Addiction Medicine Working Group on Pharmacological Management of Alcohol Withdrawal, *JAMA*, 278, 144, 1997.

34. Sellers, E.M., Naranjo, C.A., Harrison, M., Devenyi, P., Roach, C., and Sykora, K., Diazepam loading: simplified treatment of alcohol withdrawal, *Clin. Pharmacol. Ther.*, 34, 822, 1983.

35. McCrady, B., Recent research in twelve step programs, Graham, A.W., Schultz, T.K., and Wilford, B.B., Eds., *Principles of Addiction Medicine*, 2nd ed., American Society of Addiction Medicine, Chevy Chase, MD, 1998, 707.

36. Barnes, H.N., Aronson, M.D., and Delbanco, T.L., *Alcoholism: A Guide for the Primary Care Physician*, Springer-Verlag, New York, 1987.

37. American Psychiatric Association, Practice guideline for the treatment of patients with substance use disorders: alcohol, cocaine, opioids, *Am. J. Psychiatry*, 152(Suppl. 11), 1, 1995.

38. American Society of Addiction Medicine, *Patient Placement Criteria for the Treatment of Substance-Related Disorders*, 2nd ed., American Society of Addiction Medicine, Chevy Chase, MD, 1997.

39. Carroll, K.M. and Schottenfeld, R., Nonpharmacologic approaches to substance abuse treatment, *Med. Clin. North Am.*, 81, 927, 1997.

40. Saitz, R. and O'Malley, S.S., Pharmacotherapies for alcohol abuse. Withdrawal and treatment, *Med. Clin. North Am.*, 81, 881, 1997.

41. O'Connor, P.G., Farren, C.K., Rounsaville, B.J., and O'Malley, S.S., A preliminary investigation of the management of alcohol dependence with naltrexone by primary care providers, *Am. J. Med.*, 103, 477, 1997.

42. Volpicelli, J.R., Naltrexone in alcohol dependence, *Lancet*, 346, 456, 1995.

43. O'Malley, S.S., Jaffe, A.J., Chang, G., Schottenfeld, R.S., Meyer, R.E., and Rounsaville, B. ,Naltrexone and coping skills therapy for alcohol dependence. A controlled study, *Arch. Gen. Psychiatry*, 49, 881, 1992.

44. Volpicelli, J.R., Alterman, A.I., Hayashida, M., and O'Brien, C.P., Naltrexone in the treatment of alcohol dependence, *Arch. Gen. Psychiatry*, 49, 876, 1992.

45. O'Malley, S.S., Croop, R.S., Wroblewski, J.M., Labriola, D.F., and Volpicelli, J.R., Naltrexone in the treatment of alcohol dependence: a combined analysis of two trials, *Psychiatr. Ann.*, 25, 681, 1995.

15 Nervous System

Thomas Berger

OVERVIEW

Neurological disorders are common complications of acute or chronic alcohol abuse. Ethanol and its oxidative metabolite acetaldehyde may directly damage the developing and mature nervous system. Ethanol contains nonnutritive calories, so that heavy drinking is complicated by malnutrition and vitamin deficiency. Thiamine deficiency accelerates ethanol metabolism and the production of acetaldehyde. Acetaldehyde in turn reduces the activity of the thiamine-dependent enzyme transketolase by acetylation. Chronic alcohol administration potentiates the lesions of experimental thiamine deficiency and impairs the recovery of function from neural injury of diverse etiologies. Finally, genetic factors affecting the enzyme transketolase may influence the susceptibility of certain alcoholics to develop neurological complications.[1-3]

The etiological combination of direct alcohol toxicity, malnutrition, vitamin deficiency, and systemic alcohol disorders, such as chronic liver disease, generally requires a therapeutic program of alcohol abstinence, well-balanced nutrition, vitamin substitution, and neurological rehabilitation.

ACUTE INTOXICATION WITH ALCOHOL

Alcohol intoxication is so common that one might forget that it can be fatal by respiratory depression.[4-6]

Mild intoxication (0.5 to 1.5‰ for healthy and alcohol-naive individuals) is characterized by decreased psychomotoric activity, impaired concentration, behavior and self-control, "black-outs," and minimal cerebellar symptoms such as nystagmus. Although alcohol is a CNS depressant, some individuals experience paradoxical reactions upon intoxication with extreme excitement, violence, and psychotic reactions. The hangover produces headaches, malaise, nausea, vertigo, tremulousness, and lack of concentration.

Moderately intoxicated individuals (1.5 to 2.5‰) behave psychosocially uncontrolled or aggressive upon exogenous stimuli; experience euphoria, dysphoria, or depression; and show more impaired cerebellar functions such as slurred speech, ataxia, nystagmus, and vertigo. In addition, autonomic symptoms, such as tachycardia, sweating, and nausea occur.

Severe intoxication (>2.5‰) leads to disorientation, somnolence, or coma, and marked cerebellar and autonomic dysfunction. Death may occur upon fatal respiratory paralysis.

For mild to moderate intoxication, no treatment — except symptomatic — is required. Emergency management and cardiorespiratory monitoring is urgent for severe intoxication. Sedatives or tranquilizers are contraindicated because of probable additional intoxication with these substances. Haloperidol 5 to 10 mg i.v. (maximum daily dose 60 mg) can be used for extremely excited patients.

DISORDERS OF THE CENTRAL NERVOUS SYSTEM

SEIZURES

Epileptic seizures are the most frequent neurological sequelae (prevalence 20 to 35%) of alcoholism regardless of the duration of alcohol abuse.[4,7]

The pathophysiological mechanisms remain unknown, but dysregulation of potassium, magnesium, and calcium and/or neurotransmitters such as GABA and glutamate are suggested.

Alcohol intoxication as well as withdrawal are the most frequent causes for seizures in these patients. Withdrawal from alcohol for 24 to 48 hours may lead to tonic-clonic (grand mal) seizures. Clinical examination usually reveals no focal neurological signs or symptoms. EEG is normal or exhibits only nonspecific signs, such as minor EEG slowing and decreased alpha activity. In case of the first occurrence of an epileptic seizure, EEG and CT scan diagnosis is required to exclude focal brain injury. Approximately 2 to 10% of the patients develop status epilepticus and 30% of the patients with withdrawal seizures progress to delirium tremens.[8]

Focal epileptic seizures are highly indicative of focal brain injury (trauma, hemorrhage, neoplasia, encephalopathy, and metabolic disorders such as hypoglycemia and disbalance of electrolytes). Clinical examination exhibits focal neurological signs, such as cranial nerve, motor, or sensory dysfunction. Therefore, laboratory investigations, EEG, and CT scan should be performed immediately. EEG shows focal or diffuse, non-paroxysmal or paroxysmal abnormalities. Further investigations or procedures depend on detected focal brain injury. In general, hospital admission is recommended.

In addition, alcohol abuse may either provoke or unmask seizures because of pre-existing genuine epilepsy. Focal spiking may be found in EEG.

The first appearance of an epileptic seizure requires detailed differential diagnosis, but usually no acute treatment is necessary — unless status epilepticus occurs or the patient has symptomatic or genuine epilepsy.[7] If the history is uncertain, anticonvulsants can be given for a short time, but long-term treatment is not indicated for ethanol-induced seizures because of poor compliance and usually existing toxic liver disease. Alcoholics with known withdrawal seizures should receive prophylactic anticonvulsive therapy during detoxification.

CEREBRAL VASCULAR DISEASES

Chronic alcoholism increases the risk for intracerebral and subarachnoidal hemorrhages, lowers the prognosis of subarachnoidal bleedings from aneurysm, and enhances relapse risk.[9] Brain trauma, seizures, and concomitant liver disease related to alcohol abuse are additionally causative for higher incidence of acute cerebral hemorrhages or chronic sudural hematoma (Pachymeningeosis hemorrhagica interna).

Heavy drinking dramatically enhances the risk for ischemic disorders. Epidemiological investigations have demonstrated a positive correlation between the risk of hemorrhagic stroke and level of alcohol consumption, whereas ischemic stroke shows weaker relationships.[10]

Many chronic alcoholics have higher levels of blood pressure for several reasons. A daily consumption of 30 to 50 g alcohol elevates systolic and diastolic blood pressure significantly.[11] Pathological changes of plasma cortisol, renin, aldosteron, and vasopression levels, as well as changes of the adrenergic transmitter system also contribute. Alcohol intoxication as well as withdrawal or delirium tremens massively activate sympathetic events, provoking arterial hypertonia and cerebral vasospasm.[12] During withdrawal, alcoholics tend to be dehydrated with subsequent hemoconcentration. In addition, alcohol-induced hypertension and excess smoking among alcohol consumers enhance the risk of atherosclerosis. Heavy drinking is also associated with higher risk for cardioembolic ischemic stroke.[13] Other contributing factors are toxic thrombocytopenia, platelet dysfunction, abnormal fibrinogen molecules, excessive fibrinolysis, and direct toxic effects on vascular endothelium.

However, low amounts of alcohol, when taken on a regular basis, have been demonstrated to protect against cerebrovascular and cardiovascular disease.[14] Dose-dependent atherogenic and anti-atherogenic properties may constitute a main pathophysiological link between alcohol consumption and arterial disease.[15] Alcohol consumption less than once a week (occasional drinking) had no effect on atherogenesis. Light drinkers have a lower risk for incident carotid atherosclerosis (early atherogenesis) than heavy drinkers or abstainers. Moderate alcohol consumption (two drinks per day, 10 to 90 g weekly) was associated with a decreased risk of ischemic stroke in the elderly, while heavy alcohol consumption (>7 drinks per day, >300 g weekly) has deleterious effects. Protection offered by alcohol consumption of <50 g per day appeared to act through inhibition of the injurious action of high levels of LDL cholesterol, raise of HDL, and antithrombotic effects.

The data support the National Stroke Association Stroke Prevention Guidelines regarding the beneficial effects of moderate alcohol consumption. Despite these effects, it is notable that moderate alcohol consumption showed a tendency for increased risk of subarachnoidal hemorrhages[16] and that there may be ethnic differences in ethanol effects.[10]

CEREBELLAR ATROPHY

Some 30% of patients with chronic alcohol abuse develop cerebellar atrophy (atrophie cerebelleuse tardive a predomance corticale, Marie-Foix, 1922) beyond the fourth decade.[1,7] Cerebellar ataxia does not correlate with daily, annual, or lifetime consumption of ethanol; therefore, additional pathophysiological mechanisms besides direct neurotoxicity of alcohol are suggested, such as thiamine deficiency and/or electrolyte abnormalities.

The pathological hallmark is degeneration of Purkinje cells in the anterior and superior cerebellar vermis and in the cerebellar cortex.

Patients develop a slowly progressive cerebellar syndrome with gait- and standataxia, dysarthria, tremor, and nystagmus. According to the lesional topography (cerebellar vermis), lower limbs are more involved than upper. Final stages present with astasia and abasia.

Symptoms may be initially reversible in case of alcohol abstain, thiamine substitution, and physiotherapy.

ENCEPHALOPATHY AND DEMENTIA

Approximately 9% of chronic alcohol abusers have clinically manifest organic brain syndrome,[17] and up to 75% of detoxified long-term alcoholics show some degree of cognitive impairment.[18]

Alcoholic dementia is the second leading cause of adult dementia in the U.S., accounting for 10% of the cases. Wernicke encephalopathy accounts for the most cases of dementia in the western world.[2] In autopsy studies, 12.5% of diagnosed alcoholics have brain lesions characteristic for Wernicke-Korsakoff syndrome.

In 1881, Wernicke described an acute neurologic syndrome with ataxia, ophthalmoplegia, nystagmus, polyneuropathy, and a global confusional state. Shortly thereafter, Korsakoff described the chronic changes in mental status and memory he observed in patients with disorders involving polyneuropathy. Several years later (Gudden, 1896), it was realized that the symptoms described by Wernicke and Korsakoff often occur sequentially in the same patients and represent a syndrome now known as Wernicke-Korsakoff syndrome.

Long-term heavy alcohol consumption in combination with malnutrition, particularly thiamine deficiency, produces extensive brain pathology. The thiamine deficiency is primarily due to inadequate intake of vitamins, but impaired metabolism on the basis of a genetic predisposition also seems important.[3] Autopsied brain samples have been found to be severely and selectively deficient in thiamine-dependent enzymes.

Pathology consists of symmetrically punctate hemorrhagic lesions surrounding the third ventricle, aqueduct, fourth ventricle, mammillary bodies, dorsomedial thalamus, locus ceruleus, periaqueductal grey, ocular motor, and vestibular nuclei. Cerebellar changes with loss of Purkinje cells in the vermis are identical to changes found in cerebellar alcoholic degeneration.[2] Neocortical areas, especially the parietal and frontal lobes, are also involved.[19]

The typical patient shows the classical trio as of Wernicke's encephalopathy (Polioencephalitis hemorrhagica superior): mental disorder, gaze palsy, and ataxia. The onset is usually acute over hours or days in which the patient is disoriented, confused, and apathetic or somnolent. Oculomotor abnormalities are nystagmus, abducens, or conjugated horizontal gaze palsies and progress to complete external ophthalmoplegia. Gait ataxia is due to a combination of cerebellar involvement and polyneuropathy (in 82% of the cases).[2]

Once the acute confusion improves, 80% of patients present with some degree of ataxia and gaze palsy, and a severe amnesia, characteristic for Korsakoff syndrome. Patients behave passive, apathic, less affective, but the hallmark of the chronic stage is retro- and anterograde amnesia in the context of otherwise well-preserved cognitive functions. Some patients may evolve to the Korsakoff stage of the disorder without clinical evidence of an antecedent Wernicke's encephalopathy.

Diagnosis is made upon clinical and neuropsychological assessment. MRI demonstrates occasional diencephalic lesions, but in 80% a clear atrophy of the mammillary bodies.[20]

Wernicke's encephalopathy represents a neurological emergency because mortality in the acute phase ranges between 10 and 20%,[21] probably due to fatal midbrain hemorrhages. Treated adequately, neurological symptoms improve rapidly within hours to days. In addition, 46% of Korsakoff patients showed significant or complete recovery from their amnestic symptoms upon treatment.

Immediate treatment is urgently required: initially, 50 mg thiamine (vitamin B$_1$) i.v. and 50 mg thamin i.m., followed by 50 mg i.m. per day until the patient is able to perform regular nutrition. Administer additional multivitamin infusions. Parenteral thiamine application should be handled with care, because of rare anaphylactoid reactions.[22]

Hepatic encephalopathy develops in many alcoholics with liver disease and is characterized by mental alteration (psychosis, delirium, coma), frontal release signs, asterixis (flapping tremor), hyperreflexia, pyramidal signs, and occasional seizures. Patients may progress to coma and death, recover completely, or suffer recurrent or chronic episodes with dementia, dysarthria, ataxia, tremor, and choreoathetosis. Symptomatic treatment includes, among others, lactulose.

CENTRAL PONTINE AND EXTRAPONTINE MYELINOLYSIS

Although central pontine and extrapontine myelinolysis is not an exclusive disorder in alcoholics, it appears that alcoholic liver dysfunction seems to be a prerequisite. Pathophysiological mechanisms are still under debate; however, the main etiological event seems to be rapid substitution of hyponatremia with transient hypernatremia, which probably leads to osmotic damage of the vascular endothelium with release of myelinotoxic substances.[23]

The neuropathological hallmark is a triangular demyelination in the base of the pons. In addition, in 10% of the cases, extrapontine lesions are present in the grey matter of thalamus, putamen, and nucleus caudatus, as well as cerebellum and cerebral white matter.[24]

Usually, dramatic clinical symptoms occur with tetraparesis, bulbary symptoms (dysarthria and dysphagia), cerebellar ataxia, paresis of eye muscles, horizontal gaze palsy, pupillary palsy, central fever, and neurogenic bladder dysfunction. Severely affected patients may lapse to "locked-in" syndrome.

Central pontine and extrapontine myelinolysis has a poor prognosis, with a mortality of 75% and no specific treatment is available.

In light of the proposed etiology, it is recommended to treat hyponatremia very carefully. Sodium supplementation should not exceed 0.6 mmol l^{-1} per hour; the maximum daily dose is 12 mmol l^{-1}.[6] From a practical point of view, natrium substitution should be terminated at serum natrium levels of 121 to 134 mmol l^{-1}.

MOVEMENT DISORDERS

Extrapyramidal symptoms rarely occur as a sequel of chronic alcohol abuse. Transient choreiforme dyskinesias of head and limbs and Parkinson-like symptoms may occur during withdrawal of alcohol and usually reverse within weeks.[25] In rare cases, movement disorders follow pontine and especially extrapontine central myelinolysis.[26]

Another relation between alcohol and movement disorder regards essential tremor. A well-known feature of essential tremor is its dramatic suppression by small amounts of alcohol in some patients. However, the risk of tolerance and abuse makes the use of alcohol as a regular therapy for essential tremor unacceptable. On the other hand, the incidence of alcohol abuse in essential tremor is contradictory.

TOBACCO–ALCOHOL–AMBLYOPY

This bilateral demyelination of central parts of the optic nerve, chiasma opticum, and tractus opticus occurs in elderly malnourished patients with an incidence in 1 of 200 chronic alcoholics.[27]

Pathophysiology suggests cumulative neurotoxic effects of ethanol and tobacco. Tobacco smoke contains cyanides, which are insufficiently detoxified because of impaired liver function, resulting in optic nerve damage by free cyanides.[28]

Patients complain about progressive bilateral blurred vision and loss of vision. Clinical signs show bilateral central scotoma with preserved visual fields. The papilla appears initially normal; later, mild temporal pallor occurs. Visually evoked potentials are impaired.

Treatment includes alcohol and tobacco abstain and adequate nutrition with multivitamin supplementation. However, the prognosis remains poor.

MARCHIAFAVA-BIGNAMI SYNDROME

This is a very rare disorder in chronic alcoholics. *Intra vitam* clinical and radiological diagnosis is rare, more often neuropathologically postmortem. Pathology is characterized by necrosis of the corpus callosum, gliotic sclerosis of the cerebral cortex (Morell's laminar sclerosis), and histologically by diffuse chromatolysis of neurons as seen in neurological pellagra.[29,30]

Clinical symptoms and signs include initial confusion and/or clouding of consciousness, dementia, marked oppositional muscle tonus ("Gegenhalten"), seizures, spasticity, pyramidal signs, dysarthria, ataxia, astasia, and abasia. Some patients present with a syndrome called hemispheric disconnection, characterized by disassociation apraxia and dyslexia.[31]

The course is mainly acute progressive with coma and death, sometimes chronic with demented condition, and rarely with spontaneous regression. There is no treatment available.

ALCOHOL-RELATED MYELOPATHY

A progressive myelopathy with spastic paraparesis, paresthesia, and neurogenic bladder dysfunction is a rare complication of chronic alcohol abuse.

Pathology is characterized by axonomyelotropic damage and spinal tract degeneration.

Etiological factors include myelotoxicity of alcohol, malnutrition, and chronic liver disease. In case of alcohol abstain, multivitamin support, and neurorehabilitation, the prognosis is good.

SLEEP DISORDERS

Alcohol is frequently used to aid sleep (13% of adults)[32] but can also be a major cause of disruption of sleep architecture.[33]

The acute effects of alcohol include decreased latency to sleep onset, increased slow wave sleep, and decreased REM sleep during the first part of the night. During the second half of the night, REM sleep rebounds and sleep fragmentation occurs. Alcohol withdrawal is often accompanied by insomnia and may suborn the patient to continue drinking.

Alcohol consumption increases snoring; worsens sleep apnea by selective depression of genioglossal muscle activity, thus promoting upper-airway obstructive apnea; and may demask parasomnias, such as sleepwalking, enuresis, and nightmares.

In general, treatment of sleep disorders requires alcohol abstain to re-establish normal sleep behavior. Pharmacological treatment should avoid hypnotica or sedativa; low-dose tricyclic anti-depressants may be prescribed.

MYOPATHY, PERIPHERAL, AND AUTONOMIC NEUROPATHY

ALCOHOL-ASSOCIATED POLYNEUROPATHY

The incidence of alcohol-associated polyneuropathy[34,35] varies between 9 and 50%, and WHO studies suggest that after diabetes, alcohol is the second worldwide common cause for neuropathy. However, other authors warn that alcohol-induced polyneuropathy is commonly overdiagnosed, because of casually obtained patient histories and lack of detailed and intensive evaluation for other causes of polyneuropathy. Diagnosis of alcohol-associated neuropathy is suspicious if a well-nourished patient has no other organ manifestations of chronic alcohol abuse.

Chronic alcoholism and its association with peripheral nerve disease has been known for more than 200 years (Lettsom, 1787; Jackson, 1822): 100 ml ethanol per day for 3 years was the minimum amount consumed by neuropathic patients.[36] However, the pathophysiological mechanisms are still controversially discussed. Direct neurotoxic effects of alcohol, malnourishment, or both may contribute to development of damage of the peripheral nervous system.[35,36] Animal and cell culture studies failed to demonstrate a direct neurotoxic alcohol effect. On the other hand, the fact that most alcoholics with neuropathy do not improve with B vitamin substitution alone argues against a single vitamin deficiency.[36]

The typical patient with chronic alcohol abuse and neuropathy complains initially about distal, symmetric, burning, or stabbing pain in the feet. Sensory impairment progresses slowly to loss of all qualities of sensory function in a glove-and-stocking distribution. Disease progression is accompanied by painful palpation of muscles and tendons, and muscle weakness. Neurological examination provides signs of distal symmetric loss of function of sensory, motor, and autonomic fibers. Severity ranges from "burning feet" to rare cases with paraplegia and severe weakness of the upper limbs. Distal symmetric weakness and hyporeflexia occur in lower and then upper limbs as the neuropathy progresses. Gait ataxia reflects a combination of loss of joint position sense and concurrent cerebellar degeneration. Autonomic skin changes involve reddening, atrophy, hair loss, and hypohidrosis in the same distribution as the sensory loss.

Paraclinical investigations include laboratory, electrophysiological, and in rare instances neuropathological (nerve biopsy) studies. Laboratory tests exhibit common changes consistent with chronic liver disease. Chronic thiamine deficiency may be corroborated by the activity of the enzyme transketolase. Electrophysiological studies show reduction in amplitude of sensory nerve action potentials with relative preservation of conduction velocity and similar but lesser changes in compound muscle action potential amplitudes and motor nerve conduction velocities. F wave latencies of proximal motor conduction are normal. Electromyography shows typical signs of denervation. Electrophysiological changes are due to distal axonal degeneration of sensory and motor nerve fibers. Neuropathology of nerve biopsy indicates primary axonal degeneration, only scant segmental demyelination, and no signs of inflammation or vascular damage. Loss of dorsal root ganglion neurons and autonomic nerve fibers are also seen.

The major aim of treatment is withdrawal from alcohol consumption. Balanced and caloric nutrition, oral multivitamin support, and neuro-rehabilitation provide a good prognosis for recovery, although protracted over many months.

AUTONOMIC DISORDERS

A quarter of patients with high alcohol intake have various autonomic dysfunctions involving impairment of sympathetic and parasympathetic pathways.[37,38]

Usually early damage of parasympathetic fibers occurs. Impaired heart rate responses to Valsalva maneuver, deep breathing, change in posture and neck suction, as well as hoarseness and dysphagia are characteristics of severe alcoholic vagal neuropathy. Other possible manifestations of parasympathetic dysfunctions include impaired esophageal motility, abnormal pupillary reflexes, and impotence. Alcoholics with vagal neuropathy have an increased mortality rate related to autonomic cardiovascular dysfunction.

Postural hypotension is common in patients with Wernicke's encephalopathy and is the result of impaired sympathetic outflow at central or peripheral levels. Impaired thermoregulation, especially abnormal sweating responses (anhidrosis) may occur in alcoholic patients, providing evidence of involvement of postganglionic sympathetic fibers. In particular, patients with neuropathy complain about abnormal sweating. Alcohol is commonly considered to be a risk factor in the etiology of heatstroke, together with hypoglycemia, peripheral vasodilatation, impairment of behavioral thermoregulation, and misjudgment of low temperatures.

ALCOHOL-INDUCED MYOPATHIES

Alcohol affects both skeletal and cardiac muscles. The skeletal myopathies induced by alcohol abuse include subclinical, acute, chronic, and those associated with hypokalemia.[39-41] Myotoxic manifestations range from asymptomatic elevation of CK levels to fatal rhabdomyolysis. Prevalence rates are 0.8 to 3.3% for acute and hypokalemic myopathy, and 23 to 66% for chronic myopathy. Clinically important, alcohol is the most frequent drug causing rhabdomyolysis.

Several patho- and predisposing mechanisms are suggested. Muscle hyperactivity, such as epileptic seizures, cramps and physical muscle compression, and toxic vascular damage during malnutrition, cold exposure, and muscle compression may predispose for additional toxicity. Acute myopathy may result from direct toxic action of alcohol, potassium, phosphate, or magnesium depletion causing membrane instability, immune responses to acetaldehyde-protein complexes, or an increase in free radical production. Decreased actinomysin contractility, myosin ATPase activity, and calcium uptake by the sarcoplasmic reticulum are also potentially responsible.

Acute alcohol necrotizing myopathy[42] is an acute, painful myopathy with focal or general tenderness or swelling of involved muscles and often preceded by muscle cramps. Focal muscle swelling of the calf or leg may present as suggestive deep vein thrombosis. This myopathy is generally associated with chronic alcoholism exacerbated by a recent episode of unusually heavy drinking, vomiting, and diarrhea 1 to 2 days before myopathic complaints appear. Some 22% of alcoholics with liver disease had experienced acute myopathy. Blood examinations show a very marked increase in CK levels, as well as elevated LDH, aminotransferase, and aldolase levels. Myoglobinuria is responsible for brown-colored urine. Muscle biopsy show generalized fiber swelling, patchy segmental or diffuse necrosis, and hyalinization of single fibers. In general, symptoms are very mild, cramps usually resolve within 1 to 2 days, and pain, tenderness, swelling, and muscle strength improve within 1 to 2 weeks. However, acute rhabdomyolysis can be fatally masked or undiagnosed during delirium tremens. Tubular necrosis, acute renal failure, and other complications (massive muscle swellings, secondary hyperkalemia) may result. In this emergency, urgent hemodilution or faciotomy is necessary.

Alcoholic hypokalemic myopathy results from a combination of chronic alcoholism and hypokalemia/hypomagnesemia. Patients typically develop myopathic symptoms within hours to days and present severe areflexic proximal muscle weakness, sometimes muscle swellings, and marked increased CK levels. Usually, clinical symptoms do not include muscle pain, cramps, or tenderness. Following prompt potassium substitution, clinical symptoms completely resolve.[42]

Subclinical asymptomatic alcoholic myopathy involves patients with elevated CK levels, but no overt signs or symptoms of myopathy. However, some patients report previous muscle cramps or show tenderness on muscle palpation.

Chronic alcohol myopathy is a painless, slowly progressing myopathy with proximal muscle weakness and wasting, often associated with alcohol-related neuropathy. Clinically important, cardiomyopathy was found to be frequent in patients with chronic myopathy. Muscle strength is often restored within months after cessation of alcohol consumption.

REFERENCES

1. Charness, M.E., Clinical and pathologic overview of the brain disorders in alcoholics, *Alcohol-Induced Brain Damage*, Hunt, W.A., and Nixon, S.J., Eds., U.S. Department of Health and Human Services, Rockville, MD, 1993, 15.
2. Victor, M. and Adams, R.D., and Collins, G.H., *The Wernicke-Korsakoff Syndrome and Related Disorders to Alcoholism and Malnutrition*, F.A. Davies, Philadelphia, 1989.
3. Harper, C., The neuropathology of alcohol-specific brain damage, or does alcohol damage the brain? *J. Neuropath. Exp. Neurol.*, 57, 101, 1998.
4. Feuerlein, W., *Alkoholismus — Mißbrauch und Abhaengigkeit*, Thieme, Stuttgart, 1989.
5. Brust, J.C.M., Acute neurological complications of drug and alcohol abuse, *Neurologic Emergencies*, Feske, S.K. and Wen, P.Y., Eds., W.B. Saunders, Philadelphia, 1998, 503.
6. Thier P., Alkoholfolgekrankheiten, *Therapie und Verlauf neurologischer Erkrankungen*, Brandt, T., Dichgans, J., and Diner, H.C., Eds., Kohlhammer, Stuttgart, 1993, 841.
7. Victor, M., The effects of alcohol on the nervous system, *Medical Diagnosis and Treatment of Alcoholism*, Mendelson, J.H. and Mello, N.K., Eds., McGraw-Hill, New York, 1992, 201.
8. Victor, M. and Laureno, R., The neurologic complications of alcohol abuse: Epidemiologic aspects, *Advances in Neurology, Vol. 19. Neurological Epidemiology: Principles and Clinical Applications*, Schoenberg, B.S., Ed., Raven, New York, 1978, 603.
9. Juvela, S., Alcohol consumption as a risk factor for poor outcome after aneurysmal subarachnoidal hemorrhage, *Br. Med. J.*, 304, 1663, 1992.
10. Camargo, C.R., Moderate alcohol consumption and stroke: the epidemiological evidence, *Stroke*, 20, 1611, 1989.
11. Klatzky, A.L., Friedmann, G.D., Siegelaub, A.N., and Gerard, M.J., Alcohol consumption and blood pressure. Kaiser-Permanente multiphase health examination data, *N. Engl. J. Med.*, 296, 1194, 1977.
12. Calandre, L., Arenal, C., Fernandez Ortega, J., and Vallejo A., Risk factors for spontaneous cerebral hematomas. Case control study, *Stroke*, 17, 1226, 1986.
13. Hillbom, M., Juvela, S., and Karttunen, V., Mechanisms of alcohol-related strokes, *Novartis Foundation Symp.*, 216, 193, 1998.
14. Sacco, R.L., Elkind, M., and Boden-Albala, B., The protective effect of moderate alcohol consumption on ischemic stroke, *JAMA*, 281, 53, 1999.
15. Kiechl, S., Willeit, J., and Rungger, G., for the Bruneck Study Group, Alcohol consumption and artherosclerosis: What is the relation? Prospective results from the Bruneck Study, *Stroke*, 29, 900, 1998.
16. Stampfer, M.J., Colditz, G.A., Willett, W.C., Speizer, F.E., and Hennekens, C.H., A prospective study of moderate alcohol consumption and the risk of coronary disease and stroke in women, *N. Engl. J. Med.*, 319, 267, 1998.
17. Ekhardt, M.J. and Martin, P.R., Clinical assessment of cognition in alcoholism, *Alcohol. Clin. Exp. Res.*, 10, 123, 1986.
18. Verfaellie, M. and Cermak, L.S., Wernicke-Korsakoff and related nutritional disorders of the nervous system, *Behavioural Neurology and Neuropsychology*, Feinberg, T.E. and Farah, M.J., Eds., McGraw-Hill, New York, 1997, 606.
19. Kril, J.J., The cerebral cortex is damaged in chronic alcoholics, *Neuroscience*, 79, 983, 1997.
20. Charness, M.E. and DeLaPaz, R.L., Mammillary body atrophy in Wernicke encephalopathy: antemortem identification using MRI, *Ann. Neurol.*, 22, 595, 1987.
21. Reuler, J.B., Girard, D.E., and Cooney, T.G., Wernickes's encephalopathy, *N. Engl. J. Med.*, 312, 1035, 1985.
22. Thomson, A.D. and Cook, C.C., Parenteral thiamine and Wernicke's encephalopathy: the balance of risks and perception of concern, *Alcohol Alcohol.*, 32, 207, 1997.

23. Illowsky, B.P. and Laureno, R., Encephalopathy and myelinolysis after rapid correction of hyponatremia, *Brain*, 110, 855, 1987.

24. Wright, D.G., Laureno, R., and Victor, M., Pontine and extrapontine myelinolysis, *Brain*, 102, 361, 1979.

25. Neimann, J., Borg, S., and Wahlund, L.O., Parkinsonism and dyskenisias during ethanol withdrawal, *Br. J. Addict.*, 83, 437, 1988.

26. Seiser, A., Schwarz, S., Aichinger-Steiner, M.M., Funk, G., Schnider, P., and Brainin, M., Parkinsonism and dystonia in central pontine and extrapontine myelinolysis, *J. Neurol. Neurosurg. Psych.*, 65, 119, 1998.

27. Smiddy, W. and Green, W., Nutritional amblyopia, a histopathologic study with retrospective clinical correlation, *Graefes Arch. Ophthalm.*, 225, 321, 1987.

28. Aulhorn, E., Die Tabak-Alkohol-Amblyopie, *Der chronische Alkoholismus*, Schmied, H.W., Heimann, H., and Mayer, K., Eds., Gustav Fischer, Stuttgart, 1989, 163.

29. Serdaru, M., Hausser-Hauw, C., Laplane, D., Lhermitte, F., and Hauw, J.J., The clinical spectrum of alcoholic pellagra encephalopathy. A retrospective analysis of 22 cases studied pathologically, *Brain*, 111, 829, 1988.

30. Hauw, J.J., DeBaecque, C., Hausser-Hauw, C., and Serdaru, M., Chromatolysis in alcoholic encephalopathies. Pellagra-like changes in 22 cases, *Brain*, 111, 843, 1988.

31. Berek, K., Wagner, M., Chemelli, A.P., Aichner, F., and Benke, T., Hemispheric disconnection in Marchiafava-Bignami disease: clinical, neuropsychological and MRI findings, *J. Neurol. Sci.*, 123, 2, 1994.

32. Johnson, E.O., Roehrs, T., Roth, T., and Breslau, N., Epidemiology of alcohol and medication as aids to sleep in early adulthood, *Sleep*, 21, 178, 1998.

33. Obermeyer, W.H. and Benca, R.M., Effects of drugs on sleep, *Neurologic Clinics Vol. 14, Sleep Disorders II*, Aldrich, M.S., Ed., W.B. Saunders, Philadelphia, 1996, 827.

34. Windebank, A., Polyneuropathy due to nutritional deficiency and alcoholism, *Peripheral Neuropathy*, Dyck, P.J. and Thomas, P.L., Eds., W.B. Saunders, Philadelphia, 1993, 1310.

35. Shields, R.W., Alcoholic neuropathy, *Muscle Nerve*, 8, 183, 1985.

36. Behse, F. and Buchthal, F., Alcoholic neuropathy: clinical, electrophysiological, and biopsy findings, *Ann. Neurol.*, 2, 95, 1977.

37. Bannister, R. and Mathias, C.J., *Autonomic Failure. A Textbook of Clinical Disorders of the Autonomic Nervous System*, 3rd ed., Oxford University Press, Oxford, 1993.

38. Monforte, R., Estruch, R., Valls-Sole, J., Nicolas, J., Villalta, J., and Urbano-Marquez, A., Autonomic and peripheral neuropathies in patients with chronic alcoholism, *Arch. Neurol.*, 52, 45, 1995.

39. Carpenter, S. and Karpati, G., *Pathology of Skeletal Muscle*, Churchill Livingstone, New York, 1984.

40. Lane, R.J.M., Toxic and drug induced myopathies, *Handbook of Muscle Diseases*, Lane, R.J.M., Ed., Marcel Dekker, New York, 1996, 379.

41. George, K.K. and Pourmand, R., Toxic myopathies, *Neurologic Clinics Vol. 15, Acquired Neuromuscular Disease*, Pourmand, R., Ed., W.B. Saunders, Philadelphia, 1997, 731.

42. Hilton-Jones, D., Squier, M., and Taylor, D., Toxic and nutritional myopathies, *Metabolic Myopathies*, W.B. Saunders, Philadelphia, 1995, 203.

16 Liver

Rudolf E. Stauber, Michael Trauner, and Peter Fickert

OVERVIEW

Alcohol (ethanol) is directly hepatotoxic, as illustrated by epidemiologic data such as (1) the correlation between annual per capita alcohol consumption and the mortality from cirrhosis, or (2) the association of the relative risk for cirrhosis to daily alcohol consumption. The risk for cirrhosis appears to increase markedly above a threshold level of daily alcohol intake (80 g per day in men and 40 to 60 g per day in women).

Fatty liver is the most common and mildest form of alcoholic liver disease. However, with continued drinking, the development of liver cirrhosis may occur at a rate of ~2% per year. Alcoholic fatty liver is readily reversible under abstinence.

Alcoholic hepatitis develops only in about one fifth of heavy drinkers and carries a bad prognosis. Severe cases are characterized by jaundice, impairment of plasmatic coagulation, and/or hepatic encephalopathy. Glucocorticoids may interfere with self-perpetuating pathogenic immune reactions and have been shown to improve short-term survival in severe cases. Other therapeutic approaches include anabolic androgens, propylthiouracil, and insulin-glucagon infusions, none of which can be recommended for routine clinical use.

Alcoholic cirrhosis is an irreversible condition, although prognosis may be markedly improved by abstinence. Overlapping etiologies such as chronic hepatitis C may influence the clinical course to a great extent. Prognosis is conveniently determined by calculating the Child-Pugh score. Medical treatment with colchizine or hepatoprotective substances such as silymarin has no proven benefit. In case of hepatic decompensation, liver transplantation is an excellent treatment option in carefully selected patients.

EPIDEMIOLOGIC ASPECTS

Whereas the development of alcoholic liver disease was previously attributed to nutritional factors, it is now widely accepted to be directly related to hepatotoxicity of ethanol or its metabolites. Strong evidence for this assumption can be derived from epidemiologic studies.

ALCOHOL CONSUMPTION AND MORTALITY FROM LIVER CIRRHOSIS

In the U.S., liver cirrhosis was the ninth leading cause of death in 1988.[1] Deaths from liver cirrhosis dropped dramatically during the era of Prohibition and started to increase again after the repeal of Prohibition in 1933.[2] A similar relation between the availability of alcoholic beverages and the mortality from liver cirrhosis has been demonstrated in France during wine rationing in World War II.[3]

Annual per capita alcohol consumption varies widely among countries. In Europe, alcohol consumption is greater in Mediterranean than in Scandinavian countries. When alcohol consumption is plotted against mortality from liver cirrhosis (disregarding the fact that only about half of the cases of cirrhosis may be attributed to alcohol), a significant correlation is found (Figure 16.1).[3]

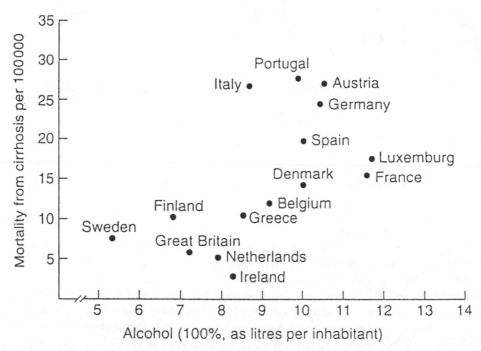

FIGURE 16.1 Relation between annual per capita alcohol consumption and mortality from cirrhosis in European countries. (From Salaspuro, M., *Oxford Textbook of Clinical Hepatology,* Oxford University Press, Oxford, 1999. With permission.)

ALCOHOL CONSUMPTION AND THE RISK FOR ALCOHOLIC LIVER DISEASE

Few studies have assessed the relation between the magnitude and/or duration of alcohol consumption and the risk for the development of alcoholic cirrhosis. In a German study, a linear relation was found between the proportion of cases with severe liver disease (alcoholic hepatitis or cirrhosis on liver histology) and the logarithm of life-long cumulative ethanol dose per kilogram body weight.[4] In a French study, patients with ascitic cirrhosis were compared with a randomly selected matched control population and an exponential increase of the relative risk for the development of cirrhosis was found with increased daily alcohol consumption (Figure 16.2).[5] For men, the risk was increased sixfold at 40 to 60 g per day and 14-fold at 60 to 80 g per day. In a subsequent study in women, the risk started to rise markedly at lower levels of alcohol intake (20 to 40 g per day).[6]

More recent data suggest that the risk for the development of cirrhosis is markedly increased above a threshold level of daily alcohol intake (80 g per day in men and 40 to 60 g per day in women), but is not further elevated by additional increments in alcohol consumption above this threshold.[7,8] In a case-control study, the relative risk for fatty liver was 50 for males consuming >80 g per day compared to males consuming <40 g per day; the risk was 8.5 for females consuming >60 g per day compared to females consuming <20 g per day.[7] In an autopsy study in 210 males, daily ingestion of 40 to 80 g of ethanol increased relative liver weight and the frequency of fatty liver, whereas the risk for bridging fibrosis and liver cirrhosis was increased only when daily ingestion exceeded 80 g.[8] Amounts of ethanol exceeding 80 g per day did not relate to further increases in the incidence of bridging fibrosis or cirrhosis. It was suggested that the risk for fibrotic liver lesions is increased above a permissive threshold level but is not directly dose related.[8] In a case-control study, the risk of hepatic decompensation was increased at a daily alcohol consumption of >125 g, but was not related to the duration of alcohol intake.[9]

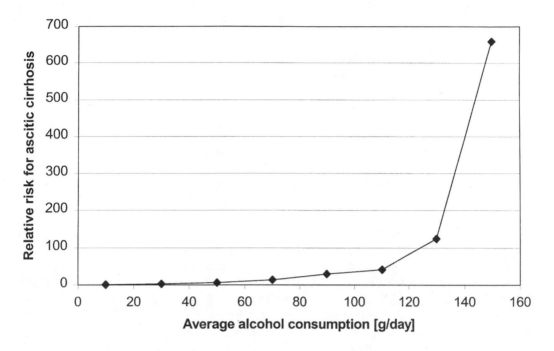

FIGURE 16.2   Relative risk for ascitic cirrhosis increases exponentially with average daily alcohol consumption. (Modified from Pequignot, G., Tuyns, A.J., and Berta, J.L., *Int. J. Epidemiol.*, 7, 113, 1978.)

ALCOHOLIC FATTY LIVER

CLINICAL FEATURES

Fatty liver is the most common alcohol-induced hepatic disorder. As symptoms are usually absent, alcoholic fatty liver is frequently detected by chance during a routine check-up, when elevated liver enzymes or an enlarged liver are noted. If abdominal symptoms are present, they are mostly related to concomitant gastritis and/or pancreatitis. Liver percussion may reveal marked hepatomegaly. Occasionally, fatty liver is complicated by icterus due to intrahepatic cholestasis or hemolysis (Zieve's syndrome).

DIAGNOSIS

Imaging Procedures

Ultrasound shows a characteristic, diffuse hyperechoic pattern. CT scan is indicated if sonographic pattern is inhomogeneous or in case of focal non-steatosis.

Laboratory Findings

Biochemical markers of chronically elevated alcohol consumption are often present, such as a marked elevation of gamma-glutamyl transpeptidase (γ-GT),[10] or macrocytosis with a mean cellular volume (MCV) >100 fl.[11] A ratio of aspartate aminotransferase (AST) to alanine aminotransferase (ALT) of >2 was found in 70% of patients with alcoholic liver disease, but also occurred in 26% of patients with postnecrotic cirrhosis.[12] A significant fall of γ-GT and/or MCV values during

TABLE 16.1
Diagnostic Accuracy of Biochemical Alcohol Markers in Patients with Liver Disease

Author	Year		γ-GT	MCV	CDT
Bell[15]	1993	Sensitivity	85%	70%	61%
		Specificity	18%	66%	92%
Stauber[16]	1995	Sensitivity	83%	45%	85%
		Specificity	16%	85%	83%
Radosavljevic[17]	1995	Sensitivity	89%	58%	90%
		Specificity	13%	79%	73%

admission may be considered as strong evidence for preceding alcohol abuse.[13] Carbohydrate-deficient transferrin (CDT) has been established as a rather sensitive and specific marker of chronically elevated alcohol consumption.[14] When CDT was evaluated in patients with chronic liver disease, its diagnostic accuracy, although far from ideal, proved to be superior to that of γ-GT or MCV (Table 16.1).[15-17]

Histology

Liver biopsy may help to discriminate alcoholic from non-alcoholic fatty liver. Histology usually reveals microvesicular steatosis, which initially shows a predominantly centrizonal, later pan-lobular distribution.[18] The presence of megamitochondria suggests recent alcohol intake.[19] Signs of alcoholic hepatitis, advanced fibrosis, and/or central vein sclerosis indicate an increased risk for the development of liver cirrhosis.[20] In a prospective study of 258 alcohol-abusing men, cirrhosis developed during a follow-up of 10 to 13 years at a rate of 2% per year.[21]

Differential Diagnosis

Fatty liver unrelated to alcohol consumption is frequently observed in patients with obesity, diabetes mellitus, or hyperlipidemia. In icteric cases with intrahepatic cholestasis, it has to be delineated from alcoholic hepatitis, which carries a much worse prognosis.

TREATMENT

Alcoholic fatty liver is readily reversible under abstinence. Hepatoprotective agents (see below) have been propagated as adjuvant treatment in toxic liver disease. In a double-blind study in 97 patients with predominantly alcoholic liver disease, silymarin administered for 4 weeks was found to accelerate the decline of liver enzymes.[22]

ALCOHOLIC HEPATITIS

CLINICAL FEATURES

As opposed to alcoholic steatosis, only ~20% of heavy drinkers develop alcoholic hepatitis. The reason for this variable susceptibility of the liver to alcoholic injury is unknown. Genetic variations in alcohol oxidizing enzymes may predispose individuals to alcoholism but do not appear to influence the development of advanced liver disease to a significant extent.[23]

Alcoholic hepatitis is characterized by jaundice, tender hepatomegaly, nausea, anorexia, fever, and leucocytosis. The clinical picture of patients with histological features of alcoholic hepatitis varies widely. Severe icteric cases with coagulopathy and/or hepatic encephalopathy have a poor prognosis. Often, acute alcoholic hepatitis is superimposed upon pre-existing chronic alcoholic liver disease.

DIAGNOSIS

Imaging Procedures

Ultrasound may reveal normal or diffuse hyperechoic pattern as in fatty liver, or may show signs of liver cirrhosis such as altered shape of the liver or signs of portal hypertension. Ultrasonographic demonstration of a "pseudoparallel channel sign," which corresponds to dilated hepatic arterial and adjacent portal venous branches, was reported to be an accurate diagnostic feature of acute alcoholic hepatitis.[24]

Laboratory Findings

Along with the alterations observed in alcoholic fatty liver (see above), hyperbilirubinemia, prolonged prothrombin time, and/or leucocytosis may be present. As opposed to acute viral hepatitis, aminotransferases are only moderately elevated, mostly with an AST:ALT ratio >2.

Histology

Liver biopsy usually yields a typical picture; however, in severe cases, it is often precluded by impaired coagulation. Alcoholic hepatitis is characterized by microvesicular steatosis, ballooning of hepatocytes, Mallory bodies, neutrophil infiltrations, and sclerosing hyaline necrosis.[18] Mallory bodies are typical for alcoholic hepatitis, but not pathognomonic. Advanced fibrosis or cirrhotic transformation is frequently present on liver histology at the time of presentation.

Differential Diagnosis

Non-alcoholic steatohepatitis (NASH) is a relatively new disease entity that cannot be discerned from alcoholic hepatitis on liver histology.[25] The most important risk factors for the development of NASH are obesity and diabetes mellitus; diagnosis is based on the exclusion of alcohol abuse by clinical and biochemical assessment. Another differential diagnosis that may be difficult to delineate in cases with superimposed infections is intrahepatic cholestasis of sepsis.

Prognosis

Severity of alcoholic hepatitis is reflected by hyperbilirubinemia, prolonged prothrombin time, and the development of hepatic encephalopathy. A prognostic score including these variables, termed "discriminant function," has been designed by Maddrey et al:[26]

$$\text{Discriminant function} = 4.6 \, (\text{Prothrombin time} - \text{Control time[s]}) + \text{Serum bilirubin [mg dL}^{-1}]$$

A discriminant function >32 and/or spontaneous hepatic encephalopathy denotes severe alcoholic hepatitis with a mortality of ~35% after 1 month.

TREATMENT

Given the significant mortality of alcoholic hepatitis, numerous therapeutic approaches have been investigated, such as corticosteroids, anabolic androgens, propylthiouracil, insulin-glucagon infusions, and various nutritional regimes.[26-36]

TABLE 16.2
Randomized Controlled Trials of Prednisolone
Treatment in Severe Alcoholic Hepatitis

Author	Year	Follow-up	Mortality: Prednisolone	Mortality: Placebo
Carithers[27]	1989	4 weeks	6%[a]	35%
Ramond[28]	1992	2 months	12%[a]	55%
Mathurin[29]	1996	1 year	31%[a]	59%
		2 years	54%	59%

[a] $p < 0.05$ vs. placebo.

Glucocorticoids

Glucocorticoids are thought to interfere with self-perpetuating immunologic mechanisms underlying the inflammatory process, that may be triggered by acetaldehyde adducts. More than 10 randomized clinical trials using prednisolone or methylprednisolone were performed, with variable results. When only trials including *severe* cases of alcoholic hepatitis (discriminant function >32 and/or spontaneous hepatic encephalopathy) are considered, methylprednisolone seems to have a beneficial effect, at least on short-term mortality (Table 16.2).[27-29]

Anabolic Androgens

Anabolic steroids might exert beneficial effects in patients with alcoholic liver disease through stimulation of protein synthesis. In a VA multicenter trial, male patients with alcoholic hepatitis (moderate, n = 132; severe, n = 131) were randomized to a glucocorticoid (prednisolone), an anabolic steroid (oxandrolone), or a placebo. Neither prednisolone nor oxandrolone significantly altered short-term survival at 30 days. Interestingly, oxandrolone reduced 6-month mortality in patients with moderately severe alcoholic hepatitis surviving the first 30 days. No such beneficial effect of oxandrolone was observed in patients with severe alcoholic hepatitis.[30]

Propylthiouracil

The rationale for using thyreostatic drugs in alcoholic liver disease is their ability to reduce the hepatic hypermetabolic state induced by ethanol. In a Canadian double-blind, randomized clinical trial, 310 patients with alcoholic liver disease of varying severity were investigated.[31] Propylthiouracil treatment significantly reduced the overall mortality rate after 2 years from 25 to 13%; in a subgroup of 160 patients with alcoholic hepatitis, mortality was reduced from 30 to 13%. A high drop-out rate of 63% was noted.

Insulin–Glucagon Infusions

Hepatic regeneration is in part under the control of hepatotrophic hormones, insulin, and glucagon. Therefore, combined infusion of insulin and glucagon has been studied in patients with alcoholic hepatitis. In a randomized study of 66 patients with alcoholic hepatitis, insulin–glucagon infusions significantly improved serum bilirubin and prothrombin time and reduced the 21-day mortality rate from 42 to 15%.[32] In contrast, in a later sequential trial, no effect on 4-week mortality rate by insulin–glucagon infusions was found in 44 patients with severe alcoholic hepatitis.[33] This treatment may be complicated by life-threatening hypoglycemia.

Nutritional Regimes

Patients with alcoholic liver disease were found to ingest approximately 50% of their calories as alcohol and thus exhibit significant protein-calorie malnutrition.[34] Therefore, it appears feasible to provide nutritional support to these patients. Various oral and parenteral nutritional regimes have been investigated in patients with alcoholic hepatitis. In 64 patients with acute alcoholic hepatitis, oral supplementation with protein or branched-chain amino acids neither affected nutritional parameters nor short-term mortality (38 vs. 32%).[35] In 54 patients with severe alcoholic hepatitis, parenteral administration of a standard amino acid solution improved nitrogen balance and prothrombin time, but again did not change short-term mortality (21 vs. 19%) or long-term mortality at 2 years (42 vs. 38%).[36]

ALCOHOLIC CIRRHOSIS

CLINICAL FEATURES

The prevalence of alcoholic cirrhosis has been underestimated due to frequent underreporting of an alcoholic etiology in death certificates. On the other hand, overlap with other etiologies of chronic liver disease may be present, such as chronic hepatitis B or C, or hemochromatosis. In particular, synergistic liver injury by alcohol and hepatitis C may lead to an accelerated course of chronic liver disease with early decompensation.[37,38]

Skin alterations such as spider angiomata or palmar erythema are frequently present. Tense ascites, subcutaneous collaterals (*caput medusae*), frank malnutrition, and various degrees of hepatic encephalopathy are typical signs of decompensated cirrhosis. The clinical course may be further complicated by bleeding from esophageal varices, infections such as spontaneous bacterial peritonitis, or the development of hepatocellular carcinoma.

DIAGNOSIS

Imaging Procedures

Ultrasound and CT scan demonstrate signs of advanced liver disease (nodular transformation of the liver) and/or portal hypertension (splenomegaly, venous collaterals, ascites). Upper GI endoscopy may reveal esophagogastric varices.

Laboratory Findings

As compared with alcoholic hepatitis, hyperbilirubinemia is less marked, but hepatic synthetic function is further diminished as reflected by decreased levels of albumin and pseudocholinesterase. Leuco- and thrombopenia are present in cases with portal hypertension as a consequence of splenomegaly and pooling.

Histology

Typically, a micronodular cirrhotic transformation is present (Laennec's cirrhosis).[18] Signs of residual alcoholic hepatitis may be present in cases with recent alcohol abuse.

Differential Diagnosis

Overlapping etiologies of chronic liver disease should be sought by appropriate laboratory tests. Positive serology indicates chronic hepatitis B or C, and elevated serum ferritin levels point to hemochromatosis. In many cases, liver biopsy is necessary to confirm or rule out these concomitant disorders.

TABLE 16.3
Child-Pugh Classification of Chronic Liver Disease

Score[a]	1	2	3
Bilirubin (mg dL^{-1})	<2	2–3	>3
Albumin (g dL^{-1})	>3.5	2.8–3.5	<2.8
Prothrombin time (s prolonged)	<4	4-6	>6
Ascites	Absent	Slight	Moderate
Hepatic encephalopathy (grade)	0	1-2	3-4

[a] Total score   Child's class
       5–6   A
       7–9   B
      10–15   C

Note: See Pugh, R.N., Murray-Lyon, I.M., Dawson, J.L., Pietroni, M.C., and Williams, R., Transection of the oesophagus for bleeding oesophageal varices, *Br. J. Surg.*, 60, 646, 1973.

Prognosis

Prognosis in patients with liver cirrhosis may be estimated using the Child-Pugh score, which is composed of simple biochemical and clinical parameters (Table 16.3).[39] Validation of this score with regard to 1-year survival yielded high sensitivity and specificity of 78% and 83%, respectively.[40] Sophisticated quantitative liver function tests, such as galactose elimination capacity or the indocyanine green clearance, had no advantage over the Child-Pugh score for assessing prognosis in liver cirrhosis.[41] Another less-cumbersome test, which measures the formation of monoethylglicinexylidide (MEGX) from lidocaine, has been reported to contain additional prognostic information independent from the Child-Pugh score.[42]

The overall probability of decompensation in patients with initially compensated cirrhosis has been reported to be 58% after 10 years.[43] The prognosis is significantly modulated by the amount of ongoing alcohol abuse. For example, in compensated cirrhotics, 5-year survival was found to be 63% in patients with continued alcohol abuse, but 89% in abstainers.[44]

MEDICAL TREATMENT OF ALCOHOLIC CIRRHOSIS

Colchizine

Experimental evidence exists that colchizine, an inhibitor of collagen synthesis, may prevent hepatic fibrogenesis and thus be beneficial in the treatment of liver cirrhosis. Mexican investigators performed a long-term placebo-controlled trial in 100 patients with liver cirrhosis of various etiologies and found a significant improvement in median survival in the colchizine-treated group from 3.5 to 11 years.[45] However, the results of this study have been questioned since irregularities in the randomization process were suspected (the baseline serum albumin was significantly higher in the verum group). Consequently, this substance has not become popular for treatment of either alcoholic or non-alcoholic liver cirrhosis.

"Hepatoprotective" Substances

Silymarin, an extract from the fruit of the milk thistle (*Silibum marianum*), contains several putative hepatoprotective flavonoids that are believed to act as free-radical scavengers. This drug has been licensed for treatment of toxic liver disease in some European countries, although its efficacy remains controversial. To date, two randomized placebo-controlled trials have assessed the effect of silymarin in alcoholic liver cirrhosis. The first trial, conducted in Austria in 170 cirrhotic patients (61% alcoholic), observed a slight trend toward increased survival in the verum group, which was significant only in a subgroup of well-compensated patients with alcoholic cirrhosis.[46] A second Spanish trial in 200 patients with alcoholic cirrhosis found no difference at all in survival for silymarin- and placebo-treated patients.[47]

Other substances with hepatoprotective effects in experimental studies include S-adenosyl-L-methionine,[48] polyunsaturated phosphatidylcholine,[49] and ursodeoxycholic acid.[50] These substances have not been assessed in controlled clinical trials.

Total Enteral Nutrition

In a study of 35 severely malnourished cirrhotics, enteral tube feeding of 2115 kcal per day as compared to an isocaloric standard hospital diet increased serum albumin levels, reduced septic complications, and improved in-hospital mortality (12 vs. 47%).[51]

LIVER TRANSPLANTATION

Liver transplantation is a highly effective treatment for decompensated alcoholic cirrhosis, provided that patients are selected carefully. Recidivism after liver transplantation has been reported in 11.5%[52] up to 31%[53] of patients, but survival was not different from non-alcoholic cirrhosis. Besides, compliance with immunosuppressive regimens was good and rejection episodes were infrequent in patients transplanted for alcoholic cirrhosis. It should be stressed that pre-transplant abstinence for at least 6 months is of utmost importance for obtaining good results.[54,55]

REFERENCES

1. Dufour, M.C., Stinson, F.S., and Caces, M.F., Trends in cirrhosis morbidity and mortality: United States, 1979–1988, *Sem. Liver. Dis.*, 13, 109, 1993.
2. DeBakey, S.F., Stinson, F.S., Grant, B.F., and Dufour, M.C., *Liver Cirrhosis Mortality in the United States, 1970–1992*, Surveillance Report No. 37, National Institute on Alcohol Abuse and Alcoholism, Division of Biometry and Epidemiology, Alcohol Epidemiologic Data System, Rockville, MD, 1995.
3. Salaspuro, M., Epidemiological aspects of alcoholic liver disease, ethanol metabolism, and pathogenesis of alcoholic liver injury, *Oxford Textbook of Clinical Hepatology*, Bircher, J., Benhamou, J.P., McIntire, N., Rizzetto, M., and Rodes, J., Eds., Oxford University Press, Oxford, 1999, 1157.
4. Lelbach, W.K., Cirrhosis in the alcoholic and its relation to the volume of alcohol abuse, *Ann. N.Y. Acad. Sci.*, 252, 85, 1975.
5. Pequignot, G., Tuyns, A.J., and Berta, J.L., Ascitic cirrhosis in relation to alcohol consumption, *Int. J. Epidemiol.*, 7, 113, 1978.
6. Tuyns, A.J. and Pequignot, G., Greater risk of ascitic cirrhosis in females in relation to alcohol consumption, *Int. J. Epidemiol.*, 13, 53, 1984.
7. Coates, R.A., Halliday, M.L., Rankin, J.G., Feinman, S.V., and Fisher, M.M., Risk of fatty infiltration or cirrhosis of the liver in relation to ethanol consumption: a case-control study, *Clin. Invest. Med.*, 9, 26, 1986.
8. Savolainen, V.T., Liesto, K., Mannikko, A., Penttila, A., and Karhunen, P.J., Alcohol consumption and alcoholic liver disease: evidence of a threshold level of effects of ethanol, *Alcohol. Clin. Exp. Res.*, 17, 1112, 1993.
9. Arico, S., Galatola, G., Tabone, M., Corrao, G., Torchio, P., Valenti, M., and De la Pierre, M., The measure of life-time alcohol consumption in patients with cirrhosis: reproducibility and clinical relevance, *Liver*, 15, 202, 1995.
10. Rosalki, S.B. and Rau, D., Serum γ-glutamyl transpeptidase activity in alcoholism, *Clin. Chim. Acta*, 39, 41, 1972.

11. Morgan, M.Y., Camilo, M.E., Luck, W., Sherlock, S., and Hoffbrand, A.V., Macrocytosis in alcohol-related liver disease: its value for screening, *Clin. Lab. Haematol.*, 3, 35, 1981.

12. Cohen, J.A. and Kaplan, M.M., The SGOT/SGPT ratio — an indicator of alcoholic liver disease, *Dig. Dis. Sci.*, 24, 835, 1979.

13. Pol, S., Poynard, T., Bedossa, P., Naveau, S., Aubert, A., and Chaput, J.C., Diagnostic value of serum gamma-glutamyl-transferase activity and mean corpuscular volume in alcoholic patients with or without cirrhosis, *Alcohol. Clin. Exp. Res.*, 14, 250, 1990.

14. Stibler, H., Carbohydrate-deficient transferrin in serum — a new marker of potentially harmful alcohol consumption reviewed, *Clin. Chem.*, 37, 2029, 1991.

15. Bell, H., Tallaksen, C., Sjaheim, T., Weberg, R., Raknerud, N., Orjasaeter, H., Try, K., and Haug, E., Serum carbohydrate-deficient transferrin as a marker of alcohol consumption in patients with chronic liver diseases, *Alcohol. Clin. Exp. Res.*, 17, 246, 1993.

16. Stauber, R.E., Stepan, V., Trauner, M., Wilders-Truschnig, M., Leb, G., and Krejs, G.J., Evaluation of carbohydrate-deficient transferrin for detection of alcohol abuse in patients with liver dysfunction, *Alcohol Alcohol.*, 30, 171, 1995.

17. Radosavljevic, M., Temsch, E., Hammer, J., Pfeffel, F., Mayer, G., Renner, F., Pidlich, J., and Mueller, C., Elevated levels of serum carbohydrate deficient transferrin are not specific for alcohol abuse in patients with liver disease, *J. Hepatol.*, 23, 706, 1995.

18. French, S.W., Nash, J., Shitabata, P., Kachi, K., Hara, C., Chedid, A., Mendenhall, C.L. and the VA Cooperative Study Group 119, Pathology of alcoholic liver disease, *Semin. Liver Dis.*, 13, 154, 1993.

19. Bruguera, M., Bertran, A., Bombi, J.A., and Rodes, J., Giant mitochondria in hepatocytes: a diagnostic hint for alcoholic liver disease, *Gastroenterology*, 73, 1383, 1977.

20. Sorensen, T.I.A., Bentsen, K.D., Eghoje, K., Orholm, M., Hoybye, G., and Christoffersen, P., Prospective evaluation of alcohol abuse and alcoholic liver injury in men as predictors of development of cirrhosis, *Lancet*, ii, 241, 1984.

21. Marbet, U.A., Bianchi, L., Meury, U., and Stalder, G.A., Longterm histological evaluation of the natural history and prognostic factors of alcoholic liver disease, *J. Hepatol.*, 4, 364, 1987.

22. Salmi, H.A. and Sarna, S., Effect of silymarin on chemical, functional, and morphological alterations of the liver: a double-blind controlled study, *Scand. J. Gastroenterol.*, 17, 517, 1982.

23. Crabb, D.W., Ethanol oxidizing enzymes: roles in alcohol metabolism and alcoholic liver disease, *Prog. Liver Dis.*, 13, 151, 1995.

24. Sumino, Y., Kravetz, D., Kanel, G.C., McHutchison, J.G., and Reynolds, T.B., Ultrasonographic diagnosis of acute alcoholic hepatitis 'pseudoparallel channel sign' of intrahepatic artery dilatation, *Gastroenterology*, 105, 1477, 1993.

25. Diehl, A.M., Goodman, Z., and Ishak, K.G., Alcohollike liver disease in nonalcoholics: a clinical and histologic comparison with alcohol-induced liver injury, *Gastroenterology*, 95, 1056, 1988.

26. Maddrey, W.C., Boitnott, J.K., Bedine, M.S., Weber, F.L., Mezey, E., and White, R.I., Corticosteroid therapy of alcoholic hepatitis, *Gastroenterology*, 75, 193, 1978.

27. Carithers, R.L., Herlong, H.F., Diehl, A.M., Shaw, E.W., Combes, B., Fallon, H.J., and Maddrey, W.C., Methylprednisolone therapy in patients with severe alcoholic hepatitis: a randomized multicenter trial, *Ann. Intern. Med.*, 110, 685, 1989.

28. Ramond, M.J., Poynard, T., Rueff, B., Mathurin, P., Theodore, C., Chaput, J.C., and Benhamou, J.P., A randomized trial of prednisolone in patients with severe alcoholic hepatitis, *N. Engl. J. Med.*, 326, 507, 1992.

29. Mathurin, P., Duchatelle, V., Ramond, M.J., Degott, C., Bedossa, P., Erlinger, S., Benhamou, J.P., Chaput, J.C., Rueff, B., and Poynard, T., Survival and prognostic factors in patients with severe alcoholic hepatitis treated with prednisolone, *Gastroenterology*, 110, 1847, 1996.

30. Mendenhall, C.L., Anderson, S., Garcia-Pont, P., Goldberg, S., Kiernan, T., Seeff, L.B., Sorrell, M., Tamburro, C., Weesner, R., Zetterman, R., et al., Short-term and long-term survival in patients with alcoholic hepatitis treated with oxandrolone and prednisolone, *N. Engl. J. Med.*, 311, 1464, 1984.

31. Orrego, H., Blake, J.E., Blendis, L.M., Compton, K.V., and Israel, Y., Long-term treatment of alcoholic liver disease with propylthiouracil, *N. Engl. J. Med.*, 317, 1421, 1987.

32. Feher, J., Cornides, A., Romany, A., Karteszi, M., Szalay, L., Gogl, A., and Picazo, J., A prospective multicenter study of insulin and glucagon infusion therapy in acute alcoholic hepatitis, *J. Hepatol.*, 5, 224, 1987.

33. Trinchet, J.C., Balkau, B., Poupon, R.E., Heintzmann, F., Callard, P., Gotheil, C., Grange, J.D., Vetter, D., Pauwels, A., Labadie, H., et al., Treatment of severe alcoholic hepatitis by infusion of insulin and glucagon: a multicenter sequential trial, *Hepatology*, 15, 76, 1992.

34. Mezey, E., Kolman, C.J., Diehl, A.M., Mitchell, M.C., and Herlong, H.F., Alcohol and dietary intake in the development of chronic pancreatitis and liver disease in alcoholism, *Am. J. Clin. Nutr.*, 48, 148, 1988.

35. Calvey, H., Davis, M., and Williams, R., Controlled trial of nutritional supplementation, with and without branched chain amino acid enrichment, in treatment of acute alcoholic hepatitis, *J. Hepatol.*, 1, 141, 1985.

36. Mezey, E., Caballeria, J., Mitchell, M.C., Pares, A., Herlong, H.F., and Rodes, J., Effect of parenteral amino acid supplementation on short-term and long-term outcomes in severe alcoholic hepatitis: a randomized controlled trial, *Hepatology*, 14, 1090, 1991.

37. Pares, A., Barrera, J.M., Caballeria, J., Ercilla, G., Bruguera, M., Caballeria, L., Castillo, R., and Rodes, J., Hepatitis C virus antibodies in chronic alcoholic patients: association with severity of liver injury, *Hepatology*, 12, 1295, 1990.

38. Marsano, L.S. and Pena, L.R., The interaction of alcoholic liver disease and hepatitis C, *Hepatogastroenterology*, 45, 331, 1998.

39. Pugh, R.N., Murray-Lyon, I.M., Dawson, J.L., Pietroni, M.C., and Williams, R., Transection of the oesophagus for bleeding oesophageal varices, *Br. J. Surg.*, 60, 646, 1973.

40. Infante-Rivard, C., Esnaola, S., and Villeneuve, J.P., Clinical and statistical validity of conventional prognostic factors in predicting short-term survival among cirrhotics, *Hepatology*, 7, 660, 1987.

41. Albers, I., Hartmann, H., Bircher, J., and Creutzfeldt, W., Superiority of the Child-Pugh classification to quantitative liver function tests for assessing prognosis of liver cirrhosis, *Scand. J. Gastroenterol.*, 24, 269, 1989.

42. Arrigoni, A., Gindro, T., Aimo, G., Cappello, N., Meloni, A., Benedetti, P., Molino, G.P., Verme, G., and Rizzetto, M., Monoethylglicinexylidide test: a prognostic indicator of survival in cirrhosis, *Hepatology*, 20, 383, 1994.

43. Gines, P., Quintero, E., Arroyo, V., Teres, J., Bruguera, M., Rimola, A., Caballeria, J., Rodes, J., and Rozman, C., Compensated cirrhosis: natural history and prognostic factors, *Hepatology*, 7, 122, 1987.

44. Powell, W.J. and Klatskin, G., Duration of survival in patients with Laennec's cirrhosis: influence of alcohol withdrawal, and possible effects of recent changes in general management of the disease, *Am. J. Med.*, 44, 406, 1968.

45. Kershenobich, D., Vargas, F., Garcia-Tsao, G., Perez Tamayo, R., Gent, M., and Rojkind, M., Colchicine in the treatment of cirrhosis of the liver, *N. Engl. J. Med.*, 318, 1709, 1988.

46. Ferenci, P., Dragosics, B., Dittrich, H., Frank, H., Benda, L., Lochs, H., Meryn, S., Base, W., and Schneider, B., Randomized controlled trial of silymarin treatment in patients with cirrhosis of the liver, *J. Hepatol.*, 9, 105, 1989.

47. Pares, A., Planas, R., Torres, M., Caballeria, J., Viver, J.M., Acero, D., Panes, J., Rigau, J., Santos, J., and Rodes, J., Effects of silymarin in alcoholic patients with cirrhosis of the liver: results of a controlled, double-blind, randomized and multicenter trial, *J. Hepatol.*, 28, 615, 1998.

48. Lieber, C.S., Casini, A., DeCarli, L.M., Kim, C.I., Lowe, N., Sasaki, R., and Leo, M.A., S-adenosyl-L-methionine attenuates alcohol-induced liver injury in the baboon, *Hepatology*, 11, 165, 1990.

49. Lieber, C.S., Robins, S.J., Li, J., DeCarli, L.M., Mak, K.M., Fasulo, J.M., and Leo, M.A., Phosphatidylcholine protects against fibrosis and cirrhosis in the baboon, *Gastroenterology*, 106, 152, 1994.

50. Neuman, M.G., Cameron, R.G., Shear, N.H., Bellentani, S., and Tiribelli, C., Effect of tauroursodeoxycholic and ursodeoxycholic acid on ethanol-induced cell injuries in the human HepG2 cell line, *Gastroenterology*, 109, 555, 1995.

51. Cabre, E., Gonzalez-Huix, F., Abad-Lacruz, A., Esteve, M., Acero, D., Fernandez-Banares, F., Xiol, X., and Gassull, M.A., Effect of total enteral nutrition on the short-term outcome of severely malnourished cirrhotics: a randomized controlled trial, *Gastroenterology*, 98, 715, 1990.

52. Kumar, S., Stauber, R.E., Gavaler, J.S., Basista, M.H., Dindzans, V.J., Schade, R.R., Rabinovitz, M., Tarter, R.E., Gordon, R., Starzl, T.E., and Van Thiel, D.H., Orthotopic liver transplantation for alcoholic liver disease, *Hepatology*, 11, 159, 1990.

53. Berlakovich, G.A., Steininger, R., Herbst, F., Barlan, M., Mittlboeck, M., and Muehlbacher, F., Efficacy of liver transplantation for alcoholic cirrhosis with respect to recidivism and compliance, *Transplantation*, 58, 560, 1994.

54. Lucey, M.R., Merion, R.M., Henley, K.S., Campbell, D.A., Turcotte, J.G., Nostrant, T.T., Blow, F.C., and Beresford, T.P., Selection for and outcome of liver transplantation in alcoholic liver disease, *Gastroenterology*, 102, 1736, 1992.

55. Lucey, M.R. and Beresford, T.P., Alcoholic liver disease: to transplant or not to transplant? *Alcohol Alcohol.*, 27, 103, 1992.

17 Gastrointestinal System and Pancreas

Rudolf E. Stauber, Michael Trauner, and Peter Fickert

OVERVIEW

Aside from liver injury, alcohol has multiple adverse effects on the digestive tract (see Table 17.1), including the induction of pancreatitis, esophagitis, and gastritis, and the development of cancers of the upper alimentary tract and the colorectum.

While about 50% of acute pancreatitis cases are caused by ethanol, chronic alcohol abuse typically leads to chronic calcifying pancreatitis. Alcohol plays an important role in the development of gastroesophageal reflux disease via altered motility of the lower esophageal sphincter. Alcoholic gastritis is the consequence of direct gastric mucosal damage by ethanol, which is further influenced by the interaction between alcohol and *Helicobacter pylori* infection.

In epidemiologic studies, alcohol was identified as a cofactor in the development of cancers of the oral cavity, oropharynx, and esophagus, and of neoplastic lesions in the colorectum, including polyps and colorectal cancer.

PANCREAS

Alcohol is the etiologic factor for about half of the cases of acute pancreatitis. In a survey of 5019 patients, acute pancreatitis was associated with alcohol abuse in 55% and with cholelithiasis in 27%.[1] Prolonged alcohol abuse typically leads to chronic, recurrent, calcifying pancreatitis.[2] After several years, the chronic inflammatory process may subside and both exocrine and endocrine pancreatic insufficiency may develop as a consequence of pancreatic atrophy.

ACUTE PANCREATITIS

The course of acute pancreatitis may be complicated by necrosis, hemorrhage, the development of pseudocysts, infection, and systemic sequelae, including multi-organ failure. The severity of acute pancreatitis may be graded according to Ranson's early prognostic signs (Table 17.2).[1]

Diagnosis

Serum amylase and lipase are highly sensitive and specific for establishing the diagnosis of acute pancreatitis.[3] Determination of serum C-reactive protein (CRP) on admission is helpful in the assessment of severity, with levels above 110 mgl^{-1} indicating necrotizing or hemorrhagic pancreatitis.[4] Abdominal ultrasound and/or computed tomography are necessary to rule out or confirm pancreatic necrosis.

Treatment

Acute pancreatitis is treated by withdrawal of food and oral fluid intake and by infusion of parenteral electrolyte solutions. These measures are usually sufficient in mild cases. Severe cases require

TABLE 17.1
Effects of Alcohol on the Gastrointestinal Tract

Pancreas
    Acute pancreatitis
    Chronic calcifying pancreatitis
Salivary glands
    Sialadenosis
Upper alimentary tract cancer
    Cancers of oral cavity and oropharynx
Esophagus
    Reflux esophagitis
    Esophageal cancer
Stomach
    Acute gastritis
    Delayed gastric emptying
Small intestine
    Increased intestinal permeability
    Malabsorption
Colon
    Diarrhea
    Colorectal polyps and cancer

TABLE 17.2
Ranson's Criteria for Estimation of Mortality or Major Complications from Acute Pancreatitis

At admission or diagnosis:
    Age > 55
    White blood cell count > 16,000 mm^{-3}
    Blood glucose > 200 mg dl^{-1}
    Serum lactic dehydrogenase > 350 Ul^{-1}
    Serum glutamic oxaloacetic transaminase >120 Ul^{-1}
During initial 48 h:
    Hematocrit fall > 10%
    Blood urea nitrogen rise > 5 mg dl^{-1}
    Serum calcium < 2 mmol l^{-1}
    paO$_2$ < 60 mmHg
    Base deficit > 4 mEql^{-1}
    Estimated fluid sequestration > 6000 ml

Number of Signs	Mortality (%)
0–2	1
3–4	16
5–6	40
7–8	100

(Modified from Ranson, J.H.C., *Am. J. Gastroenterol.*, 77, 633, 1982.)

intensive care, suction of gastric secretions via a nasogastric tube, and parenteral nutrition. Inhibition of pancreatic exocrine secretion by somatostatin or its analog, octreotide, had no effect on mortality in randomized clinical trials.[5,6] However, the need for surgical interventions was significantly reduced by infusion of somatostatin for 10 days.[5] Similarly, the protease inhibitor, gabexate mesilate, did not affect mortality but reduced the incidence of complications, as shown in a meta-analysis.[7] Somatostatin may be effective in the treatment of local complications of acute pancreatitis, such as pancreatic fistulae, or in the prevention of postoperative complications following pancreatic surgery.

In necrotizing pancreatitis, antibiotic treatment is indicated for prevention of bacterial infection of pancreatic necrosis. In randomized clinical trials, prophylactic administration of imipenem[8] or cefuroxime[9] has been shown to reduce septic complications and/or mortality in acute necrotizing pancreatitis. Necrosectomy and postoperative local lavage may be beneficial, especially in cases with infected necrosis.[10]

CHRONIC CALCIFYING PANCREATITIS

Pathogenesis

Only a small proportion of subjects abusing alcohol develop chronic pancreatitis, and there is little overlap with other somatic effects of alcohol such as liver injury. Among patients abusing alcohol, clinical pancreatitis is recognized in only 1 to 10%; therefore, additional genetic, dietary, and environmental cofactors for the development of pancreatitis have been postulated.[11]

The mechanisms leading to chronic alcoholic pancreatitis are poorly understood. One hypothesis suggested that pancreatitis resulted from excessive pancreatic secretion against increased resistance to an alcohol-induced spasm of the sphincter of Oddi. Another pathogenic factor could be increased protein secretion resulting in ductular precipitates of protein and calcium carbonate.

Clinical Features

Chronic calcifying pancreatitis is much more common in men than in women (M:F = 8:1). Upper abdominal pain is the leading symptom and may persist despite abstinence from alcohol. Exocrine pancreatic insufficiency may result in steatorrhea. Anorexia is frequently present and results from both reduced food intake due to abdominal pain and maldigestion due to exocrine pancreatic dysfunction. Endocrine pancreatic insufficiency is reflected by pathologic glucose tolerance or overt diabetes mellitus. Further complications include pancreatic pseudocysts, bile duct strictures, and splenic vein thrombosis.

Diagnosis

Plain abdominal X-ray typically shows intrapancreatic calcifications. Endoscopic retrograde cholangiopancreatography (ERCP) and, more recently, magnetic resonance cholangiopancreatography (MRCP) have been used to demonstrate irregularities of the pancreatic ducts and to rule out choledocholithiasis.[12,13]

In advanced cases, exocrine pancreatic insufficiency may be quantitated by measuring 24-hour stool fat excretion or, more conveniently, fecal chymotrypsin content. Sophisticated tests of exocrine pancreatic function, such as the secretin-cholecystokinin test or the pancreolauryl test, have not gained widespread use.

Treatment

Recurrent bouts of chronic pancreatitis are treated in a similar way as acute pancreatitis. For long-term management, abstinence from alcohol and low-fat diet are essential. Exocrine pancreatic insufficiency may be treated by substitution of microencapsulated pancreatic enzyme preparations. Theoretically, enzyme substitution should also relieve abdominal pain via feedback inhibition of pancreatic secretion, but the results of placebo-controlled trials are controversial.[14,15] Administration of opiates should be restricted because of their potential for addiction. In selected cases, insertion of stents via ERCP[16] or extracorporeal shock-wave lithotripsy of pancreatic stones[17] may be beneficial.

SALIVARY GLANDS

Ethanol decreases salivary secretion which may disturb oral homeostasis and contribute to oral disease frequently seen in alcoholics.[18] Chronic alcohol consumption may lead to sialadenosis (i.e., painless bilateral swelling of the parotids and other salivary glands). Sialadenosis probably relates to elevation of the salivary isoform of amylase seen in about 10% of alcoholics.

UPPER ALIMENTARY TRACT CANCER

Alcohol abuse has been identified as a significant risk factor for upper alimentary tract cancer, especially of the oral cavity, oropharynx, larynx, and esophagus.[19] Heavy drinking and tobacco smoking were found to be responsible for the majority of oral cancer cases among U.S. veterans.[20]

ESOPHAGUS

REFLUX ESOPHAGITIS

Ethanol impairs motility of the lower esophageal sphincter and thereby causes gastroesophageal reflux.[21] There is a wide spectrum of gastroesophageal reflux disease from occasional reflux episodes to various degrees of erosive esophagitis, which may be further complicated by ulcer formation, stricture, or columnar epithelial metaplasia (Barrett's esophagus).

Proton pump inhibitors are highly effective in induction of healing of erosive esophagitis, but recurrence rate is high (80% at 1 year) unless maintenance therapy is instituted.[22] Patients in whom conservative treatment fails may benefit from antireflux surgery (i.e., Nissen fundoplication).[23]

ESOPHAGEAL CANCER

Consumption of more than 21 alcoholic drinks per week was found to increase the risk for esophageal *squamous cell carcinoma* about tenfold as compared to consumption of less than 7 drinks per week.[24] Smoking of >80 pack-years likewise increased this risk (OR = 17 compared to non-smokers). There is a much weaker association between *adenocarcinomas* of the esophagus and gastric cardia to either alcohol or smoking. Adenocarcinomas have been increasing over the last 2 decades and appear to be linked to obesity.[24]

Chronic esophageal inflammation induced by alcohol predisposes to the development of esophageal cancer in several ways. Acetaldehyde formation by alcohol dehydrogenase present in esophageal mucosa may alter normal DNA repair mechanisms and thus contribute to carcinogenesis. Furthermore, induction of cytochrome P450 2E1 by ethanol may activate dietary carcinogens such as nitrosamines. Smoking is a frequent cofactor in esophageal carcinogenesis.

STOMACH

INTERACTION BETWEEN ALCOHOL AND *HELICOBACTER PYLORI*

Alcohol is a frequent cause of acute gastritis. With respect to the role of *Helicobacter pylori (H. pylori)* in gastroduodenal ulcers or non-ulcer dyspepsia, much interest has emerged in examining the role of *H. pylori* in alcoholic gastritis. Eradication of *H. pylori* but not abstinence from alcohol led to resolution of histologic gastritis and improvement of dyspeptic symptoms.[25] In a Swedish study, the prevalence of *H. pylori* was reported to be equal in alcoholics and controls.[26] However, in a larger study in 451 patients among Finnish military personnel, the presence of *H. pylori* infection was related to alcohol consumption in a dose-dependent fashion.[27] Taken together, these findings suggest a predominant role of *H. pylori* infection rather than the toxic effects of alcohol *per se* in the pathogenesis of alcoholic gastritis.

Gastric alcohol dehydrogenase (ADH) contributes little to overall ethanol metabolism but may play an important role in the pathogenesis of gastritis by generating toxic metabolites from ethanol. As *H. pylori* possesses ADH,[28] it has the potential to enhance gastric alcohol metabolism. In contrast, the presence of *H. pylori* infection with chronic active gastritis has been found to lower the activity of gastric mucosal ADH activity in the antrum.[29] Thus, the net effect of *H. pylori* infection on gastric mucosal alcohol metabolism remains uncertain. More importantly, the ADH content of *H. pylori* may contribute to gastric mucosal injury via generation of acetaldehyde from ethanol.[28]

ACUTE GASTRITIS

Clinical Features

Vomitus matutinus is a typical symptom of alcoholism and relates to various degrees of acute gastritis. Hematemesis may result from severe hemorrhagic gastritis. Heavy vomiting is thought to be the cause of Mallory-Weiss tears, that is, mucosal tears at the gastroesophageal junction, which may also lead to significant upper gastrointestinal hemorrhage.

Diagnosis

Given the high rate of spontaneous healing of acute gastritis, endoscopy is only indicated if symptoms persist for more than a week. Upper gastrointestinal hemorrhage necessitates emergency endoscopy.

Treatment

In most cases, no treatment is necessary as acute gastritis heals spontaneously after a few days. Antacids and/or sucralfate may be useful in patients with a prolonged course. In healthy volunteers, sucralfate was able to prevent gastric mucosal injury by ethanol.[30] In acute hemorrhagic gastritis, intravenous proton pump inhibitors (PPIs) are given for a few days and thereafter switched to oral PPIs. In Mallory-Weiss tear, PPIs are equally effective; in addition, hemostasis can be achieved during endoscopy by intramucosal injection of adrenaline. In patients with relapsing bouts of gastritis, eradication of *H. pylori* by antibiotics may be considered.[31]

INTESTINES

ALCOHOL-INDUCED DYSMOTILITY AND MALABSORPTION

Alcohol causes intestinal dysmotility and accelerates small intestinal transit.[32] These alterations of intestinal motility may contribute to alcohol-induced diarrhea. Considerable experimental evidence has accumulated for alcohol-induced malabsorption as ethanol inhibits uptake and utilization of many nutrients, including vitamins and essential elements.[33]

Bacteriocolonic Pathway for Ethanol Oxidation

Colonic bacteria containing ADH have been shown to metabolize alcohol to acetaldehyde in the colonic lumen, which might lead to carcinogenesis locally in the colorectum.[34] Experiments in rats treated with ciprofloxacin suggest that this bacteriocolonic pathway for ethanol oxidation may significantly contribute to total ethanol elimination.[35]

Intestinal Permeability

Alcohol has been shown to disrupt the intestinal barrier function as measured by various permeability markers, such as polyethylene glycols or disaccharides. Increased intestinal permeability may play a role in the pathogenesis of a putative alcohol enteropathy, which might contribute to intestinal blood and protein loss.[36]

Colorectal Polyps and Cancer

Apart from other risk factors, such as excess energy intake relative to requirements, intake of red meat and refined sugar, lack of dietary vegetables and fruits, and smoking, alcohol appears to increase the risk for colorectal cancer.[37] Alcohol consumption of >30 g per day, especially in combination with a diet low in folate and methionine, was found to increase the risk for several types of neoplastic lesions in the distal colorectum (hyperplastic polyps, adenomas, and carcinomas).[37,38] Of interest, the increased risk for colorectal cancer by alcohol and low dietary methyl supply has been linked to genetic variants in methylenetetrahydrofolate reductase polymorphism.[39]

REFERENCES

1. Ranson, J.H.C., Etiological and prognostic factors in human acute pancreatitis: a review, *Am. J. Gastroenterol.*, 77, 633, 1982.
2. Sarles, H., Chronic calcifying pancreatitis — chronic alcoholic pancreatitis, *Gastroenterology*, 66, 604, 1974.
3. Ventrucci, M., Pezzilli, R., Gullo, L., Plate, L., Sprovieri, G., and Barbara, L., Role of serum pancreatic enzyme assays in diagnosis of pancreatic disease, *Dig. Dis. Sci.*, 34, 39, 1989.
4. Puolakkainen, P., Valtonen, V., Paananen, A., and Schroder, T., C-reactive protein (CRP) and serum phospholipase A_2 in the assessment of the severity of acute pancreatitis, *Gut*, 28, 764, 1987.
5. Planas, M., Perez, A., Iglesia, R., Porta, I., Masclans, J.R., and Bermejo, B., Severe acute pancreatitis: treatment with somatostatin, *Intensive Care Med.*, 24, 37, 1998.
6. McKay, C., Baxter, J., and Imrie, C., A randomized, controlled trial of octreotide in the management of patients with acute pancreatitis, *Int. J. Pancreatol.*, 21, 13, 1997.
7. Messori, A., Rampazzo, R., Scroccaro, G., Olivato, R., Bassi, C., Falconi, M., Pederzoli, P., and Martini, N., Effectiveness of gabexate mesilate in acute pancreatitis, *Dig. Dis. Sci.*, 40, 734, 1995.
8. Pederzoli, P., Bassi, C., Vesentini, S., and Campedelli, A., A randomized multicenter clinical trial of antibiotic prophylaxis of septic complications in acute necrotizing pancreatitis with imipenem, *Surg. Gynecol. Obstet.*, 176, 480, 1993.
9. Sainio, V., Kemppainen, E., Puolakkainen, P., Taavitsainen, M., Kivisaari, L., Valtonen, V., Haapiainen, R., Schroder, T., and Kivilaakso, E., Early antibiotic treatment in acute necrotizing pancreatitis, *Lancet*, 346, 663, 1995.
10. Beger, H.G., Buchler, M., Bittner, R., Block, S., Nevalainen, T., and Roscher, R., Necrosectomy and postoperative local lavage in necrotizing pancreatitis, *Br. J. Surg.*, 75, 207, 1988.
11. Malagelada, J.R., The pathophysiology of alcoholic pancreatitis, *Pancreas*, 1, 270, 1986.

12. Niederau, C. and Grendell, J.H., Diagnosis of chronic pancreatitis, *Gastroenterology*, 88, 1973, 1985.

13. Lomanto, D., Pavone, P., Laghi, A., Panebianco, V., Mazzocchi, P., Fiocca, F., Lezoche, E., Passariello, R., and Speranza, V., Magnetic resonance-cholangiopancreatography in the diagnosis of biliopancreatic diseases, *Am. J. Surg.*, 174, 33, 1997.

14. Isaksson, G. and Ihse, I., Pain reduction by an oral pancreatic enzyme preparation in chronic pancreatitis, *Dig. Dis. Sci.*, 28, 97, 1983.

15. Mossner, J., Secknus, R., Meyer, J., Niederau, C., and Adler, G., Treatment of pain with pancreatic extracts in chronic pancreatitis: results of a prospective placebo-controlled multicenter trial, *Digestion*, 53, 54, 1992.

16. Smits, M.E., Badiga, S.M., Rauws, E.A., Tytgat, G.N., and Huibregtse, K., Long-term results of pancreatic stents in chronic pancreatitis, *Gastrointest. Endosc.*, 42, 461, 1995.

17. Delhaye, M., Vandermeeren, A., Baize, M., and Cremer, M., Extracorporeal shock-wave lithotripsy of pancreatic calculi, *Gastroenterology*, 102, 610, 1992.

18. Proctor, G.B. and Shori, D.K., The effects of ethanol on salivary glands, *Alcohol and the Gastrointestinal Tract*, Preedy, V.R. and Watson, R.R., Eds., CRC Press, Boca Raton, FL, 1996, 111.

19. Seitz, H.K., Poschl, G., and Simanowski, U.A., Alcohol and cancer, *Recent Dev. Alcohol.*, 14, 67, 1998.

20. Mashberg, A., Boffetta, P., Winkelman, R., and Garfinkel, L., Tobacco smoking, alcohol drinking, and cancer of the oral cavity and oropharynx among U.S. veterans, *Cancer*, 72, 1369, 1993.

21. Vitale, G.C., Cheadle, W.G., Patel, B., Sadek, S.A., Michel, M.E., and Cuschieri, A., The effect of alcohol on nocturnal gastroesophageal reflux, *JAMA*, 258, 2077, 1987.

22. Chiba, N., Proton pump inhibitors in acute healing and maintenance of erosive or worse esophagitis: a systematic overview, *Can. J. Gastroenterol.*, 11 (Suppl. B), 66B, 1997.

23. Isolauri, J., Luostarinen, M., Viljakka, M., Isolauri, E., Keyrilainen, O., and Karvonen, A.L., Long-term comparison of antireflux surgery versus conservative therapy for reflux esophagitis, *Ann. Surg.*, 225, 295, 1997.

24. Vaughan, T.L., Davis, S., Kristal, A., and Thomas, D.B., Obesity, alcohol, and tobacco as risk factors for cancers of the esophagus and gastric cardia: adenocarcinoma versus squamous cell carcinoma, *Cancer Epidemiol. Biomarkers Prev.*, 4, 85, 1995.

25. Uppal, R., Lateef, S.K., Korsten, M.A., Paronetto, F., and Lieber, C.S., Chronic alcoholic gastritis: roles of alcohol and *Helicobacter pylori*, *Arch. Intern. Med.*, 151, 760, 1991.

26. Hauge, T., Persson, J., and Kjerstadius, T., *Helicobacter pylori*, active chronic antral gastritis, and gastrointestinal symptoms in alcoholics, *Alcohol. Clin. Exp. Res.*, 18, 886, 1994.

27. Paunio, M., Hook-Nikanne, J., Kosunen, T.U., Vainio, U., Salaspuro, M., Makinen, J., and Heinonen, O.P., Association of alcohol consumption and *Helicobacter pylori* infection in young adulthood and early middle age among patients with gastric complaints: a case-control study on Finnish conscripts, officers and other military personnel, *Eur. J. Epidemiol.*, 10, 205, 1994.

28. Kaihovaara, P., Salmela, K.S., Roine, R.P., Kosunen, T.U., and Salaspuro, M., Purification and characterization of *Helicobacter pylori* alcohol dehydrogenase, *Alcohol. Clin. Exp. Res.*, 18, 1220, 1994.

29. Thuluvath, P., Wojno, K.J., Yardley, J.H., and Mezey, E., Effects of *Helicobacter pylori* infection and gastritis on gastric alcohol dehydrogenase activity, *Alcohol. Clin. Exp. Res.*, 18, 795, 1994.

30. Cohen, M.M., Bowdler, R., Gervais, P., Morris, G.P., and Wang, H.R., Sucralfate protection of human gastric mucosa against acute ethanol injury, *Gastroenterology*, 96, 292, 1989.

31. Lieber, C.S., Gastric ethanol metabolism and gastritis: interactions with other drugs, *Helicobacter pylori*, and antibiotic therapy (1957–1997) — a review, *Alcohol. Clin. Exp. Res.*, 21, 1360, 1997.

32. Keshavarzian, A. and Fields, J.Z., Gastrointestinal motility disorders induced by ethanol, *Alcohol and the Gastrointestinal Tract*, Preedy, V.R. and Watson, R.R., Eds., CRC Press, Boca Raton, FL, 1996, 235.

33. Thomson, A.D., Heap, L.C., and Ward R.J., Alcohol-induced malabsorption in the gastrointestinal tract, *Alcohol and the Gastrointestinal Tract*, Preedy, V.R. and Watson, R.R., Eds., CRC Press, Boca Raton, FL, 1996, 203.

34. Jokelainen, K., Roine, R.P., Vaananen, H., Farkkila, M., and Salaspuro, M., *In vitro* acetaldehyde formation by human colonic bacteria, *Gut*, 35, 1271, 1994.

35. Jokelainen, K., Nosova, T., Koivisto, T., Vakevainen, S., Jousimies-Somer, H., Heine, R., and Salaspuro, M., Inhibition of bacteriocolonic pathway for ethanol oxidation by ciprofloxacin in rats, *Life Sci.*, 61, 1755, 1997.

36. Bjarnason, I. and Macpherson, A., Alcohol and small intestinal permeability, *Alcohol and the Gastrointestinal Tract*, Preedy, V.R. and Watson, R.R., Eds., CRC Press, Boca Raton, FL, 1996, 219.

37. Giovannucci, E. and Willett, W.C., Dietary factors and risk of colon cancer, *Ann. Med.*, 26, 443, 1994.

38. Kearney, J., Giovannucci, E., Rimm, E.B., Stampfer, M.J., Colditz, G.A., Ascherio, A., Bleday, R., and Willett, W.C., Diet, alcohol, and smoking and the occurrence of hyperplastic polyps of the colon and rectum (United States), *Cancer Causes Control*, 6, 45, 1995.

39. Chen, J., Giovannucci, E., Kelsey, K., Rimm, E.B., Stampfer, M.J., Colditz, G.A., Spiegelman, D., Willett, W.C., and Hunter, D.J., A methylenetetrahydrofolate reductase polymorphism and the risk of colorectal cancer, *Cancer Res.*, 56, 4862, 1996.

18   Cardiovascular System

Kurt Stoschitzky

OVERVIEW

There is general agreement that heavy alcohol consumption may be deleterious to the cardiovascular system as a whole. However, mild to moderate drinking may have different effects (see Table 18.1). On the one hand, low daily doses of alcohol (i.e., up to 30 g ethanol in men and up to 20 g in women) reduce the risk of coronary heart disease and ischemic stroke. On the other hand, even drinking of less than 30 g alcohol in men and less than 20 g in women may cause hypertension, alcoholic cardiomyopathy, arrhythmias, and sudden cardiac death, as well as intracerebral and subarachnoidal hemorrhages. Usually, chronic drinking is more hazardous to the cardiovascular system than acute or binge drinking of equal amounts of ethanol. Particularly because of the decreased risk of coronary heart disease, myocardial infarction, and ischemic stroke with low doses of alcohol, the association of alcohol intake and total mortality is a J-shaped function with a low point between 20 and 40 g ethanol per day in men and between 15 and 30 g in women (see Figure 18.1). However, it must be emphasized that the low point of this J-shaped curve strongly depends on the underlying risk of coronary heart disease of the individual. Although one drink per day generally appears to be safe, counseling must be individualized and all other medical and psychosocial problems of the patient should be taken into account.

ALCOHOL AND THE MYOCARDIUM

Alcohol has acute negative inotropic effects mediated by direct interaction with cardiac muscle cells.[1] Chronic consumption of ethanol may result in alcoholic cardiomyopathy (ACM), which is the major cause of secondary, non-ischemic cardiomyopathy in the Western world. ACM appears to be caused predominantly by the following two mechanisms: (1) a direct toxic effect of ethanol and/or its metabolites (e.g., protein-acetaldehyde adducts) on the myocardium; and (2) nutritional effects (e.g., thiamine deficiency). Acute as well as chronic intake of ethanol may depress myocardial contractility, even when ingested by non-alcoholic individuals. ACM most commonly occurs in men 30 to 50 years of age who have consumed large amounts of ethanol for more than 1 decade,[2] and women appear to be markedly more sensitive to the toxic effects of alcohol than men.[3] From the clinical as well as from the histological point of view, ACM and dilated cardiomyopathy (DCM) are almost identical.[4] The most frequent findings in patients with ACM are dilated heart chambers as well as deterioration of systolic (reduced ejection fraction) and diastolic (increased stiffness of the myocardium) function. Clinical features are those of congestive heart failure with decreased workload, dyspnea even at low effort, peripheral edema, and jugular venous distention, frequently combined with tachyarrhythmias (atrial fibrillation), gallop sounds, and systolic murmur due to relative mitral regurgitation.[2]

Cardiac dysfunction caused by ethanol may be reversible even when abstinence is resumed after years of harmful alcohol consumption. Although the length of alcohol exposure as well as the mechanisms responsible for the transition from reversible to permanent myocardial damage are still unclear, people with manifest ACM who continue to drink have a 40 to 50% probability of dying within 3 to 6 years. Therefore, it has to be emphasized that immediate and total abstinence as early as possible remains the only causal therapy and the key to treatment of ACM.[2]

TABLE 18.1
Different Effects of Alcohol on the
Cardiovascular System

Chronic moderate alcohol consumption (i.e., up to 30 g
of ethanol per day in men and up to 20 g in women) **may:**

Prevent	Cause
Coronary heart disease	Alcoholic cardiomyopathy
Myocardial infarction	Cardiac arrhythmias
Ischemic stroke	Sudden cardiac death
	High blood pressure
	Hemorrhagic stroke
	Subarachnoidal hemorrhage

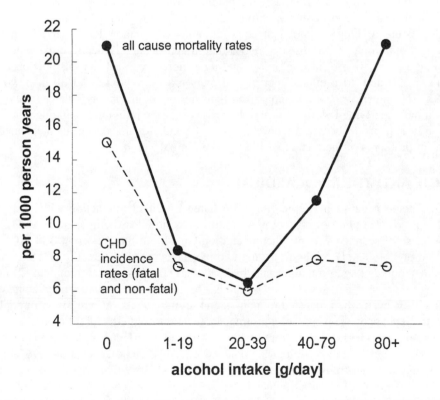

FIGURE 18.1 Association of chronic daily alcohol intake with total mortality and incidence of fatal and non-fatal coronary heart disease (CHD). (From Keil, U., Chambless, L.E., Doering, A., Filipiak, B., and Stieber, J., The relation of alcohol intake and all-cause mortality in a beer-drinking population, *Epidemiology, 8*, 150, 1997. Used with permission.)

ALCOHOL, CORONARY HEART DISEASE, AND MYOCARDIAL INFARCTION

It is well known that heavy ethanol intake increases the risk of death from all causes. However, it has been found that average daily alcohol consumption is inversely related to risk of non-fatal and fatal coronary heart disease (CHD) and myocardial infarction, reducing the risk by up to 30 to

40%.[5,6] Taken together, light to moderate alcohol intake (i.e., up to 30 g ethanol per day in men and up to 20 g in women) may substantially reduce mortality from CHD and myocardial infarction without dramatic increases in other causes of death.[7,8] Thus, the association of chronic daily alcohol consumption with total mortality behaves like a J-shaped curve with its low point between 20 and 40 g of daily ethanol (Figure 18.1);[9] that is, the risk of mortality of people who drink 20 to 40 g alcohol per day appears to be significantly lower than that of non-drinkers or heavy drinkers. However, it should be kept in mind that there is no general agreement as to depth, width, and the precise low point of this J-shaped curve. In addition, the low point of the J-shaped curve of the association of ethanol intake with total mortality lies about one third lower in women than in men since the former usually have a lower body weight and a better resorption of ethanol. Therefore, it has to be emphasized that people with a high risk of CHD may gain considerable benefit from regular light to moderate alcohol consumption (i.e., up to 30 g ethanol per day in men and up to 20 g in women), whereas those with a low risk of CHD may not benefit at all. Thus, any recommendations must also take into account the psychiatric, non-psychiatric medical, and psychosocial effects of alcohol.[6,8] Furthermore, please keep in mind that drinking alcohol does not compensate for the increase in risk produced by other risk factors such as smoking.[7]

The mechanism by which alcohol reduces the risk of CHD has not yet been entirely clarified. The most important beneficial effect of ethanol appears to be an increase in total high density lipoprotein (HDL) cholesterol as well as in HDL_2 and HDL_3.[6,8] In addition, there is some evidence that alcohol may reduce platelet aggregation and enhance the clot-dissolving system.[10]

There is also ongoing debate about the potential benefit of the type of beverage on CHD and mortality. It has been repeatedly postulated that antioxidant substances such as flavonoids and polyphenols, which are particularly present in red wine, may substantially contribute to the beneficial effects of ethanol because they may protect LDL cholesterol against oxidation. However, evidence from available observational data does not clearly suggest benefit for wine compared with other alcoholic beverages (see Chapter 20 on the immune system).[8,11]

The *French Paradox* — a lower mortality rate from CHD in France compared to other industrialized countries despite a similar level of risk factors including serum cholesterol and HDL concentrations — may act as a good example for the beneficial effects of ethanol on CHD since it appears to be best explained by the high regular consumption of wine in France resulting in an inhibition of platelet reactivity.[12] On the other hand, the French paradox is associated with a higher mortality from accidents and cancer, which may also be a result of the consumption of higher amounts of wine in France.[13]

ALCOHOL, ARRHYTHMIAS, AND SUDDEN CARDIAC DEATH

Acute and, particularly, chronic intake of high amounts of ethanol may facilitate the induction of supraventricular as well as ventricular arrhythmias. Possible arrhythmogenic mechanisms of ethanol include toxic heart muscle injury, prolongation of ventricular repolarization, sympathetic stimulation, reduced vagal tone, electrolyte disturbances (particularly hypokalemia; see Chapter 19 on electrolyte disturbances), worsening of sleep apnea, and worsening of myocardial ischemia.[14] The most common arrhythmias caused by ethanol are atrial flutter or fibrillation, which is usually found together with alcoholic cardiomyopathy, frequently as the initial finding. However, acute ethanol intake may also predispose to atrial flutter or fibrillation.[2] Furthermore, ventricular tachycardia and ventricular fibrillation may also occur and are the main causes of alcohol-induced sudden cardiac death (SCD). In addition, prolonged conduction times in the His-Purkinje system (AV-block, bundle-branch-block) have been observed.[14] The fact that alcohol has induced these disturbances does not have any bearing on the treatment of these arrhythmias.

Alcohol-dependent patients as well as non-alcoholic persons without evidence of other heart disease often develop uncomfortable palpitations, typically following a binge of alcohol consumption on a weekend — the *holiday heart syndrome* — which is usually caused by atrial fibrillation or flutter and frequent ventricular premature beats. SCD, most frequently caused by ventricular fibrillation, is not uncommon in this context, even in younger alcoholics,[2] whereas alcohol-induced arrhythmias usually disappear within a couple of days of complete abstinence in non-alcoholic persons. On the other hand, men consuming more than six drinks (i.e., >84 g ethanol) daily have a relative risk of SCD of 1.7, and up to one fourth of chronic alcohol abusers die from SCD by ventricular arrhythmias degenerating into ventricular fibrillation.[14] Similar to alcoholic cardiomyopathy, immediate and total abstinence as early as possible is the key to treatment.[2] In addition, beta-blockers may be given and electrolyte disturbances (particularly hypokalemia) should be compensated when they occur.

ALCOHOL AND BLOOD PRESSURE

Alcohol can exert different effects on blood pressure. Acute ethanol intake causes peripheral vasodilation, together with an acute reduction in myocardial contractility, resulting in a decrease of blood pressure and a compensatory increase in heart rate and cardiac output due to elevation of sympathetic tone. In addition, chronic drinking of low daily doses of alcohol also may cause a mild drop in blood pressure. No clear mechanism has so far been reported for these effects for alcohol on blood pressure.[15,16] In contrast, chronic intake of more than 30 to 60 g alcohol per day clearly increases blood pressure, but the amount of rise of blood pressure individually varies within wide ranges. At present, heavy chronic alcohol drinking is the second most important risk factor for hypertension in the Western world — closely after overweight.

Blood pressure further rises within hours or days when alcohol is acutely withdrawn from very heavy drinkers due to an increase in plasma catecholamines, renin activity, aldosterone, and cortisol.[17] On the other hand, high blood pressure usually returns to normal within a few weeks of abstinence.[16] Thus, the contrary effects of low and high chronic doses of alcohol on blood pressure are in keeping with those on coronary artery disease shown in Figure 18.1. In addition to complete abstinence from alcohol, hypertension should be treated according to the recommendations of the Joint National Committee (JNC-VI)[20] and the World Health Organization/International Society of Hypertension,[21] preferably with beta blockers (beta-adrenoceptor antagonists), diuretics, ACE inhibitors, calcium antagonists (calcium channel blockers) and/or alpha blockers (alpha-adrenoceptor antagonists).

ALCOHOL AND STROKE

Intake of large amounts of alcohol (i.e., more than 40 to 60 g per day) increases the risk of both ischemic and hemorrhagic stroke. However, the correlation between alcohol consumption and the risk of hemorrhagic stroke is linear, whereas that of ischemic stroke is J-shaped similar to that of coronary heart disease shown in Figure 18.1. Thus, light to moderate alcohol consumption (i.e., up to 30 g ethanol per day in men and up to 20 g in women) may be beneficial with respect to prevention of ischemic stroke but not of hemorrhagic stroke. The association of alcohol and subarachnoid hemorrhage appears to be similar to that of alcohol and intracerebral hemorrhage.[18]

TERATOGENIC EFFECTS OF ALCOHOL
ON THE CARDIOVASCULAR SYSTEM

Alcohol is the most common teratogen to which embryos and fetuses are exposed in the Western world. The period of greatest risk is the first trimester. Most common defects are ventricular and atrial septal defects, tetralogy of Fallot, aortic coarctation, endocardial cushion defect, and absence of a pulmonal artery. These defects can usually be observed as a part of the fetal alcohol syndrome (i.e., alcoholic embryopathy), which occurs in 30 to 50% of the offspring of chronic alcoholic women, the risk of alcoholic embryopathy being clearly correlated with the total amount of alcohol consumed. Therefore, total abstinence has to be recommended to pregnant women.[2]

EFFECTS OF ALCOHOL WITHDRAWAL ON THE CARDIOVASCULAR SYSTEM

Acute withdrawal of alcohol after a long period of chronic ethanol intake may cause a marked increase of sympatho-adrenergic activity, resulting in tachycardia, blood pressure increase, myocardial ischemia, and cardiac arrhythmias.[19] Beta-blockers should be used as treatment of first choice, and electrolyte disturbances (particularly hypokalemia) should be generously compensated when they occur.

REFERENCES

1. Thomas, A.P., Rozanski, D.J., Renard, D.C., and Rubin, E., Effects of ethanol on the contractile function of the heart: a review, *Alcohol. Clin. Exp. Res.,* 18, 121, 1994

2. Braunwald, E., Ed., *Heart Disease*, W.B. Saunders, Philadelphia, 1998.

3. Urbano-Marquez, A., Estruch, R., Fernandez-Sola, J., Nicholas, J.M., Pare, J.C., and Rubin, E., The greater risk of alcoholic cardiomyopathy and myopathy in women compared with men, *JAMA*, 274, 149, 1995.

4. Richardson, P.J., Patel, V.B., and Preedy, V.R., Alcohol and the myocardium, *Alcohol and Cardiovascular Diseases*, Chadwick, D.J. and Goode, J., Eds., John Wiley & Sons, Chichester, 1998, 35.

5. Rimm, E.B., Giovanucci, E.L., Willett, W.C., Colditz, G.A., Ascherio, A., Rosner, B., and Stampfer, M.J., Prospective study of alcohol consumption and risk of coronary disease in men, *Lancet*, 338, 464, 1991.

6. Gaziano, J.M., Buring, J.E., Breslow, J.L., Goldhaber, S.Z., Rosner, B., Vandenburgh, M., Willett, W., and Hennekens, C.H., Moderate alcohol intake, increased levels of high-density lipoprotein and its subfractions, and decreased risk of myocardial infarction, *N. Engl. J. Med.,* 329, 1829, 1993.

7. Thun, M.J., Peto, R., Lopez, A.D., Monaco, J.H., Henley, B.A., Heath, C.W. Jr., and Doll, R., Alcohol consumption and mortality among middle-aged and elderly U.S. adults, *N. Engl. J. Med.,* 337, 1705, 1997.

8. Gaziano, J.M. and Buring, J.E., Alcohol intake, lipids and risk of myocardial infarction, *Alcohol and Cardiovascular Diseases*, Chadwick, D.J. and Goode, J., Eds., John Wiley & Sons, Chichester, 1998, 208.

9. Keil, U., Liese, A., Filipiak, B., Swales, J.D., and Grobbee, D.E., Alcohol, blood pressure and hypertension, *Alcohol and Cardiovascular Diseases*, Chadwick, D.J. and Goode, J., Eds., John Wiley & Sons, Chichester, 1998, 125.

10. Hendriks, H.F.J. and van der Gaag, M.S., Alcohol, coagulation and fibrinolysis, *Alcohol and Cardiovascular Diseases*, Chadwick, D.J. and Goode, J., Eds., John Wiley & Sons, Chichester, 1998, 111.

11. Klatsky, A.L., Armstrong, M.A., and Friedman, G.D., Red wine, white wine, liquor, beer, and risk for coronary artery disease hospitalization, *Am. J. Cardiol.,* 80, 416, 1997.

12. Renaud, S. and de Lorgeril, M., Wine, alcohol, platelets, and the French paradox for coronary heart disease, *Lancet*, 339, 1523, 1992.

13. Renaud, S. and Gueguen, R., The French paradox and wine drinking, *Alcohol and Cardiovascular Diseases*, Chadwick, D.J. and Goode, J., Eds., John Wiley & Sons, Chichester, 1998, 208.

14. Kupari, M. and Koskinen, P., Alcohol, cardiac arrhythmias and sudden death, *Alcohol and Cardiovascular Diseases*, Chadwick, D.J. and Goode, J., Eds., John Wiley & Sons, Chichester, 1998, 68.

15. Klatsky, A.L., Alcohol and hypertension, *Clin. Chim. Acta*, 246, 91, 1996.

16. Fauci, A.S., Braunwald, E., Isselbacher, K.J., Wilson, J.D., Martin, J.B., Kasper, D.L., Hauser, S.L., and Longo, D.L., *Harrisons's Principles of Internal Medicine*, McGraw-Hill, New York, 1998.

17. Keil, U., Chambless, L.E., Doering, A., Filipiak, B., and Stieber, J., The relation of alcohol intake and all-cause mortality in a beer-drinking population, *Epidemiology*, 8, 150, 1997.

18. Hillbom, M., Juvela, S., and Karttunen, V., Mechanisms of alcohol-related strokes, *Alcohol and Cardiovascular Diseases*, Chadwick, D.J. and Goode, J., Eds., John Wiley & Sons, Chichester, 1998, 193.

19. Denison, H., Jern, S., Jagenburg, R., Wendestam, C., and Wallerstedt, S., ST-segment changes and catecholamine-related myocardial enzyme release during alcohol withdrawal, *Alcohol Alcohol.*, 32, 185, 1997.

20. The sixth report of the Joint National Committee on prevention, detection, evaluation, and treatment of high blood pressure, *Arch. Intern. Med.*, 157, 2413, 1997.

21. World Health Organization–International Society of Hypertension, Guidelines for the Management of Hypertension, Guidelines Subcommittee, *J. Hypertens.*, 1, 151, 1999.

19 Kidney and Electrolyte Disturbances

Michael Joannidis and Lloyd Cantley

OVERVIEW

Ingestion of ethanol is associated with a variety of fluid, electrolyte, and acid-base disturbances. In hospitalized alcoholic patients, hypophosphatemia and hypomagnesemia are the most frequent electrolyte disorders, followed by hypokalemia, hypocalcemia, and hyponatremia. Renal involvement is mainly restricted to reversible renal tubular functional changes.[12] Ethanol ingestion itself does not lead to manifest renal damage as long as patients do not have pronounced liver disease. The only exceptions to this are renal failure secondary to severe rhabdomyolysis, some rare cases of uric acid nephropathy, and occasional reports of acute renal failure in chronic alcoholic patients taking nonsteroidal anti-inflammatory agents (NSAIDs).[36,64,69] In patients with advanced liver disease, abnormalities of renal function are nearly inevitable.

ACID-BASE DISTURBANCES

The acid-base disorders described below may be found in alcoholic patients as a single acid-base disorder or mixed acid-base disorder (i.e., a combination of two or more disturbances) (Table 19.1). The exact prevalence of acid-base disorders is still undetermined. An Italian study reported 36% (from a total of 61 alcoholic patients) with a simple or mixed acid-base disorder.[12] Alcoholic ketoacidosis (AKA) is described as the most frequent disturbance, followed by the combinations AKA plus metabolic alkalosis, AKA plus respiratory alkalosis, and finally a triple disorder of AKA plus metabolic and respiratory alkalosis.[12,72]

ALCOHOLIC KETOACIDOSIS (AKA)

Pathophysiology

AKA occurs in the setting of decreased carbohydrate intake (fasting) plus alcohol-induced inhibition of gluconeogenesis. This leads to low insulin levels that promote lipolysis from adipose tissue, increasing levels of free fatty acids and compensatory glucagon secretion. Glucagon excess increases hepatic beta-oxidation of free fatty acids resulting in enhanced ketone body production (beta-hydroxybutyrate ≫ acetoacetate). Release of catecholamines in alcoholic patients due to either intravascular volume depletion or alcohol withdrawal contributes to the ketoacidosis by inhibiting insulin secretion and stimulating glucagon release. The sequential hepatic metabolism of ethanol into acetaldehyde and then acetic acid also contributes to the enhanced acid production.

Clinical Presentation

Patients with AKA typically present with a history of binge drinking with decreased or absent food intake during the last 24 to 72 hours. Patients may present with abdominal pain, nausea, or evidence of dehydration (hypotension, tachycardia, orthostatic changes in blood pressure).

TABLE 19.1

Most Common Acid Base Disorders in Alcoholic Patients (in order of prevalence)

Acid-base disorder	Characteristic labs	Treatment	Remarks
Alcoholic ketoacidosis	AG > 16; ↑ ketones in urine/plasma	Normal saline if hypovolemia present; If hypoglycemia; 100 ml glucose 33%; Glucose 5% at 150 ml h^{-1} (add potassium phosphate as necessary)	Lactic acidosis (often combined); Check potassium phosphate levels repeatedly
Lactic acidosis	AG > 16; serum lactate ↑	Normal saline for correction of hypovolemia	AKA (often combined)
Metabolic alkalosis	HCO$_3^-$ ↑; Urine chloride <10 meq l^{-1} if volume depletion	Normal saline; H$_2^-$ receptor antagonists/H$^+$ pump inhibitors i.v.	After volume repletion, metabolic alkalosis will cease
Respiratory alkalosis: Acute Chronic	pCO$_2$ ↓; HCO$_3^-$ ↓ HCO$_3^-$ ↓↓	If withdrawal, sedate pt. (e.g., oxazepam); No treatment for chronic respiratory alkalosis	

Laboratory values indicative of AKA consist of an increased anion gap (AG) acidosis (normal AG [Na-Cl-HCO$_3$] = 12±4 meq l^{-1}), with pH levels are usually between 7.1 and 7.4; in rare cases, pH < 7.0 has been observed (less than 10% of the patients)[72]; reduced serum bicarbonate levels (mean value 13 mmol L^{-1}); presence of ketones in the urine; and/or increased serum acetoacetate levels. It is important to know that the nitroprusside test used for detection of ketones primarily reacts with acetoacetate and does not detect beta-hydroxybutyrate at all. Thus, a few patients with AKA show only normal or modestly elevated levels.[12,72] Normal alcohol levels do not rule out diagnosis of AKA. Plasma blood glucose levels may be low, normal, or modestly elevated. At plasma glucose levels > 250 mg dl^{-1}, the patient should be monitored for hyperglycemia after correction of ketosis.

Treatment

Hypoglycemia, defined as blood glucose levels below 60 mg dl^{-1} can be found in about 12% of patients with AKA.[72] Usually, they are malnourished. The altered mental status in those patients can be corrected by 33 g to 50 g glucose administered as a 33% or 50% solution. Hemodynamic instability or volume depletion are treated with appropriate fluid replacement as normal saline. Unless the patient is hyperglycemic, intravenous administration of 5% glucose at a rate 150 ml h^{-1} usually terminates ketosis and reverses acidosis of AKA within 12 to 24 hours.[47] To avoid Wernicke's encephalopathy or acute beriberi in the alcoholic patient, 50 to 100 mg thiamine should be given intravenously. Alcoholic patients are usually hypokalemic and hypophospatemic. Since administration of glucose triggers the release of insulin with enhanced cellular uptake of potassium and phosphate, cautious administration of potassium phosphate may be warranted if serum levels are low. Potassium and phosphate levels must be monitored and substituted if necessary (usually 20 to 40 mmol potassium per liter glucose 5%).

LACTIC ACIDOSIS

Pathophysiology

If the patient is hypotensive or comatose, organ perfusion may be reduced leading to anaerobic glycolysis and enhanced lactic acid production (this form of acidosis is a complication in 50% of patients with AKA).[72] Diagnosis is based on the presence of a high AG acidosis with elevated lactate levels in blood. Reestablishing organ perfusion is the main goal (see Chapter 5 on the emergency management of alcohol intoxication).

METABOLIC ALKALOSIS

Pathophysiology

Metabolic alkalosis usually occurs from the loss of acid or gain of alkali. A frequent cause of metabolic alkalosis in alcoholic patients is vomiting with loss of hydrogen ions (together with sodium, chloride, and potassium). As long as renal perfusion and glomerular filtration rate (GFR) are normal, metabolic alkalosis will not be sustained because bicarbonate generated is excreted in the urine. However, in the setting of volume depletion, salt conservatory mechanisms in the kidney result in reabsorption of sodium bicarbonate and persistent alkalosis even if vomiting has stopped.

Clinical Presentation

Alcoholic patients usually present with a history of prolonged vomiting, showing evidence of volume depletion (hypotension, tachycardia, orthostatic changes in blood pressure). Respective laboratory values are elevated serum bicarbonate, hypochloremia, and hypokalemia. Arterial pCO_2 may be elevated due to respiratory compensation. Elevated blood urea nitrogen-to-creatinine ratio (>20) indicates prerenal azotemia. Urine chloride is low (<10 meq l^{-1}).

Treatment

Patients showing signs of volume depletion should be repleted with normal saline (up to 2 to 4 liters). Intravenous addition of H_2-receptor antagonists (ranitidine, cimetidine) or proton pump inhibitors (e.g., omeprazole, lansoprazole, pantoprazole) will diminish acid losses. Most patients need potassium replacement (see hypokalemia).

RESPIRATORY ALKALOSIS

Pathophysiology

Acute respiratory alkalosis is common in patients withdrawing from alcohol.[55] Alcohol withdrawal is frequently accompanied by a relative hypermetabolic state characterized by tachycardia, central nervous system hyperactivity, and tachypnea. Increased catecholamine release from the adrenal medulla, but also psychological disturbances like anxiety and craving for alcohol, are supposedly responsible for these disturbances.[55]

Chronic respiratory alkalosis is a frequent finding in 25 to 50% patients with cirrhosis.[54] Increased respiratory drive in these patients may result from cerebral irritation by accumulating endogenous toxins and metabolites (e.g., progesterone, estradiol) secondary to reduced clearance by the cirrhotic liver.

Clinical Presentation

The patient with acute withdrawal syndrome hyperventilates (tachypnea and hyperpnea). Arterial pH is elevated (usually pH between 7.5 and 7.6) with an arterial pCO_2 often reduced below 20 mmHg. Mild hypokalemia and/or hypophosphatemia (3.0 to 3.5 meq l^{-1} and 0.6 to 0.9 mmol l^{-1}, respectively) is usually associated with respiratory alkalosis and does not necessarily represent total body potassium or phosphate depletion. In non-withdrawing patients (mostly patients with cirrhosis), hyperventilation may not be so prominent. Since compensation takes place in these patients, pH is only moderately elevated (7.45 to 7.5) and serum bicarbonate is decreased.

TABLE 19.2

Most Common Electrolyte Disorders in Alcoholic Patients (in order of prevalence)

Electrolyte disorder	Symptoms	Characteristic labs	Treatment	Remarks
Hypophosphatemia	Muscle weakness; respiratory failure Rhabdomyolysis	0.32–0.64 mmol l^{-1}; <0.32 mmol l^{-1}	Oral repletion i.v. phospate (max. 2.5 mg kg^{-1} body weight over 6 h)	Often precipitated by respiratory alkalosis; ↑ risk of rhabdomyolysis
Hypomagnesemia	Seizures; Arrhythmias	0.4–0.75 mmol l^{-1}; <0.4 mmol l^{-1} and symptoms	p.o. 300–600 mg Mg/day 4–8 mmol Mg^{++} i.v. over 5–10 min followed by 25–50 mmol/day (max. 50 mmol/day)	Cautious substitution if renal function is impaired
Hypocalcemia	Tetany; Seizures; Trousseau/Chvostek signs	<1.8 mmol	Acute hypocalcemia: 10–20 ml Ca-gluconate 10% over 4–8 min, followed by a Ca-gluconate drip (see text) Chronic hypocalcemia: 1000–2000 mg calcium/day plus vit D 500–1000 IU/day	Check magensium levels and substitute if <0.75 mmol l^{-1}
Hypokalemia	Muscle cramps; Confusion; Cardiac arrythmias	3.0–3.5 mmol l^{-1}; <3.0 mmol l^{-1}	Oral supplements (potassium chloride/ actetate/bicarbonate) Oral + i.v. supplements (potassium chloride)	Dangerous arrhythmias in patients receiving digitalis
Hyponatremia	Somnolence; Confusion	<135 mmol l^{-1}	Water restriction; Withhold diuretics if possible	

Treatment

Benzodiazepines given in sedative doses are the treatment of choice during acute withdrawal. They are given over 3 to 5 days, followed by tapering (e.g., oxazepam 15 to 30 mg q6-8h p.o.; further treatment, see Chapter 6 on the treatment of alcoholic withdrawal syndrome). There is no effective way to treat chronic hyperventilation in patients with severe liver disease.

ELECTROLYTE DISTURBANCES (Table 19.2)

HYPOPHOSPHATEMIA

Pathophysiology

Hypophosphatemia in alcoholic patients is due to underlying chronic phosphate depletion, complicated by acute shifts of phosphate into the cellular compartment. Chronic phosphate depletion occurs from poor dietary intake of phosphate and vitamin D, from chronic diarrhea, and from increased renal phosphate excretion due to tubular dysfunction and secondary hyperparathyroidism. Infusion with dextrose can result in stimulation of insulin secretion and a further decrease in phosphate levels due to a shift of phosphate into the cell. This effect may be enhanced by respiratory alkalosis due to withdrawal. Re-feeding may aggravate hypophosphatemia, as new protein synthesis and glucose transport into the cells increase demand for phosphate.

Prevalence and Clinical Presentation

Hypophosphatemia is present in 30 to 40% of hospitalized alcoholic patients on admission.[3,12,17,58,72] In about 50% of the patients, hypophosphatemia can be observed within 12 to 36 hours after admission. Profound hypophosphatemia (serum levels $\leq$ 0.32 mmol l^{-1} [= 1 mg dl^{-1}]) was reported in about 1% of hospitalized alcoholic patients[8] and may be associated with symptoms of metabolic encephalopathy and muscle weakness. These symptoms may occur even with higher serum phosphate levels (0.32 to 0.64 mmol l^{-1}) when longstanding hypophosphatemia is present. Associated respiratory muscle weakness may be of importance for patients with underlying COPD. Alcoholic patients with hypophosphatemia are at serious risk for clinically significant rhabdomyolysis.[36,64]

Treatment

Keep plasma phosphate levels above 0.32 mmol l^{-1}, oral supplementation is preferred (dose 15 to 20 mg per kg body weight per day), usually as sodium- or potassium phosphate. Intravenous application carries the risk hypocalcemia and should be reserved for patients with severe symptomatic hypophosphatemia, who do not tolerate oral supplementation. Maximal substitution rate is of 2.5 mg per kg body weight over 6 hours until a serum level of 0.65 mmol l^{-1} is achieved.[68,73]

HYPOMAGNESEMIA

Pathophysiology

Hypomagnesemia occurs due to excessive urinary magnesium excretion, reflecting alcohol-induced tubular dysfunction which is reversible within 4 weeks of abstinence.[12] Other factors include dietary deficiency, acute pancreatitis, and diarrhea.

Prevalence and Clinical Manifestations

Alcoholism is the most common cause of hypomagnesemia, with about 28 to 32% of alcoholic patients admitted to the hospital exhibiting some degree of magnesium depletion.[12,16,39] Symptoms of hypomagnesemia are often not very pronounced and are usually confined to the neuromuscular system, such as generalized weakness, muscle fasciculations, tremors, and positive Trousseau's and Chvostek's signs. These symptoms can be attributed to hypocalcemia secondary to hypomagnesemia, since hypomagnesemia causes both reduced PTH secretion and skeletal resistance to parathyroid hormone. Severe hypomagnesemia may lead to ECG changes such as PR time prolongation and wide QRS complexes; in the worst cases, ventricular arrythmias may occur. It is has been reported that total body magnesium depletion may be possible in the presence of normomagnesemia. Thus, magnesium depletion should be considered as a possible cause of refractory hypokalemia or hypocalcemia in this group of patients.[59]

Treatment

Magnesium should be supplemented by oral route (preferred method, usually 300 mg per day magnesium; in severe cases, up to 600 mg per day in divided doses over a period of 2 to 4 weeks[1]). A frequent side effect with high doses is diarrhea. In severe cases (e.g., patients with tetany, seizures, or arrhythmias), an intravenous bolus of 4 to 8 mmol magnesium over 5 to 10 min should be given, followed by 25 to 50 mmol per day (e.g., 6 to 12 ml 50% $MgSO_4$ to 1 liter glucose 5% and administering this solution over 12 to 24 hours maximal total Mg^{2+} dose of 50 mmol per day) aiming at keeping serum magnesium levels above 0.4 mmol l^{-1}.[1,68] If renal function is impaired, magnesium should be administered cautiously with frequent monitoring of the serum magnesium concentration.

Hypocalcemia

Pathophysiology

Hypocalcemia in alcoholic patients can be attributed to three causes:

1. Magnesium depletion, resulting in parathyroid hormone (PTH) resistance (S-Mg < 0.4 mmol l^{-1}) and decreased PTH secretion
2. Reduced dietary intake/malabsorption of calcium and vitamin D, resulting in hypovitaminosis[52]
3. Transitory hypoparathyroidism caused by ethanol ingestion itself [41]

Prevalence and Clinical Presentation

Hypocalcemia can be found in about 20 to 26% of admitted alcoholic patients,[12,16,39] although clinically significant hypocalcemia is a rare complication (about 9% of alcoholic patients).[15] Symptoms are usually confined to the neuromuscular system, such as generalized weakness, muscle fasciculations, tremors, tetany, and positive Trousseau's and Chvostek's signs. In about 50% of hypocalcemic patients hypomagnesemia can be found.[59]

Treatment

If acute symptoms are present, intravenous calcium gluconate can be given. This is usually done by injecting 10 to 20 ml 10% solution of Ca-gluconate slowly over 3 to 6 min (10 ml 10% Ca-gluconate = 2.2 mmol Ca), followed by a drip (10 ampoules 10% Ca-gluconate added to 900 ml of glucose 5% at an infusion rate of 50 ml h^{-1}).[7] In chronic hypocalcemia, calcium and vitamin D should be substituted until oral intake has normalized (calcium 1000 to 2000 mg per day p.o., vitamin D_3 500 to 1000 IU per day). Additionally, oral magnesium supplementation should be considered in alcoholic patients with unexplained hypocalcemia even if their magnesium levels are not decreased.[59]

Hypokalemia

Pathophysiology

Hypokalemia is often associated with total body potassium depletion as a result of dietary potassium deficiency, gastrointestinal (vomiting or diarrhea) or renal losses. However, hypokalemia may also be observed when total body content is only slightly reduced as a result of potassium shift into the cells. This is observed during respiratory alkalosis in withdrawal or liver cirrhosis, beta-adrenergic stimulation due to elevated epinephrine levels during withdrawal, or may be induced by insulin, which is released when the starved alcoholic is re-fed, or by exaggerated release of insulin in response to hyperglycemia resulting from hypophosphatemia.

Prevalence and Clinical Presentation

Hypokalemia occurs in 13 to 23% of hospitalized withdrawing alcoholics.[12,39,42] In most cases, hypokalemia is mild (e.g., in respiratory alkalosis) and not symptomatic unless serum levels are less than 3 meq l^{-1}. Hypokalemia results in hyperpolarization of the cell, making it more difficult to initiate cellular action potentials. This may result in mental depression or confusion, which may be followed by agitation and limb-girdle weakness. In case of profound hypokalemia, frank paralysis and apnea may occur. Furthermore, hypokalemia prevents the necessary rise in muscle blood flow during exercise, which can result in rhabdomyolysis. Cardiac arrhythmias are the most dangerous complications of hypokalemia, especially in patients receiving digitalis. Renal effects of hypokalemia (i.e., decreased renal blood flow and filtration rate, renal hypertrophy) normally do not have a major impact on the overall well-being of the patient and need a prolonged period of hypokalemia to be established.

Treatment

As a general rule of thumb, a decrease in plasma potassium of 1 meq l^{-1} with a normal pH represents a decrease in total body potassium of 300 meq l^{-1}. Potassium supplements can be given as intravenous chloride or phosphate salts or oral preparations of chloride, bicarbonate or acetate salts. The oral route for potassium is generally safer. Administration via peripheral veins should not exceed 20 to 40 meq l^{-1}. Potassium should be administered with extreme caution to azotemic or oliguric patients, since urinary excretion of potassium depends on GFR and urinary flow rate to the distal convoluted tubule.

HYPONATREMIA

Pathophysiology

Hyponatremia in alcoholism typically occurs as a result of effective circulating volume depletion, leading to increased secretion of antidiuretic hormone (ADH). This is usually found in patients with advanced liver disease or with volume depletion secondary to diuretic therapy (see paragraph on pre-renal azotemia). A second mechanism of hyponatremia is water intoxication in the setting of the "beer drinker's syndrome" (for further details, see hyponatremia).

Prevalence and Clinical Presentation

Hyponatremia has been reported in about 17% of alcoholic patients.[15] Pseudohyponatremia due to alcohol-induced hypertrigylceridemia is frequent. Hyponatremia in patients with liver cirrhosis develops slowly and thus does not usually produce symptoms but may exacerbate hepatic encephalopathy at very low sodium levels.

Treatment

Water restriction will improve hyponatremia but relies on patient compliance, which often is poor due to excessive thirst in this setting. Diuretics should be withheld.

FLUID DISTURBANCES

HYPONATREMIA DUE TO WATER INTOXICATION

Pathophysiology

Ingestion of huge amounts of beer (i.e., more than 5 to 10 l of beer per day) by alcoholics whose diet contains almost no additional solute (e.g., Na^+, K^+, proteins) for excretion into the urine, may lead to retention of free water and, thus, to hyponatremia and water intoxication. Maximal dilution of the urine in a normal subject is approximately 50 mosm per kilogram of water, meaning that the patient needs to excrete 500 mosm solute to excrete a 10-l water load. As there is virtually no solute in beer, ingestion of large quantities of beer in combination with poor protein intake and consequently little urinary urea excretion will lead to inability to excrete the water load and severe hyponatremia. In addition, despite the ability of the kidney to limit urinary sodium loss to about 5 meq per day, chronic absence of salt from the diet will eventually lead to total body sodium depletion and worsen the hyponatremia.

Prevalence and Clinical Presentation

The so-called Beer drinker's syndrome occurs in alcoholics with a history of ingestion of large amounts of beer without any other dietary intake.[32] Prevalence is unknown because the syndrome is based on occasional reports. The symptoms of hyponatremia depend on the speed of sodium decrease in serum. A drop of 10 meq l[-1] over a few hours may produce profound neurologic symptoms, while serum sodium levels as low as 110 meq l[-1] may be well tolerated if reached slowly.[13]

Treatment

Water restriction will correct hyponatremia in this setting. In severe hyponatremia with mental status changes, administration of hypertonic saline may be warranted. Correction of the serum sodium can be performed at a rate of 1.5 to 2.0 meq l[-1] h[-1] for the first 1 to 2 hours (until symptoms improve), but should then be slowed so as to avoid a correction rate of more than 12 meq l[-1] per day.[11,65]

WATER DIURESIS

Pathophysiology

It is well known that ethanol induces a marked diuresis associated with a decreased release of antidiuretic hormone (ADH): The ADH-suppressing action is only observed while blood levels of ethanol are rising.[30]

Prevalence and Clinical Presentation

Water diuresis and enhanced thirst are typical manifestations of alcohol ingestion.

Treatment

No intervention is necessary; simply make water available to the patient.

RENAL DISTURBANCES

RENAL TUBULAR DYSFUNCTION AND HYPERURICEMIA

Pathophysiology

Chronic alcoholism seems to be associated with renal tubular functional changes which normalize within a few weeks after withdrawal. These changes are characterized by phosphaturia, increased excretion of magnesium, and urate retention.[12] A significant correlation between alcohol (especially beer) consumption and the prevalence of hyperuricemia and gout has been demonstrated.[61] In alcohol intoxication, hyperuricemia may be attributed to elevated serum lactate concentrations resulting from metabolism of ingested alcohol. Lactate interferes with tubular secretion of uric acid, resulting in hyperuricemia. In patients with alcoholic ketoacidosis, the production of beta-hydroxybutyrate and acetoacetate contributes to an additional uric acid retention. Excessive urate overproduction is also observed in alcohol-induced rhabdomyolysis secondary to the release of purine precursors from damaged muscle.

Clinical Manifestation

Renal tubular dysfunction contributes to the electrolyte disturbances mentioned above such as hypophosphatemia, hypomagnesemia, and hypokalemia. Hyperuricemia is associated with increased risk of gout attacks; uric acid nephropathy is rarely observed.[18]

Treatment

Renal tubular dysfunction is reversible within weeks of alcohol abstinence and thus does not require special therapy. Hyperuricemia is usually not treated unless gout attacks do occur. In that case, allopurinol (300 mg per day) is the therapy of choice. However, serious side effects of allopurinol (rash, leukopenia, thrombocytopenia, drug fever) should be considered.

RHABDOMYOLYSIS ASSOCIATED ACUTE RENAL FAILURE

Pathophysiology

Muscle necrosis in the setting of alcoholism can occur due to hypophosphatemia, seizures (especially in the setting of hypokalemia), coma-induced pressure necrosis, and traumatic or direct toxic muscle injury.[35] This results in release of myoglobin. Myoglobin is a small monomeric protein (MW = 17,000) that does not bind to plasma proteins and is thus rapidly filtered and excreted. Renal failure results from different mechanisms: obstructing intratubular pigment casts; concurrent volume depletion secondary to fluid sequestration into the injured muscle and renal hypoperfusion (myoglobin may inhibit the vasodilator effect of nitric oxide); and proximal tubular injury from free chelatable iron from myoglobin.

Clinical Presentation

Alcoholism is a leading cause of rhabdomyolysis,[21] especially in the presence of pronounced hypophosphatemia.[35] Prevalence has been reported as up to 5% of patients.[46]

Marked overproduction of hemoglobin or myoglobin typically leads to red or brown urine, unless pigment excretion is limited because of a low glomerular filtration rate or clearance from the plasma by extrarenal mechanisms. Patients with rhabdomyolysis present with the triad of pigmented granular casts in the urine, red to brown color of the urine supernatant, and marked elevation in the plasma level of creatinine kinase (CK). The serum levels of CK do not always predict the development of renal failure. However, 58% of patients who developed acute renal failure had peak CK levels greater than 16,000 U l^{-1} compared to only 11% in those who did not develop acute renal failure.[67] Additional laboratory signs may be hyperkalemia, hyperphosphatemia, hypocalcemia, and hyperuricemia. It must be noted that hyperphosphatemia may be absent if hypophosphatemia is the cause for rhabdomyolysis.

Treatment

Effectiveness depends on the early initiation of therapy. Therapy consists of two major approaches: initial hydration and forced diuresis.[6,19]

Hydration should be done initially with physiological saline to re-establish renal perfusion and urine flow. Based on experience with victims of crush injury, about 12 liters of fluid per day are recommended as long as renal function is sufficient.[6]

Based on the same studies, *forced diuresis* and alkalinization by a mannitol-alkaline solution should be performed until myoglobinuria has stopped (e.g., addition of 10 g mannitol and 40 meq sodium bicarbonate to 1 l of 0.5 N saline).[6,19] Urine output should be maintained about 300 ml h^{-1} and urine pH should be raised above 6.5 to increase solubility of heme pigments and thus prevent tubular cast formation. The protective effect of mannitol may be due to decreased intratubular myoglobin deposition and possibly due to its free radical-scavenger properties, thereby minimizing cell injury. During mannitol therapy, it is critical to monitor serum osmolarity to prevent hyperosmolar states. This is particularly important in the setting of reduced GFR since mannitol may accumulate in the serum. It has been reported that forced saline diuresis with furosemide also may be effective in traumatic and nontraumatic rhabdomyolysis.[37,62]

RENAL DISTURBANCES IN ALCOHOLIC PATIENTS
WITH LIVER CIRRHOSIS

SODIUM RETENTION AND EDEMA FORMATION

Pathophysiology

Increased sodium retention does occur early in the course of liver cirrhosis, even before ascites appear or glomerular filtration rate is impaired.[10,34] Although the exact mechanism is still unclear, sodium retention seems to occur mainly by enhanced reabsorption in the proximal tubule.[70] A hepatorenal reflex has been postulated in which hepatic disease should directly stimulate Na retention.[43] This early retention of sodium and, consequently, fluid is part of the *overflow* hypothesis used for the explanation of ascites formation in patients with liver cirrhosis.[45] The second mechanism for sodium retention is *underfilling* (i.e., depletion of effective circulating volume),[63] and is the more important mechanism in advanced liver cirrhosis. The development of effective circulating volume depletion occurs by two mechansims, splanchnic vasodilatation[25] (most likely mediated by the vasodilator nitric oxide[66] and vasodilatory prostaglandins[25]) and third-spacing of fluid into the abdominal cavity. As liver disease progresses, ascites develops by exudation of lymph from the surface of the liver as well as from transudation from intestinal and mesenteric capillaries. These fluid losses result in activation of the renin-angiotensin-aldosterone system as well as the sympathetic nervous system.[4,31] Patients at this stage present with a decrease in peripheral vascular resistance and blood pressure, with a compensatory increase in cardiac output.[27] Sodium retention at this stage can clearly be attributed to underfilling and is a normal response of the kidney.

Clinical Presentation

The main symptom is edema formation which may accumulate over a period of several days or weeks. Edema often starts in the lower extremities but may rapidly generalize. Ascites is usually present by the later stages of cirrhosis. Abdominal ultrasound is the most sensitive examination for ascites (which is found initially around the liver), while amounts larger than 1 liter are detectable by routine physical examination. Most patients present with other signs of cirrhosis as well, including spider nevi, palmar erythema, jaundice, gonadal atrophy, and gynecomastia.

Treatment

Treatment is usually based on three main modalities: salt restriction, diuretic therapy, and paracentesis. If salt restriction alone is insufficient to control edema, then diuretic therapy should be added. This combination is successful in about 90% of patients.

Salt Restriction

Patients with mild to moderate edema typically present with a sodium excretion of about 40 meq per day. Thus, restriction of sodium intake below this value should lead to a reduction in Na content of the body and edema. This correlates with a diet containing about 2 g sodium chloride per day, which is at the limit of practicability outside the hospital.[56] Additional natriuresis can be achieved by bed rest, which mobilizes the edema into the circulatory space, increasing effective vascular volume.

Diuretic Therapy

The aldosterone antagonist spironolactone is the initial therapy of choice.[51] In patients not responding to spironolactone alone, a combination with furosemide has proven successful. Usually, a once daily application of spironolactone (100 mg) with a twice daily application of furosemide (40 mg) is sufficient; doses may be increased to 400 mg per day and 160 mg per day, respectively.[56] The most serious side effect of spironolactone is the development of gynecomastia.

Caution

Ascites and edema reside in different compartments and fluid mobilization does occur at a different rates. The maximum rate in patients who have only ascites has been found to be 900 ml per 24 hours. Thus, the maximum fluid removal in this group of patients should be around 500 to 700 ml per day. Higher rates may result in intravascular volume depletion and prerenal azotemia.[53] Thus, if rapid removal of ascites is warranted, paracentesis should be performed instead of trying to force diuresis. In patients with peripheral edema, removal of larger amounts of fluid should be safe; orthostatic changes in blood pressure, serum sodium, BUN, and creatinine should be monitored regularly. Hyokalemia should be avoided.

Paracentesis

Based on recent controlled trials, large-volume paracentesis may be regarded as a safe procedure in patients with tense ascites.[23,24,26] Serial large-volume paracentesis is useful in patients who have become diuretic resistant.[57] The efficacy and choice of colloid replacement to prevent hypotension and pre-renal azotemia is still a matter of debate, although patients receiving albumin (10 g per liter of ascites removed) show better hemodynamic stability and less activation of the renin-angiotensin system.[23,26]

In patients who cannot be adequately treated with the above modalities, portasystemic shunting, transjugular intrahepatic portasystemic shunt (TIPS), and finally liver transplantation must be considered (see Chapter 16 on liver cirrhosis).

PRE-RENAL AZOTEMIA IN PATIENTS WITH LIVER CIRRHOSIS

Pathophysiology

As liver disease progresses, the loss in peripheral vascular resistance is compensated for by vasoconstriction with reduced renal perfusion, resulting in enhanced renal sodium reabsorption and worsening of the edema and ascites. The vigorous use of diuretics to manage the edema and ascites can lead to additional intravascular volume depletion and further reduction in GFR. Despite this fall in GFR, serum creatinine and BUN are frequently normal or only slightly elevated because urea and especially creatinine production are reduced in these patients secondary to the liver disease, reduced muscle mass, and decreased meat and protein intake. Thus, these patients may present with a normal serum creatinine but already have a reduced glomerular filtration rate.[50] Even 24-hour clearance measurements may overestimate GFR due to tubular secretion of creatinine.[9] Patients in this stage have elevated renin-aldosterone levels and activated sympathetic nervous system, followed by activation of ADH in the final stages of cirrhosis resulting in impaired water excretion and hyponatremia.[4] At this stage of the disease mean life expectancy of patients is already reduced to 5 to 6 months.

Clinical Presentation

Pre-renal azotemia in patients with liver cirrhosis is often the consequence of diuretic overtreatment, gastrointestinal fluid losses, or nonsteroidal antiinflammatory drugs (NSAIDs), which decrease renal perfusion by inhibiting vasodilator prostaglandins.[20,40] Common findings are oliguria, benign urinary sediment, urinary sodium concentration below 10 meq l^{-1}, and increases in plasma creatinine and BUN.

Treatment

Renal function usually recovers after withholding diuretics and NSAIDs. A trial of fluid repletion with normal saline should be included.

HEPATORENAL SYNDROME (HRS)

Pathophysiology

This syndrome usually characterizes the end-stage of reduced renal perfusion resulting in acute renal failure.[20] HRS is mostly seen in patients with cirrhosis but can also be observed with acute hepatitis or fulminant hepatic failure. HRS is a diagnosis of exclusion when other causes of renal failure (in patients with liver cirrhosis, this is mostly pre-renal azotemia) have been ruled out. The exact mechanism is still a matter of investigation, but it is likely that marked cortical ischemia in the setting of reduced peripheral vascular resistance (mostly due to splanchnic vasodilatation and compensatory renal vasoconstriction) plays a critical role.[20] Investigations of patients with HRS showed that small liver size, activated renin-angiotensin-aldosteron system, and elevated vasopressin levels are predictive for the development of HRS.[22] Other potential mediators of HRS that have been examined are endotoxin (which might cause renal vasoconstriction as well as peripheral arterial vasodilatation), vasoconstrictor thromboxanes, and endothelin.[20,60]

Clinical Presentation

Symptoms and diagnosis are similar to pre-renal azotemia, so the following criteria have been proposed:[5] plasma creatinine > 1.5 progressing over days to weeks in patients with severe acute or chronic liver disease with portal hypertension; the absence of any other cause for renal failure; urinary sodium < 10 meq l^{-1}; and lack of improvement in renal function after volume repletion and withholding of diuretics or NSAIDs, if applicable.

Treatment

Hepatorenal syndrome is a diagnosis of exclusion. Thus, ATN (see below) or a pre-renal form of renal failure must be excluded. Withhold diuretics, give volume if possible. HRS is typically irreversible as long as liver function does not improve. Experimental therapeutic approaches include the combination of an ADH analog (such as ornipressin) with volume expansion using albumin infusion.[29,44] The transjugular intrahepatic portosystemic shunt (TIPS) seems to improve glomerular filtration but is associated with a higher incidence of encephalopathy.[28] If renal function does not recover, treatment with dialysis or continuous hemofiltration may be initiated, although survival using this therapeutic regimen depends on the reversibility of liver failure. Recovery of renal function after successful liver transplantation is the rule.

ACUTE TUBULAR NECROSIS (ATN) IN PATIENTS WITH LIVER CIRRHOSIS

Pathophysiology

ATN may develop in patients with liver cirrhosis after exposure to radiocontrast agents, aminoglycoside therapy, massive bleeding, or sepsis.

Clinical Presentation

Diagnosis may be difficult because the usual diagnostic criteria for ATN (i.e., muddy brown casts, fractional sodium excretion >2%) may not be applicable in liver cirrhosis.[14] A rapid increase in plasma creatinine and oligo-/anuria may be present in either ATN or hepatorenal syndrome. In the setting of an appropriate clinical insult, ATN should be assumed and appropriate supportive measures instituted.

Treatment

There is no specific treatment for ATN. After removal of the triggering agent (aminogylcosides, etc.), recovery is possible. Renal replacement therapy must be initiated to bridge the time until recovery of renal function.

GLOMERULONEPHRITIS IN PATIENTS WITH LIVER CIRRHOSIS

Pathophysiology

Morphologic glomerular pathologies are a frequent finding in patients with liver cirrhosis (in more than 50% of biopsies/autopsies performed, patients with liver cirrhosis revealed some glomerular abnormality).[49] The predominant form appears to be mesangial and/or glomerular deposition IgA, which is found in up to one third of the patients. Although some investigators found enhanced prevalence of renal IgA deposition in patients with alcoholic liver cirrhosis, this has not been generally accepted.[71] Also, serum IgA levels are elevated in more than 90% of patients with liver cirrhosis. The most likely explanation is impaired removal of IgA-containing immune complexes by hepatic Kupffer cells.[2] Increased intestinal permeability leading to increased IgA production appears to be an additional factor in alcoholic patients.[38]

Clinical Presentation

Most patients with alcoholic cirrhosis do not show specific signs of a glomerular diesease, although some may present with proteinuria, hematuria, and nephritic urinary sediment.[48,49]

Treatment

At present, there is no distinctive therapy proven effective in randomized trials.

REFERENCES

1. Abbott, L.G. and Rude, R.K., Clinical manifestations of magnesium deficiency, *Miner. Electrolyte Metab.*, 19, 314, 1993.
2. Amore, A., Coppo, R., Roccatello, D., Piccoli, G., Mazzucco, G., Gomez, C.M., Lamm, M.E., and Emancipator, S.N., Experimental IgA nephropathy secondary to hepatocellular injury induced by dietary deficiencies and heavy alcohol intake, *Lab. Invest.*, 70, 68, 1994.
3. Angeli, P., Gatta, A., Caregaro, L., Luisetto, G., Menon, F., Merkel, C., Bolognesi, M., and Ruol, A., Hypophosphatemia and renal tubular dysfunction in alcoholics. Are they related to liver function impairment? [see comments], *Gastroenterology*, 100, 502, 1991.
4. Arroyo, V., Bosch, J., Gaya-Beltran, J., Kravetz, D., Estrada, L., Rivera, F., and Rodes, J., Plasma renin activity and urinary sodium excretion as prognostic indicators in nonazotemic cirrhosis with ascites, *Ann. Intern. Med.*, 94, 198, 1981.
5. Arroyo, V., Gines, P., Gerbes, A.L., Dudley, F.J., Gentilini, P., Laffi, G., Reynolds, T.B., Ring-Larsen, H., and Scholmerich, J., Definition and diagnostic criteria of refractory ascites and hepatorenal syndrome in cirrhosis. International Ascites Club, *Hepatology*, 23, 164, 1996.
6. Better, O.S. and Stein, J.H., Early management of shock and prophylaxis of acute renal failure in traumatic rhabdomyolysis [see comments], *N. Engl. J. Med.*, 322, 825, 1990.
7. Bushinsky, D.A. and Monk, R.D., Calcium [see comments], *Lancet*, 352, 306, 1998.
8. Camp, M.A. and Allon, M., Severe hypophosphatemia in hospitalized patients, *Miner. Electrolyte Metab.*, 16, 365, 1990.

9. Caregaro, L., Menon, F., Angeli, P., Amodio, P., Merkel, C., Bortoluzzi, A., Alberino, F., and Gatta, A., Limitations of serum creatinine level and creatinine clearance as filtration markers in cirrhosis, *Arch. Intern. Med.,* 154, 201, 1994.

10. Chaimovitz, C., Szylman, P., Alroy, G., and Better, O.S., Mechanism of increased renal tubular sodium reabsorption in cirrhosis, *Am. J. Med.,* 52, 198, 1972.

11. Cluitmans, F.H. and Meinders, A.E., Management of severe hyponatremia: rapid or slow correction? [see comments], *Am. J. Med.,* 88, 161, 1990.

12. De, M.S., Cecchin, E., Basile, A., Bertotti, A., Nardini, R., and Bartoli, E., Renal tubular dysfunction in chronic alcohol abuse — effects of abstinence. *N. Engl. J. Med.,* 329, 1927, 1993.

13. Demanet, J.C., Bonnyns, M., Bleiberg, H., and Stevens-Rocmans, C., Coma due to water intoxication in beer drinkers, *Lancet*, 2, 1115, 1971.

14. Diamond, J.R. and Yoburn, D.C., Nonoliguric acute renal failure associated with a low fractional excretion of sodium, *Ann. Intern. Med.,* 96, 597, 1982.

15. Elisaf, M., Merkouropoulos, M., Tsianos, E.V., and Siamopoulos, K.C., Acid-base and electrolyte abnormalities in alcoholic patients, *Miner. Electrolyte Metab.,* 20, 274, 1994.

16. Elisaf, M., Merkouropoulos, M., Tsianos, E.V., and Siamopoulos, K.C., Pathogenetic mechanisms of hypomagnesemia in alcoholic patients, *J. Trace Elem. Med. Biol.,* 9, 210, 1995.

17. Elisaf, M.S. and Siamopoulos, K.C., Mechanisms of hypophosphataemia in alcoholic patients, *Int. J. Clin. Pract.,* 51, 501, 1997.

18. Emmerson, B.T. and Ravenscroft, P.J., Abnormal renal urate homeostasis in systemic disorders, *Nephron*, 14, 62, 1975.

19. Eneas, J.F., Schoenfeld, P.Y., and Humphreys, M.H., The effect of infusion of mannitol-sodium bicarbonate on the clinical course of myoglobinuria, *Arch. Intern. Med.,* 139, 801, 1979.

20. Epstein, M., Hepatorenal syndrome: emerging perspectives of pathophysiology and therapy [editorial], *J. Am. Soc. Nephrol.,* 4, 1735, 1994.

21. Gabow, P.A., Kaehny, W.D., and Kelleher, S.P., The spectrum of rhabdomyolysis, *Medicine (Baltimore)*, 61, 141, 1982.

22. Gines, A., Escorsell, A., Gines, P., Salo, J., Jimenez, W., Inglada, L., Navasa, M., Claria, J., Rimola, A., and Arroyo, V., Incidence, predictive factors, and prognosis of the hepatorenal syndrome in cirrhosis with ascites [see comments], *Gastroenterology*, 105, 229, 1993.

23. Gines, A., Fernandez-Esparrach, G., Monescillo, A., Vila, C., Domenech, E., Abecasis, R., Angeli, P., Ruiz-Del-Arbol, L., Planas, R., Sola, R., Gines, P., Terg, R., Inglada, L., Vaque, P., Salerno, F., Vargas, V., Clemente, G., Quer, J.C., Jimenez, W., Arroyo, V., and Rodes, J., Randomized trial comparing albumin, dextran 70, and polygeline in cirrhotic patients with ascites treated by paracentesis [see comments], *Gastroenterology*, 111, 1002, 1996.

24. Gines, P., Arroyo, V., Quintero, E., Planas, R., Bory, F., Cabrera, J., Rimola, A., Viver, J., Camps, J., and Jimenez, W., Comparison of paracentesis and diuretics in the treatment of cirrhotics with tense ascites. Results of a randomized study, *Gastroenterology*, 93, 234, 1987.

25. Gines, P., Fernandez-Esparrach, G., Arroyo, V., and Rodes, J., Pathogenesis of ascites in cirrhosis, *Semin. Liver Dis.*, 17, 175, 1997.

26. Gines, P., Tito, L., Arroyo, V., Planas, R., Panes, J., Viver, J., Torres, M., Humbert, P., Rimola, A., and Llach, J., Randomized comparative study of therapeutic paracentesis with and without intravenous albumin in cirrhosis, *Gastroenterology*, 94, 1493, 1988.

27. Groszmann, R.J., Hyperdynamic circulation of liver disease 40 years later: pathophysiology and clinical consequences [editorial; comment], *Hepatology*, 20, 1359, 1994.

28. Guevara, M., Gines, P., Bandi, J.C., Gilabert, R., Sort, P., Jimenez, W., Garcia-Pagan, J.C., Bosch, J., Arroyo, V., and Rodes, J., Transjugular intrahepatic portosystemic shunt in hepatorenal syndrome: effects on renal function and vasoactive systems [see comments], *Hepatology*, 28, 416, 1998.

29. Guevara, M., Gines, P., Fernandez-Esparrach, G., Sort, P., Salmeron, J.M., Jimenez, W., Arroyo, V., and Rodes, J., Reversibility of hepatorenal syndrome by prolonged administration of ornipressin and plasma volume expansion, *Hepatology*, 27, 35, 1998.

30. Helderman, J.H., Vestal, R.E., Rowe, J.W., Tobin, J.D., Andres, R., and Robertson, G.L., The response of arginine vasopressin to intravenous ethanol and hypertonic saline in man: the impact of aging, *J. Gerontol.*, 33, 39, 1978.

31. Henriksen, J.H., Bendtsen, F., Gerbes, A.L., Christensen, N.J., Ring-Larsen, H., and Sorensen, T.I., Estimated central blood volume in cirrhosis: relationship to sympathetic nervous activity, beta-adrenergic blockade and atrial natriuretic factor, *Hepatology*, 16, 1163, 1992.

32. Hilden, T. and Svendsen, T.L., Electrolyte disturbances in beer drinkers. A specific "hypo-osmolality syndrome," *Lancet*, 2, 245, 1975.

33. Hirsch, D.J., Jindal, K.K., Trillo, A., and Cohen, A.D., Acute renal failure after binge drinking [letter] [see comments], *Nephrol. Dial. Transplant.*, 9, 330, 1994.

34. Klingler, E.L.J., Vaamonde, C.A., Vaamonde, L.S., Lancestremere, R.G., Morosi, H.J., Frisch, E., and Papper, S., Renal function changes in cirrhosis of the liver. A prospective study, *Arch. Intern. Med.*, 125, 1010, 1970.

35. Knochel, J.P., Mechanisms of rhabdomyolysis, *Curr. Opin. Rheumatol.*, 5, 725, 1993.

36. Knochel, J., The pathophysiology and clinical characteristics of severe hypophosphatemia, *Arch. Intern. Med.*, 137, 203, 1977.

37. Knottenbelt, J.D., Traumatic rhabdomyolysis from severe beating — experience of volume diuresis in 200 patients, *J. Trauma*, 37, 214, 1994.

38. Kohler, H., [Alcohol and IgA in the kidney], *Klin. Wochenschr.*, 63, 959, 1985.

39. Koide, T., Ozeki, K., Kaihara, S., Kato, A., Murao, S., and Kono, H., Etiology of QT prolongation and T wave changes in chronic alcoholism, *Jpn. Heart J.*, 22, 151, 1981.

40. Laffi, G., Daskalopoulos, G., Kronborg, I., Hsueh, W., Gentilini, P., and Zipser, R.D., Effects of sulindac and ibuprofen in patients with cirrhosis and ascites. An explanation for the renal-sparing effect of sulindac, *Gastroenterology*, 90, 182, 1986.

41. Laitinen, K., Lamberg-Allardt, C., Tunninen, R., Karonen, S.L., Tahtela, R., Ylikahri, R., and Valimaki, M., Transient hypoparathyroidism during acute alcohol intoxication, *N. Engl. J. Med.*, 324, 721, 1991.

42. Lamminpaa, A. and Vilska, J., Acid-base balance in alcohol users seen in an emergency room, *Vet. Hum. Toxicol.*, 33, 482, 1991.

43. Lang, F., Tschernko, E., Schulze, E., Ottl, I., Ritter, M., Volkl, H., Hallbrucker, C., and Haussinger, D., Hepatorenal reflex regulating kidney function [see comments], *Hepatology*, 14, 590, 1991.

44. Lenz, K., Hortnagl, H., Druml, W., Reither, H., Schmid, R., Schneeweiss, B., Laggner, A., Grimm, G., and Gerbes, A.L., Ornipressin in the treatment of functional renal failure in decompensated liver cirrhosis. Effects on renal hemodynamics and atrial natriuretic factor, *Gastroenterology*, 101, 1060, 1991.

45. Lieberman, F.L., Overflow theory of ascites formation [letter], *Gastroenterology*, 96, 274, 1989.

46. Martin, F., Ward, K., Slavin, G., Levi, J., and Peters, T.J., Alcoholic skeletal myopathy, a clinical and pathological study, *Q. J. Med.*, 55, 233, 1985.

47. Miller, P.D., Heinig, R.E., and Waterhouse, C., Treatment of alcoholic acidosis: the role of dextrose and phosphorus, *Arch. Intern. Med.*, 138, 67, 1978.

48. Nakamoto, Y., Iida, H., Kobayashi, K., Dohi, K., Kida, H., Hattori, N., and Takeuchi, J., Hepatic glomerulonephritis. Characteristics of hepatic IgA glomerulonephritis as the major part, *Virchows Arch. [Pathol. Anat.]*, 392, 45, 1981.

49. Newell, G.C., Cirrhotic glomerulonephritis: incidence, morphology, clinical features, and pathogenesis, *Am. J. Kidney Dis.*, 9, 183, 1987.

50. Papadakis, M.A. and Arieff, A.I., Unpredictability of clinical evaluation of renal function in cirrhosis. Prospective study, *Am. J. Med.*, 82, 945, 1987.

51. Perez-Ayuso, R.M., Arroyo, V., Planas, R., Gaya, J., Bory, F., Rimola, A., Rivera, F., and Rodes, J., Randomized comparative study of efficacy of furosemide versus spironolactone in nonazotemic cirrhosis with ascites. Relationship between the diuretic response and the activity of the renin-aldosterone system, *Gastroenterology*, 84, 961, 1983.

52. Pitts, T.O. and Van, T.D., Disorders of divalent ions and vitamin D metabolism in chronic alcoholism, *Recent. Dev. Alcohol*, 4, 357, 1986.

53. Pockros, P.J. and Reynolds, T.B., Rapid diuresis in patients with ascites from chronic liver disease: the importance of peripheral edema, *Gastroenterology*, 90, 1827, 1986.

54. Prytz, H. and Thomsen, A.C., Acid-base status in liver cirrhosis. Disturbances in stable, terminal and portal-caval shunted patients, *Scand. J. Gastroenterol.*, 11, 249, 1976.

55. Roelofs, S.M., Hyperventilation, anxiety, craving for alcohol: a subacute alcohol withdrawal syndrome, *Alcohol*, 2, 501, 1985.

56. Runyon, B.A., Care of patients with ascites [see comments], *N. Engl. J. Med.*, 330, 337, 1994.

57. Runyon, B.A., Management of adult patients with ascites caused by cirrhosis, *Hepatology*, 27, 264, 1998.
58. Ryback, R.S., Eckardt, M.J., and Pautler, C.P., Clinical relationships between serum phosphorus and other blood chemistry values in alcoholics, *Arch. Intern. Med.*, 140, 673, 1980.
59. Ryzen, E., Nelson, T.A., and Rude, R.K., Low blood mononuclear cell magnesium content and hypocalcemia in normomagnesemic patients, *West. J. Med.*, 147, 549, 1987.
60. Sacerdoti, D., Balazy, M., Angeli, P., Gatta, A., and McGiff, J.C., Eicosanoid excretion in hepatic cirrhosis. Predominance of 20-HETE, *J. Clin. Invest.*, 100, 1264, 1997.
61. Saker, B.M., Tofler, O.B., Burvill, M.J., and Reilly, K.A., Alcohol consumption and gout, *Med. J. Aust.*, 1, 1213, 1967.
62. Scherrer, P. and Perret, C., [Prevention of acute renal insufficiency due to nontraumatic rhabdomyolysis], *Schweiz. Med. Wochenschr.*, 116, 572, 1986.
63. Schrier, R.W., Arroyo, V., Bernardi, M., Epstein, M., Henriksen, J.H., and Rodes, J., Peripheral arterial vasodilation hypothesis: a proposal for the initiation of renal sodium and water retention in cirrhosis [see comments], *Hepatology*, 8, 1151, 1988.
64. Singhal, P., Kumar, A., Desroches, L., Gibbons, N., and Mattana, J., Prevalence and predictors of rhabdomyolysis in patients with hypophosphatemia [see comments], *Am. J. Med.*, 92, 458, 1992.
65. Sterns, R.H., Cappuccio, J.D., Silver, S.M., and Cohen, E.P., Neurologic sequelae after treatment of severe hyponatremia: a multicenter perspective, *J. Am. Soc. Nephrol.*, 4, 1522, 1994.
66. Vallance, P. and Moncada, S., Hyperdynamic circulation in cirrhosis: a role for nitric oxide? *Lancet*, 337, 776, 1991.
67. Ward, M.M., Factors predictive of acute renal failure in rhabdomyolysis, *Arch. Intern. Med.*, 148, 1553, 1988.
68. Weisinger, J.R. and Bellorin-Font, E., Magnesium and phosphorus [see comments], *Lancet*, 352, 391, 1998.
69. Wen, S.F., Parthasarathy, R., Iliopoulos, O., and Oberley, T.D., Acute renal failure following binge drinking and nonsteroidal antiinflammatory drugs, *Am. J. Kidney Dis.*, 20, 281, 1992.
70. Wong, F., Massie, D., Hsu, P., and Dudley, F., Renal response to a saline load in well-compensated alcoholic cirrhosis, *Hepatology*, 20, 873, 1994.
71. Woodroffe, A.J., IgA, glomerulonephritis and liver disease, *Aust. N.Z. J. Med.*, 11, 109, 1981.
72. Wrenn, K.D., Slovis, C.M., Minion, G.E., and Rutkowski, R., The syndrome of alcoholic ketoacidosis, *Am. J. Med.*, 91, 119, 1991.
73. Lentz, R.D., Brown, D.M., and Kjellstrand, C.M., Treatment of severe hypophosphatemia, *Ann. Intern. Med.*, 89, 194, 1978.

20   Immune System

Michael Schirmer, Christian Wiedermann,
and Guenther Konwalinka

OVERVIEW

Abuse of alcohol has multiple effects on both cellular and humoral immune responses. Alcohol-induced immunodeficiency is related to an increased risk for infectious diseases and certain cancers. Several rheumatic diseases can be triggered by alcohol consumption. The risks of systemic lupus erythematosus and rheumatoid arthritis, however, appear reduced in women with low daily consumption of alcohol. Alcohol intake increases the risk of gastrointestinal bleeding after administration of nonsteroidal antiinflammatory drugs. Chronic alcohol intake also increases methotrexate hepatotoxicity.

INTRODUCTION

It is an old clinical experience that alcoholics have an increased incidence and severity of infectious diseases. Today we know that alcohol depresses cell-mediated immunity as well as the primary antibody response to neoantigens. Thus, alcoholics should be considered immunosuppressed individuals. This chapter presents major effects of alcohol on the immune system and the course and treatment of rheumatic diseases.

PHYSIOLOGICAL EFFECTS OF ALCOHOL ON THE IMMUNE SYSTEM

CELL-MEDIATED AND HUMORAL IMMUNE RESPONSES

Alcohol has a variety of short- and long-term effects on cellular and humoral immune responses. Abnormalities of the immune system include leucopenia with alterations of lymphocyte subsets and decreased T-cell mitogenesis, alterations of immunoglobulin production, and dysfunction of neutrophils.

Infections such as tuberculosis and listeriosis in alcoholics indicate defective functioning of cellular immunity. In humans, the data on counts of lymphocyte subsets are controversial.[1] In patients with alcoholic liver disease, it has been shown that total lymphocyte numbers are rather decreased relative to normal. Some studies showed that the numbers of suppressor (CD8+) T-cells are more reduced than helper (CD4+) T-cells in patients with alcoholic liver disease, resulting in an increase in the CD4:CD8 ratio. The lack of suppressor T-cells expressed as an increase in the CD4:CD8 ratio may account for high susceptibility to infections. In addition, the lymphocyte function, including the response to mitogens *in vitro*, and clinical estimation of delayed hypersensitivity after intradermal antigenic challenge are strongly impaired in alcoholics. Thus, peripheral blood (PB) mononuclear cells of alcoholics — independent of liver disease progression — are significantly less responsive than PB mononuclear cells of controls to phytohemagglutinin (PHA), concanavalin A (ConA), or pokeweed mitogen (PWM).[2] Concerning delayed hypersensitivity as measured by skin induration after injection of intradermal antigen, it is reported that this immune reaction is also significantly depressed in alcoholics.[3]

Alcoholics have elevated levels of circulating immunoglobulins, and immunoglobulin levels might even rise with increasing severity of cirrhosis.[4] Whether this increased antibody production is a direct effect of ethanol or a consequence of the associated protein-energy malnutrition usually present in alcoholics remains open. Exposure to alcohol decreases the expression of MHC class II proteins on B-cells and macrophages,[5] which may be related to an alcohol-induced increase in endogenous glucocorticoids. This down-regulation of MHC class II proteins might interfere with the primary antibody response to neoantigens and thus explain why the increased levels of antibodies do not protect alcoholics against infection. Besides the qualitative defect of the humoral immune response, the number of B-cells is also significantly reduced in patients with chronic alcohol abuse.[6] These changes are not related to age, nutritional status, or the presence of other alcohol-related diseases.

The neutrophil dysfunction in alcoholic patients is well established and another reason for their increased risk of infections, as these hemopoietic cells are most important for killing invading bacteria.[7] In alcoholics with advanced cirrhosis, phagocytic capacity and chemotaxis, bacterial phagocytosis, and killing were strongly impaired.

CYTOKINE SECRETION IN ALCOHOLICS

Cytokines are responsible for the communication between immunocompetent cells and are mostly produced by T-cells and macrophages. In this tightly regulated cytokine system, any change in the concentrations of various soluble mediators can result in immune alterations that modify resistance to infections and even cancer. Therefore, the influence of alcohol consumption on cytokine secretion has been studied extensively.

Increased plasma concentrations of tumor necrosis factor-alpha (TNF-α) have been observed in chronic alcoholic liver disease during alcohol abuse.[8] Interestingly, such increased levels of TNF-α have also been related to decreased long-term survival in patients with severe alcoholic hepatitis:[9] 14 of 17 patients with elevated plasma TNF-α died at a median time of 8 months after discharge from hospital, whereas all six patients with normal TNF-α levels survived. In alcoholics without liver disease, however, TNF-α production after stimulation of PB lymphocytes with interleukin (IL)-2 and interferon (IFN)-α was significantly reduced.[10]

Another recently characterized cytokine, IL-12, has been postulated as the major cytokine involved in initiation and restoration of cell-mediated immune response, and therefore this cytokine is responsible for the differentiation of T-cells to the Th-1 type, which is responsible for the cellular immune reaction. Interestingly, the plasma levels of IL-12 were not depressed but significantly increased after active alcohol consumption, both in patients with and without liver disease.[11] The Th-1 response is also expressed by the increased IFN-γ serum levels found in patients with alcoholic liver cirrhosis. Thus, much evidence exists that the increased levels of IL-12 measured in these patients are related to alcohol.

ANTIOXIDANT EFFECTS

Moderate wine consumption is reported to exert a protective effect against coronary heart disease (see Chapter 18). A possible mechanism of this potential health benefit may be an antioxidant effect of compounds within the alcoholic beverage (e.g., polyphenolic constituents).[12] Wine, especially red wine, contains a range of polyphenols counteracting the pro-oxidant effects of ethanol. Therefore, the net effect of such beverages depends on the balance of these pro- and antioxidant effects. It is interesting that the *in vivo* measured antioxidant plasma capacity not only increased after the ingestion of 113 ml red wine, but also after the same amount of alcohol-free red wine containing polyphenols.[13] Alcohol-free white wine and water had no effect. Based on these data, it was suggested that the polyphenols in red wine are absorbed in the upper gastrointestinal tract and are responsible for the beneficial antioxidant effects.

CLINICAL ASPECTS

Alcohol-Induced Immunodeficiency

Chronic alcoholics have an increased susceptibility to bacterial pneumonia, tuberculosis, and other infectious diseases. In a 14-year follow-up study with more than 6000 alcohol-dependent persons, alcoholics had a three to seven times greater rate of death from pneumonia than the population as a whole.[14] Even relatively small amounts of alcohol, such as two alcoholic drinks daily (about 26 g ethanol), can induce an altered immune regulation, resulting also in an increased risk of cancer.[15] In a case-control study of upper aerodigestive tract tumors, 546 patients with cancer of the oral cavity and pharynx, 410 with cancer of the esophagus, 388 with cancer of the larynx, and 2263 controls were included.[16] The results showed that the odds ratios for female and male drinkers with a consumption of more than 42 drinks per week (i.e., >546 g per week or 78 g per day) were increased to 3.8 and 4.5 for cancer of the oral cavity and pharynx, 4.7 and 3.0 for cancer of the esophagus and 2.0 and 2.6 for cancer of the larynx, respectively, as compared to the controls. For breast cancer, a 10% greater risk was reported in association with one alcoholic drink daily (about 13 g ethanol).[17] In contrast, recently published data from the Framingham Study found no association between the risk of breast cancer and the *light* consumption of alcohol.[18]

Based on the high risk of infections and cancer, a reversal of the immunocompromised status is desirable. This aim, however, can only be achieved by abstinence, which has previously been shown to normalize the number of helper and suppressor T-cell subsets and natural killer cells after 9 months, at least in patients without liver disease.[19]

Alcohol, Autoimmunity, and Rheumatic Diseases

More than 80% of patients with alcoholic liver disease have circulating autoantibodies directed against nuclei, smooth muscle, and mitochondria (see Chapter 28 in this book). For these immune reactions, new antigens might be responsible. These may be derived by cytosolic proteins modified by ethanol metabolites. It is therefore interesting that a reduced risk for autoimmune diseases like systemic lupus erythematosus (SLE) and rheumatoid arthritis (RA) was found in women who consume alcohol on a regular basis. In a recent retrospective case-control study, the odds ratio of SLE for patients who drank more than three units of alcohol per week (i.e., >39 g per week) was less than 0.5; and with 0.3, the odds ratio was even more reduced in those patients who drank more than ten units of alcohol (i.e., >130 g per week).[20] However, if SLE was manifest, regular alcohol intake plus lower socioeconomic status correlated with higher morbidity, including increased functional disability and organ damage.[21] In two independent studies, the risk of RA was half in women with regular alcohol consumption compared to normal controls.[22,23]

It is commonly suggested that gout attacks occur frequently in alcoholics. One study has raised the question of whether there is a difference between chronic alcoholics and nonalcoholics in frequency or severity of acute gouty flares as well as serum urate levels. This study concludes that the frequency of attacks is equal, but on presentation with acute arthritis, the index serum urate values were significantly lower than in nonalcoholics (8 ± 1 vs. 10 ± 1; $p < 0.01$).[24] For other rheumatic diseases like osteoporosis, osteonecrosis, and myopathy, alcohol must also be considered as a serious independent risk factor.[25]

Alcohol Allergy and Intolerance

In general, self-reported food allergy and intolerance are more frequent than objectively confirmable by double-blind, placebo-controlled food challenge (12% vs. 2%).[26] Even in those subjects with confirmed food allergy, clinical symptoms of allergy and intolerance to wine, champagne, or beer are rare. These symptoms might be explainable by histamine intolerance or sulfite sensitivity. Intolerance to histamine can present with sneezing, flush, headache, diarrhea, skin itch, and shortness of breath.[27] The patients develop these symptoms after not more than one glass of wine, and administration of antihistaminic drugs is obligatory. It seems that in alcoholics, histamine degradation is diminished, which might be based on a deficiency of diamine oxidase.

THERAPEUTIC CONSIDERATIONS IN ALCOHOLICS WITH RHEUMATIC DISEASES

When prescribing drugs for alcoholics with rheumatic diseases, one should be aware of some interactions occurring between alcohol and antirheumatic drugs. This holds true not only for patients with alcohol-related liver disease, but also in all other patients with chronic alcohol consumption. The most common complications are observed after intake of nonsteroidal anti-inflammatory drugs and methotrexate.

Nonsteroidal antiinflammatory drugs (NSAIDs) are among the most frequently used drugs in many countries.[28] They are often used in rheumatic diseases because of their analgesic plus antiphlogistic properties, primarily for symptoms associated with osteoarthritis, rheumatoid arthritis, and other non-inflammatory and inflammatory musculosceletal conditions. Many studies have shown that NSAIDs increase the risk of peptic ulcer complications by three- to fivefold, and it has been estimated that 15 to 35% of all peptic ulcer complications are due to NSAIDs. Therefore, it is important to note that alcohol further increases the risk of gastrointestinal ulcers, bleeding, or perforation. Advanced age and smoking are other independent risk factors for such gastrointestinal side effects. If the hypothesis holds true that NSAIDs specifically inhibiting the pain-related COX-2 enzyme have less gastrointestinal side effects, then these drugs should be preferred in alcoholics.

During treatment with methotrexate (MTX), hepatotoxicity is the major adverse reaction.[29] MTX is an immunosuppressive agent widely used for treatment of autoimmune diseases like rheumatoid arthritis (RA) and psoriatic arthritis. Alcoholics have an additional risk for such hepatic injury by MTX.[30] RA patients who drank more than 100 g ethanol per week were more likely to have advanced changes on liver biopsy (18% vs. 5%) and to show histologic progression (73% vs. 26%) under long-term administration of MTX. Patients with psoriasis even showed advanced changes on liver biopsy in 8% (vs. 3% of controls; $p < 0.01$) and histologic progression in 33% (vs. 24%; $p = 0.02$). Therefore in patients with chronic alcoholism, MTX should not be used and patients treated with MTX must avoid alcoholic beverages.

REFERENCES

1. Cook, R.T., T cell modulations in human alcoholics, *Alcohol, Drugs of Abuse, and Immune Functions,* Watson, R.R., Eds., CRC Press, Boca Raton, FL, 1995, 57.
2. Mutchnick, M.G. and Lee, H.H., Impaired lymphocyte proliferative response to mitogen in alcoholic patients. Absence of a relation to liver disease activity, *Alcohol. Clin. Exp. Res.*, 12, 155, 1988.
3. Gluckman, S.J., Dvorak, V.C., and MacGregor, R.R., Host defenses during prolonged alcohol consumption in a controlled environment, *Arch. Intern. Med.*, 137, 1539, 1977.
4. Thompson, R.A., Carter, R., Stokes, R.P., Geddes, A.M., and Goodall, J.A.D., Serum immunoglobulins, complement component levels and autoantibodies in liver disease, *Clin. Exp. Immunol.*, 14, 335, 1973.
5. Weiss, P.A., Collier, S.D., and Pruett, S.B., Effect of ethanol on B cells expression of major histocompatibility class II proteins in immunized mice, *Immunopharmacology,* 39, 61, 1998.
6. Sacanella, E., Estruch, R., Gaya, A., Fernandez-Sola, J., Antunez, E., and Urbano-Marquez, A., Activated lymphocytes (CD25+ CD69+ cells) and decreased CD19+ cells in well nourished chronic alcoholics without ethanol-related diseases, *Alcohol. Clin. Exp. Res.*, 22, 897, 1998.
7. Liu, Y.K., Effects of alcohol on granulocytes and lymphocytes, *Semin. Hematol.*, 17, 130, 1980.

8. Santos-Perez, J.L., Diez-Ruiz, A., Luna-Casado, L., Soto-Mas, J.A., Wachter, H., Fuchs, D., and Gutierrez-Gea, F., T-cell activation, expression of adhesion molecules and response to ethanol in alcoholic cirrhosis, *Immunol. Lett.,* 50, 179, 1996.
9. Felver, M.E., Mezey, E., McGurie, M., Mitchell, M.C., Herlong, H.F., Veech, G.A., and Veech, R.L., Plasma tumor necrosis factor alpha predicts decreased long-term survival in severe alcoholic hepatitis, *Alcohol. Clin. Exp. Res.,* 14, 255, 1990.
10. Laso, F.J., Lapena, P., Madruga, J.I., San Miguel, J.F., Orfao, A., Iglesias, M.C., and Alvarez-Mon, M., Alterations in tumor necrosis factor-alpha, interferon-gamma, and interleukin-6 production by natural killer cell-enriched peripheral blood mononuclear cells in chronic alcoholism: relationship with liver disease and ethanol intake, *Alcohol. Clin. Exp. Res.,* 21, 1226, 1997.
11. Laso, F.J., Iglesias, M.C., Lopez, A., Ciudad, J., San Miguel, J.F., and Orfao, A., Increased interleukin-12 serum levels in chronic alcoholism, *J. Hepatol.,* 28, 771, 1998.
12. Soleas, G.J., Diamandis, E.P., and Goldberg, D.M., Wine as a biological fluid: history, production, and role in disease prevention, *J. Clin. Lab. Anal.,* 11, 287, 1997.
13. Serafini, M., Maiani, G., and Ferro-Luzzi, A., Alcohol-free red wine enhances plasma antioxidant capacity in humans, *J. Nutr.,* 128, 1003, 1998.
14. Schmidt, W. and de Lint, J., Causes of death of alcoholics, *Q. J. Stud. Alcohol.,* 33, 171, 1972.
15. Longnecker, M.P. and Enger, S.M., Epidemiologic data on alcoholic beverage consumption and risk of cancer, *Clin. Chim. Acta,* 246, 121, 1996.
16. Franceschi, S., Bidoli, E., Negri, E., Barbone, F., and La Vecchia, C., Alcohol and cancers of the upper aerodigestive tract in men and women, *Cancer Epidemiol. Biomarkers Pre.,* 3, 299, 1994.
17. Longnecker, M.P., Alcoholic beverage consumption in relation to risk of breast cancer: meta-analysis and review, *Cancer Causes Control,* 5, 73, 1994.
18. Zhang, Y., Kreger, B.E., Dorgan, J.F., Splansky G.L., Cupples L.A., and Ellison, R.C., Alcohol consumption and risk of breast cancer: The Framingham Study revisited, *Am. J. Epidemiol.,* 149, 93, 1999.
19. Laso, F.J., Madruga, J.I., San Miguel, J.F., Ciudad, J., Lopez, A., Alvarez Mon, M., and Orfao, A., Long lasting immunological effects of ethanol after withdrawal, *Cytometry,* 26, 275, 1996.
20. Hardy, C.J., Palmer, B.P., Muir, K.R., Sutton, A.J., and Powell, R.J., Smoking history, alcohol consumption, and systemic lupus erythematosus: a case-control study, *Ann. Rheum. Dis.,* 57, 451, 1998.
21. Lotstein, D.S., Ward, M.M., Bush, T.M., Lambert, R.E., van Vollenhoven, R., and Neuwelt, C.M., Socioeconomic status and health in women with systemic lupus erythematosus, *J. Rheumatol.,* 25, 1720, 1998.
22. Hazes, J.M., Dijkmans, B.A., Vandenbroucke, J.P., de Vries, R.R., and Cats, A., Lifestyle and the risk of rheumatoid arthritis: cigarette smoking and alcohol consumption, *Ann. Rheum. Dis.,* 49, 980, 1990.
23. Voigt, L.F., Koepsell, T.D., Nelson, J.L., Dugowson, C.E., and Daling, J.R., Smoking, obesity, alcohol consumption, and the risk of rheumatoid arthritis, *Epidemiology,* 5, 525, 1994.
24. Vandenberg, M.K., Moxley, G., Breitbach, S.A., and Roberts, W.N., Gout attacks in chronic alcoholics occur at lower serum urate levels than in nonalcoholics, *J. Rheumatol.,* 21, 700, 1994.
25. Al-Jarallah, K.F., Shebab, D.K., and Buchanan, W.W., Rheumatic complications of alcohol abuse, *Semin. Arthr. Rheum.,* 22, 162, 1992.
26. Jansen, J.J., Kardinaal, A.F., Huijbers, G., Vlieg-Boerstra, B.J., Martens, B.P., and Ockhuizen, T., Prevalence of food allergy and intolerance in the adult Dutch population, *J. Allergy Clin. Immunol.,* 93, 446, 1994.
27. Wantke, F., Gotz, M., and Jarisch, R., The red wine provocation test: intolerance to histamine as a model for food intolerance, *Allergy Proc.,* 15, 27, 1994.
28. Griffin, M.R., Epidemiology of nonsteroidal anti-inflammatory drug-associated gastrointestinal injury, *Am. J. Med.,* 104, 23S, 1998.
29. West, S.G., Methotrexate hepatotoxicity, *Rheum. Dis. Clin. North. Am.,* 23, 883, 1997.
30. Whiting-O'Keefe, Q.E., Fye, K.H., and Sack, K.D., Methotrexate and histologic hepatic abnormalities: a meta-analysis, *Am. J. Med.,* 90, 711, 1991.

21 Endocrine System

Michael Trauner, Barbara Obermayer-Pietsch,
Peter Fickert, and Rudolf E. Stauber

OVERVIEW

Alcohol (ethanol) can impair the function of several parts of the endocrine system. Clinically important examples include hypogonadism in alcohol-dependent men and women, alcohol-induced hypoglycemia, pseudo-Cushing's syndrome, low-T_3 syndrome, hypoparathyroidism, and osteopenia. Most of these syndromes result from a direct effect of alcohol (ethanol) and its metabolites (e.g., acetaldehyde) on hormone-producing cells, and can be observed before the manifestation of alcohol-induced liver disease.

INTRODUCTION

Acute and chronic ingestion of alcohol (ethanol) profoundly alters the normal function of various parts of the endocrine system, including the hypothalamic-pituitary-gonadal (HPA) axis, adrenals, thyroid, parathyroids, bone metabolism, and endocrine pancreas (Table 21.1). While some of these changes give rise to clinically overt disease, others may cause only asymptomatic laboratory abnormalities which, however, need to be interpreted correctly. With respect to hormone levels, the reader is referred to Table 21.2 for general orientation in regard to the range of changes to be expected. Most studies have been conducted in chronic alcohol-dependent patients and are subject to confounding variables such as coexisting liver disease and nutritional deprivation commonly encountered in these individuals. Conversely, some of these endocrine changes may have an important impact on liver disease, whereas others might contribute to patterns of addiction and withdrawal symptoms in alcohol-dependent patients.

HYPOTHALAMIC-PITUITARY-GONADAL AXIS

Chronic alcohol abuse can result in severe disturbances of the hypothalamic-pituitary-gonadal axis with gonadal failure in both men and women.[1] Most endocrine changes observed in chronic alcohol-dependent patients are the result of ethanol toxicity per se, rather than an indirect consequence of alcohol-induced liver disease.[1]

MEN

Acute alcohol ingestion in normal male volunteers induces a rapid fall in plasma testosterone levels consistent with an acute gonadotoxic effect of alcohol.[2,3] Plasma luteinizing hormone (LH) levels are markedly elevated, apparently as an intact feedback response to lowered circulating testosterone levels. Chronic alcohol exposure (over 5 to 22 days) also decreases plasma testosterone levels, whereas plasma LH and follicle stimulating hormone (FSH) concentrations remain inappropriately low for the degree of gonadal failure, suggesting a combined gonadal and hypothalamic-pituitary toxic effect of ethanol and its metabolites (e.g., acetaldehyde).[1,2,4] Androgen deficit ("hypoandrogenization") in chronic alcohol-dependent men frequently results in testicular atrophy and cessation

TABLE 21.1
Effects of Alcohol on the Endocrine System

System	Effect
Hypothalamic-pituitary-gonadal axis	Hypogonadism
Hypothalamic-pituitary-adrenal axis	Pseudo-Cushing's syndrome
Thyroid gland	Low-T_3 syndrome
Parathyroid glands	Hypoparathyroidism
Bone metabolism	Osteopenia
Endocrine pancreas	Hypoglycemia

of spermatogenesis (in 50% of patients), as well as reduced libido and erectile impotence (60 to 80%).[1] Semen of alcoholics often shows abnormalities, including decreased numbers and motility of spermatozoa, and increased proportions of abnormal forms.[5]

In addition to "hypoandrogenization," feminization ("hyperestrogenization") is also observed in chronic alcohol-dependent men — although less common than hypoandrogenization, which usually precedes feminization.[6] Clinical features of feminization include a loss of body hair (in 60% of patients), palmar erythema (40%), spider angiomata (35%), and gynecomastia (20%).[1,6] Hyperestrogenization results from a combination of moderately increased plasma estrogen levels (e.g., estradiol, estrone) in the presence of reduced plasma androgen levels (e.g., testosterone, 5-α-dihydrotestosterone).[1,7] Increased levels of plasma estrogens are formed by conversion (aromatization) of androgens in peripheral tissues (e.g., fat, muscle) where aromatase activity is up-regulated by alcohol. Adrenal overproduction of weak androgens and estrogen precursors has been observed in chronic alcohol-dependent men, probably as a result of direct stimulation of the adrenal cortex by ethanol and acetaldehyde.[1,8] In addition, in patients with liver cirrhosis and portosystemic shunting, androgens may escape from the enterohepatic into the systemic circulation, where they undergo increased peripheral aromatization to estrogens.[1] Finally, part of the estrogenization may be due to the ingestion of exogenous, plant-derived phytoestrogens contained in alcoholic beverages (e.g., Bourbon whiskey, beer).[1,6]

Treatment with high doses of nonaromatizable androgens may result in long-term rehabilitation with return of sexual function in only 25% of patients.[9,10] Alcohol abstinence is the only rational approach, and cessation of alcohol consumption has been reported to increase sperm output and motility.[11] It must be kept in mind that drugs used for the treatment of complications of alcoholic liver disease such as spironolactone (an aldosterone antagonist and K^+-sparing diuretic) can also cause gynecomastia and impotence.

WOMEN

Acute alcohol administration has no effect in nonalcoholic women, but chronic ethanol abuse disturbs hypothalamic-pituitary-gonadal function.[1,6] Alcohol-dependent women are not "superfeminized" (or "hyperestrogenized") as might be expected from the findings in alcohol-dependent men, but instead are "defeminized" and show hypogonadism with ovarian atrophy, paucity of developing follicles and few or no corpora lutea, oligomenorrhea, loss of breast and pelvic fat accumulation, and infertility.[1,6] Hypogonadism in women is caused by similar mechanisms as in men (see above) and is characterized by reduced plasma levels of estradiol and progesterone, with inadequately increased plasma FSH and LH levels, and a loss of the midcycle ovulatory gonadotropin (LH, FSH) peak.[1,6] In addition, chronic alcohol-dependent women can show two- to fourfold elevations of serum prolactin levels throughout the menstrual cycle, which may also contribute to oligo/amenorrhea.[6] The frequency of menstrual disturbances, spontaneous abortions, and miscarriages increases with the level of drinking.[12]

In contrast, moderate drinking (i.e., less than two alcoholic drinks per day) increases estrogen levels (up to twofold) in postmenopausal women.[13] This could contribute to the increased risk of

TABLE 21.2
Clinical Picture and Clinically Relevant Hormonal Changes in Alcohol-Dependent Patients

Disease	Clinical Features	Laboratory Values	Clinically Relevant Change
Male hypogonadism	Testicular atrophy, reduced libido, erectile impotence, loss of body hair, palmar erythema, spider angiomata, gynecomastia	LH ↑ FSH ↑ Testosterone ↓ Estradiol ↑	>20 U l^{-1} (1.2–2.2-fold increase) >20 U l^{-1} (1.5–3.2-fold increase) <3 µg l^{-1} (1.3–2.5-fold decrease) >55 pg ml^{-1} (1.3–4-fold increase)
Female hypogonadism	Ovarian atrophy, oligo/amenorrhea, infertility, loss of breast and pelvic fat	LH ↑ FSH ↑ Estradiol ↓ *But:* moderate drinking after menopause –estradiol ↑ PRL ↑	Basal >25 U l^{-1} (premenopausal) Decreased midcycle peak (normal 25–100 U l^{-1}) Basal >20 U l^{-1} (premenopausal) Decreased midcycle peak (normal 12–30 U l^{-1}) Basal <30 pg ml^{-1} (premenopausal) Decreased midcycle peak (normal >200 pg ml^{-1}) >55 pg ml^{-1} (postmenopausal) >20.8 ng ml^{-1} (2–4-fold increase)
Pseudo-Cushing's syndrome	Truncal obesity, bull's neck, peripheral muscle wasting, easy bruising, facial erythema, moon face, arterial hypertension, osteopenia	ACTH (8 a.m.) ↑ Cortisol (8 a.m.) ↑ Urinary cortisol ↑	>52 ng l^{-1}, loss of diurnal variation >250 µg l^{-1}, loss of diurnal variation >100 µg d^{-1}
Low-T$_3$ syndrome	None	Basal TSH →/↑ Free T$_3$ ↓ Free T$_4$ → Reverse T$_3$ ↑	Normal (0.1–4 mU l^{-1}) or mildly elevated <3 pmol l^{-1} normal (9–23 pmol l^{-1}) >0.61 nmol l^{-1}
Impaired bone and mineral metabolism	Osteopenia, bone pain, fractures	Osteocalcin ↓ PTH ↓ Ionized serum calcium ↓ Urinary calcium ↑	<3 µg l^{-1} <10 ng l^{-1} <1.12 mg dl^{-1} >8 mg g^{-1} creatinine
Hypoglycemia	Tremor, palpitations, sweating, dizziness, disorientation, personality changes, fits, loss of consciousness	Fasting glucose ↓ Insulin ↑ C-peptide ↑	<50 mg dl^{-1} >20 mU l^{-1} >5.4 µg l^{-1}

breast cancer in these individuals.[14,15] Conversely, potentially beneficial effects of these findings on the prevention of atherosclerosis and osteoporosis remain to be determined.[16]

HYPOTHALAMIC-PITUITARY-ADRENAL AXIS

Acute alcohol exposure in nonalcoholic males has no effect on plasma adrenocorticotropic hormone (ACTH) or cortisol levels,[17] but stimulates ACTH and cortisol secretion in chronic alcohol-dependent patients.[18] Chronic alcohol-dependent patients can rarely develop a syndrome (in up to 18% of patients) which is clinically and biochemically similar to Cushing's syndrome and therefore was termed "pseudo-Cushing's syndrome."[19] These patients present with peripheral muscle wasting, truncal obesity, easy bruising, glucose intolerance, arterial hypertension, facial erythema, and moon face, all of which are clinical features characteristic of Cushing's syndrome.[6,19-22] Laboratory features in these patients include elevated serum ACTH and cortisol levels, sometimes with loss of diurnal variation, and elevated 24-hour urinary free cortisol,[19,23] similar to Cushing's syndrome. Increased plasma ACTH and cortisol levels can be suppressed by overnight high-dose (8 mg) dexamethasone, but not by low-dose (1 mg) dexamethasone.[19,23,24] Therefore, this syndrome can be indistinguishable from true Cushing's syndrome, with the only exception that pseudo-Cushing's syndrome reverts after drinking is interrupted.[5]

Pseudo-Cushing's syndrome is caused by increased hypothalamic corticotropin-releasing hormone (CRH) secretion as a result of central stress, resulting in excessive pituitary ACTH secretion, followed by adrenal hyperplasia and increased cortisol production.[22,25-27] In contrast to true Cushing's syndrome, pseudo-Cushing's syndrome causes only intermittent and modest hypercortisolism since negative feedback inhibition of ACTH release by cortisol is still intact. However, the hypertrophied adrenal glands continue to produce excessive glucocorticoids in response to ACTH. Another important pathogenic factor is the direct stimulatory effects of ethanol and acetaldehyde on the adrenal cortex (see above). Specific glucocorticoid-suppressive therapy is not justified because all clinical and laboratory features disappear once the patient has stopped drinking.[21] ACTH and cortisol plasma levels usually normalize within a few days at the same rate or parallel with the decrease in serum γ-glutamyl transferase levels.[19,23] However, this syndrome may recur with resumption of alcohol abuse.

Experimental data suggest that corticosteroids might also stimulate alcohol consumption and drinking behavior.[28,29] Alcohol withdrawal in chronic alcohol-dependent patients who develop an abstinence syndrome is associated with a marked activation of the stress hormone cascade with elevations in cortisol secretion, particularly during the initial phase of withdrawal,[30] changes that might contribute to the behavioral and neurological changes associated with withdrawal.

Alcohol itself has no direct effect on adrenal aldosterone production, but secondary hyperaldosteronism resulting from peripheral vasodilation with activation of the renin-angiotensin-aldosterone system amd impaired hepatic aldosterone metabolism is a typical finding in alcohol-induced liver cirrhosis.

THYROID GLAND

Acute and chronic alcohol consumption results in increased oxygen consumption, a state resembling hyperthyroidism.[21] Since increased oxygen demand may contribute to alcohol-induced liver damage — particularly in central zones of the liver lobule that are most sensitive to anoxia — antithyroid drugs have been tested clinically in the treatment of alcoholic hepatitis (see Chapter 16 in this book). Thyroid function tests in patients with alcoholic hepatitis and liver cirrhosis may show a "low T_3 syndrome" characterized by decreased hepatic conversion of T_4 to T_3, but without clinical evidence of hypothyroidism.[6,21] On the other hand, serum levels of reverse T_3 produced at extrahepatic sites may be increased in this setting. Male patients with pronounced feminization can have high total T_4 levels due to estrogen-induced induction of thyroid-binding globulin, resulting in decreased hepatic clearance of the molecule.[31] However, free T_4 serum levels are normal.[6]

PARATHYROID GLANDS

Acute alcohol administration to normal volunteers reduces secretion and plasma levels of PTH, increases urinary excretion of calcium, and decreases ionized calcium levels in serum.[32] Chronic alcoholism is frequently associated with hypocalcemia, although it has not been shown that this is due to hypoparathyroidism.[33] Parathyroid function is not markedly disturbed in chronic alcohol-dependent patients, although hypomagnesemia secondary to increased urinary magnesium loss can result in parathormone resistance.[5,34]

BONE METABOLISM

Acute toxic effects of alcohol consumption on bone metabolism are linked to the parathyroid gland in the sense of a negative calcium balance.[35] Chronic alcohol ingestion has a direct toxic effect on osteoblasts and, therefore, decreases bone formation,[36] whereas bone resorption as measured by urinary hydroxyprolin excretion[37] and the renal phosphate threshold may be increased.[32] This uncoupling of osteogenic cells is suggested to be reversible after alcohol withdrawal[38] and specific therapy is not justified. Additional factors for the development of secondary osteopenia are nutritional deficiencies frequently encountered in alcoholics, especially in vitamin D metabolism, hypogonadism, and finally liver damage (see above).[1] Supplementation of calcium (1 g per day) and vitamin D (400 U per day) may be justified in patients with nutritional deficits. Bone loss was found to correlate with duration of alcohol drinking history[37] and may cause severe osteopenia with subsequent bone fractures.[39]

ENDOCRINE PANCREAS

Alcohol inhibits gluconeogenesis and causes hypoglycemia when glycogen stores are depleted. Typically, alcohol-induced hypoglycemia follows consumption of even moderate amounts of alcohol by 6 to 36 hours in chronically malnourished persons or healthy individuals who have not been eating food for one or more days.[40,41] Children (e.g., in the setting of inadvertent/accidental alcohol ingestion) are especially susceptible to ethanol-induced hypoglycemia. Alcohol potentiates the hypoglycemic actions of insulin and, when combined with sucrose ingestion (e.g., in certain cocktail drinks such as gin/tonic), may produce hyperinsulinism and thereby postprandial hypoglycemia in some individuals.[40] Inhibition of pituitary growth hormone (GH) secretion through alcohol could also contribute to alcohol-induced hypoglycemia.[5] Alcohol-induced hypoglycemia is an important differential diagnosis in alcohol-dependent patients presenting with altered mental state and confusion. It is important to keep in mind that blood alcohol levels may no longer be elevated when the patient is hypoglycemic.

On the other hand, patients with chronic alcohol-induced liver disease have varying degrees of glucose intolerance, ranging from asymptomatic postprandial elevations of blood glucose to frank insulin-dependent diabetes mellitus. However, the extent to which insulin-dependent diabetes is a consequence of liver disease, rather than an associated condition, is still controversial.[42] Alcohol abuse per se is not a risk factor for the developement of diabetes mellitus.

REFERENCES

1. Van Thiel, D.H., Stone, B.G., and Schade, R.R., The liver and its effect on endocrine function in health and disease, *Diseases of the Liver*, 7th ed., Schiff, L. and Schiff, E.R., Eds., J.B. Lippincott, Philadelphia, 1987, 129.
2. Gordon, G.G., Altman, K., Southren, A.L., Rubin, E., and Lieber, C.S., Effect of alcohol (ethanol) administration on sex-hormone metabolism in normal men, *N. Engl. J. Med.*, 295, 793, 1976.
3. Van Thiel, D.H., Ethanol: its adverse effects upon the hypothalamic-pituitary-gonadal axis, *J. Lab. Clin. Med.*, 101, 21, 1983.
4. Van Thiel, D.W., Lester, R., and Sherins, R.J., Hypogonadism in alcoholic liver disease: evidence for a double effect, *Gastroenterology*, 67, 1188, 1974.
5. Caballeria, J. and Pares, A., Extrahepatic manifestations of alcoholism, *Oxford Textbook of Clinical Hepatology*, 1st ed., McIntyre, N., Benhamou J.P., Bircher, J., Rizzetto, M., and Rodes, J., Eds., Oxford University Press, Oxford, 1991, 856.
6. Smanik, E.J., Barkoukis, H., Mullen, K.D., and McCullough, A.J., The liver and its effect on endocrine function in health and disease, *Diseases of the Liver*, 7th ed., Schiff, L. and Schiff, E.R., Eds., J.B. Lippincott, Philadelphia, 1373, 1993.

7. Wright, H.I., Gavaler, J.S., and Van Thiel, D.H., Effects of alcohol on the male reproductive system, *Alcohol Health Res. World,* 15, 110, 1991.

8. Cobb, C.F. and Van Thiel, D.W., Mechanism of ethanol-induced adrenal stimulation, *Alcoholism,* 6, 202, 1982.

9. Van Thiel, D.W., Gavaler, J.S., and Sanghvi, A., Recovery of sexual function in abstinent alcoholic men, *Gastroenterology,* 84, 677, 1982.

10. Korenman, S.G., Sexual function and dysfunction, *Williams Textbook of Endocrinology,* 9th ed., Wilson, J.D., Foster, D.W., Kronenberg, H.W., and Larsen P.R., Eds., W.B. Saunders, Philadelphia, 1998, 927.

11. Brzek, A., Alcohol and male fertility (preliminary report), *Andrologia,* 19, 32, 1987.

12. Mello, N.K., Mendelsohn, J.H., and Teoh, S.K., An overview of the effects of alcohol on neuroendocrine function in women, *Alcohol and the Endocrine System,* NIAA Research Monograph No. 23, NIH Pub. No. 93-3533, Zakhari, S., Ed., Bethesda, MD, 1993, 139.

13. Gavaler, J.S. and Van Thiel, D.H., The association between moderate alcoholic beverage consumption and serum estradiol and testosterone levels in normal postmenopausal women: relationship to the literature, *Alcohol. Clin. Exp. Res.,* 16, 87, 1992.

14. Schatzkin, A., Jones, D.Y., Hoover, R.N., Taylor, P.R., Brinton, L.A., Ziegler, R.G., Harvey, E.B., Carter, C.L., Licitra L.M., and Dufour, M.C., Alcohol consumption and breast cancer in the epidemiologic follow-up study of the first national health and nutrition examination survey, *N. Engl. J. Med.,* 316, 1169, 1988.

15. Lippman, M.E., Endocrine-responsive cancer, *Williams Textbook of Endocrinology,* 9th ed., Wilson, J.D., Foster, D.W., Kronenberg, H.W., and Larsen P.R., Eds., W.B. Saunders, Philadelphia, 1998, 1675.

16. Gavaler, J.S., Effects of alcohol on female endocrine function, *Alcohol Health Res. World,* 15, 104, 1991.

17. Ida, Y., Tsujimaru, S., Nakamaura, K., Shirao, I., Mukasa, H., Egami, H., and Nakazawa, Y., Effects of acute and repeated alcohol ingestion on hypothalamic-pituitary-gonadal and hypothalamic-pituitary-adrenal functioning in normal males, *Drug Alcohol Depend.,* 31, 57, 1992.

18. Elias, A.N., Meshkinpour, H., Valenta, L.J., and Grossman, M.K., Pseudo-Cushing's syndrome: the role of alcohol, *J. Clin. Gastroenterol.,* 4, 137, 1982.

19. Kirkman, S. and Nelson, D.H., Alcohol-induced pseudo-Cushing's disease: a study of prevalence with review of the literature, *Metabolism,* 37, 390, 1988.

20. Rees, L.H., Besser, G.M., Jeffcoate, W.J., Goldie, D.J., and Marks, V., Alcohol-induced pseudo-Cushing's syndrome, *Lancet,* 1, 726, 1977.

21. Johnson P.J., The effects of liver disease on the endocrine system, *Oxford Textbook of Clinical Hepatology,* 1st ed., McIntyre, N., Benhamou J.P., Bircher, J., Rizzetto, M., and Rodes, J., Eds., Oxford University Press, Oxford, 1991, 1214.

22. Orth, D.N. and Kovacs, W.J., The adrenal cortex, *Williams Textbook of Endocrinology,* 9th ed., Wilson, J.D., Foster, D.W., Kronenberg, H.W., and Larsen P.R., Eds., W.B. Saunders, Philadelphia, 1998, 927.

23. Lamberts, S.W., Klijn, J.G., de Jong, F.H., and Birkenhager, J.C., Hormone secretion in alcohol-induced pseudo-Cushing's syndrome. Differential diagnosis with Cushing disease, *JAMA,* 242, 1640, 1979.

24. Kapcala, L.P., Alcohol-induced pseudo-Cushing's syndrome mimicking Cushing's disease in a patient with an adrenal mass, *Am. J. Med.,* 82, 849, 1987.

25. Proto, G., Barberi, M., and Bertolissi, F., Pseudo-Cushing's syndrome: an example of alcohol-induced central disorder in corticotropin-releasing factor-ACTH release? *Drug Alcohol Depend.,* 16, 111, 1985.

26. Nieman, L.K. and Cutler, G.B., Cushing's syndrome, in *Endocrinology,* 3rd ed., DeGroot, L.J., Ed., W.B. Saunders, Philadelphia, 1995, 1741.

27. Groote Veldman, R. and Meinders, A.E., On the mechanisms of alcohol-induced pseudo-Cushing's syndrome, *Endocr. Rev.,* 17, 262, 1996.

28. Piazza, P.V., Maccari, S., Deminiere, J.M., Moal, M.L., Mormede, P., and Simon, H., Corticosterone levels determine individual vulnerability to amphetamine self-administration, *Proc. Natl. Acad. Sci. U.S.A.,* 88, 2088, 1991.

29. Piazza, P.V. and Moal, M.L., The role of stress in drug self-administration, *Trends Pharmacol. Sci.,* 19, 67, 1998.

30. Adinoff, B., Risher-Flowers, D., De Jong, J., Ravitz, B., Bone, G.H.A., Nutt, D.J., Roehrich, L., Martin, P.R., and Linnoila, M., Disturbances of hypothalamic-pituitary-adrenal axis functioning during ethanol withdrawal in six men, *Am. J. Psychiatry,* 148, 1023, 1991.

31. Borst, G.C., Eil, C., and Burman, K.D., Euthyroid hyperthyroxinemia, *Ann. Intern. Med.,* 98, 366, 1983.

32. Laitinen, K., Lamberg-Allardt, C., Tunninen, R., Karonen, S.L., Tahtela, R., Ylikahri, R., and Valimaki, M., Transient hypoparathyroidism during acute alcohol intoxication, *N. Engl. J. Med.,* 324, 721, 1991.

33. Fitzpatrick, L.A., and Arnold, A., Hypoparathyroidism, *Endocrinology,* 3rd ed., DeGroot, L.J., Ed., W.B. Saunders, Philadelphia, 1995, 1123.

34. Noth, R.H. and Walter, R.M., The effects of alcohol on the endocrine system, *Med. Clin. North Am.,* 68, 133, 1984.

35. Garcia-Sanchez, A., Gonzales-Calvin, J.L., Diez-Ruiz, A., Casalc, J.L., Gallego-Rojo, F., and Salvatierra, D., Effect of acute alcohol ingestion on mineral metabolism and osteoblastic function, *Alcohol Alcohol.,* 30, 449, 1995.

36. Pepersack, T., Fuss, M., Otero, J., Bergmann, P., Valsamis, J., and Corvilain, J., Longitudinal study of bone metabolism after ethanol withdrawal in alcoholic patients, *J. Bone Miner. Res.,* 7, 383, 1992.

37. Laitinen, K., Lamberg-Allardt, C., Tunninen, R., Harkonen, M., and Valimaki, M., Bone mineral density and abstention-induced changes in bone mineral metabolism in noncirrhotic male alcoholics, *Am. J. Med.,* 93, 642, 1992.

38. Lindholm, J., Steiniche, T., Rasmussen, E., Thamsborg, G., Nielsen, I.O., Brockstedt-Rasmussen, H., Storm, T., Hyldstrup, L., and Schou, C., Bone disorders in men with chronic alcoholism: a reversible disease? *J. Clin. Endocrinol. Metab.,* 73, 118, 1991.

39. Gonzales-Calvin, J.L., Garcia-Sanchez, A., Bellot, V., Munoz-Torres, M., Raya-Alvarez, E., and Salvatierra-Rios, D., Mineral metabolism, osteoblastic function and bone mass in chronic alcoholism, *Alcohol Alcohol.,* 28, 571, 1993.

40. Cryer, P.E., Glucose homeostasis and hypoglycemia, *Williams Textbook of Endocrinology,* 6th ed., Wilson, J.D. and Foster, D.W., Eds., W.B. Saunders, Philadelphia, 1985, 989.

41. Service, F.J., Hypoglycemia, including hypoglycemia in neonates and children, in *Endocrinology,* 3rd ed., DeGroot, L.J., Ed., W.B. Saunders, Philadelphia, 1995, 1605.

42. Kruszynska, Y.T. and Boloux, P.M., The effects of liver disease on the endocrine system, *Oxford Textbook of Clinical Hepatology,* 2nd ed., McIntyre, N., Benhamou J.P., Bircher, J., Rizzetto, M., and Rodes, J., Eds., Oxford University Press, Oxford, 1999, 1748.

22 Vitamin Deficiencies, Zinc Deficiency, and Anaphylactic Reactions

Norbert Reider

OVERVIEW

Vitamin deficiencies are frequent problems in alcoholics. Skin manifestations present infrequently and are often nonspecific. Therapy consists of vitamin replacement. The same applies for zinc deficiency. Acute reactions that present the symptoms of anaphylaxis might be due to histamine or additives in the alcoholic beverages or to the alcohol itself. Treatment consists of avoidance on the one hand and therapy of acute anaphylactic symptoms on the other.

ZINC DEFICIENCY [1-3]

Zinc belongs to the essential trace elements. Wine, beer, and spirits contain very low amounts of zinc. Subjects receiving less than 0.2 mg zinc daily (recommended daily intake, 16 mg) develop clinical manifestations within 2 to 3 months. Systemic symptoms comprise mental disorders, photophobia, diarrhea, and sepsis. On the skin, the finger flexural creases and the palms show grey flat blisters surrounded by a red-brown erythema. Periorificial areas show eczematous eruptions. In chronic cases, skin lesions typically present on areas exposed to pressure, such as ankles, elbows, and knees with well-demarcated, thickened, and brownish lesions. On the face, seborrheic-like changes may occur. Particularly in alcoholics, a reticulate, scaly dermatitis on the trunk has been described.

Zinc deficiency is diagnosed by the clinical picture and low serum zinc and alkaline phosphatase levels. As plasma albumin binds 70% of zinc, hypoalbuminemia may lead to false negative zinc levels.

For treatment, 30 to 50 mg zinc is given two to three times a day (p.o. or i.v.). Clinical improvement of diarrhea should occur within a few days, and healing of skin lesions can be expected within weeks.

VITAMIN DEFICIENCIES[4]

VITAMIN B

Isolated deficiencies of B vitamins are uncommon; in most cases, the whole group ($B_{1,3,6,12}$) is involved. The clinical pictures resemble each other.

Vitamin B_1 (Thiamine, Aneurin)

Unpolished rice, cereals, and yeast are rich in thiamine. In Southeast Asia, a thiamine deficiency may result if *polished* rice is used as the staple food. In the U.S. and Europe, more commonly

0-8493-7801-X/00/$0.00+$.50
© 2000 by CRC Press LLC

insufficient nutrition from alcoholism may lead to the clinical picture of beriberi, which is characterized by symmetrical polyneuritis, weakness, anorexia, cardiac insufficiency, and edemas most pronounced at the ankles, hands, and face.[5] Another manifestation of thiamine deficiency frequently associated with alcohol abuses is the Wernicke-Korsakoff syndrome, which does not typically go along with skin manifestations.

For treatment, 2 to 3 mg — in severe cases, up to 15 mg thiamine — are given three times daily. Beer is relatively rich in thiamine.

Vitamin B₃

Pellagra[6,7] is caused by an inadequate dietary supplement of niacin (nicotinic acid, vitamin B₃) and tryptophan. In industrial countries, it is only rarely encountered nowadays, mainly in chronic alcoholics, patients with gastrointestinal diseases and psychiatric disorders, and in subjects treated with isoniazid or hydantoin.

The clinical features comprise diarrhea, dermatitis, and neuropathological symptoms like depression, disorientation, restlessness, and peripheral neuritis. Skin lesions typically present as well-marginated redness and scaling on the front of the neck (Casal's necklace), a symmetrical "butterfly" eruption on the face, and dermatitis on areas exposed to sunlight, heat, or friction. The changes resemble sunburn, and re-exposure to sun is followed by exacerbation. Mucosal involvement is a frequent finding and presents as stomatitis, glossitis, or vulvitis. A pellagra-like dermatosis can be observed in Pacific Islanders using a psychoactive beverage called Kava.[8]

The diagnosis of pellagra may be complicated by the absence of skin lesions in the majority of cases. Pellagrans may show decreased zinc levels in plasma and urine.[9] Histology is not diagnostic.

In severe cases, niacin can be administered intravenously in doses of 50 to 100 mg once or twice a day, or 500 mg per day orally. A response can be seen within a few days.

Vitamin B₁₂ (Cyanocobalamin)

This vitamin is found mainly in meat, liver, milk, and eggs. Deficiency may occur in alcoholics, vegetarians, and — due to the lack of "intrinsic factor" — in pernicious anemia. Skin lesions present as hyperpigmentation pronounced in the flexures and on the knuckles.[10] Another characteristic finding is an enlarged, red tongue. As a supplement, administration of 2 mg cobalamin orally, or 1 mg i.m. on a monthly basis, are equally effective.[11]

Folic Acid

Folic acid is present in meat, liver, milk, and vegetables. The conversion to the biologically active form, biotinic acid, requires the presence of vitamin C. No constant cutaneous changes have been described, although a greyish-brown hyperpigmentation similar to that of vitamin B₁₂ deficiency may occur.

Vitamin C

While vitamin C deficiency is due to limited availability of fresh fruits in many parts of the world, the main cause in Europe is alcoholism. Skin changes of scurvy[12] comprise follicular keratosis and a purpuric rash on trunk, upper arms, and lower extremities. Stomatitis, epistaxis and bleeding gums may occur.

A daily dose of 500 to 1000 mg vitamin C for several weeks leads to a fast clinical response.

FLUSHING AND ANAPHYLACTIC REACTIONS

Flushing after intake of alcohol may occur in certain genetic disturbances, mainly the oriental flushing syndrome:[13] A majority of people of Asian descent develop extensive flushing after alcohol intake due to a deficiency of liver aldehyde dehydrogenase (ALDH), which results in an increase of the alcohol metabolite acetaldehyde. The diagnosis can be confirmed by use of an ethanol patch test, which shows erythema due to accumulation of acetaldehyde in the ethanol-treated skin.

The chlorpropamide-alcohol flush[14] occurs mainly in non-insulin-dependent diabetics receiving chlorpropamide as an oral antidiabetic drug. This disorder is predominantly inherited, but release of prostaglandins also seems to be involved, as aspirin is able to block the flush.

Alcohol intolerance is well known in subjects with a deficiency of diaminoxidase,[15] which is involved in the metabolism of histamine. The prevalence of this disorder is estimated to be about 10% in Western populations. Patients develop flushing, headache, soft stools, and gastrointestinal cramping after ingestion of histamine-rich beverages like red wine, beer, champagne, cheese, seafoods, and dried spices.

Moreover, alcohol itself has been shown to induce histamine release from mast cells and basophilic granulocytes. Food allergies can be aggravated or provoked by concomitant consumption of alcohol.

Apart from that, rare cases of severe anaphylactic reactions, including urticaria, angioedema, and asthma, shortly after intake of small amounts of alcohol have been described. It has been suggested that a type I allergic reaction[16] is involved in these subjects, as specific IgE against acetaldehyde-protein adducts were detected in the serum of patients. Skin prick tests with acetic acid (but not with alcohol) may be positive.

As most anaphylactoid reactions associated with alcohol intake are not severe and self-limited, therapy in most cases consists of the application of antihistamines (e.g., loratadine or cetirizine 10 mg p.o.; chlorpheniramine maleate 10 to 20 mg i.v.; dimetinden maleate 4 mg i.v.), corticosteroids (e.g., hydrocortisone 250 mg i.v. and 100 mg every 6 hours); in severe cases, adrenalin 0.5 to 1 mg s.c., i.v., i.m.

REFERENCES

1. Weismann, K., Zinc metabolism and the skin, *Recent Advances in Dermatology*, Churchill Livingstone, Vol. 5, 1980.
2. Ecker, R.I. and Schroeter, A.L., Acrodermatitis and aquired zinc deficiency, *Arch. Dermatol.*, 114, 937, 1978.
3. Gibson, R.S. and Ferguson, E.L., Nutrition intervention strategies to combat zinc defciency in developing countries, *Nutr. Res. Rev.*, 11, 115, 1998.
4. Cook, C.C., Hallwood, P.M., and Thomson, A.D., B vitamin deficiency and neuropsychiatric syndromes in alcohol misuse, *Alcohol Alcohol.*, 33, 317, 1998.
5. Sauberlich, H.E., Herman, Y.F., Stevens, C.O., and Herman, R.H., Thiamine requirement of the adult human, *Am. J. Clin. Nutr.*, 32, 2237, 1979.
6. Findlay, G.H., Pellagra, kwashiorkor and sun exposure, *Br. J. Dermatol.*, 77, 666, 1965.
7. Rook, Wilkinson, and Ebling, Eds., *Textbook of Dermatology*, Blackwell Science, 1998.
8. Ruze, P., Kava-induced dermopathy: a niacin deficiency? *Lancet*, 335, 1142, 1990.
9. Vanucchi, H., Favaro, R.M., Cunha, D.F., and Marchini, J.S., Assessment of zinc nutritional status of pellagra patients, *Alcohol Alcohol.*, 30, 297, 1995.
10. Noppakun, N. and Swasdikul, D., Reversible hyperpigmentation of skin and nails with white hair due to vitamin B_{12} deficiency, *Arch. Dermatol.*, 122, 896, 1986.
11. Kuzminski, A.M., Del-Giacco, E.J., Allen, R.H., Stabler, S.P., and Lindenbaum, J., Effective treatment of cobalamin deficiency with oral cobalamin, *Blood*, 92, 1191, 1998.
12. Ghorbani, A.J. and Eichler, C., Scurvy, *J. Am. Acad. Dermatol.*, 30, 881, 1994.
13. Wolff, P.H., Ethnic differences in alcohol sensitivity, *Science*, 175, 449, 1972.
14. Wiles, P.G. and Pyke, D., The chlorpropamide alcohol flush, *Clin. Sci.*, 67, 375, 1984.
15. Jarisch, R. and Wantke, F., Wine and headache, *Int. Arch. Allergy Immunol.*, 110, 7, 1996.
16. Sticherling, M., Brasch, J., Bruening, H., and Christophers, E., Urticarial and anaphylactic reactions following alcohol intake, *Br. J. Dermatol.*, 132, 464, 1995.

23 Skin

Alfred Grassegger

OVERVIEW

Ethanol intake plays a considerable but often underestimated role in dermatologic diseases. It may not only affect severity, duration, and even onset of skin diseases, but also is involved in pharmacologic aspects of dermatologic treatments.

DERMATOLOGIC CONDITIONS THAT MAY BE PROVOKED BY ETHANOL INTAKE INCLUDE

- Porphyrias, especially porphyria cutanea tarda[1-3]
- Psoriasis vulgaris[1,2,4,6] and interaction with the
- Metabolism of retinoic acid (etretinate, acitretine)[5-8]
- Rosacea[1,2]
- Acquired zinc deficiency[1,2] (see Chapter 22)
- Cancer of the oral mucosa [1,2,9-13]
- Perniones[1, 2]
- Ecthymata[1, 2]
- Epizoonoses[1, 2]
- Pellagra (see Chapter 22)
- Allergic and pseudoallergic reactions[9] (see Chapter 22)

HEPATIC PORPHYRIAS

PORPHYRIA CUTANEA TARDA (PCT)

Hepatic porphyrias include porphyria cutanea tarda, acute intermittent porphyria, and porphyria variegata. *Porphyria cutanea tarda* (PCT) is the most important hepatic porphyria seen by dermatologists. The prevalence among adults between the ages of 40 and 70 years is about 1%. Males are more often affected than females (ratio, 2:1). Alcohol consumption is an important — but not the only — trigger of hepatic porphyrias (see below).

Porphyria cutanea tarda is biochemically characterized by deficiency of the enzyme uroporphyrinogen III decarboxylase. Thus, porphyrin content is increased in tissues, especially in skin. Exogen factors such as alcohol consumption are needed for the development of clinical symptoms. One should look for the following:

- Alcoholic beverages, barbiturates, and benzodiazepines
- Antiphlogistic compounds (pyrazolone derivatives)
- Opioid and NSAID analgesics
- Anticonvulsants
- Estrogens
- Tolbutamide, chloropropamide

- Antimicrobials (sulfonamides, griseofulvine, chloramphenicol, anthelminthics)
- Ergotamine, methyl-DOPA, and theophylline

Skin changes, hepatic impairment, and porphyrinuria are the clinical features of the disease. On sun-exposed areas such as the face, dorsum of the hands, and nape of the neck, there are bullous erosions and tense blisters on noninflammatory skin developing in response to minor traumata such as pressure or contusion. Hemorrhagic crusts are frequently present. Healing occurs with slight atrophy and scarring, sometimes with depigmentation or hyperpigmentation. Milia formation (post-bullous scarring) is seen within scars, representing an important diagnostic sign.

Further characteristic features include hypertrichosis in the eyebrows and cheek area. Darkening of hairs is frequently found and sometimes associated with solar elastosis and comedones (Favre-Racouchot syndrome). In rare cases, scleroderma-like thickening of the skin might occur, resembling diffuse progressive sclerosis (i.e., a pseudosclerosis condition termed "scleroporphyria").

Red-brown urine shows red fluorescence under UV-A light (Wood's light) due to elevated uroporphyrin concentrations. Hepatic transaminases are elevated in serum. Another feature is hypersiderinemia, and development of hemochromatosis has been described.

Avoidance of sun exposure (using protective clothes and sun protection creams in the UV-B *and* UV-A range) and avoidance of toxic agents (alcohol, oral contraceptives, drugs) are important. Phlebotomy (300 to 500 ml weekly) is recommended to reduce serum iron levels until serum hemoglobin level of 12 g dl^{-1} is reached. If control of the disease is not achieved, chloroquine is given in low doses (i.e., 125 mg once weekly). High doses of chloroquine are dangerous because liver cell necrosis might occur. Chloroquine is contraindicated if serious liver damage is already present (requires cooperation with hepatologist).

ERYTHROPOETIC PROTOPORPHYRIA

Exogenic triggers are **not** necessary for the clinical manifestation of erythropoetic porphyria. This is a relatively rare (1:100,000 in the general population) hereditary disorder of the porphyrin metabolism characterized by sensitivity to light. The genetic basis of the disease is a deficiency of the mitochondrial enzyme ferrochelatase. The disease starts in early childhood. Protoporphyrin concentration is increased in erythrocytes.

After sun exposure, there is a burning sensation of the skin with erythema, but not blister formation. Cholecystolithiasis is an associated feature in adults, occasionally accompanied by liver cirrhosis. It is important to know that excessive alcohol intake can lead to acute hepatic failure in this disease!

Currently, only symptomatic treatment is available. Beta-carotene as an antioxidant is recommended at a dosage of 100 to 300 mg daily. Sun protection measures are recommended (e.g., sun block; wearing long sleeves, trousers, and a hat).

PSORIASIS VULGARIS[1,2]

Apart from antimalarial drugs, beta-blocking agents, and lithium, alcohol is an important exogenic trigger that may be responsible for the exacerbation of preexisting psoriasis. Approximately 2 to 5% of the population are genetically predisposed to psoriasis vulgaris. HLA association is found, in that HLA-Cw6 is associated with type I psoriasis with early manifestation (before age 40) but not with type II psoriasis (late onset psoriasis). HLA-B27 is associated with psoriatic arthropathy.

The manifestation of psoriasis needs exogenic provocation factors such as physical or chemical traumata to the epithelial integrity (Koebner phenomenon), focal infection, or certain medications. Hypocalcemia and pregnancy might be additional triggers. T-cell stimulation by streptococcal or staphylococcal superantigens was recently emphasized to be important in eliciting psoriasis.

MAIN CLINICAL CHARACTERISTICS OF PSORIASIS

Skin lesions can be extremely variable. The primary lesion is a red, squamous plaque (Figures 23.1A and 23.1B), mainly located on the extensor sites of the extremities, capillitium, sacrum. Generalization can occur with tiny erythematous plaques (psoriasis guttata) or even erythroderma with sterile pustular eruption (psoriasis pustulosa). This generalized pustular variant is life-threatening. There is an intertriginous variant of psoriasis (psoriasis inversa) that might be confused with, for example, perianal eczema or submammary candidosis. A serious clinical association is psoriatic arthropathy, which is present in about 5% of all psoriatic patients. Psoriatic monoarthritis or oligoarthritis is typical. Small joints are not always often heavily involved, and mutilation and ancylosing arthritis including spondylitis can occur.

ALCOHOL AND PSORIASIS

The percentage of heavy drinkers is higher in patients with psoriasis compared to the normal population. Alcohol consumption might aggravate psoriasis. *In vitro* studies have shown that ethanol induces IL-6, IFN-γ and TGF-α expression in keratinocytes of psoriatic patients (see also Chapter 22 on the immune system).[7] The pharmacologic interaction of ethanol and retinoid therapy is described later.

TREATMENT OF PSORIASIS

Treatment implies topical and systemic measures. Corticosteroids, tar products, anthralin, calcipotriol ointments, and UV-B irradiation are often used topically. Systemic corticosteroids are contraindicated because a rebound phenomenon after discontinuation is common. Retinoids have brought a tremendous benefit to psoriatic patients. The aromatic retinoid etretinate and its metabolite acitretin are used. Retinoids are able to control the pathologic keratinization and stop proliferation

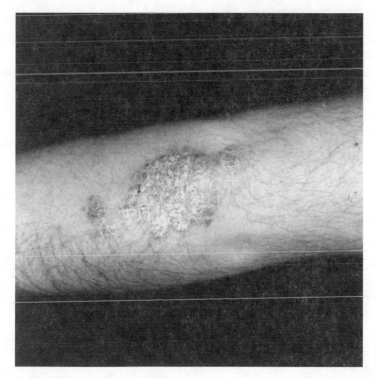

FIGURE 23.1A   Psoriasis vulgaris (plaque type).

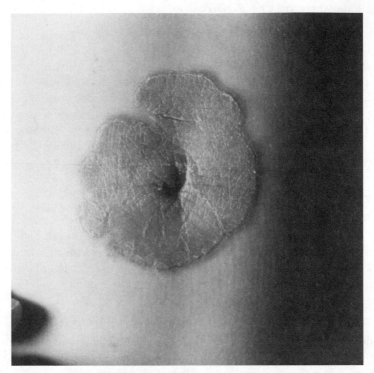

FIGURE 23.1B   Psoriasis vulgaris (periumbilical region).

and inflammatory reaction. Side effects are common, including dry cheilitis, conjunctivitis, hair loss, hyperlipidemia, and impairment of liver function. Cheilitis is found in almost every patient taking retinoids, thus serving as an indicator for a patient's treatment compliance. Retinoids are teratogenic; therefore, women of child-bearing age must use reliable contraception during and for at least 2 years after use of etretinate.

Psoralen with UV-A irradiation (PUVA-treatment) is another treatment option. Topically applied psoralens combined with UV-A treatment minimize side effects (balneo-photochemotherapy).

RETINOIDS AND ALCOHOL INTAKE

Table 23.1 lists the main retinoids in clinical use at present.

TABLE 23.1
The Main Retinoids in Clinical Use

Retinoid	Use
all-trans-Retinoic acid	Topical treatment of acne comedonica, premature photoaging, hyperpigmentation
13-*cis*-Retinoic acid	Systemic treatment of severe acne or acne conglobata
Etretinate	Systemic treatment of, for example, psoriasis, lichen planus, pityriasis rubra pilaris, palmoplantar hyperkeratosis
Acitretin	Metabolite of etretinate with a shorter biological half-life
Adapalene	Chemically derived from tretinoin with antiinflammatory properties
Tazarotene	Derived from etretinate for topical treatment, e.g., of psoriasis

As mentioned, retinoids are teratogenic compounds. Therefore, women of child-bearing age are at risk during systemic medication. Topical treatment is considered not risky unless treatment is extensive or involves larger areas of the body. However, this author would not recommend topical retinoic acid treatment during pregnancy.

Acitretin, the metabolite of etretinate, has a shorter (1 to 2 days) biologic half-life than etretinate, which was shown to have a half-life of 3 months during chronic application. As with etretinate, however, a 2-year period of contraception is necessary for acitretin because it converts back to etretinate in the presence of small amounts of ethanol.[5,6] In addition, toxic effects of ethanol and retinoic acid on liver function are likely to be additive, and severe liver damage may occur. Thus, during retinoid therapy, alcohol intake should be strictly avoided; in fact, chronic alcoholism is an absolute contraindication for retinoid therapy. Decreased efficacy of isotretinoin has also been described during acute alcohol intake.[8]

ROSACEA ("FACIES ETHYLICA")

Rosacea (Figures 23.2 and 23.3) is an acne-like disease characterized by papules, teleangiectasia and, in later stages, sebaceous gland hyperplasia that results in rhinophyma. The etiology of rosacea is unknown. Unlike acne, hair follicles are not primary involved. Besides a genetic predisposition, exogenic provocation factors such as cold weather, heat, extensive sun exposure, and ethanol consumption are frequently found. The saprophyte *Demodex folliculorum* plays a possible, although unproven role in rosacea.[2] Thus, roseaca is not necessarily due to harmful alcohol consumption. Despite this fact, rosacea might still erroneously be referred to as the "alcoholic face" (i.e., facies ethylica). It should be emphasized here that without proper diagnosis of alcohol abuse or dependence, the clinical picture might simply be misleading. On the positive side, one can liberate a rosacea patient from a very strong social stigma by effective therapy of his/her non-alcoholic rosacea.

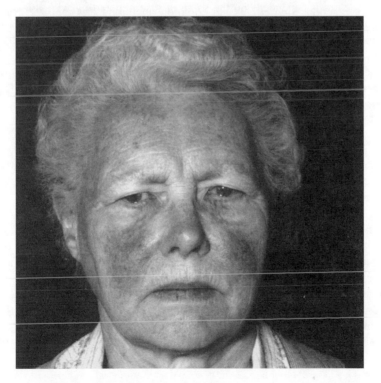

FIGURE 23.2   Rosacea (stadium teleangiectaticum).

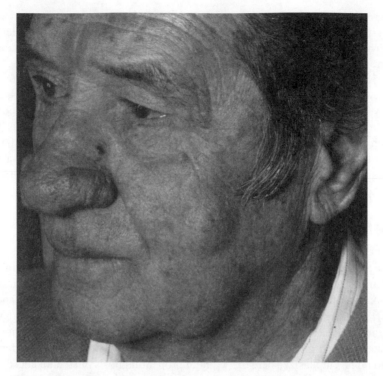

FIGURE 23.3   Rosacea (Rhinophyma).

The clinical picture is dependent on the stage of disease, starting with teleangiectasias of the face, followed by papules and pustules. Exacerbations are known after excessive alcohol drinking. Conjunctivits and iritis are associated, and keratitis is a possible complication that might lead to blindness when left untreated.

Tetracyclines with their antiinflammatory properties (inhibition of peroxide formation) are the mainstay of therapy. Alternatively, isotretinoin was also shown to be effective. Topical treatment with 0.5% metronidazol emulsions has been shown to be effective.

ACQUIRED ZINC DEFICIENCY SYNDROME

Zinc belongs to the essential trace elements and is required in the synthesis of metalloproteins (lactate dehydrogenase, alkaline phosphatase, superoxide dismutase) and DNA, and RNA polymerases and transcription factors. Thus, it plays a key role in development, growth, and metabolism. Deficiency of zinc leads to cutaneous and intestinal inflammatory symptoms.

Besides the hereditary zinc deficiency syndrome (acrodermatitis enteropathica) — which is an autosomal recessive disorder leading to decreased zinc resorption and malnutrition — parenteral nutrition without zinc supplementation, malabsorption, catabolic conditions, and chronic alcoholism are major causes of the acquired variant.

Skin changes are characterized by periorificial or acral dermatitis (perleche, acral erythema, vesicular and crusted anular lesions, persistent paronychia), diffuse effluvium, diarrhea, weight loss, anorexia, weakness, and lethargy. Plasma levels of zinc are below 70 mg dl^{-1}.

Skin changes improve within weeks if zinc sulfate or zinc chloride is substituted orally or intravenously (30 to 50 mg molecular zinc).

CANCER OF THE ORAL MUCOSA

Alcoholism has long been recognized to be associated with oral cancer.[9] When combined with heavy smoking a synergistic effect was found.[10] Besides immunosuppression of continued exposure to large amounts of alcohol, it is currently supposed that toxic effects of ethanol and/or acetaldehyde on oral mucosa play a significant role in tumor promotion, maybe due to increased lipid peroxidation and eicosanoid metabolism.[11, 12]

Clinically, the initial lesion is a painless lump or ulcer in the oral cavity. The delay of initial symptom and examination is 4 to 6 months. Early diagnosis is mandatory to achieve a favorable outcome. For example, the 5-year survival rate for all tongue cancers is 35 to 45%.[13] Treatment of choice is surgery combined with irradiation if lymph nodes are involved.

OTHER SKIN CHANGES

SKIN CHANGES SOMETIMES FOUND IN ALCOHOL-DEPENDENT INDIVIDUALS OF LOW SOCIOECONOMIC STATUS

The following describes skin lesions typical for patients of very low socioeconomic status (i.e., the homeless). This is *not* to mean that homeless people are necessarily alcohol dependent. However, alcohol-dependent patients may eventually find themselves in a very low socioeconomic position; this section explains how to give them proper care.

Perniones

Perniones are characterized by erythematous or bluish-red edematous, circumscribed, or diffuse inflammatory swelling that is painful on warming. The lesions get bright red at room temperature due to heat-induced hyperemia. Pathogenetically, temperatures just above 0°C with high humidity play a major role. Acrozyanosis or hyperhidrosis may coexist as a symptom of autonomic dysregulation. People working in humd, cold environments are predisposed for perniones. Theoretically, alcoholism might also predispose to this disorder due to the vasodilatory effect of ethanol, especially on cutaneous vessels. In addition, ethanol impairs central thermoregulation.

Treatment should promote circulation with vasodilating agents, such as pentoxifyllin or cinnarizin. Protection from moist and cold environmental conditions is mandatory. If more severe inflammatory signs are present, topical corticosteroids are recommended.

ECTHYMATA

This disease resembles streptococcal impetigo but extends deeper into the skin, forming superficial ulcers, predominantly on the lower extremities. Poor hygiene and cold exposure (circumstances that might be found in chronic alcoholism) contribute significantly to pathogenesis. Group A streptococci are the major pathogens found in the lesions. Autoinoculation and poststreptococcal sequela (e.g., glomerulonephritis) are possible complications. Systemic antibiotics for several weeks, combined with antiseptic topical measurements, are the treatment of choice.

Epizoonoses

Epizoonoses are disorders caused by external parasites (ectoparasites). These implicate scabies (mites), pediculosis (lice), cimicosis (bugs), pulicosis (fleas), and in a wider sense, insect bites and stings. Because body (clothes) lice are sometimes found in vagabonds, skin findings (scratch marks) are sometimes called "cutis vagantium." Therapy for scabies and pediculosis mainly consists of local application of hexachlorocyclohexane or permethrine emulsions.

REFERENCES

1. Fritsch, P., *Dermatologie und Venerologie,* Springer-Verlag, Berlin, 1998.
2. Braun-Falco, O., Plewig, G., Wolff, H.H., and Winkelmann, R.K., *Dermatology,* Springer-Verlag, Berlin, 1991.
3. Bonkovsky, H.L. and Schned, A.R., Fatal liver failure in protoporphyria. Synergism between ethanol excess and the genetic defect, *Gastroenterology,* 90, 191, 1986.
4. Ockenfels, H.M., Keim-Maas, C., Funk, R., Nussbaum, G., and Goos, M., Ethanol enhances the IFN-gamma, TGF-alpha and IL-6 secretion in psoriatic co-cultures, *Br. J. Dermatol.,* 135, 746, 1996.
5. Almond-Roesler, B. and Orfanos, C.E., *trans*-Acitretin is metabolized back to etretinate. Importance for oral retinoid therapy, *Hautarzt,* 47, 173, 1996.
6. Larsen, F.G., Jakobsen, P., Knudsen, J., Weismann, K., Kragballe, K., and Nielsen, K.F., Conversion of acitretin to entretinate in psoriatic patients is influenced by ethanol, *J. Invest. Dermatol.,* 100, 623, 1993.
7. Merk, H.F. and Bickers, D.R., *Dermatopharmakologie und Dermatotherapie,* Blackwell Wissenschafts-Verlag, Berlin, 1992.
8. Soria, C., Allegue, F., Galiana, J., and Ledo, A., Decreased isotretinoin efficacy during acute alcohol intake, *Dermatologica,* 182, 203, 1991.
9. Binnie, W.H., Rankin, K.V., and Mackenzie, I.C., Etiology of oral squamous cell carcinoma, *J. Oral Pathol.,* 12, 29, 1983.
10. Mashberg, A., Garfinkel, L., and Harris, S., Alcohol as a primary risk factor in oral squamous carcinoma, *CA Cancer J. Clin.,* 31, 146, 1981.
11. Mufti, S.I., Nachiappan, V., and Eskelson, C.D., Ethanol-mediated promotion of oesophageal carcinogenesis: association with lipid peroxidation and changes in phospholipid fatty acid profile of the target tissue, *Alcohol Alcohol.,* 32, 221, 1997.
12. Mufti, S.I., Darban, H.R., and Watson, R.R., Alcohol, cancer, and immunomodulatio, *Crit. Review. Oncol. Hematol.,* 9, 243, 1989.
13. Ildstad, S.T., Bigelow, M.E., and Remensnyder, J.P., Squamous cell carcinoma of the tongue: a comparison of the anterior two thirds of the tongue with its base, *Am. J. Surg.,* 146, 456, 1983.
14. Sticherling, M., Brasch, J., Bruning, H., and Christophers, E., Urticarial and anaphylactoid reactions following ethanol intake, *Brit. J. Dermatol.,* 132, 464, 1995.

24 Alcohol Embryopathy: Symptoms, Course, and Etiology

Frank Majewski

OVERVIEW

Main features of alcohol embryopathy (AE); which is often imprecisely referred to as *fetal alcohol syndrome* (FAS), include intrauterine growth retardation, microcephaly, mental retardation (mean IQ = 66 in children with AE III), typical face and various internal malformations, especially congenital heart defects and genitourinary tract malformations. We examined 230 children with AE and graded the severity of AE from mild to severe (AE I–III) according to dysmorphologic appearance. Internal malformations, mental and statomotor development, as well as maternal history of alcohol consumption correlated to the relative degree of AE phenotype.

A positive correlation was found between the degree of AE and the frequency of congenital heart defects (10% in AE I, 19% in AE II, and 63% in AE III), other internal malformations and genital anomalies, and the degree of mental retardation (mean IQ was 91 in AE I, 79 in AE II, and 66 in AE III).

While the degree of mental retardation and microcephaly remains rather stable, there is some catch-up growth in height and more in weight, especially in female patients. The face also changes: the shortened nose and mandible normalize or even change to a prominent chin in adults with AE.

The stage of maternal alcohol illness, but not the daily (mostly excessive, mean 171 g) maternal alcohol consumption, significantly influenced the degree of AE. All mothers of children with AE were alcohol dependent. In the chronical stage, significantly more children with AE III were born than in the critical stage. The frequency of AE among the offspring was also related to the increasing stage of maternal alcohol illness. In the critical stage, there were 21%, and in the chronical stage 41% (42% in all three internationally available studies) of the children affected with AE. The pathogenesis of AE is still unclear, but prevention by successful withdrawal treatment is possible, as some healthy children of formerly addicted mothers with affected children have shown. Excessive alcohol abuse during pregnancy can cause severe damage in the offspring, which can vary from minimal cerebral disturbances to severe mental and physical handicap. The combination of intrauterine and postnatal growth retardation, dysmorphias/malformations, and mental retardation is referred to as alcohol embryopathy (AE) or fetal alcohol syndrome (FAS). The term "fetal alcohol effects" (FAE) describes mild behavioral and mental disturbances, without physical abnormalities.

DEFINITIONS

ALCOHOL EMBRYOPATHY

Main symptoms of AE are intrauterine growth retardation (IUGR), microcephaly, motor and mental retardation, muscular hypotonia, hyperactivity, a characteristic face (rounded forehead, short upturned nose, nasolabial furrows, small lips, retrogenia), and a variety of internal malformations, especially of the heart and genitals (Table 24.1). The diagnosis of AE is likely if all or most of these symptoms, as well as a history of maternal alcohol abuse during pregnancy, are present. Other (rare) syndromes with IUGR and microcephaly should be excluded.

TABLE 24.1

Frequencies of Symptoms in 230 Children with AE

Points	Symptoms	AE III (%)	AE II (%)	AE I (%)	Total (%)
4	Intrauterine growth retardation	95	81	77	84
—	Postnatal growth retardation	96	87	72	84
4	Microcephaly	88	76	71	77
2/4/8	Statomotor/mental retardation	98	92	69	84
4	Hyperactivity	81	79	58	72
2	Muscular hypotonia	72	58	45	57
2	Epicanthic folds	52	54	37	46
2	Ptosis	46	22	14	25
2	Blepharophimosis	35	42	12	29
—	Antimongol. palpebral fissures	48	26	21	29
—	Strabism	25	18	11	17
—	Dysplastic ears	41	32	15	29
3	Short upturned nose	69	56	39	53
1	Nasolabial furrows	88	64	54	65
1	Small lips	79	69	48	64
4	Cleft palate	17	5	0	7
2	High arched palate	41	20	15	24
—	Hypoplasia of maxilla	2	3	3	2
2	Hypoplasia of mandible	89	79	33	65
3	Anomalous palmar creases	87	71	48	67
2	Brachyclinodactyly V	48	39	23	36
2	Camptodactyly	25	11	5	12
1	Hypoplasia of endphalanges	26	8	7	12
2	Limited supination	21	6	6	10
2	Hip dislocation	13	9	9	10
—	Flat feet	33	62	30	41
—	Pectus excavatum	20	18	24	21
—	Pectus carinatum	12	7	5	8
4	Congenital heart defect	63	19	10	27
—	Hemangiomas	24	15	8	15
2/4	Genital anomalies	61	38	27	40
1	Sacral dimple	63	53	33	48
2	Hernias	22	8	8	11
4	Genitourinary malformations	16	9	0	7

AE I   (n = 83): 10–29 points
AE II   (n = 83): 30–39 points
AE III   (n = 64): >40 points

Lemoine et al.[27] were the first to report on children with AE. They reported on the characteristics in 127 children of alcoholic parents. They noted a recognizable craniofacial anomaly, that is, microcephaly, a short and upturned nose, small lips, and retrogenia. The facial anomalies were "typical during the first two years … and changed with age …". Most of their patients exhibited marked pre- and postnatal growth retardation, underweight, mental retardation (IQ around 70), and various malformations (e.g., heart defects, microphthalmia, cleft palate, hip dislocation, and visceral anomalies. Because this paper appeared in a *local* French medical journal, there was international interest only in the papers of Jones et al., which were published in the *Lancet*.[21,22] Jones' first report described 11 children of alcoholic mothers. All exhibited growth retardation, underweight, and microcephaly. All showed motor and mental developmental delay. Characteristic dysmorphic facial features included ptosis of upper lids, epicanthic folds, short upturned nose, small vermillion border of upper lip, and retrogenia. Furthermore, some children suffered from congenital heart defect, anomalous palmar creases, and limited supination. In their second paper,[21] Jones et al. examined 26 offspring of 23 chronic alcoholic mothers. The perinatal mortality was 17%; 32% of surviving children showed symptoms of AE. After these publications, numerous case reports appeared worldwide that confirmed the specific clinical picture of AE.[2-5,7,8,11-14,16,23,24,26,29,31,33-35,37,40-42,45,47,48,51-53,56,63-65]

FETAL ALCOHOL EFFECTS

Because the development of the brain can be disturbed during the entire pregnancy, the symptoms of this "embryotoxic encephalopathy"[31] are various. Therefore, the definition of alcohol effects is somewhat weak and seems to be nonspecific. These effects are observed as developmental delay — especially of speech, attention deficits, hyperactivity, learning disabilities, and emotional and social adaptive disturbances, without the typical morphological abnormalities of AE.[1,57] The effects on the offspring of mild or moderate alcohol consumption during pregnancy are mostly mild, and they are often difficult to verify.

Streissguth et al.[55,58] prospectively examined 500 children; 250 of the mothers had consumed alcohol moderately to heavily during pregnancy, and 250 had consumed little or none. Newborns of mothers who drank more than one ounce daily (29.6 g) during pregnancy showed delayed reactions to the stimuli of a light, a rattle, and a bell. At the ages of 8 months and 4 years, these children had some behavioral disturbances, especially attentional deficits. At a mean age of 7.5 years all of the 482 reexamined children were healthy, but there was a decrease in IQ of 7 points in 30 children whose mothers had consumed more than one ounce of alcohol per day. Mentally subnormal children were only observed among the offspring of mothers who had consumed more than two ounces (59 g) of absolute alcohol per day during pregnancy. Olson et al.[42] reported on the follow-up of 458 children at age 11 years by questionnaires mailed to their classroom teachers. A wide variety of classroom-related problems, including attention, activity, information-processing, and academic difficulties were salient for prenatal exposure. Maternal binge drinking ("five or more drinks per occasion") and drinking during very early pregnancy were particularly salient for the poorer school performance of these children. In contrast, Autti-Raemoe and Granstroem[4] observed no influence of first trimester "moderate to heavy drinking" on 21 children at the age of 1.5 years compared to nonexposed controls.

DIAGNOSIS, CLASSIFICATION, AND CLINICAL SYMPTOMS OF AE

No single symptom is specific for AE. The diagnosis is probable only if various characteristics are present together with a history of maternal alcohol abuse during pregnancy. The ascertainment of cases and the clinical description varies from author to author. In some studies, only severely affected children were examined; in others, only milder forms were examined. In the latter, internal malformations are rare or lacking. Therefore, a direct comparison of the frequencies of clinical symptoms in the different studies is not meaningful. The following summarizes the clinical symptoms of 230 children who manifested three degrees of severity of AE (see below). These children were examined by the author over a period of 20 years. Because most other investigators came to the same results, only gross differences will be discussed.

The degree of AE is highly variable. Although there is a continuum from severe to mild damage, a classification into three degrees of severity is meaningful for prognosis.[35] In the left column of Table 24.1, 25 symptoms were scored on a scale from 1 to 4; only extremely severe brain damage was graded with a score of 8. The sum of each case allowed a classification, given at the bottom. It should be emphasized that this scoring system allows a comparable classification into the degrees I to III, but not the initial diagnosis of AE (e.g., a child with the recessively inherited Dubowitz syndrome can easily reach a score of AE III). Furthermore, this classification is possible only during the first years of life because later on, the facial anomalies change (see below). This classification was followed by most German authors. Dehaene et al.[12] also used a classification into 3, and Streissguth et al.[53] into 5 degrees, but their criteria involved clinical judgments only.

AE III: The severe type of AE is characterized by marked pre- and postnatal growth retardation, microcephaly, and mental retardation. The face is so typical that the diagnosis of maternal alcoholism during pregnancy can be deduced: the forehead is rounded, there may be short palpebral fissures (blepharophimosis), the nose is short and upturned, the philtrum is flat, the vermillion border of the lips (mainly the upper) is very narrow, the mandible is hypoplastic. Children with AE III frequently suffer from internal malformations (Table 24.1). Mental impairment is always severe and most children are hypotonic and hyperactive (Figure 24.1a and b).

AE II: Patients with the moderate type of AE are growth retarded as well as microcephalic. Their mental retardation is not as severe as in AE III. The face is dysmorphic (Figure 24.2) but without proven maternal alcoholism, the diagnosis can only be suspected. However, hyperactivity and muscular hypotonia may be of diagnostic help. Internal malformations are not as frequent as in AE III (Table 24.1).

AE I: The mild form of AE is characterized by pre- and postnatal growth retardation, underweight, and microcephaly. Mental development is normal or only slightly subnormal. The faces of most children are normal (Figure 24.3), and there are few or no internal malformations (Table 24.1). Diagnosis is only possible by verification of severe maternal alcoholism during pregnancy.

If the diagnosis by facial anomalies is questionable, the examiner should look at the crying baby: the skin of the rounded forehead is wrinkled, the nasolabial furrows are increased, and the lateral parts of the lower lips are turned down. Furthermore, hyperexcitability and restless spontaneous movements may help in the diagnosis of questionable cases.

In Table 24.1, the frequencies of 34 common symptoms of 230 children with different degrees of AE are listed. In the following, the various dysmorphic features of AE are described.

FACE

The face in patients with AE III is characterized by rounded forehead, antimongoloid slant to palpebral fissures (48%), blepharophimosis (35%), short upturned nose (69%), deep nasolabial furrows (88%), and hypoplastic mandible (89%). All symptoms may be also present in milder forms, but with lower frequency. We observed hypoplasia of maxilla in only 2 to 3% of our cases, whereas other authors (e.g., Spohr et al.[52]) observed this symptom in 19%. This difference is probably caused by a higher proportion of milder cases in the cohort.[52] Mid-face hypoplasia was mentioned by other authors, but the frequency was not given.[60] The impression of small palpebral fissures is caused by ptosis and epicanthic folds, whereas blepharophimosis is defined by horizontally shortened palpebral fissures. We have measured the length of palpebral fissures[37] and observed blepharophimosis in only 29% of our cases with all degrees of severity. In our patients of AE III, we observed blepharophimosis in 35% (Table 24.1). Blepharophimosis was noted by Clarren and Smith[8] in more than 80% of their cases and by Spohr et al.[52] in 41% at the initial examination of their 71 cases and in 29% at the follow-up examination.

Facial appearance changes with age. In older patients, the nose is no longer short and upturned, the lips are no longer thin, and the chin often becomes rather prominent (Figure 24.4a and b). The same changes of facial apperarance were noted by several authors.[27,28,34,52,56,60] Because retrogenia changes to progenia, the impression of hypoplastic maxilla may be more frequent in older cases. The only unchanged features in all cohorts are small palpebral fissures and microcephaly. In older patients, baby-age photos often serve as a necessary diagnostic tool. The face in severely affected children is so characteristic that the diagnosis can be delineated from photos alone (Figure 24.1a and b); 6 out of 7 expert clinicians were able to accurately identify most of the 21 7-year-old children who had been prenatally exposed to high levels of alcohol.[10]

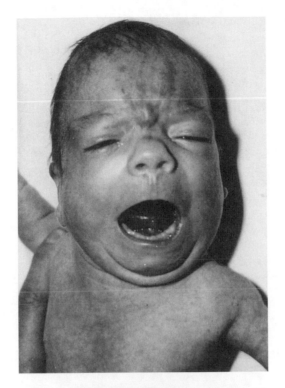

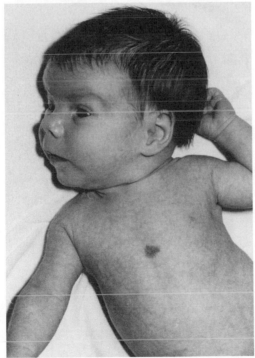

FIGURE 24.1   (a) Face of a newborn with AE III; (b) profile of a newborn with AE III.

With time, further symptoms turned out to be typical of AE (not listed in Table 24.1); for example, flat philtrum (95% in the cohort of Loeser et al.[33]), small teeth (31% in the series by Spohr[51]), and thick and brittle hair.

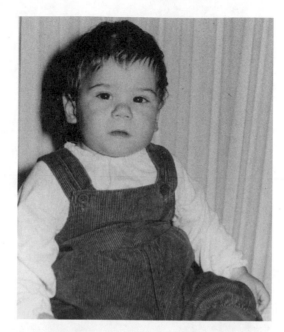

FIGURE 24.2   Face of a boy with AE II.

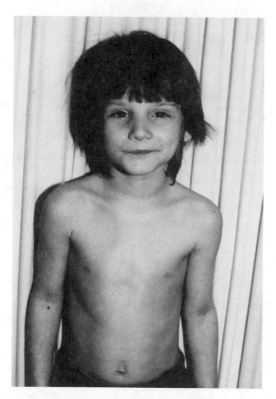

FIGURE 24.3   Aspect of a boy with AE I.

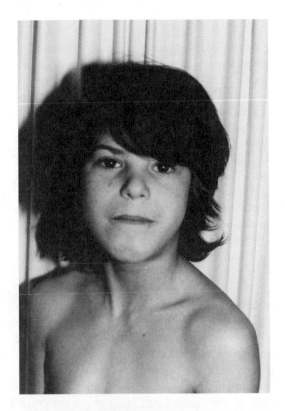

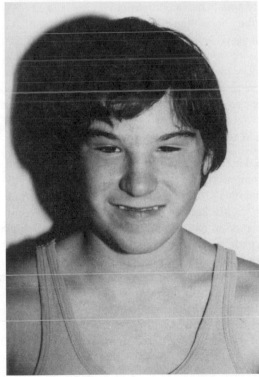

FIGURE 24.4 (a) Face of a girl with AE III at age 10 years; (b) appearance of a boy with AE II at age 12 years.

Malformations

In our patients, 84% manifested intrauterine and postnatal growth retardation, 77% were micro-cephalic, and 84% were mentally retarded; 27% of all patients suffered from congenital heart defects, mostly septal defects. In addition, we observed more complex heart defects, such as transposition of great vessels, pentalogy of Fallot, and aplasia of one lung artery. A nearly identical percentage (29%) of congenital heart defects was observed by Loeser et al.[33] in their sample of 216 cases of AE. They observed septal defects in 47 out of 63 patients with heart defects. The frequency of congenital heart defects in our patient group was related to the degree of AE; it amounted to 63% in patients with AE III, 19% in those with AE II, and 10% in patients with AE I. Some 40% of all patients exhibited mostly minor anomalies of external genitalia (i.e., hypospadias, cryptorchism, hypoplasia of labia minora) and at least 7% suffered from malformations of the genitourinary tract (diverticulas of bladder, hypoplastic kidney, polycystic kidney, megaureter, and hydronephrosis). Genital anomalies also correlated with the degree of AE; they were present in 61% of children with AE III, in 38% of children with AE II, and in 27% of children with AE I. Spina bifida was present in 2% of our cohort. Most of these frequencies are in concordance with other larger series.[8,33,51]

We observed tortuosity of retinal vessels in about 10%, and milder anomalies (e.g., myopia and strabism) infrequently. Significant hypoplasia of the optic nerve disc was found in only one patient. Stroemland[62] was the first to report ocular involvement in AE (i.e., myopia, strabism, hypoplasia of optic nerve disc, and increased tortuosity of retinal vessels) in nearly 90% of her 30 patients, but this figure may be elevated due to ascertainment bias in an ophthalmological clinic.

Furthermore, less frequently observed symptoms were cleft palate (7%), clinodactyly V (36%), camptodactyly (12%), hypoplasia of endphalanges (12%), limited supination (10%), in some cases due to radioulnar synostosis, pectus excavatum (21%) or carinatum (8%), sacral dimple (48%), hernias (11%), and (mostly small) hemangiomas (15%).

Frequencies of symptoms according to the different degrees of AE are given in Table 24.1. Although the classification of AE was initially based on dysmorphic criteria, it appeared that nearly all clinical features were more frequent in AE III than in AE II, and they were rare in AE I. Except for cleft palate, genitourinary malformations, and spina bifida, all features were also observed in cases of AE I, but were less frequent and mostly of milder degree than in cases of AE II or III. In cases of AE II, the frequencies of nearly all symptoms lie between those of AE III and I.[38]

Morphological and Functional Disturbances of the CNS

There are only 16 published brain dissections.[9,21,36,44,67,69] The malformations observed ranged from microdysplasias and heterotopias (63%) to severe brain malformations (31%). These malformations included hydrocephalus internus (19%)[9,44], hypoplasia of cerebellum (25%)[9,44,69], and agenesis of corpus callosum (19%)[9,44,69]. Marked hydrocephalus internus e vacuo and agenesis of corpus callosum were further observed in patient no. 181 with AE III (unpublished). The severest malformations were observed in patient no. 18:[44] agenesis of corpus callosum, hypoplasia of cerebellum, hydrocephalus internus et externus, and a porencephalic cyst. In a few cases, holoprosencephaly has been reported as a possible pathogenic consequence of heavy maternal alcohol abuse.[6,46]

Four of our patients suffered from neural tube defects. The frequency of spina bifida in our series was 2%; compared to the general population, this is a 20-fold increase. Friedman[15] also suggested an increased frequency of neural tube defects in children with AE.

Approximately 10% of our patients suffered from convulsions, and 72% demonstrated hyper-excitability, hyperactivity, and ataxia. In most children, these symptoms decreased after the age of 2 to 3 years. Muscular hypotonia was observed in 57% of our patients. The degree of mental retardation was related to the physical abnormalities in the children. The mean IQ of patients with AE III was 66, whereas it was 79 in patients with AE II, and 91 in patients with AE I.[37]A similar correlation between the degree of morphological abnormalities and mental retardation was observed by Streissguth et al.[54] in 20 cases. In a follow-up study of eight children, the initial mean IQ of these children was 56; 10 years later at follow-up, it was 61.[56]

After several years, Loeser and Ilse[31] re-examined 22 patients aged 14 to 20 years with AE of different degrees. Four patients were able to attend a regular school, two attended a school for children with learning disabilities, two a special school for children with physical handicaps, nine a school for the mentally handicapped, and one patient was unable to be educated. Unfortunately, no figures for the degree of AE in 15 patients are given, but all 7 patients with AE III attended a school for the mentally handicapped.

Streissguth et al.[60] reexamined adolescents and adults with AE (mean age 18 years; range 12 to 40 years). The average IQ of these patients was 66 (range 30 to 90). Arithmetic deficits were most characteristic. Maladaptive behaviors such as poor judgment, distractibility, and difficulty perceiving social cues were common. None of the adults were able to live on their own.

Most children with AE are impaired in their cognitive, emotional, and behavioral development. In early childhood, they are hyperexcitable and hyperactive. They show delay of speech and language, attention deficits, and/or specific learning disorders such as dyslexia, dyscalculia, and poor achievement in motor skills and in logic and planning abilities. They tend to act impulsively and lack personal distance and/or recognition of danger.

GROWTH

The mean birth weight of 124 children with AE born at term was 2355 g. This weight corresponds to the 50th percentile of children born in the 34½ week of gestation. Mean head circumference (31.97 cm) and length (46.05 cm) were similarly retarded by 5 to 5½ weeks. In most newborns with AE, there was a proportionate retardation of all three parameters and no relative microcephaly (i.e., OFC related to length).

There was a decrease in the mean values of weight, length, and head circumference from Degree I to Degree II to Degree III (Table 24.2).

Postnatally, most children with AE grew below, but parallel to, the third centile. Weight gain is more retarded than height gain, especially in the first years of life. The last examination of our oldest female patient with AE III was at age 18 years. Her final height was 145 cm. She had a normal puberty, normal female proportions, and was slightly overweight, but she was still microcephalic and mentally retarded. Carpal bone age was nearly normal. After the age of 12 years, weight gain was faster than height gain. Typically, the most impaired parameter was head circumference. The same catch-up growth for weight was observed by Streissguth et al.[56] and Spohr et al.[52] in their adolescent or adult female patients. The predicted final height of our oldest male patient with AE III will be 160 cm. Streissguth et al.[60] reported on 31 adolescent or adult patients with

TABLE 24.2

Auxiological Data of 124 Children with AE I, II, and III Born at Term

	Mean Weight (g)		Mean Length (cm)		Mean OFC (cm)	
	m	f	m	f	m	f
AE I (n = 42)	2.545	2.676	48.3	48.1	32.9	33.1
AE II (n = 49)	2.371	2.329	46.0	46.0	32.0	31.5
AE III (n = 33)	2.125	1.955	44.4	43.8	31.5	31.0
Healthy newborn	3.460	3.300	52.0	51.0	35.0	34.0

OFC = occipito-frontal circumference; m = male; f = female.

AE. The mean growth retardation corresponded to −2.1 SD (range, −6 to 0 SD), head circumference to −1.9 SD (range, −5 to +2 SD), and weight to −1.4 SD (−4 to 0 SD). Weight deficiency, which is typical for young children with AE, was less marked in these adolescents and adults; 25% of the patients with AE did not suffer from underweight. The mean weight:height proportion was 48% (range, 3 to 90%). The time of onset of puberty in all patients was within normal limits.

DIFFERENTIAL DIAGNOSIS

In each child with intrauterine and postnatal growth retardation, microcephaly, and a dysmorphic face, the tentative diagnosis of AE is the most probable because AE is rather frequent (1:200–1:3000), and all other types of intrauterine growth retardation (except of trisomy 18, frequency 1:3000) are rare (1:20,000 or less) or very rare (a few published cases only). All structural and numerical chromosomal aberrations should be excluded, as well as de Lange syndrome, Dubowitz syndrome, Silver-Russell syndrome, and some further 20 types of IUGR.

PATHOGENESIS AND EPIDEMIOLOGY

All mothers of our patients with AE were alcohol dependent. We and Loeser et al.[34] have never seen a child with AE due to a mother's social drinking or even binge drinking (more than five "drinks" per occasion). Streissguth et al.[59] observed psychological disturbances after prenatal exposure to binge drinking, but no case with AE. We are often asked by pediatricians to examine children of mothers with varying degrees of alcohol abuse during pregnancy. In no case, except for maternal alcohol addiction, did we notice features of AE. Most of the mothers with children suffering from AE drank more than 150 g absolute alcohol per day during pregnancy (mean, 171 g in 48 mothers explored by us). Mothers of children with AE III had no higher daily alcohol intake in the first trimester than mothers of children with AE I (Figure 24.5). Loeser et al.[30] reported on eight children prenatally exposed to excessive amounts of alcohol (i.e., more than 180 g per day). One child exhibited no disturbances, three children presented with alcohol effects, and four with a very mild degree of AE. They concluded that the severity of disturbance in the outcome does not depend on the amounts of alcohol. In this study, 43 mothers of children with AE I consumed an average amount of 175 g alcohol per day during pregnancy.[34] This is nearly the same amount as in 19 mothers of children with AE I (161 g per day, Figure 24.5). Loeser[34] was able to calculate the amounts of daily intake during pregnancy in 103 mothers. In this detailed investigation, he found no linear correlation between the amounts of alcohol consumption and the degree of AE among the offspring. Nearly identical to our study group (n = 48, mean 171 g), the 103 mothers of affected children had an average alcohol intake of 176 g daily. If the mother drank less than 50 g daily, no child showed symptoms of AE. In our study group, all the mothers of affected children also drank more than 50 g daily. These identical data in two different study groups may be due to chance, but the relatively high numbers of mothers (48 and 103, respectively) favor the reliability of these data. If they are realistic, they show that AE is the consequence of excessive maternal drinking during pregnancy.

In 72 mothers, we could classify the stage of alcohol illness according to Jellinek.[20] In the prodromal stage, alcohol intake is excessive, but there is no loss of control. With the loss of control, drinkers are in the critical stage, which leads to psychological and physical dependence. In the chronical stage, mothers drink compulsively and begin drinking in the morning. This stage leads to organic illness and psychosis, and to psychological and physical ruin. Mothers in the chronical stage during pregnancy had significantly more children with AE than those in the critical stage, and mothers in the critical stage had significantly more children with AE I than those in the chronical stage (Table 24.3). In the prodromal stage, only one child was born with mild AE.

This correlation of maternal stage of alcohol illness and degree of damage in the offspring is supported by our observations in 38 siblings (Table 24.4). Mostly (with one exception in family Br.), the younger sibling was more severely impaired than the older one (Figure 24.6). In the

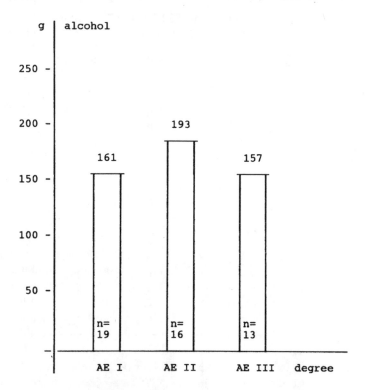

FIGURE 24.5 Correlation between degree of AE and maternal alcohol consumption.

TABLE 24.3
Correlation Between the Degree of AE in the Offspring (n = 72) and the Stage of Maternal Alcohol Illness

| Stage | Children | | |
of Mothers	AE I	AE II	AE III
Prodromal	1	—	—
Critical	15	10	7
Chronical	9	12	18

Note: According to Reference 20.

families Mue. and Sch, the first two children (dizygotic twins in family Mue.) showed fetal alcohol effects, whereas the third child suffered from AE I and II. From our study, it is evident that extremely high daily alcohol intake and an increased stage of maternal alcohol illness are prerequisites for AE. Hanson et al.[18] and other authors suggested that moderate alcohol intake and social drinking during pregnancy can cause embryonic damage. However, the two children in their study who exhibited symptoms of AE were born to *heavily* alcoholic mothers. Sulaiman et al.[63] correlated the maternal alcohol intake with the perinatal outcome. Before pregnancy, more than 90% consumed alcohol and 53% smoked. In the first 4 months of pregnancy, the proportion of alcohol-consuming women decreased to 57% and that of smoking women to 44%. There was no negative influence

TABLE 24.4
Degree of Severity of AE I-III in 17 Families
with Several Affected Children

Family	Sibling 1		Sibling 2	Sibling 3
Li.	I		II	
Ha.	I		II	III
Sp.	I		II	III
Ci.	I		II	
Ko.	I		I	
Fe.	I		II	
Ba.	I		II	
Be.	III		III	
Roe.	I		I	
Cr.	I		II	
Da.	I		II	
Eb.	II		III	
Fa.	I		II	
Ma.	I		I	III
Mue.	FAE	/	FAE	I
Sch.	FAE		FAE	II
Br.	II		I	

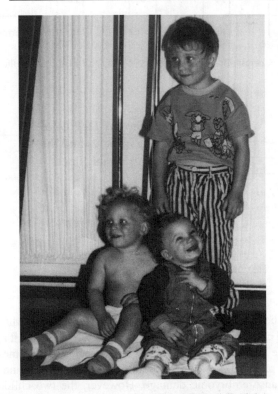

FIGURE 24.6 Three siblings, the younger ones with AE I (left) and II (right).

on the newborn if the mothers consumed less than 14 g alcohol per day during pregnancy. Among the newborns of mothers who consumed 14 to 17 g daily, there was a decrease of birth weight by 109 g, and of head circumference by 13 mm (not significant). There was a significant decrease in weight, length, head circumference, and Apgar scores among the newborns of mothers who drank more than 17 g per day (without an upper limit). But after correction with respect to smoking, social class, maternal height, and other variables, only the decrease in Apgar scores (−0.23 points) and duration of gestation (−2 weeks) remained significant. This is not in contradiction to our observations: there is only a major risk to the offspring if the mother is alcohol addicted and drinks excessively during pregnancy. Larsson et al.[25] prospectively examined and followed 40 children who all were prenatally exposed to various amounts of alcohol. The children of women with chronic alcohol illness exhibited significant growth retardation. Three out of six children prenatally exposed to excessive amounts presented with symptoms of AE. None of the children of mothers who stopped drinking during pregnancy exhibited growth retardation or symptoms of AE; but 12 out of 13 children of alcoholic mothers suffered from psychological or behavioral disturbances, even if the mother reduced or stopped alcohol abuse during pregnancy.

Autti-Raemoe and Gramstroem[4] examined 53 children prenatally exposed to alcohol of various duration at 1½ years of age. The mothers drank moderate (28 to 150 g per week) or heavy (more than 150 g per week) amounts during the first trimester (group I), heavy during the first and second trimester (group II), and heavy during the whole pregnancy (group III). There were no developmental differences between group I children and non-exposed controls. The children of groups II and III showed significantly lower scores in language and total mental assessment. The percentage of retarded children grew with increasing duration of prenatal alcohol exposure. In group II, there was one child with AE; and in group III, 5/19 (38%).

We examined 27 children of 24 mothers who asked for genetic counseling because of alcohol problems during early pregnancy. These mothers mostly asked for termination of the pregnancy, which was recommended in no case. Nearly all mothers reduced their alcohol intake after genetic counseling. All 24 children of the non-addicted mothers and one child of a mother in the critical stage of alcohol illness were healthy. Two mothers in the critical stage gave birth to children with AE I and AE II; the latter child exhibited no intrauterine growth retardation, possibly due to maternal abstinence during the second and third trimester of pregnancy.

From these observations, one might hypothesize that some secondary factors related to alcohol illness may increase embryonic damage; for example, hypoglycemia, elevated levels of acetaldehyde,[66] methanol,[1] and deficiencies of zinc,[65] vitamins, or folate.

DEGREE OF AE AND FAE IN TWINS

The twin study by Streissguth and Dehaene[61] demonstrated that the teratogenic effects of maternal alcoholism may be influenced by genetic factors. The authors described 16 sets of twins with a history of maternal alcoholism or alcohol abuse during the target pregnancy. All five monozygotic twins were equally affected. In two pairs, both twins had AE; in one pair, both had FAE; and in two pairs, neither twin was affected. By contrast, only 7 of 11 dizygotic twin pairs were concordant: in two pairs, one twin had AE and one had FAE; in two further pairs, one twin had FAE and the other was not affected. Among the twins concordant for diagnosis, there was one pair with AE, whereas only one child had a cleft lip and palate. We observed a possibly dizygotic pair of male twins who were similarly affected by FAE; the younger sister had AE I (family Mue. in Table 24.4).

FREQUENCY OF AE AMONG THE OFFSPRING

In two further studies, we examined 81 children of 69 mothers who had undergone withdrawal treatment. All mothers had been alcohol-addicted before and during pregnancy. From these studies, we learned that the frequency of AE among the offspring is influenced by the stage of maternal alcohol illness. In the prodromal stage only one child exhibited mild symptoms of AE; in the critical stage, 21%; and in the chronical stage, 41% of the offspring had symptoms of AE (Table 24.5).

TABLE 24.5
**Frequency of AE in the Offspring in Relation
to the Stage of Maternal Alcohol Illness**

Stage	Prodromal	Critical	Chronical
Frequency	1/16	8/38	11/27
	(6%)	21%	41%

TABLE 24.6
**Frequency of AE among the Offspring
of Chronic Alcoholic Women**

Frequency			
%	n	Country	Ref.
43	10/23	U.S.	22
43	15/35	Ireland	17
41	11/27	Germany	38
42.3	**36/85**		**Total**

Similar to that demonstrated in Table 24.3, there were higher degrees of AE in the chronical stage than in the critical stage.

In the literature, there are no similar studies. Only Jones et al.[21] in the U.S. and Halliday et al.[17] in Ireland studied the frequencies of AE among the offspring of chronically or heavily alcoholic mothers. Both observed a frequency of 43% of children with AE. Summing up all comparable studies, 42% of offspring of mothers with chronic alcohol illness suffered from AE (Table 24.6). Since all three studies came to similar results, this percentage seems to be realistic.

PREVALENCE OF AE IN THE GENERAL POPULATION

Abel and Sokol[2] calculated the frequency of AE in the "Western world" at 0.33 per 1000, but the French data were not included. Dehaene et al.[11] prospectively observed 45 new cases of AE within 3 years. They[12] observed a frequency of all types of AE of 1/208 and of AE with severe manifestation at 1/820 in the maternity hospital of Roubaix, France. These data indicate that AE at the present time is the most frequent type of intrauterine and postnatal growth retardation and one of the most frequently recognizable causes of mental retardation, exceeding the prevalence of trisomy.[21]

In a prospective epidemiological study, Kaminsky et al.[23] observed no correlation between maternal alcohol consumption and major malformations in the offspring; but they did find increased frequencies of prematurity and stillbirths, as well as decreased birth weights, when the mothers drank more than 40 ml wine or the equivalent of other alcoholic beverages per day. Plant[45] carried out a prospective study on 1012 newborns. While 92% of the mothers drank mostly moderate amounts of alcohol during pregnancy, no cases of AE were observed in the offspring. These prospective studies further indicate that AE is not induced by mild or moderate maternal alcohol consumption.

PREVENTION

From our study, it is evident that the majority of children of chronic alcoholic mothers are severely affected (see also Chapter 13 on special therapeutic considerations concerning women). From these results, termination of pregnancy may seem justified in pregnant women with chronic alcohol illness. However, a better method of prevention is dissemination of information to the population and provision of withdrawal treatment for alcoholic women. As in Huddinge, Sweden,[26] all pregnant women should be asked about their alcohol intake; and if the pregnant woman has alcohol problems, treatment should be offered. Prevention programs and strategies are reviewed by Weiner and Morse[68] and elsewhere in this book

We are aware of two mothers who had children after successful withdrawal treatment. Before withdrawal, one mother was in the chronical stage and gave birth to a child with AE III; the other one was in the critical stage and also had a child with AE III. After withdrawal treatment, both of them became pregnant again and gave birth to normal and healthy children.

REFERENCES

1. Abel, E.L., Prenatal effects of alcohol, *Drug Alcohol Depend.,* 14, 1, 1984.
2. Abel, E.L. and Sokol, R.J, A revised conservative estimate of the incidence of fetal alcohol syndrome and its economic impact, *Alcohol. Clin. Exp. Res.,* 15, 514, 1991.
3. Aronson, M., Kyllerman, M., Sabel, K.-G., Sandin, B., and Olegard, R, Children of alcoholic mothers, *Acta Paediatr. Scand.,* 74, 27, 1985.
4. Autti-Raemoe, I. and Granstroem, M.L., The effect of intrauterine alcohol exposition in various durations on early cognitive development, *Neuropediatrics,* 22, 203, 1990.
5. Beattie, J.O., Day, R.E., Cockburn, F., and Gary, R.A. Alcohol and the fetus in the west of Scotland, *Br. Med. J.,* 287, 17, 1983.
6. Boennemann, C. and Meinecke, P., Holoprosencephaly as a possible embryonic alcohol effect: another observation, *Am. J. Med. Genet.,* 37, 431, 1990.
7. Cahuana, A. and Gairi, J.M., Sindrome alcoholico fetal en Espana, *Sindrome Alcoholico Fetal,* Jornadas Internationales, Fundacion Valgrande, Madrid, 1985, 163.
8. Clarren, S.K. and Smith, D.W., The fetal alcohol syndrome. Experience with 65 patients and a review of the world literature, *N. Engl. J. Med.,* 298, 1063, 1978.
9. Clarren, S.K., Alvord, E.C., Sumi, S.M., Streissguth, A.P., and Smith, D.W., Brain malformations related to prenatal exposure to ethanol, *J. Pediatr.,* 92, 64, 1978.
10. Clarren, S.K., Sampson, P.D., Larsen, J., Donnell, D.J., Barr, H.M., Bookstein, F.L., Martin, D.C., and Streissguth, A.P., Facial aspects of fetal alcohol exposure: assessment by photographs and morphometric analysis, *Am. J. Med. Genet.,* 26, 651, 1987.
11. Dehaene, P., Crépin, G., Delahousse, G., Querleu, D., Walbaum, R., Titran, M., and Samaille-Vilette, C., Aspects epidémiologiques du syndrome d'alcoolisme foetal. 45 observations en 3 ans, *Nouv. Presse Méd. (Paris),* 10, 2639, 1981.
12. Dehaene, P., Samaille-Vilette, C., Boulanger-AEquelle, P., Subtil, D., Delahousse, G., and Crepin, G, Diagnostique et prévalence du syndrome d'alcoolisme foetal en maternitée, *Nouv. Presse Méd. (Paris),* 20, 1002, 1991.
13. Dupuis, C., Dehaene, P., Deroubaiy-Tella, P., Blanc-Garin, A.P., Rey, C., and Carpentier-Courault, C., Les cardiopathies des enfants nées des mères alcooliques, *Arch. Malad. Coeur Vaisseaux (Paris),* 71, 565, 1978.
14. Florey, C. du V., Taylor, D., Bolumar, F., Kaminski, M., and Olsen, J., Eds. EUROMAC: A European Concerted Action: Maternal Alcohol Consumption and its relation to the outcome of pregnancy and child development at 18 months, *Int. J. Epidemiol.,* 21 (Suppl. 1), 1992.
15. Friedman, J.M., Can maternal alcohol ingestion cause neural tube defects? *J. Pediatr.,* 101, 232, 1982.
16. Grisolia, D.S., Ed., Sindroma alcoholico fetal, *Jornadas Internationales, Serie Cientifica,* Fundacion Valgrande, Madrid, 1985.
17. Halliday, H.C., Reid, M.M., and McClure, G., Results of heavy drinking in pregnancy, *Br. J. Obstet. Gynecol.,* 89, 892, 1982.
18. Hanson, J.W., Streissguth, A.P., and Smith, D.W., The effects of moderate alcohol consumption during pregnancy on fetal growth and morphogenesis, *J. Pediatr.,* 92, 457, 1978.

19. Hennekam, R.C.M., Tilanus, M., Hamel, B.C.J., Voshart-van Heeren, H., Mariman, E.C.M., van Beersum, S.E.C., van den Boogaard, M.-J. H., and Breuning, M.H., Deletion at chromosome 16q13.3 as a cause of Rubinstein-Taybi syndrome: clinical aspects, *Am. J. Hum. Genet.*, 52, 255, 1993.

20. Jellinek, E.M., Phases in the drinking history of alcoholics: analysis of a survey conducted by the official organ of AA, *Q. J. Stud. Alcohol*, 7, 1, 1946.

21. Jones, K.L., Smith, D.W., Ulleland, C., and Streissguth, A.P., Pattern of malformations in offspring of chronic alcoholic mothers, *Lancet I*, 1267, 1973.

22. Jones, K.L., Smith, D.W., Streissguth, A.P., and Myrianthopoulos, N.C., Outcome in offspring of chronic alcoholic women, *Lancet I*, 1076, 1974.

23. Kaminski, M., Franc, M., Lebouvier, M., du Mazaubrun, C., and Rumeau-Rouquette, C., Moderate alcohol use and pregnancy outcome, *Neurobehav. Toxicol. Teratol.*, 3, 173, 1981.

24. Kyllerman, M., Aronsson, A., Karlberg, E., Olegard, R., Sabel, K.-G., Sandin, B., Johansson, P.R., Carlsson, C., and Iversen, K., Epidemiologic and neuropediatric aspects of the fetal alcohol syndrome, *Neuropaediatr.*, Suppl. 10, 435, 1979.

25. Larsson, G., Bohlinger, A.B., and Tunell, R., Prospective study of children exposed to variable amounts of alcohol *in utero*, *Arch. Dis. Childhood*, 60, 316, 1985.

26. Larsson, G., Program for early identification and treatment of pregnant abusers, *Die Alkoholembryopathie*, F. Majewski, Ed., Umwelt und Medizin, Frankfurt, 1987, 189.

27. Lemoine, P., Harousseau, H., Borteyru, J.P., and Menuet, J.C., Les enfants des parents alcooliques. Anomalies observées à propos de 127 cas, *Quest. Médical*, 21, 476, 1968.

28. Lemoine, P. and Lemoine, Ph., Avenir des enfants des méres alcooliques (étude de 105 cas retrouvés à l'âge adulte) et quelques constations d'intérêt prophylactique, *Ann. Pediatr.*, 39, 226, 1992.

29. Loeser, H., Herzfehler und toxische Herzmuskelschaeden bei Alkoholembryopathie, *Die Alkoholembryopathie*, F. Majewski, Ed., Umwelt und Medizin, Frankfurt, 1987, 124.

30. Loeser, H., Graevinghoff, K., and Rustemeyer, P., Schwachformen der Alkoholembryopathie nach exzessivem Alkoholgenuß, *Monatschr. Kinderheilk.*, 137, 764, 1989.

31. Loeser, H. and Ilse, R., Koerperliche und geistige Langzeitentwicklung bei Kindern mit Alkoholembryopathie, *Sozialpaediatr. Prax. Klin.*, 13, 8, 1991.

32. Loeser, H., Alkoholeffekte und Schwachformen der Alkoholembryopathie, *Dtsch. Aerztebl.*, 88, 1921, 1991.

33. Loeser, H., Pfefferkorn, J.R., and Themann, H., Alkohol in der Schwangerschaft und kindliche Herzschaeden, *Klin. Paediat.*, 204, 335, 1992.

34. Loeser, H., *Alkoholembryopathie und Alkoholeffekte*, Fischer, Stuttgart, 1995.

35. Majewski, F., Bierich, J.R., Loeser, H., Michaelis, R., Leiber, B., and Bettecken, F., Zur Klinik und Pathogenese der Alkoholembryopathie (Bericht ueber 68 Patienten), *Muench. Med. Wschr.*, 118, 1635, 1976.

36. Majewski, F., Fischbach, H., Peiffer, J., and Bierich, J.R., Zur Frage der Interruptio bei alkoholkranken Frauen, *Dtsch. Med. Wschrift.*, 103, 895, 1978.

37. Majewski, F., Alcohol embryopathy: some facts and speculations about pathogenesis, *Neurobehav. Toxicol. Teratol.*, 3, 129, 1981.

38. Majewski, F., Teratogene Schaeden durch Alkohol, *Psychiatrie der Gegenwart*, K.P. Kisker et al., Eds., Springer, Berlin, 1987, 243.

39. Majewski, F., Die Alkoholembryopathie — eine haeufige und vermeidbare Stoerung, *Die Alkoholembryopathie*, F. Majewski, Ed., Umwelt und Medizin, Frankfurt, 1987, 109.

40. Majewski, F., Alcohol embryopathy: experience in 200 patients, *Dev. Brain Dysfunct.*, 6, 248, 1993.

41. Nestler, V., Spohr, H.-L., and Steinhausen, H.-C., *Die Alkoholembryopathie*, Enke, Stuttgart, 1981.

42. Olegard, R., Sabel, K.G., Aronsson, M., Sandin, B., Johannsson, P.R., Carlsson, C., Kyllerman, M., Iversen, K., and Hrbek, A., Effects on the child of alcohol abuse during pregnancy. Retrospective and prospective studies, *Acta Paediatr.*, Scand. (Suppl.), 275, 112, 1979.

43. Olson, H.C., Sampson, P.D., Barr, H., Streissguth, A.P., and Bookstein, F.L., Prenatal exposure to alcohol and school problems in late childhood: a longitudinal prospective study, *Dev. Psychopathol.*, 4, 341, 1992.

44. Peiffer, J., Majewski, F., Fischbach, H., Bierich, J.R., and Volk, B., Alcohol embryopathy. Neuropathology of 3 children and 3 fetuses, *J. Neurol. Sci.*, 41, 125, 1979.

45. Plant, M., *Women, Drinking, and Pregnancy*, Tavistock, London, 1985.

46. Ronen, G.M. and Andrews, W.L., Holoprosencephaly as a possible embryonic alcohol effect, *Am. J. Med. Genet.*, 40, 151, 1991.

47. Spohr, H.-L., Majewski, F., and Nolte, R., EEG-examination of children with fetal alcohol syndrome, paper presented at the *7th Conf. Eur. Teratol. Soc.*, Herzlia, Israel,1979.

48. Spohr, H.-L. and Steinhausen, H.-C., Der Verlauf der Alkoholembryopathie, *Mschr. Kinderheilk.*, 132, 844, 1984.

49. Spohr, H.-L., Die Alkoholembryopathie — Aspekte zur Entwicklung praenatal alkoholgeschaedigter Kinder, *Oeffentl. Gesundheitswes.*, 47, 430, 1985.

50. Spohr, H.-L., Neurologische und psychiatrische Befunde bei praenataler Alkoholexposition, *Die Alkoholembryopathie*, F. Majewski, Ed., Umwelt und Medizin, Frankfurt, 1987, 134.

51. Spohr, H.-L., Das fetale Alkoholsyndrom — die Alkoholembryopathie — ein klinischer ueberblick, *Alkohol in der Schwangerschaft und die Folge fuer das Kind*, M. Steiner, Ed., Fischer, Frankfurt, 1990.

52. Spohr, H.-L., Willms, J., and Steinhausen, H.-C., Prenatal alcohol exposure and long-term developmental consequences, *Lancet I*, 907, 1993.

53. Steinhausen, H.C., Willms, J., and Spohr, H.-L., Correlates of psychopathology and intelligence in children with fetal alcohol syndrome, *J. Child Psychol. Psychiatr. Allied Discipl.*, 35, 323,1994.

54. Streissguth, A.P., Herman, C.S., and Smith, D.W., Intelligence, behavior and dysmorphogenesis in the fetal alcohol syndrome: a report on 20 patients, *J. Paediatr.*, 92, 363,1978.

55. Streissguth, A.P., Martin, J.C., Martin, D.C., and Barr, H.M., The Seattle longitudinal prospective study on alcohol and pregnancy, *Neurobehav. Toxicol. Teratol.*, 3, 323, 1981.

56. Streissguth, A.P., Clarren, S.K., and Jones, K.L., Natural history of the fetal alcohol syndrome: a 10-year follow-up of 11 patients, *Lancet II*, 85, 1985.

57. Streissguth, A.P., Fetal alcohol syndrome and fetal alcohol effects: teratogeneic cause of mental retardation and developmental disabilities, *Die Alkoholembryopathie*, F. Majewski, Ed., Umwelt und Medizin, Frankfurt, 1987, 143.

58. Streissguth, A.P., Barr, H.M., and Sampson, P.D., Moderate prenatal alcohol exposure: effects on child IQ and learning problems at age 7½ years, *Alcohol. Clin. Exp. Res.*, 14, 662, 1990.

59. Streissguth, A.P., Bookstein, F.L., Sampson, P.D., and Barr, H.M., Neurobehavioral effects of prenatal alcohol. III. Partial least squares analysis of neuropsychologic tests, *Neurotoxicol. Teratol.*, 11, 493, 1989.

60. Streissguth, A.P., Aase, J.M., Clarren, S.K., Randels, S.P., LaDue, R.A., and Smith, D.F., Fetal alcohol syndrome in adolescents and adults, *JAMA*, 265, 1961, 1991.

61. Streissguth, A.P. and Dehaene, P., Fetal alcohol syndrome in twins of alcoholic mothers: concordance of diagnosis and IQ, *Am. J. Med. Genet.*, 47, 857, 1993.

62. Stroemland, K., Ocular involvement in the fetal alcohol syndrome, *Survey Ophthalmol.*, 31, 277, 1987.

63. Sulaiman, N.D., Florey, E.V., Taylor, D.J., and Ogston, S.A., Alcohol consumption in Dundee primigravidas and its effects on outcome of pregnancy, *Br. Med. J.*, 296, 1500, 1988.

64. Tanaka, H., Arima, M., and Suzuki, N., The fetal alcohol syndrome in Japan, *Brain Dev.*, 3, 305, 1981.

65. Tanaka, H., Nakazawa, K., Suzuki, N., and Arima, M., Prevention possibility for brain dysfunction in rat with the fetal alcohol syndrome — low-zinc-status and hypoglycemia, *Brain Dev.*, 4, 429, 1982.

66. Véghelyi, P.V., Osztovics, M., Kardos, G., Leisztner, L., Szaszovensky, E., Igali, S., and Imrei, J., The fetal alcohol syndrome: symptoms and pathogenesis, *Acta Paediatr. Hungarica*, 19, 171, 1978.

67. Volk, B., Klinisch-neuropathologische Befunde und experimentelle Untersuchungen zur Alkoholembryopathie, *Die Alkoholembryopathie*, F. Majewski, Ed., Umwelt und Medizin, Frankfurt, 1987, 89.

68. Weiner, L. and Morse, B.A., Fetal alcohol syndrome: a framework for successful prevention, H.-L. Spohr and H.-C. Steinhausen, Eds., *Alcohol, Pregnancy and the Developing Child*, University Press, Cambridge, 1996, 269.

69. Wisniewski, K., Dambska, M., Shev, J.H., and Quazi, Q., A clinical neuropathological study of the fetal alcohol syndrome, *Neuropediatrics*, 14, 197, 1983.

Section II

Research

25 Epidemiology

Michael Fleming and Linda Baier Manwell

OVERVIEW

The prevalence of alcohol use disorders is variable. The highest levels of use are in Europe and the former Soviet Bloc countries. The population at greatest risk is young Caucasian men; however, the increasing levels of drinking among U.S. college students and pregnant women are a major concern.

Differences in rates of harm vary and are related to patterns of use, social and economic issues, public policy, enforcement of appropriate laws, and overall health of the country. Primary care settings, emergency departments, and hospitals continue to have higher rates of alcohol problems compared to general population samples.

The evidence presented in this chapter is compelling. Alcohol is one of the world's major public health problems. Health care professionals in every country need to learn all they can about this devastating problem. Establishment of systematic screening methods and intervention programs may prevent alcohol-related morbidity and mortality. The medical community can no longer stand by and watch so many people, families, and communities be destroyed by the excessive use of alcohol.

RELEVANCE TO HEALTH CARE PROVIDERS

At-risk, harmful, and dependent drinking are among the most common and important problems facing health care systems and society worldwide. Health care providers need to know the prevalence of these disorders in both their patient and community populations. They need to understand that these prevalence rates will vary by gender, age, social environment, and community.

Current research indicates that the natural history of alcohol use disorders does not follow a traditional disease model. These disorders have high rates of spontaneous recovery and many persons with alcohol problems stop drinking with minimal intervention and treatment. Health care providers need to understand the natural history of these problems to provide effective treatment.

A dose-response relationship between alcohol and health has been demonstrated. Providers need to switch their focus from a psychiatric disease model to a public health harm reduction model. Interventions must focus not only on the treatment of alcoholism, but also on reductions in levels of alcohol use. This means changing the behavior of individual patients as well as influencing consumption norms in the community.

A high rate of comorbidity exists between alcohol use and other medical problems such as hypertension, diabetes, sexually transmitted diseases, partner and family violence, trauma, nicotine addiction, depression, anxiety, and thought disorders. Health care providers need to understand the relationship between these problems and alcohol.

Alcohol interacts with many medications and treatments. Many medications used in the treatment of hypertension, diabetes, and depression are affected by alcohol. Health care providers need to advise patients who are using these medications to avoid alcohol.

RISK AND THE NEW PUBLIC HEALTH PARADIGM

The alcohol field is moving toward a public health harm reduction paradigm and away from an exclusive focus on the identification and treatment of alcoholism and abstinence-based endpoints. The harm reduction paradigm focuses on reducing alcohol use to low-risk levels. This shift is based on three observations. First, most problems related to alcohol use occur in persons who are not alcoholic. Second, the natural history of recovery is very complicated and does not fit a single model. Third, the use of a new term, "at-risk drinking," has emerged in place of the terms "hazardous" or "heavy" drinking. The term "risk" is intended to place heavy alcohol use in the context of other health risks such as high blood pressure, elevated cholesterol, or high blood sugar levels.

ALCOHOL CONSUMPTION IN THE GENERAL POPULATION

Table 25.1 presents alcohol consumption in seven areas of the world: Western Europe, European Union, Eastern Europe, Latin America, North America, Australia, and other parts of the world (Algeria, China, Iceland, Israel, Japan, Malaysia, Morocco, Singapore, South Africa, Thailand, Ukraine, and Vietnam). The table, which reports consumption in liters of pure alcohol (LPA) per adult per area, illustrates a 2 to 8% decrease in alcohol use between 1990 and 1995 except in Latin America and the "Rest of World" category. The lowest rates of alcohol use were in countries located in Latin America (3.95 LPA), and the highest were in countries residing within the European Union (9.29 LPA). The 64% increase in alcohol use in the "Rest of World" category suggests a true increase in alcohol use in these countries. The total use in these countries, however, even with this increase, is very low compared to most European countries.

Table 25.2 summarizes alcohol use in 40 countries in Europe, the Middle East, and in the former Soviet Bloc. The consumption is primarily derived from sales tax information. This data was collected in 1995 by the European Office of the World Health Organization located in Copenhagen, Denmark. We obtained the data from its *Country Profiles* Web Site.[1] The data set includes sociodemographic characteristics of the population in each country, life expectancy at birth, infant

TABLE 25.1
Alcohol Consumption in 1990 and 1995 in Seven Areas of the World

Region	Number of Countries Included	Total Alcohol Consumption per Capita 1990 (LPA)[b]	Total Alcohol Consumption per Capita 1995 (LPA)[b]	Percentage Change 1990–1995
Western Europe	19	8.56	8.12	–5.2
European Union	16	9.76	9.29	–4.9
Eastern Europe	8	5.92	5.79	–2.1
Latin America	10	3.85	3.95	2.7
North America	2	7.35	6.74	–8.4
Australia	2	7.98	7.5	–6.1
Rest of World[a]	12	2.45	4.02	64.4
World Total	53	4.39	5.07	15.5

Notes: These figures, limited by available data, are based on countries featured in the *World Drink Trends* 1996 book.

[a] Algeria, China, Iceland, Israel, Japan, Malaysia, Morocco, Singapore, South Africa, Thailand, Ukraine, and Vietnam.
[b] LPA: Liter(s) of pure alcohol.
Source: *World Drink Trends*, NTC Publications, Farm Road, Henley on Thames, Oxon R69.

TABLE 25.2
Alcohol Consumption and Alcohol-Related Harm in 40 Countries in Europe, the Middle East, and the Former Soviet Bloc

Country	Alcohol Consumption (liters)		Alcohol-Related Harm (per 100,000)		
	1980	1992–1993	Liver Cirrhosis	Injury/ Poisoning	Motor Vehicle Accidents
Armenia	2.2	2.8	15.3	73.2	13.8
Austria	10.9	10.8	25.9	56.7	14
Belarus	10.2	7.9	7.7	135.75	16.8
Belgium	10.8	9.1	11.3	57.7	16.6
Bulgaria	8.3	8.3	16.5	63.1	11.8
Czech Republic	9	9.2	16.5	78.4	13.6
Denmark	9.2	10	13.5	60.6	9.8
Estonia	11.2	6.7	9.2	180.8	24.2
Finland	6.3	6.7	9.9	79.3	8.3
France	14.9	11.5	15.6	68	14.6
Georgia	7	3.5	25.1	63.6	19.3
Germany	Unavailable	12.1	21.5	44.7	11.4
Greece	6.7	9.2	8.2	38.1	17.9
Hungary	11.8	10.2	78.9	111.8	16.9
Iceland	3.1	3.3	0.3	41.1	7.8
Ireland	7.2	8.3	3.1	39.9	11.9
Israel	2	2	8.3	42.7	6.7
Italy	13	8.6	22	44.7	15.1
Kyrgystan	Unavailable	1.9	32.1	101.9	21.6
Latvia	11.3	6.4	13.2	233.3	35
Lithuania	11.1	4.3	13.4	191	21.8
Luxembourg	10.9	12.6	16.5	62.6	19.2
The Netherlands	8.8	7.9	5.1	32.1	7.9
Norway	4.6	3.8	4.5	48.2	6.3
Poland	8.7	6.8	12.6	76.4	17.8
Portugal	10	10.4	26.4	57.7	23.2
Republic of Moldova	6.8	3.2	68.2	130	13.3
Romania	8	8	44.7	76.3	13.9
Russian Fed.	10.5	4.9	15.7	225.7	25.1
Slovak Republic	10.7	9.3	37.5	73	10.5
Slovenia	11.9	9.3	36.1	102.1	27.7
Spain	13.6	10	18.7	44.4	18.5
Sweden	5.7	5.3	6.4	44.2	7.3
Switzerland	11	9.7	8.3	57.5	9.2
Turkey	0.7	0.8	1.2[a]	4.9[a]	10.5[a]
Turkmenistan	4.3	1.9	17.7	59.1	18.8
Ukraine	6.3	2	16.1	128.5	19.3
United Kingdom	7.5	7.3	5.8	30.6	7.6

[a] Unstandardized rate.

Source: Table compiled from data from on the World Health Organization Regional Office for Europe Web Site. *Country Profiles,* 1995, http://www.who.dk/hp/adt/acountry.htm#Profiles.

mortality, economic and employment issues, alcohol consumption, alcohol-related harm, national policy, taxation and prevention and regulations, labeling, and alcohol prevention programs. The data presented in Table 25.2 is limited to alcohol consumption and frequency of alcohol-related harm.

Table 25.2 illustrates a significant variability in consumption patterns. The numbers are reported in liters of pure alcohol (LPA) per adult in each country. The lowest rates of alcohol use reported in 1992–1993 were in Turkey (0.8 LPA), Israel (2.0 LPA), Turkmenistan (1.9 LPA), and Krygystan (1.9 LPA). Many countries in Western Europe reported large reductions in use between 1980 and 1992–1993: France (14.9 to 11.5), Italy (13 to 8.6), Spain (13.6 to 10). Other countries such as Ireland (7.2 to 8.3) and Portugal (10 to 10.4) demonstrated mild increases in use. The significant decrease in alcohol use in the former Soviet Bloc countries may reflect economic changes, increases in homemade alcohol, and unreported alcohol sales.

Table 25.3 reports data from a more recent survey that compares consumption data for 1993 and 1995 for 38 selected countries. Countries reporting the highest use were primarily European countries. Ten countries reported greater than 9 LPA per year. Lowest rates of alcohol use were in countries located primarily in North Africa, Southeast Asia, and Latin America. Many of these countries reported less than 1 LPA per adult per year.

Of interest are rates of alcohol use disorders in Japan and persons of Japanese ancestry who moved to the U.S.. Table 25.4 compares alcohol use among four groups, each divided into persons who report a flush response to alcohol and those who do not. The oriental flushing reflex encompasses a variety of symptoms, including rapid heartbeat, nausea, feeling itchy, perspiring, and headache, which is more common among those of Asian descent than those of Caucasian descent. Overall, Japanese who reside in Japan drink more severely regardless of flush status than Japanese Americans and Caucasians residing in the U.S. The frequency of a flushing response in Japanese adults living in Japan is 42%. The frequency of the flush response in Caucasians living in Santa Clara, California, is 4% (a tenfold difference). Rates of heavy alcohol use (>21 oz. alcohol per day in the last 2 weeks) is highest in Japanese living in Japan who do not have the flush response (23%) and lowest in Japanese adults who have the flush response and live in Oahu, Hawaii, or Santa Clara (1%). While rates of heavy alcohol use and frequent episodes of intoxication are lower in persons who have the flush response in all four groups, the rates of alcohol use are surprisingly high in Japanese with a flush response who live in Japan. The flush response does not appear to protect Japanese who live in Japan from at-risk drinking.[2]

Table 25.5 reports responses to questions regarding alcohol-related problems. Again, the Japanese living in Japan had much higher rates of problems with control, blackouts, morning drinking, and health care professional intervention than Japanese living in the U.S. Blackouts, for example, were reported by 18% of the sample living in Japan and only 5 to 6% of Japanese living in the U.S. Morning drinking occurred in 8% of the Japan sample and 1% in the Oahu and Santa Clara subjects. Alcohol use appears to be a major problem in Japan, with acculturation of Japanese residing in the U.S. resulting in lower levels of alcohol use and alcohol-related problems. More recent data is not available (personal communication with Dr. Michie Hesselbrock, University of Connecticut, and Dr. Higuchi of the Kuiihama National Hospital, February 5, 1999).

FREQUENCY OF AT-RISK USE, HARMFUL DRINKING, AND ALCOHOL DEPENDENCE IN THE GENERAL POPULATION

The worldwide prevalence of at-risk drinking, harmful drinking, and alcohol dependence is not known. While many countries conduct national surveys to estimate prevalence rates, there is a great deal of variability in sampling strategies, interview techniques, research instruments, and diagnostic criteria. It is difficult to make comparisons across countries.

TABLE 25.3
A Comparison of Alcohol Consumption in 1993 and 1995 in 38 Selected Countries

Country	Liters of Pure Alcohol	
	1993	1995
Luxembourg	12	11.6
France	11.5	11.5
Portugal	10.7	11
Hungary	10.2	10.2
Spain	9.9	10.2
Czech Republic	9.6	10.1
Denmark	9.7	10
Germany	10.4	9.9
Austria	10.1	9.8
Switzerland	10	9.4
Republic of Ireland	8.3	9.2
Belgium	9.6	9.1
Greece	9.2	9.0
Romania	8	9.0
Italy	8.7	8.8
Bulgaria	8.3	8.1
The Netherlands	7.9	8.0
Cyprus	7.6	7.9
Slovak Republic	8.4	7.8
Australia	7.5	7.6
Argentina	7.2	7.3
New Zealand	7.3	7
U.S.	6.7	6.8
Japan	6.6	6.6
Venezuela	5.9	5.3
South Africa	4.5	4.9
China	3.2	Unavailable
Cuba	3.8	3.8
Brazil	3.4	3.6
Mexico	3.3	3.3
Singapore	1.5	1.7
Peru	1.1	1.2
Thailand	0.4	0.6
Malaysia	0.5	0.6
Tunisia	0.5	0.5
Algeria	0.3	0.3
Morocco	0.3	0.3
Vietnam	0.2	0.2

Source: World Drink Trends, NTC Publications, Farm Road, Henley on Thames, Oxon R69.

AT-RISK DRINKING

Reports listing the frequency of at-risk drinking in the general population were not available for many countries because national surveys are in progress and not yet reported. A recurring problem

TABLE 25.4

A Comparison of Japanese, Japanese Americans, and Caucasians: Flushers and Non-flushers among Current Drinkers

| | Japanese | | Japanese American | | | | Caucasian | |
	Japan		Oahu, HI		Santa Clara, CA		Santa Clara, CA	
Reaction to Alcohol	NF	F	NF	F	NF	F	NF	F
Number and percent of non-	(536)	(385)	(264)	(113)	(289)	(120)	(419)	(19)
flushers and flushers	58%	42%	70%	30%	71%	29%	96%	4%
Amount of alcohol in last								
2 weeks of drinking								
<7 oz.	54%	63%	74%	88%	82%	94%	73%	(14)
7–21 oz.	23%	23%	19%	11%	14%	5%	23%	(2)
>21 oz.	23%	14%	7%	1%	4%	1%	4%	(0)
Frequency of drinking any								
alcohol beverages								
1 time per month	14%	23%	28%	53%	34%	43%	15%	35%
1–3 times per month	20%	26%	22%	26%	24%	31%	23%	38%
1–2 times per week	16%	15%	24%	13%	19%	15%	25%	19%
3 or more × per week	50%	36%	26%	9%	23%	10%	36%	10%
Frequency of getting drunk								
Never	44%	50%	53%	67%	49%	65%	56%	(10)
Not in last 12 months	15%	14%	13%	17%	20%	18%	7%	(1)
1–11 times per year	26%	26%	25%	11%	25%	14%	28%	(3)
Once a month or more	14%	10%	9%	6%	5%	3%	10%	(1)

Source: Alcohol Comsumption Patterns and Related Problems in the United States and Japan: Summary Report of a Joint United States-Japan Alcohol Epidemiological Project. National Institute on Alcohol Abuse and Alcoholism and the National Institute on Alcoholism, Kurihama National Hospital, Rockville, MD, NIAAA, 1991.

in the reports that have been published is the variation in levels of alcohol consumption used to define heavy drinking, at-risk use, or hazardous drinking. For example, at-risk or heavy drinking was defined as 21 drinks, 14 drinks, or 7 drinks per week; binge drinking was defined as 4, 5, or 6 drinks per occasion. Frequency of binge drinking was reported at once per week to once per month. The amount of alcohol per standard drink was also not defined in many reports. Studies have found alcohol content ranging from 8 to 14 grams of alcohol per drink, varying by country and region.

The Scottish Health Survey, conducted in 1995, reported that 33% of men drank more than 21 drinks per week and 8% drank more than 50 drinks per week,[3] while 12% of the women in the study drank more than 14 drinks per week. Predictors of heavy use included younger age (16 to 24), employment as a manual laborer, and lower social class. A similar study in Great Britain found that 27% of the men drank more than 21 drinks per week and 11% of the women drank more than 14 drinks per week. A WHO-sponsored study in Macedonia in 1992 suggested that 16% of the population were heavy drinkers. A prevalence study conducted in Japan in 1997 reported that 5% of the population of drinkers consumed 150 ml or more per day.

The National Household Survey is conducted annually in the U.S.[4] Binge use is defined as five or more drinks on the same occasion at least once in the past month, and heavy use is defined as five or more drinks on the same occasion on at least five different days in the past month. The 1997 survey found that 15% (31 million people) engaged in binge drinking and 5% (11.2 million people) were heavy drinkers. The level of alcohol use was strongly associated with illicit drugs; 30% of the heavy drinkers had used illicit drugs in the past month, whereas only 5% of low-risk

TABLE 25.5

A Comparison of Japanese, Japanese Americans, and Caucasians: Rates of Drinking Problems Among Current Drinkers by Study Site and Gender

		Japanese	Japanese American		Caucasian
		Japan	Oahu	Santa Clara	Santa Clara
In the previous 12 months					
Felt that you should cut down	Male	24%	18%	15%	22%
on your drinking or stop altogether	Female	10%	10%	10%	17%
	Total	**18%**	**14%**	**12%**	**19%**
Sometimes got drunk even when	Male	5%	7%	3%	4%
there was an important reason to	Female	2%	4%	4%	1%
stay sober	**Total**	**4%**	**6%**	**3%**	**3%**
Awakened the next day not being	Male	27%	8%	8%	13%
able to remember some of the	Female	5%	2%	5%	7%
things you had done while drinking	**Total**	**18%**	**5%**	**6%**	**10%**
Took a drink first thing when you	Male	13%	2%	1%	5%
got up in the morning	Female	1%	0%	1%	1%
	Total	**8%**	**1%**	**1%**	**3%**
Been told by a health worker that	Male	9%	1%	0%	3%
the amount you were drinking was	Female	3%	1%	0%	0%
having an effect on your health	**Total**	**7%**	**1%**	**0%**	**2%**
Been ashamed of something you did	Male	10%	3%	2%	6%
while drinking	Female	5%	1%	2%	6%
	Total	**7%**	**2%**	**2%**	**6%**
Regularly have a drink instead of a	Male	6%	2%	2%	1%
meal	Female	3%	2%	1%	1%
	Total	**4%**	**2%**	**1%**	**1%**

Source: Alcohol Comsumption Patterns and Related Problems in the United States and Japan: Summary Report of a Joint United States-Japan Alcohol Epidemiological Project. National Institute on Alcohol Abuse and Alcoholism and the Nationsl Institute on Alcoholism, Kurihama National Hospital, Rockville, MD, NIAAA, 1991.

drinkers had used illicit drugs. Rates vary by gender, race, and educational level. Caucasian men between the ages of 18 and 25 who had not attended college had the highest rates of binge use and heavy drinking. African Americans had the lowest rates of binge use and heavy drinking. While persons with a college degree had higher rates of overall use, they had lower rates of at-risk use.

HARMFUL DRINKING AND DEPENDENCE

The most recent study to assess the prevalence of alcohol abuse and alcohol dependence was the National Longitudinal Alcohol Epidemiological Survey. This survey, conducted in 1992, involved a multistage random sampling of the U.S. household population, yielding a sample size of 42,861 respondents 18 years of age and older. Using data from this survey, Grant reported a combined prevalence of alcohol abuse and alcohol dependence of 7%. The percent of persons who were alcohol dependent was 4%.[5]

Persons at greatest risk for meeting criteria for alcohol dependence were young men with less than a high school education who began drinking before the age of 15. Persons who were separated from their spouse, or who had never married, had twice the rate of dependence as persons who were married and living with their spouse. Persons living in the Pacific Northwest and Mountain region of the U.S. were nearly twice as likely to be alcohol dependent as persons living in other parts of the country. A limited number of studies in western European countries using ICD-9 criteria found similar rates of alcohol dependence of 3 to 5%. Reliable estimates for most other countries are not available.

SPECIAL POPULATIONS

PREGNANT WOMEN

The Behavioral Risk Factor Surveillance System (BRFSS) Survey, developed by the U.S. Centers for Disease Control, utilizes a standardized questionnaire to collect information on self-reported health habits and risk factors that contribute to the development of chronic diseases. The alcohol use data provides important information on the frequency of heavy drinking in women of child-bearing age. In 1995, the study surveyed 26,000 women between the ages of 18 and 44. Results indicate that 21% had consumed five or more drinks on one occasion in the last 30 days; 3% had consumed 31 to 69 drinks in the last 30 days; and 2% drank more than 60 drinks in the past 30 days. Of the 1067 pregnant respondents, 3.5% reported drinking two or more drinks per day or five or more drinks in the last month.[6] This is a twofold increase in the frequency of at-risk drinking in pregnancy since the previous survey done in 1990. If the data are generalizable to all births in the U.S., it suggests that 165,000 children born in 1995 were exposed to potentially harmful effects of alcohol. Wilsnack performed an analysis of 15 other surveys and found that partner drinking, depression, and unwanted sexual experiences were predictive for heavy alcohol use in women.[7]

YOUTHS

Monitoring the Future is an annual survey conducted among U.S. high school students to assess their level of tobacco, alcohol, and other drug use.[8] The 1997 survey found a slight increase in overall alcohol use in 12th graders (age 18) from 72 to 75%. The frequency of binge drinking (defined as five or more drinks on at least one occasion in the last 2 weeks) was 14% in 8th graders (age 14), 24% for 10th graders (age 16), and 31% for students in the 12th grade. There was no significant change between 1991 and 1998 in rates of binge drinking. The study found a decrease in the frequency of 8th graders who became intoxicated in the last 30 days — from 10 to 8%.

Beginning in 1991, cohorts of students were queried annually about their perceptions regarding the harmful effects of a number of drugs. There was a dramatic across-the-board decrease in the students' perception of risk from alcohol and illicit drugs. In 1991, 60% of 8th, 10th, and 12th graders felt that five or more drinks one or more times each weekend was potentially harmful. In 1998, this number had dropped to 42%. The change in marijuana risk perception went from 40% in 1991 to 16% in 1998.

The *Youth Risk Behavior Surveillance System* is another national survey conducted in the U.S.[9] The 1997 survey found that 37% of high school students had ridden in a car with an intoxicated driver. Hispanic students were the most likely to engage in this behavior (43%) and African American students the least likely (34%); 17% of the students surveyed reported they drove a vehicle after drinking alcohol. This survey also found that 33% of the students reported drinking five or more drinks at least once in the previous 30 days. Caucasian and Hispanic male students in the 11th and 12th grades were the heaviest drinking group. Males were twice as likely to use alcohol prior to intercourse as female students (31 vs. 19%).

Another survey assessed student drinking patterns in Scotland, Wales, and Northern Ireland.[10] The survey found that 37% of boys ages 15 years and older in Scotland drank at least once per week; 51% of boys ages 15 years and older in Wales drank at least once per week; and 42% of boys ages 15 years and older in Northern Ireland drank at least once per week. The figures for girls were 25, 44, and 28%, respectively. Approximately 51% of the total sample had been "drunk" at least twice in their lifetime.

UNIVERSITY STUDENTS

Researchers from the Harvard University School of Public Health conducted nationwide surveys of U.S. university students in 1993 (n = 15,013) and 1997 (n = 14,521).[11] They found some of the highest rates of alcohol use ever found in a large national survey in any country. They conducted mailed surveys with a random sample of students at 130 public and private universities. The study found that 24% of men and 19% of women were frequent binge drinkers; 25% of men and 20% of women were occasional binge drinkers; 33% of men and 42% of women were non-binge drinkers; and 18% of men and 19% of women reported no alcohol use.

Binge drinking was defined as five drinks in a row for men or four drinks in a row for women during the 2 weeks prior to completing the questionnaire. Frequent binge drinking was defined as three or more episodes of binge drinking in the past 2 weeks. Abstinence was defined as no alcohol use in the past year. The study also found that 81% of students who belonged to fraternities or sororities were binge drinkers. Asian students showed the greatest increase in binge drinking between the 1993 and 1997 surveys. This study suggests that university students in the U.S. have some of the highest rates of at-risk drinking of any group in the world.

OLDER ADULTS

Older adults are one of the fastest growing populations in the world. In the past, health care providers have assumed that the frequency of alcohol use disorders in this population is very low and that alcohol-related problems are uncommon. Recent studies, however, suggest a different situation. A prevalence study, conducted in an urban area in upstate New York, interviewed 2325 adults over the age of 60 using a telephone random digit dialing method. At-risk drinkers were defined as persons who drank two or more drinks per day in the past 12 months. The study found that 12% of men and 2% of women met criteria for at-risk drinking.[12] Another study found that alcohol-related hospitalizations is one of the most common reasons for inpatient care in this population.[13] These studies suggest that alcohol use is common and may contribute to serious medical problems in older people.

FREQUENCY OF AT-RISK USE, HARMFUL DRINKING, AND ALCOHOL DEPENDENCE IN CLINICAL SAMPLES

PRIMARY CARE SAMPLES

The prevalence data presented in Tables 25.6 and 25.7 are from two studies conducted between 1992 and 1994. The subjects were obtained from the practices of 110 family physicians and general internists in 22 clinics located in ten counties in Wisconsin. The clinics were located in both rural and urban areas. The subjects were asked to complete an alcohol questionnaire as they waited to see their physician for a routine visit.[14-16] These studies are the largest prevalence surveys conducted in community-based primary care settings in the U.S.

Table 25.6 reports alcohol use, frequency of binge drinking, and prevalence of at-risk, harmful, and dependent drinking in the past 90 days for 19,372 adults ages 18 to 60. As noted, 18% of men reported two or more drinks per day, and 8% of men reported frequent binge use in the past 90 days. The overall frequency of at-risk drinking was 9.4%, harmful drinking 8.0%, and dependent drinking 5.2%. Rates of dependent drinking were 2.5 times higher for men than women.[15]

The prevalence of alcohol use disorders in older adults is illustrated in Table 25.7. The study found that 15% of men over the age of 60 drank 15 or more drinks per week.[14] Rates were much lower in women. Almost 9% of the men reported positive responses to two or more CAGE questions in this sample.[17] Rates of alcohol use in this older adult population were much higher than expected and were similar to levels of alcohol use in the data presented in Table 25.6 for persons ages 18 to

TABLE 25.6
Frequency of Alcohol Use, Binge Drinking, At-Risk Harmful and Dependent Drinking in a Primary Care Sample Located in the U.S.

	Men (n = 7144)	Women (n = 12,228)	Total (n = 19,372)
Alcohol use in previous 90days			
0 drinks/week	32.3%	43.0%	39.1%
1–7 drinks/week	28.8%	37.7%	34.5%
8–14 drinks/week	21.1%	13.5%	16.3%
15 or more drinks/week	17.7%	5.7%	10.2%
Binge drinking (number of times consuming 6 or more drinks per occasion in past 90 days)			
0	64.7%	83.8%	76.8%
1–2 times	18.6%	11.7%	14.2%
3–5 times	8.4%	2.9%	4.9%
>5 times	8.2%	1.6%	4.1%
Abstainers	30.5%	43.5%	39.6%
Low risk	45.2%	35.1%	37.7%
At-risk	4.6%	12.0%	**9.4%**
Harmful	11.6%	6.1%	**8.0%**
Dependent	8.4%	3.4%	**5.2%**

Note: Data collected from 1992 to 1994 in a sample of 19,372 adults ages 18 to 60.

Source: Fleming, M.F., Manwell, L.B., Barry, K.L., and Johnson, K., *Am. J. Public Health,* 88, 90, 1998. With permission.

TABLE 25.7
Alcohol Use, Binge Drinking, Self-Reported Drinking Problem, and CAGE Responses in a U.S. Primary Care Sample of Older Adults

	61–65 years		66–75 years		>75 years	
	Men	Women	Men	Women	Men	Women
Sample size	(794)	(972)	(1163)	(1323)	(300)	(473)
Mean drinks/wk						
<1	40.3	58.5	49.8	70.3	57.3	80.5
1–7	24.8	26.0	21.1	18.9	18.0	10.4
8–14	18.1	11.3	14.7	7.3	13.7	6.1
15–21	5.5	1.8	5.5	1.6	4.3	1.5
>21	11.2	2.5	8.8	1.9	6.7	1.5
Binge drinking, 6 or more drinks per occasion	14.1	3.0	8.8	1.3	4.6	0.9
Self-reported drinking problem	11.6	3.8	10.8	3.6	11.2	3.1
One + CAGE	22.2	10.4	18.5	7.9	16.7	6.6
Two + CAGE	10.5	3.9	7.8	2.9	7.5	2.1

Note: Data collected from 1993 to 1994 in a sample of 5065 older adults ages 61 to 85.

Source: Adams, W.L., Barry, K.L., and Fleming, M.F., *JAMA,* 276, 1964, 1996. With permission.

60. This finding may reflect an older-adult retired population with the financial resources and good health to continue to consume large amounts of alcohol.

The data presented in Tables 25.6 and 25.7 suggest that primary health care providers in the U.S. who have 2000 adult patients in their practice can expect to have 188 at-risk, 160 harmful, and 110 dependent drinkers in their practices. The prevalence is likely to vary from this estimate, depending on the percent of female patients and the age distribution of the patient population. The greater the number of women and older adults in the practice, the lower the number of persons who will meet criteria for at-risk, harmful, or dependent drinking. These numbers reflect the observation that alcohol use disorders are at least as common as other disorders seen in most primary care practices, such as high blood pressure, elevated lipids, and diabetes.

EMERGENCY DEPARTMENTS AND HOSPITALS

Rates of patients with alcohol use disorders seen in emergency departments and hospital populations vary by specialty service and type of hospital. Emergency departments located in major trauma centers report that up to 50% of patients seen in these facilities have positive blood alcohol levels or report recent at-risk alcohol use.[18-20] A recent study in the emergency departments of three hospitals in a large city in Mexico found similar rates of alcohol problems as those found in surveys conducted in the U.S.[21]

Surveys in general medical and psychiatric units find that 10 to 25% of the patients meet criteria for harmful or dependent alcohol use.[22,23] The highest rates of alcohol-related problems are found in trauma services and in intensive care units. Comorbid disorders such as tobacco and drug addiction, chronic mental illness, and medical problems complicate the clinical course of many of these patients. Unfortunately, many patients continue to experience severe withdrawal symptoms during their hospitalization due to the lack of early identification of their alcohol problem and the absence of appropriate pharmacological intervention.

These findings suggest that emergency departments and hospitals need to establish screening procedures and appropriate intervention strategies. Inpatient alcohol and drug consultation services, combined with strong community treatment programs, and mutual-help programs can make a difference in reducing readmissions and the frequency of alcohol-related harm.

ALCOHOL-RELATED HARM

Alcohol affects many organ systems and is often associated with accidents and injuries. Common organ systems affected include the brain, cardiovascular system, liver, pancreas, upper and lower gastrointestinal tract, and immune system.[24] There is also the issue of exposure to multiple toxins and the interactive effects of alcohol and tobacco on the esophagus, oral mucosa, and upper respiratory tract, as well as the developing fetus. Another issue focuses on the differences in the toxicity of alcohol by gender, race, and age.[25]

Three measures of alcohol-related harm that have been collected in many national surveys include death rates from liver cirrhosis, rates of injury and/or poisonings, and rates of motor vehicle accidents. National studies to determine the frequency of alcohol-related harm to the brain, cardiovascular system, and immune system are not generally available. Questions such as the prevalence of alcohol use disorders in hypertensive patients or diabetics have yet to be addressed in large-scale national studies. Table 25.2 compares the rates of cirrhosis, injury/poisoning, and motor vehicle accidents per 100,000 population in 1992–1993 for 40 countries. This data was collected by the World Health Organization Regional Office for Europe by questionnaire and direct inquiry.[1]

Rates of death from liver cirrhosis vary from a low of 0.3 in Iceland to 79 in Hungary. The highest rates were reported in countries in Eastern Europe, such as Hungary, Romania, Georgia, the Slovak Republic, and Slovenia. Countries in Western Europe with the highest rates included Austria (26), Germany (22), and Portugal (26). While the rates of liver cirrhosis have decreased in most countries since the 1980s, there are many exceptions to this observation, especially in Eastern Europe and in some Latin American countries.

Rates of cirrhosis for the Americas and Caribbean countries also vary widely; examples not shown in Table 25.2 include Mexico (49), Chile (46), Venezuela (19), U.S. (12), Cuba (12), and Canada (9).[26] Rates of cirrhosis have increased significantly in Mexico, Brazil, and the Andean countries. Cirrhosis is the sixth leading cause of death among males in Mexico. Rates have declined in the U.S., Canada, and English-speaking Caribbean countries.[27] Explanations for the high rates of cirrhosis in Eastern Europe and Latin America include frequent episodes of heavy binge drinking, poor nutrition, infectious agents, and type of alcoholic beverage consumed.

A second measure of alcohol-related harm used in the WHO survey was alcohol deaths due to injury and/or poisoning. This category does not include motor vehicle accidents. While this category may have some variability as to how it was defined in each country, it does allow for comparison and correlates with economic, political, and social changes occurring in many of these countries. The highest rates were in the Baltic countries of Latvia (233), Lithuania (191), Estonia (181), and the Russian Federation (226). The majority of countries in Western Europe reported rates of 40 to 60 deaths per 100,000 population for this category of alcohol-related harm. The lowest rates were reported in The Netherlands and the United Kingdom. The higher rates in certain countries may be related to heavy drinking in high-risk situations, such as drinking in the workplace, drinking outside in the wintertime or in unheated habitats, or drinking homemade alcohol that may be contaminated with methanol and other toxins. For example, Austria's rural areas produce large amounts of apple cider. The distilling process results in significant amounts of methanol, which may explain the higher rates of cirrhosis in Austria.

A third measure of alcohol-related harm is motor vehicle accidents. As with the other categories, the frequency of these events varies by country. The data presented in Table 25.2 includes *all* deaths from motor vehicle accidents. Most countries estimate that 40 to 50% of these deaths are alcohol related. The highest reported rates were in Latvia (35), Estonia (24), and Slovenia (28). The Nordic countries (7), Israel (7), Iceland (8), and the United Kingdom (8) had the lowest rates. These differences are most likely related to road conditions and highway safety issues, public policy, legal penalties, enforcement of drunk driving laws, and social norms.

Countries with very strict drunk-driving laws have much lower rates of alcohol-related motor vehicle accidents than countries that tolerate driving under the influence of alcohol. While not listed in Table 25.2, the frequency of alcohol-related motor vehicle accidents in the U.S. has decreased over the last 10 years as a direct result of policy changes such as raising the legal drinking age to 21, increased penalties for drunk driving, mandatory alcohol assessments, zero tolerance for under-age drinking and driving, and active prevention programs. There has been a slight increase, however, in the number of deaths from motor vehicle accidents in the last 2 years as a result of increased speed limits on major highways.

The issue of the protective effect of alcohol on the prevention of ischemic heart disease remains controversial.[26,28] Some public health leaders, such as those in Scotland, advocate the use of one to two drinks of alcohol per day for men over the age of 40 or postmenopausal women.[3] Others take a counter-view, predicting an increase in overall morbidity and mortality as a result of advocating daily alcohol use.[29] A recent thoughtful review of the evidence by Drs. Hanna, Chou, and Grant does not support the J-shaped curve that has been proposed by a number of researchers.[30] Although they did confirm that the current data supports the notion that 1 to 2 drinks per day may have a mild protective effect for some populations, the question is far from resolved.[31,32] The next logical step is to conduct a randomized trial with low-dose alcohol to determine if overall mortality is reduced.

The relationship between alcohol and depression is now well established. One of the current questions of interest is the dose-response effect of alcohol and mood. Rowe conducted a study of a sample of 2500 adults in a primary care clinic and found that persons drinking four or more drinks per day (>48 g) had significantly higher rates of depression.[33] Persons drinking lesser amounts did not have an increased frequency of depression compared to a group of persons who were abstinent. This dose-response is similar to the effect of alcohol on other organ systems.

FREQUENCY OF COMORBID MENTAL HEALTH DISORDERS

Alcohol use is associated with a number of mental health problems, including thought disorders, depression, anxiety, post-traumatic stress disorders, and addiction to tobacco products and other mood-altering drugs. A study conducted in 17 community-based mental health centers for the chronically mentally ill found that 50% of persons with a diagnosis of chronic schizophrenia had a current alcohol or drug problem.[34] A study in a primary care sample of adult problem drinkers participating in a brief intervention trial found the following rates of comorbidity: the frequency of lifetime depression was 28% for men and 49% for women; the rates of current depression were 9% for men and 21% for women; the rates of antisocial personality disorders were 11% in men and 6% in women; and tobacco use rates were 52% for men and 58% for women.[35]

NATURAL HISTORY OF RECOVERY

Traditionally, alcohol and drug disorders were thought to follow a natural progression from early signs and symptoms through end-stage disease. Affected persons would develop progressively chronic disease and either die from their disease or begin the long process of recovery. Alcoholics Anonymous and specialized treatment were felt to be essential in order to achieve long-term sobriety. Many health care providers have seen patients in withdrawal or in the emergency department who fit this model. However, most patients seen in primary care with alcohol-related problems do not fit this classic model of progression.

The clinical course of alcohol and drug disorders is complex and variable.[36-38] Patients may experience periods of harmful use, punctuated by periods of non-use or non-problematic use.[39,40] Some individuals are heavy alcohol users throughout most of their adult lives, periodically experiencing some minor problems, but never escalating to more severe symptoms. Others drink heavily once or twice a year, are involved in a serious motor vehicle accident, and stop drinking on their own. Still others escalate to multiple consequences involving negative family, work, and social situations. Unfortunately, there are also those drinkers who develop rapid progression of their addictive disorders and die after 5 to 10 years of heavy use.

Recovery can be just as variable. Some persons stop their use of the chemical on their own and are never seen in the treatment system.[41,42] Some reach treatment through family, work and/or their health care provider. Most people, however, experience relapse — perhaps several times — before they achieve long-term sobriety.

SPONTANEOUS RECOVERY WITH NO TREATMENT

Case study: *Elizabeth is a 45-year-old lawyer who had a history of heavy alcohol use in college, but reduced her consumption during law school. Upon completion of law school, she resumed her previous pattern of use and began to experiment with cocaine. She became completely abstinent while pregnant, but resumed her alcohol use pattern after the birth of her son. Elizabeth's consumption soon escalated and she began drinking daily and became intoxicated at least once a week. Seven years ago, her family and colleagues confronted her with their concerns about her drinking. At that time, she stopped drinking on her own and has remained abstinent for 6 years.*

PARTIAL RECOVERY WITH MINOR RELAPSES

Case study: *John is a 48-year-old salesman who started using alcohol to feel comfortable at parties when he was in his teens. He had difficulty controlling his use from the first drink. He was unable to leave a drink unfinished and became intoxicated on most occasions when he drank. John drinks heavily five nights a week. At his last company physical exam, his GGT and blood pressure were elevated. He also reported persistent abdominal pain. He was arrested for driving under the influence of alcohol on two occasions. His father recently died from cirrhosis. At his wife's insistence, he periodically stops drinking for periods of up to 3 months. John was confronted by his employer for performance problems and entered an outpatient alcohol treatment program. In the last 5 years, he has had four relapses that lasted 1 to 2 months, but he has returned to AA meetings and has had long periods of sobriety between the relapses.*

PROGRESSIVE DISEASE WITH A FATAL OUTCOME

Case study: *Jerek was a 55-year-old seasonally employed construction worker who began drinking at the age of 13. His father, grandfather, and two uncles drank heavily. One uncle died at age 25 in an alcohol-related auto accident. His father died in prison while Jerek was still in high school. When he was in his early 30s, Jerek had periods of controlled drinking and was able to maintain employment and family responsibilities. He later began to lose construction jobs because he was unable to come to work after binge drinking on weekends. He was divorced at age 42 and had no contact with his three children. He often drank in the morning to counteract withdrawal symptoms. He was suicidal on a number of occasions but was always too afraid to try. He received treatment at the county detoxification unit four times and participated in a 28-day treatment program twice. Jerek was most recently seen in the emergency department after vomiting blood and experiencing severe abdominal pain. Shortly after admission, he suffered a cardiopulmonary arrest and died.*

REFERENCES

1. World Health Organization Regional Office for Europe, *Country Profiles.* 1995, http://www.who.dk/hp/adt/acountry.htm#Profiles.
2. National Institute on Alcohol Abuse and Alcoholism, Cultural Influences and Drinking Patterns: A Focus on Hispanic and Japanese Populations, U.S. Department of Health and Human Services, Public Health Service, Alcohol, Drug Abuse, and Mental Health Administration, DHHS publication no. (ADM) 88-1563, 1988.
3. Scotland's Health: Scottish Health Survey, 1995, Scottish Office, Department of Health, 1997, http://www.official-documents.co.uk/document/scottish/shealth/shhm.htm.
4. U.S. Department of Health and Human Services, *National Household Survey on Drug Abuse,* Washington, D.C., DHHS, Public Health Service, Substance Abuse and Mental Health Services Administration, 1998, http://www.health.org/pubs/97hhs/httoc.htm.
5. Grant, B.F., DSM-IV, DSM-III-R, and ICD-10 alcohol and drug abuse/harmful use and dependence, United States, 1992: a nosological comparison, *Alcohol. Clin. Exp. Res.,* 20, 1481, 1996.
6. MMWR, Alcohol and Other Drug Related Birth Defects Awareness Week May 11–17, 1997, *MMWR Morb. Mortal Wkly. Rep.,* 46, 346, 1997.
7. Wilsnack, S.C. and Wilsnack, R.W., Drinking and problem drinking in U.S. women, Patterns and recent trends, *Rec. Devel. Alcohol.,* 12, 29, 1995.
8. Monitoring the Future Study, Conducted at the Institute for Social Research, University of Michigan. Supported by research grants from the National Institute on Drug Abuse, 1998 data tables: http://www.isr.umich.edu/src/mtf/.
9. Centers for Disease Control and Prevention, Youth Risk Behavior Surveillance United States, 1997. Atlanta, GA, Division of Adolescent and School Health, National Center for Chronic Disease Prevention and Health Promotion, Centers for Disease Control and Prevention, 1997. http://www.cdc.gov/nccd-php/dash/yrbs/youth97.htm.
10. King, A., Wold, B., Smith, C.T., and Harel, Y., The health of youth: a cross-national survey, WHO Regional Publications, European Series no. 69, 1996.

11. Wechsler, H., Dowdall, G.W., Maenner, G., Glendhill-Hoyt, J., Lee, H., Changes in binge drinking and related problems among American college students between 1993 and 1997. Results of the Harvard School of Public Health College Alcohol Study, *J. Am. College Health*, 47, 57, 1998.

12. Mirand, A.L. and Welte, J.W., Alcohol consumption among the elderly in a general population, Erie County, New York, *Am. J. Public Health*, 86, 978, 1996.

13. Adams, W.L., Yuan, Z., Barboriak, J.J., and Rimm, A.A., Alcohol-related hospitalizations of elderly people. Prevalence and geographic variation in the United States, *JAMA*, 270, 1222, 1993.

14. Adams, W.L., Barry, K.L., and Fleming, M.F., Screening for problem drinking in older primary care patients, *JAMA*, 276, 1964, 1996.

15. Manwell, L.B., Fleming, M.F., Johnson, K., and Barry, K.L., Tobacco, alcohol, and drug use in a primary care sample: 90-day prevalence and associated factors, *J. Addict. Dis.*, 17, 67, 1998.

16. Fleming, M.F., Manwell, L.B., Barry, K.L., Johnson, K.L., and Johnson, K., At-risk drinking in an HMO primary care sample: prevalence and health policy implications, *Am. J. Public Health*, 88, 90, 1998.

17. Ewing, J.A., Detecting alcoholism: the CAGE questionnaire, *JAMA*, 252, 1905, 1984.

18. Chang, G. and Astrachan, B.M., The emergency department surveillance of alcohol intoxication after motor vehicle accidents, *JAMA*, 260, 2533, 1988.

19. Cherpitel, C.J., Breath analysis and self-reports as measures of alcohol-related emergency room admissions, *J. Stud. Alcohol.*, 50, 155, 1989.

20. Cherpitel, C.J., Alcohol use among HMO patients in the emergency room, primary care and the general population, *J. Stud. Alcohol.*, 56, 272, 1995.

21. Borges, G., Cherpitel, C.J., Medina-Mora, M.E., Mondragon, L., and Casanova, L., Alcohol consumption in emergency room patients and the general population: a population based study, *Alcohol. Clin. Exp. Res.*, 22, 1986, 1998.

22. Cleary, P.D., Miller, M., Bush, B.T., Warburg, M.M., Delbanco, T.L., and Aronson, M.D., Prevalence and recognition of alcohol abuse in a primary care population, *Am. J. Med.*, 85, 466, 1988.

23. Moore, R.D., Bone, L.R., Geller, G., Mamon, J.A., Stokes, E.J., and Levine, D.M., Prevalence, detection and treatment of alcoholism in hospitalized patients, *JAMA*, 261, 403, 1989.

24. National Institute on Alcohol Abuse and Alcoholism. Alcohol's effects on organ function, *Alcohol Health Res. World*, 21, 1, 1997.

25. Urbano-Marquez, A., Estruch, R., Fernandez-Sola, J., Nicolas, J.M., Pare, J.C., and Rubin, E., The greater risk of alcoholic cardiomyopathy and myopathy in women compared with men, *JAMA*, 274, 149, 1995.

26. Edwards, G., et al., *Alcohol Policy and the Public Good*, Oxford University Press, Oxford, 1994.

27. Pan American Health Organization, *Health in the Americas*, Vol. 1. Pan American Sanitary Bureau, Regional Office of the World Health Organization, Washington, D.C., 1998, http://www.paho.org/english/HIA1998/HealthVol1.pdf.

28. Hanna, E.Z., Dufour, M., Elliot, E.F., and Hartford, T., Dying to be equal: women, alcohol and cardiovascular disease, *Br. J. Addict.*, 87, 1593,1992.

29. Stampfer, M.J., Rimm, E.B., and Walsh, D.C., Commentary: alcohol, the heart, and public policy, *Am. J. Public Health*, 83, 801, 1992.

30. Hanna, E.Z., Chou, S.P., and Grant, B.F., The relationship between drinking and heart disease morbidity in the United States: results from the National Health Interview Survey, *Alcohol. Clin. Exp. Res.*, 21, 111, 1997.

31. Klatsky, A.L., Armstrong, M.A., and Friedman, G.D., Alcohol and mortality, *Ann. Intern. Med.*, 117, 646, 1992.

32. Ridker, P.M., Vaughan, D.E., Stampfer, M.J., Glynn, R.J., and Hennekens, C.H., Association of moderate alcohol consumption and plasma concentration of endogenous tissue-type plasminogen activator, *JAMA*, 272, 929, 1994.

33. Rowe, M.G., Fleming, M.F., Barry, K.L., Manwell, L.B., and Kropp, S., Correlates of depression in primary care, *J. Fam. Pract.*, 41, 551, 1995.

34. Barry, K.L., Fleming, M.F., Greenley, J.R., Kropp, S., and Widlak, P., Characteristics of persons with severe mental illness and substance abuse in rural areas, *Psychiatr. Serv.*, 47, 88, 1996.

35. Barry, K.L., Fleming, M.F., Manwell, L.B., and Copeland, L.A., Conduct disorder and antisocial personality in adult primary care patients, *J. Fam. Pract.*, 45, 151, 1997.

36. Vaillant, G., *The Natural History of Alcoholism Revisited,* Harvard University Press, Cambridge, MA, 1995.
37. Temple, M.T. and Leino, E.V., Long-term outcomes of drinking: a 20-year longitudinal study of men, *Br. J. Addict.,* 84, 889, 1989.
38. Humphreys, K., Moos, R.H., and Finney, J.W., Two pathways out of drinking problems without professional treatment, *Addict. Behav.,* 20, 427, 1995.
39. Cunningham, J.A., Sobell, L.C., Sobell, M.B., and Kapur, G., Resolution from alcohol problems with and without treatment: reasons for change, *J. Subst. Abuse,* 7, 365, 1995.
40. Cunningham, J.A., Sobell, L.S., and Sobell, M.B., Are disease and conceptions of alcohol abuse related to beliefs about outcome and recovery? *J. Appl. Soc. Psychol.,* 26, 773, 1996.
41. Sobell, L.C., Cunningham, J.A., and Sobell, M.B., Recovery from alcohol problems with and without treatment: prevalence in two populations surveys, *Am. J. Public Health,* 86, 966, 1996.
42. Sobell, L.C., Sobell, M.B., and Toneatto, T., Recovery from alcohol problems without treatment, *Self-Control and the Addictive Behaviors,* Heather, N., Miller, W.R., and Greeley, J., Eds., Maxwell MacMillan, New York, 1992, 198.

26 Comorbidity

Ulrich W. Preuss and Wie Mooi Wong

OVERVIEW

This chapter reviews the theories and prevalence of comorbidity between alcoholism and several psychiatric disorders. The term "comorbidity"[1] was introduced to assess concurrent disorders that may affect treatment outcome. Evaluated through epidemiological studies or ascertained from individuals entering treatment, at least two thirds of alcoholic individuals show substanstial comorbidity of anxiety, sadness, manic-like conditions, other substance use disorders, and severe and pervasive antisocial behavior.

Several hypotheses have been proposed to explain a high concurrence between two comorbid diseases. Reviewing the relevant literature, the theory that psychiatric symptomatology among alcoholics may reflect long-term major psychiatric disorders is not widely supported, nor is the hypothesis that alcoholism may reflect an effort to "self-medicate" preexisting psychiatric symptoms, which is only true for acute alcohol effects. A genetic link or some common environmental factors shared between alcoholism and some comorbid disorders can only be supported for concurrent substance abuse, but not for other psychiatric disorders. The confounding factors that might arise from research methodology have a major impact on study results of comorbidity. The hypothesis that alcoholism itself elicits or aggravates some psychiatric symptoms is, in large part, supported. Keeping these perspectives in mind, comorbidity between alcoholism and anxiety disorders, affective disorders, eating disorders, schizophrenia, and substance abuse is reviewed and evaluated in this chapter.

INTRODUCTION

The term "comorbidity" was introduced as a reminder to clinical trial investigators to assess concurrent disorders that may affect treatment outcome.[1] Several hypotheses have been proposed to help explain the high concurrence between alcoholism and psychiatric disorders. These include:

1. The psychiatric symptomatology observed among alcoholics may reflect long-term major psychiatric disorders.[2-6]
2. These psychiatric symptoms among alcoholics reflect an effort to "self-medicate" preexisting psychiatric symptoms through the use of high doses of alcohol.[6,7]
3. There might be a genetic linkage with alcoholism for at least some disorders such as manic depression, schizophrenia, or the antisocial personality disorders.[12]
4. The concurrence of major psychiatric disorders and alcohol dependence is a consequence of research methodology, that is, an individual with more than one psychiatric disorder will be more likely to be identified as a clinical case and be included in a study.[8]
5. Alcoholism itself elicits or aggravates some psychiatric symptoms.

The National Comorbidity Survey (NCS)[4] reported that there is a much stronger evidence for lifetime concurrence of psychiatric disorders with alcohol dependence than alcohol abuse. The concurrence was stronger among women than men. Alcoholism disorders and psychiatric disorders have significantly higher rates of comorbidity in clinical samples than in community samples.[11]

The following reviews comorbidity between alcoholism and major psychiatric disorders such as anxiety, bipolar, personality, eating, substance abuse, depressive disorders, as well as schizophrenia and suicidal behavior.

ANXIETY DISORDERS AND ALCOHOLISM

Diagnostic systems such as ICD-10 and DSM-IV subgroup anxiety disorders into four major groups: as: agoraphobia with and without panic disorders, social phobias, generalized anxiety disorder possibly related to depressive disorders, and post-traumatic stress disorder (PTSD).

Main symptoms of anxiety disorders are the unexpected occurrence of anxiety and affective tensions, combined with a number of psychovegetative symptoms such as tremors, shortness of breath, tachycardia, sweating, paresthesias, nausea, and other abdominal disturbances. *However*, all these symptoms may also occur in alcohol withdrawal.

Epidemiological and clinical studies consistently revealed a high prevalence of social phobia[10-12] among alcoholics. Concurrence of alcoholism and social phobia has consistently been noted in both males and females from community surveys and family studies.[13-16] Recent reviews have concluded that the association between anxiety disorders and alcoholism could be attributed chiefly to phobic disorders, rather than panic or generalized anxiety states.[12,17]

Previous studies have discussed this association of alcoholism and anxiety disorders under the "tension reduction" or "self-medication" theory.[6,7]

The "tension reduction" theory proposes that alcohol reduces emotional tension and that people drink in order to experience relief from tension. Because anxiety includes the experience of tension, self-application of alcohol might be a consequence. In patients with anxiety, alcohol may be used in order to cope with feared situations.[19,20] Some investigations showed that anxiety disorders preceded symptoms of alcoholism in 65% of those persons with both disorders.[21]

However, the relationship between alcoholism and anxiety disorders is likely to be more complex. Another study showed that in a huge number of patients, the onset of alcoholism precedes the onset of anxiety disorders.[24] Among twins, the results of an investigation of concordance suggested that anxiety and depression are more likely to be consequences rather than causes of alcoholism.[23] Some studies have reported that preexisting anxiety and other psychiatric symptomatology rarely improve, and often even intensify with heavy drinking.[7,14] For example, there is evidence that even modest doses of alcohol are associated with increases — not decreases — in physiological measures associated with tension, as well as with subjective feelings of anxiety.[24] Therefore, little evidence exists to corroborate the theory that a substantial proportion of alcoholics might develop anxiety disorders in attempting to seek out possible tension-reducing properties of a brain depressant such as alcohol.

Nonetheless, an impressive correlation between alcoholism and severe anxiety syndromes comes from the observation of anxiety in alcoholic withdrawal. The development of physical dependence to any brain depressant results in acute abstinence syndrome, lasting about 4 to 5 days. Symptoms include tremors, tension, restlessness, and insomnia. This is often followed by a secondary or protracted abstinence syndrome, lasting months, and characterized by anxiety, emotional instability, autonomic overactivity, restlessness, and sleep impairment.[15,25] Almost all symptoms of anxiety among alcoholics were observed during the first several weeks of abstinence.[26]

High rates of drinking and substance abuse among primary anxiety disorder patients were also revealed — up to 20% in clinical investigations[27] compared to 1 to 5% in general population samples.[101] However, the strength of association between anxiety disorders and alcoholism in recent large-scale epidemiological studies suggests that comorbidity between these two disorders is not attributable only to an increased frequency of treatment-seeking among those with comorbidity.[3,4]

EPIDEMIOLOGY

Recent studies involving large samples reinvestigated comorbidity of alcoholism and anxiety disorders.

In the NCS[11], a U.S.-nationally representative household survey involving 1142 persons, a comorbidity rate for alcoholism and any anxiety disorders was 36% in men and 61% in woman (Table 26.1). Anxiety and affective disorders constituted the largest proportion of lifetime concurrent cases among women. However, diagnosis in this survey was mainly made by non-clinicians and the results were based on retrospective reports.

In the Epidemiological Catchment Area (ECA) Study,[4] strong associations between alcohol abuse (or dependence) and phobic disorders (odds ratio = relative risk compared to controls 2.4), panic disorder (odds ratio 4.3), and anxiety disorder (odds ratio 1.5) were revealed.

In the Collaborative Study on the Genetics of Alcoholism (COGA, s. Table 26.1),[35,71] the lifetime rate for independent anxiety disorders was significantly higher among 2713 alcoholics compared to 919 controls (9 vs. 4%). Most of the difference was attributed to panic disorder (4 vs. 1%) and social phobia (3 vs. 1%), but no significant group differences were revealed for agoraphobia or obsessive-compulsive disorder.

A family study on 165 probands selected for alcoholism and anxiety disorders, involving 61 controls and 1053 first-degree relatives, investigated the patterns of familial aggregation, comorbidity of alcoholism, and anxiety disorders.[28] The findings indicated that alcoholics were associated with relatives suffering from anxiety disorders, particularly among females. Both alcoholism and anxiety disorders were highly familial, and the familial aggregation of alcoholism was attributable to alcohol dependence rather than to alcohol abuse, particularly among male relatives. Aggregation of alcohol dependence and anxiety disorders in families differed according to the subtype of anxiety disorders. Evidence showed a partly shared diathesis underlying panic disorders and alcoholism, whereas social phobia and alcoholism aggregated independently. Onset of social phobia also tended to precede that of alcoholism in this study, whereas other studies showed equal proportions of subjects with comorbid panic disorders reporting the onset of panic earlier, simultaneously, or later than the onset of alcoholism.[29] Subjects with panic disorder were far less likely to report using alcohol for self-medication of anxiety. Panic attacks may instead be precipitated by physiological changes resulting from alcoholism.[28]

In summary, anxiety disorders may coexist in alcoholics more often than in control samples. Recent evidence shows that panic disorders and alcoholism may, at least in part, share a common genetic background. Recent studies also show that specific subtypes of anxiety and alcoholism reveal greater association than others (i.e., phobic disorders more than panic or generalized anxiety states and alcohol dependence more than abuse).[28]

However, not all studies support these findings and despite progress in comorbidity research, the nature of the association between these disorders remains unclear, largely because of the heterogeneity of both disorders and partly as a result of the disparate methodologies employed among the studies that have been conducted thus far.

POSTTRAUMATIC STRESS DISORDER (PTSD) AND ALCOHOLISM

In PTSD, alcohol use might, theoretically, be involved in so-called high-risk behaviors, which subsequently increase their risk for experiencing a traumatic event that could lead to PTSD. Conversely, alcohol users might themselves be more susceptible to PTSD after traumatic exposure. Among Vietnam veterans seeking treatment for PTSD, 60 to 80% exhibit concurrent diagnoses of drug/alcohol abuse or dependence, more common among veterans with high combat exposure. Vietnam veterans with PTSD and alcoholism had an earlier age of onset for alcoholism, and alcoholism preceded PTSD by 3.1 years.[95] In a sample of WWII veterans, alcoholism followed 6.9 years after the onset of PTSD.[97]

TABLE 26.1
Psychiatric Comorbidity of Alcohol Dependence and Control Samples in Epidemiological Studies

	Alcohol dependence												Control Samples	
	NSA n = 1212[11]				COGA: n = 2713[35]				ECA: n = 2653[4,100]				ECA[101]	Bavarian Study[101]
	Males		Females		Males		Females		Males		Females			
	Total %	OR	Total %	OR	Total %	OR	Total %	OR	Total %	OR	%	OR	%	%
Alcohol dependence													4.7	5.1
Anxiety														
GAD	8.6	3.86	15.7	3.01	3.9	5.53	7.7	5.91	2.0					
Panic	3.6	2.27	12.0	2.98					2.0	2.00	7.0	3.50	0.8	0.4
Agoraphobia	6.5	1.82	18.5	2.53	2.4	6.00	4.8	2.54						
Social phobia	19.3	2.41	30.3	2.62	3.0	4.33	6.8	3.21						
Simple phobia	13.9	3.11	30.7	2.63					13.0	1.44	31.0	1.93	7.7	1.1
PTSD	10.3	3.20	26.2	3.60										
Any	35.8	2.22	60.7	3.08	9.3	3.92	16.6	3.40					8.8	1.6
Affective														
Depression	24.3	2.95	48.5	4.05	38.4	4.13	49.7	2.23	5.0	1.66	19.0	2.71	3.0	1.4
Dysthymia	1.2	3.81	20.9	3.63	2.2	11.0	6.3	3.70					3.3	5.4
Mania	6.2	12.0	6.8	5.30	2.7	3.85	5.9	4.53	1.0	3.33	4.0	10.00	0.5	0.1
Any	28.1	3.16	53.5	4.36	39.7	4.31	52.1	2.14						
Schizophrenia													0.8	0.4
Drug abuse	11.1	2.97	12.4	5.16										
Drug dependence	29.5	9.81	34.7	15.75										
Any	40.6	7.73	47.1	14.12					19.0	2.71	31.0	6.2	1.9	0.7
Other														
Somatization									0.07	3.50	0.87	4.35	0.1	0.0
OCD					2.5	2.50	2.5	9.14					1.5	0.1
Conduct disorder	41.6	4.29	22.8	5.83										
Antisocial disorder	24.5	7.16	7.8	17.1					15.0	3.75	10.0	12.34		
Bulimia[54]		0.7		6.10		3.46	1.26							
Anorexia[54]					0.0									
Any:	27.1	8.34	28.9	6.10										

Note: OCD, obsessive compulsive disorder; OR = odds ratio = relative risk compared to each control population; GAD, generalized anxiety disorder.

The relationship between alcohol use and PTSD might be noncausal. Furthermore, an antisocial personality and conduct disorder, as well as major depression, have been linked to traumatic exposure, PTSD, and other drug abuse disorders. A comorbidity of these disorders might predispose persons to alcohol abuse and PTSD, thereby accounting for the observed association between PTSD and alcoholism. The self-medication and tension reduction models have shown little evidence in this comorbity case and have no empirical basis.[96]

AFFECTIVE DISORDERS AND ALCOHOLISM

Depression is a constellation of signs and symptoms that includes depressed mood or interest/drive, anhedonia, psychomotor disturbance, sleep disturbance, appetite disturbance, changes in diurnal variation, suicidal intention or behavior, and decreased self-esteem.[27]

Epidemiological studies have convincingly shown that lifetime diagnoses of affective disorders and alcoholism occur more frequently than a concurrence of both disorders expected by chance.[33] Estimates of sadness among alcoholics range from 28 to 98%.[34] Such a wide range must reflect a variety of factors including diagnostic heterogeneity of the patients and differences in instruments used to measure depressive symptoms, as well as the impact of recent drinking.[26,35,36]

When two disorders coexist frequently, causal associations must be considered. Alcoholism may cause major depression … and major depression may cause alcoholism. The sadness-inducing effects of alcohol are especially likely to be observed with falling blood alcohol concentrations, during periods of sustained intoxication and during protracted periods of drinking or withdrawal.[24] Community studies reported that a lifetime history of major depression increased four-fold the likelihood of an alcohol disorder.[36,37]

As to the "self-medication"-hypothesis, which poses that patients drink because they are depressed, there is little convincing data indicating that a substantial proportion of individuals with major depressive disorders are likely to go on to develop alcohol dependence.[38] Furthermore, if alcohol were used as an antidepressant, then alcohol intake should be abolished or at least alleviated by bona fide antidepressants in alcoholics with clinical depression.

Differentiations among affective states in alcoholics have focused on a primary vs. secondary distinction based on the chronology of development of the syndromes.[26] In this approach, the psychiatric disorder with onset at the earliest age is labeled as primary and subsequent conditions are noted as secondary. But this might be too restrictive because independent depressive episodes, with their need for longer-term treatments, might develop during periods of abstinence but still be labeled as secondary. Recent evidence has indicated that 70% or more of alcohol-dependent patients report at least one period of abstinence lasting 3 or more months in the course of their alcohol dependence and there is an average of two such occurrences in which the mean duration exceeds 12 months.[39]

In treatment outcome, a comorbid depression has been shown to be of predictive relevance in both women and men. While associated with poor outcome in men, women with depression showed improved results.[40]

In the assumption of a common genetic background for both alcoholism and depression, one would expect high rates of depression in offsprings of alcoholics and vice versa. However, family studies showed that sons of alcoholics compared with carefully matched controls demonstrated that, at least by the early 30s, the two groups did not differ significantly on their rates of major depressive disorders.[41] Individuals with major depressive disorders are as likely to develop alcohol dependence as the general population.[38] Thus, except for an aggregation of affective disorders among relatives of alcoholics, there is little evidence for a common genetic background of alcoholism and depression up to now.

Family studies reported[10] that depressives without alcoholism did not pass on alcoholism within their families, and probands with depression and alcoholism tended to pass on both depression and alcoholism. This supports the hypothesis that depression and alcoholism are not manifestations of the same underlying disorder.

EPIDEMIOLOGY

The rate of severe depression in the course of alcohol abuse or alcoholism is at least 30 to 40%.[24] Depressive symptoms are reported to be more likely in female than male alcoholics.[42]

As an example, the Epidemiological Catchment Area (ECA) Study reported excess comorbidity between affective disorders and alcoholism with an odds ratio (relative risk compared to control population) of 6.2.[4] Another study found that a lifetime history of major depression increased fourfold the likelihood of an alcohol disorder.[37]

In a clinical study,[26] 42% of 191 alcoholics studied showed clinically significant levels of depression with Hamilton Depression Scale scores greater than 20. Only 6% remained depressed at week 4 after first interview. Mood-related symptoms constituted the largest portion of presenting depression and abated most rapidly. Autonomic symptoms remained the most prevalent type of depressive symptoms at the end of investigation.

On the one hand, a number of family studies has shown that primary alcoholism plays an etiological role in some secondary depressions.[43-46] On the other hand, primary depression apparently is familial if it clearly precedes the onset of alcoholism.[47-49]

In 2945 alcohol-dependent subjects of the COGA Study,[35,71] a timeline method for determining the type of depressive disorder among probands' relatives and comparison subjects was employed.[39] The individuals were compared with regard to the primary and secondary depression approach. Major depressive episodes with an onset before the development of alcohol dependence or during a subsequent long abstinence period were observed in 15% of the alcoholics, while 26% reported at least one substance-induced depressive episode. Subjects with independent — as compared to substance-induced — major depressive episodes were more likely to be married, Caucasian, female, to have had experience with fewer drugs and less treatment for alcoholism, to have attempted suicide, and to have more relatives with a major mood disorder.

Other studies also showed that among relatives of alcoholics, a higher rate of major depression is found.[9] Alcoholism in depressed females even appeared to increase the familial risk for depression, particularly among female relatives.[51]

However, a recent family-based study[13] reported that unipolar depression and alcoholics may segregate independently in families. Additionally, no effect from the concurrence of unipolar depression and alcoholism in probands was found on the recurrence risks in relatives. The nonfamilial components of unipolar depression and alcoholism correlated positively in this study.

Depression may also influence the degree of treatment participation[41] and has been reported to be associated with poorer drinking outcome following treatment for alcoholism.[42]

BIPOLAR DISORDERS AND ALCOHOLISM

Mania is, together with depression, the major feature of bipolar disorders. It is characterized by elevated, expansive, or irritable mood plus a number of other signs and symptoms, including grandiosity, elation, racing thoughts, pressured speech, distractibility, decreased need for sleep, increased activity, and impulsive behavior.[52]

Data from the ECA study[4] showed that more than 60% of bipolar I patients have a lifetime history of substance abuse. Of these patients, alcohol abuse alone represents 33%, and alcohol and drug abuse 43%. Substance abuse is slightly less common in bipolar II patients: 49% have a history of substance abuse, with alcohol abuse being present in the histories of about 80% of these patients. Conversely, the prevalence of mania in alcoholics showed low rates of 2 to 4%. However, increased abuse of alcohol may be more likely during manic phases.

Bipolar disorders and alcoholism are both familial, each with a strong genetic component. Overlap between the familial components was observed in relatives of alcoholics and bipolar disorder patients.[13]

A four-fold increase in risk for alcoholism among relatives of male patients with bipolar disorder was reported.[13] In the aforementioned family study,[26] a modest covariation of familial components of bipolar disorder and alcoholism was suggested. Alcoholism may occur in most of the comorbid cases as a secondary complication.

EATING DISORDERS AND ALCOHOLISM

Alcoholism has been linked to major eating disorders, that is, anorexia nervosa and bulimia nervosa or problems with the control of appetitive behaviors.

Some reports with small sample size noted that between 14% and over 50% of bulimic individuals might meet criteria for alcohol dependence,[55-56] and 7 to 33% of patients with anorexia reported substance abuse or dependence, including alcohol.[57,58] Conversely, 15% of 143 alcoholic woman in treatment showed some type of eating disorder,[59] although the eating problems were more related to use of stimulants, not alcohol. In a metastatistical study, comorbidity rates of alcoholism among bulimics were reported to range between 11 and 89%.[60] Among anorectics, comorbidity rates between 9 and 34% were found. On average, greater alcohol use among bulimic rather than anorectic women was found.

The rate of crossover of eating disorders and substance use disorders within families indicated prevalence rates between 7 and 60% for substance use disorders among relatives of individuals with eating disorders.[61] Evidence from studies suggests that a sizable proportion of bulimic women (i.e., 34%) have a comorbid alcohol or substance use disorder, whereas between 8 to 41% of women with substance abuse disorders or alcoholism have a current or past history of bulimia nervosa.[57]

Within the COGA sample[54] (see Table 26.2), 2283 women and 1982 men were interviewed regarding alcoholism, anorexia, and bulimia.

Lifetime rates for anorexia and bulimia were 1 and 6%, respectively, for the alcoholic woman. Bulimia was also observed in 1% of the alcoholic men. After controlling for other psychiatric diagnosis, anorexia was seen in only 16% of woman with primary alcoholism and none of the alcoholic men. The rates for bulimia were 3 and 1%, respectively. However, no strong familial crossover between alcoholism and anorexia or bulimia was revealed in this study. These results are supported by twin studies reporting that most of the genetic variation influencing vulnerability to alcoholism in women was unrelated to the genetic factors influencing liability for bulimia.[85,92] Thus, although bulimia, anorexia nervosa, and alcoholism frequently coexist within individuals and within families, they do not appear to be alternative manifestations of a common underlying etiology.[43,64]

So, if there is little evidence for a common underlying etiology for both eating disorders and alcoholism, the existence of a common "addictive personality" is doubtful. It may follow that certain individuals may be predisposed to both kind of disorders.

The "self-medication" theory is also inconclusive in this kind of comorbidity. Some eating disorders have been successfully treated with antidepressive medication, which did not improve drinking in other studies.[57,91]

An important factor in the etiology in eating disorders is dysfunctional family interaction, which might aggravate a preexisting psychological or physiological problem.[58]

Because of the aggregation of alcoholism in families, it has been suggested that a predisposition to alcoholism is genetically transmitted. Twin studies have also found genetic links for both anorexia nervosa and, to a lesser extent, bulimia nervosa.[56] However, based on the COGA results, there might be independent genetic and environmental factors in the etiology of both disorders.

PERSONALITY DISORDERS AND ALCOHOLISM

While prospective studies showed that personality states do not predict the onset of drinking, personality disorders may play an important role in the pathogenesis and prognosis of alcoholism.

A growing number of studies addresses the whole spectrum of Axis II comorbidity in alcoholic inpatients. Prevalence rates range from 57 to 78% and seem to differ with the instruments used. Greatest prevalence rates were found for paranoid (7 to 44%), antisocial (3 to 47%), borderline (16 to 32%), histrionic (6 to 34%), avoidant (2 to 32%), and dependent personality disorders (4 to 29%).[73] This more recent study[73] reported at least one personality disorder diagnosed in one third (34%) of the patients, two personality disorders in 9%, and three in 4%.

A special focus in this area was the comorbidity of alcoholism and antisocial personality disorder (ASPD). Major characteristics of ASPD are an impairment in the ability to form meaningful relationships with others and an engagement in behaviors that deviate from social norms.[68] ASPD frequently coexists with alcoholism.[74] Traits related to antisociality have been repeatedly shown to be robust predictors of both alcoholism and ASPD, but are not necessarily either causal or integrating.[68]

Alcoholics with ASPD have an earlier age of onset for problem drinking or alcoholism, or first intoxication, more alcohol-related arrests and occupational consequences of drinking, more social consequences of drinking, higher average daily alcohol consumption, and a higher likelihood of drug abuse or dependence.[73-80]

ASPD is considered to be important both in the development of alcoholism and its clinical course. Alcoholics with ASPD or major depression had poorer 1-year drinking outcomes than did alcoholics who had neither comorbid diagnosis.[74]

Family studies of alcohol and drug dependence have consistently found elevated rates of ASPD in relatives.[75] The association between ASPD and problematic alcohol use is so close that alcoholism has often been considered to be a part of the syndrome or a complication of ASPD rather than being a distinct entity.[79,80] The ECA Study[4] reported an extremely high rate of 90% lifetime substance use disorders among prisoners diagnosed with ASPD.

Alcohol is often thought to be reinforcing for its ability to alter affective problems, and individuals with ASPD are, according to the "self-medication" approach, prone to experience relief by drinking. However, violent acts and impulsive aggression showed a high coincidence with alcohol use, and impulsive violence is often followed by high alcohol intake, not vice versa.

On the basis of adoption studies, evidence was found for an independent genetic inheritance of alcoholism and ASPD.[78] Cloninger[79,80] suggested that at least two more homogeneous subforms of alcoholism exist. Analysis of records on 862 men and 93 women born in Stockholm between 1930 and 1949, of known paternity and adopted by nonrelatives at an early age, revealed two patterns of alcohol abuse. Type 1 alcoholics, characterized by later onset of alcohol-related difficulties, guilt over drinking, alcoholic liver disease, and loss of control over drinking, tended to have alcohol abuse, but not criminality, in their biological parents. Prolonged hospitalization prior to adoption and low socioeconomic status in the adoptive parents appeared to be risk indicators for severity. Without such exacerbating factors, course of illness tended to be mild. Daughters of biological fathers with Type 1 background tended to have an increase in alcohol abuse, but not criminality or other psychiatric disorders.

Characteristics of Type 2 alcoholics, which showed a significant overlap with ASPD, include early onset of alcohol problems, fighting while intoxicated, troubles while drinking, and inability to abstain from alcohol. Their biological fathers tended to have a background of both treatment for alcoholism and significant criminality. Mothers had no excess of either. Regardless of postnatal environment, their adopted-away sons had a ninefold increase in risk of alcohol abuse, yielding an estimate of 90% heritability of this form of alcohol abuse in men. Unlike the daughters of Type 1 men, daughters of Type 2 men showed no increase in either alcohol abuse or criminality, but did have a significant increase in somatoform disorders.

Thus, both alcoholism and ASPD have a protracted and insidious onset, with behavioral antecedents, appearing in childhood and adolescence,[68] and their relationship is not yet fully clarified.

SCHIZOPHRENIA AND ALCOHOLISM

Clinical[66,67] and epidemiomologic[4,101] investigations have shown a high coincidence of alcoholism and substance abuse in patients with schizophrenia.

However, alcohol abuse and alcoholism may themselves elicit psychotic symptoms, as they occur in alcohol delirium and alcohol hallucinosis. While these alcohol-induced disorders and schizophrenia show a very similar psychopathological profile, they are sometimes difficult to differentiate from schizophrenia because chronic courses of alcohol-induced hallucinosis similar to schizophrenia have been reported.[62]

Twin studies[102] showed that both disorders are more common in monozygotic twins (MZ) than in dizygotic twins (DZ), suggesting that individuals suffering from schizophrenia and alcoholism have a genetic predisposition to both disorders, which is of the same nature as that which causes the disorders when they occur alone. In this study's twins, the diagnoses of schizophrenia and alcoholism were uncorrelated, supporting the hypothesis that the specific environmental and heriditary factors of causal importance in the two disorders are not closely related.

The hypothesis regarding the role played by genes and environment in individuals suffering from both disorders are similar to alcoholism comorbid cases in depression and most of the anxiety disorders. Individuals suffering from both have only a genetic predisposition to schizophrenia, and alcoholism would be viewed as developing in certain schizophrenics for reasons unrelated to the individual's genotype. For environmental reasons, some schizophrenics may learn to abuse alcohol to reduce the anxiety associated with their psychotic symptoms. The second hypothesis is that individuals suffering from both schizophrenia and alcoholism have a genetic predisposition only to alcoholism. Schizophrenia would then be viewed as having developed for environmental reasons in a subgroup of alcoholics, which is very unlikely.

However, the impact of alcohol use and abuse on the course and prognosis of schizophrenia is ambiguous.[61] One group of researchers reported positive and beneficial effects, others an earlier onset and more positive symptoms in schizophrenics with alcohol abuse or alcoholism.[63]

Thus, schizophrenia has a very low prevalence in the common population (about 0.5 to 1%)[101] compared to the prevalence of alcoholism (up to 14%)[101] in common population. Schizophrenia among alcoholics is very rare, whereas alcoholism among schizophrenia patients shows a high incidence.

EPIDEMIOLOGY

Alcohol is the most abused substance in schizophrenics, even if some researchers also reported a high prevalence of stimulant use and abuse among these patients.[63]

Very few studies reported systematic research on the comorbidity of schizophrenia and alcoholism. In 150 inpatient schizophrenics, 22% were found to be alcoholics.[65] Higher rates were reported from a schizophrenic sample of 149 patients showing a rate of 33% alcohol abuse and alcoholism.[64] In a 1975 review article,[32] rates of 3 to 63% of schizophrenic patients were reported to be alcoholic.

Recent research of several groups reported prevalence rates for alcoholism in schizophrenic samples between 12 and 43%.[62]

Larger German samples of 447 and 183 schizophrenic inpatients in Munich revealed an alcoholism lifetime prevalence of 35 and 18%, respectively.[66,67] Patients with first psychotic episodes showed a comorbidity of more than 69%. Alcoholism was antecedent in over 80% of the patients.[67]

A number of studies analyzed the frequency of alcohol use disorders in different samples of schizophrenics. In two U.S. samples, between 20 and 48% of the patients had alcohol or substance abuse disorders.[86,87] Similar rates were found in a German sample. Between 12 and 24% of the patients with schizophrenia showed alcohol abuse disorders.[88]

The ECA study[4] reported an odds ratio of more than 4 for schizophrenics suffering from alcoholism, compared to healthy controls and patients with major depression. A community sample study of 2144 persons revealed 20 persons diagnosed as schizophrenics. Alcoholism was present in more than 61% of these patients.[88]

SUICIDAL BEHAVIOR AND ALCOHOLISM

Like alcoholism, suicide risk also runs in families.[94] High mortality rates in alcoholics are not only caused by somatic disorders following high alcohol intake; a high suicide rate is also observed in alcoholics. Lifetime risk for suicide in alcoholics was reported to be 11 to 15%[73] compared to 3% in the general population.[103] Thus, alcoholics have a 60 to 120 times higher risk of suicide than normal control and may contribute to 25% of all suicides. Parasuicidal attempts are noted to be more common among alcoholics than committed suicides.[27]

The association between alcohol consumption and suicide has been investigated in 13 nations (2 from America, 10 from Europe, and 1 from Australia/Pacific Ocean).[89] The results showed that in 9 out of 13 of these nations, increased alcohol consumption is related to higher rates of suicide and homicide.

In the U.S., suicide rates were specifically associated with sales of spirits, age composition per capita land area, unemployment, and religious preferences over time. Whereas the suicide rate increased significantly as a function of increased spirit sales, beer and wine sales were not associated with suicide rates. The effect of spirit sales remained significant in the presence of correlated effects with regard to possible covariates like age, gender, ethnic group distributions, population pressure, economic measures, and measures of religious participation.[90]

SUBSTANCE ABUSE AND SMOKING

Alcoholism and substance abuse frequently coexist. Several studies reported rates of substance abuse among alcoholics between 20 and 40%[9,14] compared to 1 to 2% in general population samples.[102]

The COGA study[35,69] investigated 1212 alcoholics and 2755 siblings for marijuana and cocaine consumption as well as smoking. Alcohol, marijuana, nicotine, and cocaine use were found to be elevated in families of alcoholics. There is evidence that both common and specific addictive factors are transmitted in these families.[77] In a study of 3372 twin pairs, evidence for a shared vulnerability factor that underlies the abuse of several sedatives stimulants and other substance groups[82] was found. Conversely, increased rates of alcohol dependence were also found in relatives of opiate dependants.[70]

In the aforementioned National Comorbidity Survey,[11] substance abuse disorders, conduct disorders, and antisocial personality disorders were reported to account for the majority of lifetime concurrent psychiatric disorders among men.

NICOTINE

The close association of nicotine addiction and alcoholism is well established. As many as 80% of alcoholics smoke and up to 30% of smokers are reported to be alcohol abusers or alcoholics,[99] compared to about 26% smokers in a normal German population.[72] Only recently has attention been focused on the role of tobacco in abstinent alcoholics. Both disorders are reported to have high mortality rates. In a retrospective study of 85 treated alcoholics, the cause of mortality, as determined from death certificates from 1972 to 1983, revealed that nonsmoking alcoholics had a risk of dying three times higher and in smoking alcoholics over four times higher than that of the nonalcoholic, nonsmoking controls.[98]

COMMENT ON IMPORTANT ALCOHOL TYPOLOGIES AND COMORBIDITY

A vast number of alcohol typologies have been developed over the past 150 years. Various factors were used to distinguish between different alcoholic subgroups, including personality characteristics and coexisting psychiatric disorders aside from gender and alcohol consumption patterns.[79,104,105]

Along with more descriptive therapies[104] that did not significantly recognize psychiatric comorbidity among alcoholics, two newer typology concepts were pubished in the last 2 decades — named after Cloninger[79] and Babor[106] — which made psychiatric comorbidity an integral part of their theories.

Cloninger's typology identified two subtypes from a study of alcoholism and other relevant characteristics in a large number of Swedish adoptees and their biological and adoptive parents. This typology was recently replicated.[107]

Type I alcoholics are suggested to show a later onset of alcohol problems, develop psychological rather than physical dependence, and report feelings of guilt and depression about their alcohol use. Type II (male-limited) alcoholics, which manifest alcohol problems at an early age, exhibit spontaneous alcohol-seeking behavior and are socially disruptive when drinking. Heritable personality characteristics such as antisocial traits are suggested to be an integrative part of this alcoholic subgroup.

Babor's typology[106] is based on the assumption that the heterogeneity among alcoholics is attributable to a complex interaction between genetic, biological, psychological, and sociocultural factors. Hence, 17 factors — including age of onset, severity of dependence, and family history of alcoholism — were included to characterize two subtypes using statistical cluster analysis techniques.

One subgroup, designated as type A alcoholics, was characterized by later onset of alcoholism, fewer childhood risk factors (such as attention deficit hyperactivity disorder, ADHD), less severe alcohol dependence, fewer alcohol-related problems, and less intensive psychiatric problems. The other subgroup, called type B alcoholics, showed more childhood risk factors, a family history of alcoholism, early onset of alcohol-related problems, greater severity of dependence, and multiple drug abuse.

However, the usefulness of these typologies in clinical practice with alcoholic in- and outpatients has been questioned.[108]

The variety and manifestation of alcoholism are very heterogenous, but they were reduced into two broad groups in both typologies mentioned above. In clinical practice, several studies could not subgroup a significant number of alcoholics using Cloninger's criteria.[109-112] Evidence for at least a possible third type of alcoholism was raised from research on alcoholic twins.[110]

In two recent studies of alcoholics in Australia and Spain,[111,112] the investigators failed to classify these alcoholics and problem drinkers according to Cloninger's criteria. In the first of these, Cloninger's typology did not predict gender differences in symptoms of alcohol dependence, family history, or personality.[111]

One of the major objections to Cloninger's typology was found in a study with sons of alcoholic fathers.[113] The results did not support any consistent trend in the correlation between the fathers' alcoholic characteristics and the sons' problem picture, which was expected to be higher in sons of type II alcoholics. It was concluded that type II alcoholics might represent a separate diagnostic entity — the antisocial personality disorder — and not alcoholism itself.

The hypothesis that type II alcoholics are more likely to have primary antisocial personality disorder was recently supported.[112]

Better evaluations were found with Babor's classification of alcoholics. Initially, Babor focused on subtyping inpatient alcoholics and found equal numbers of patients classified as type A and B. Two subsequent investigations[114,115] applied this typology to their samples and reported a higher number of type A alcoholics. The number of subgrouping criteria was reduced from 17 to 5. Thus, this typology may be more useful for subtyping inpatient and outpatient samples of alcoholics on a theoretical basis and also with regard to comorbidity. However, it remains difficult to subgroup alcoholics according to these criteria and there is a large overlap between Cloninger's type I/II and Babor's type A/B. The Babor typology was also used in clinical trials comparing psychotherapeutical and pharmacotherapeutical treatment strategies and may have prognostic importance.[116,117]

So, for clinical practitioners and researchers, the typology suggested by Babor et al. may be more useful to subgroup alcoholics with regard to comorbidity and treatment prognosis. First, it was evaluated in a prospective and longitudinal trial of inpatient and outpatient alcoholics; and second, compared to the Cloninger typology, it showed more positive results in subtyping alcoholics in subgroups also with regard to comorbidity.

However, even Babor's multidimension-based typology might be too narrow because it may not show sufficient therapeutic strategies for, for example, type B alcoholics, and it does not include important biological dimensions, such as a profile of candidate genes, neurotransmitter systems, or physiological reactivity, as suggested by Cloninger.[79]

Thus, the question for a more comprehensive typology for alcoholics with regard to comorbidity still remains open.

CONCLUSION

Despite the reported high prevalence rates of several psychiatric disorders and alcoholism, their interrelationships are not yet very clear. Several hypotheses were proposed to clarify these relationships of comorbidity.

The "self-medication" hypothesis, in which alcohol and drug use are motivated by and dependent on another condition or state, and that alcoholism is not the primary or independent condition, is contradicted by most experimental and clinical studies: depression or anxiety in alcoholics is often elicited through alcoholism itself or it precedes these disorders. While subclinically anxious and depressive syndromes may be relieved through alcohol, this may happen as an acute alcohol effect. However, these symptoms are intensified during a longer period of drinking, repeated withdrawal, and may result in clinical symptomatology and inpatient treatment as a consequence.

If alcoholism and other psychiatric disorders were dependent on each other or have a major common etiological factor, it would be expected that two comorbid disorders show a genetic and familial relationship, and that alcoholism be part of the spectrum of depression, anxiety, schizophrenia, and other diseases.

However, most of adoption, twin, and high-risk studies reported alcohol abuse and alcoholism to be mainly genetically independent of other psychiatric disorders (e.g., eating disorders, depression, or schizophrenia).

The primary vs. secondary disease scheme remains descriptive and has little to contribute to clarification of the relationships among comorbid diseases.

Research methodology used in studies about comorbidity showed large variability and may contribute to the very different numbers and percentages of comorbidity rates reported in the literature on this field. Furthermore, several studies, especially the older ones, did not use common classification schemes or unbiased samples. Epidemiological data were influenced by many factors, such as population sample selected, method or design employed, biases of the examiners, length of the study, and treatment intervention, especially in clinical samples.

Other reasons for the different results in comorbidity research include the different study approaches and samples investigated. For example, cross-sectional designs are likely to inflate rates of psychiatric comorbidity in alcoholics, for example, through overlapping diagnostic criteria in DSM-IV Axis II diagnosis. Clinical populations mostly yield much higher comorbidity rates than the general population, inpatient treatments higher rates than outpatient, public investigations higher than private samples.[98]

Thus, more efforts are needed to unify research methods in epidemiological, outpatient, and clinical samples, as already suggested by the COGA study group. These efforts may contribute to further clarification of the relationship and differences between comorbid alcoholism and psychiatric disorders.

REFERENCES

1. Feinstein, A.R., The pre-therapeutic classification of comorbidity in chronic disease, *J. Chronic Dis.,* 23, 455, 1970.
2. George, D.T., Nutt, D.J., Dwyer, B.A., and Linnoila, M., Alcoholism and panic disorder: is the comorbidity more than coincidence? *Acta Psychiatr. Scand.,* 91, 97, 1990.
3. Kushner, M.G., Sher, K.J., and Breitman, B.D., The relationship between alcohol problems and the anxiety disorders, *Am. J. Psychiatry,* 147, 685, 1990.
4. Regier, D.A., Farmer, M.E., Rae, D.S., Locke, B.Z., Keith, S.J., Judd, L.L., and Goodwin, F.K., Comorbidity of mental disorders with alcohol and other drug abuse: results from the Epidemiologic Catchment Area (ECA) study, *JAMA,* 264, 2511, 1990.
5. Maier, W., Minges, J., and Lichtermann, D., Alcoholism and panic disorder: co-occurrence and co-transmission in families, *Eur. Arch. Psychiatry Clin. Neurosci.,* 243, 205, 1993.
6. Conger, J.J., Alcoholism: theory problem and challenge. II. Reinforcement theory and the dynamics of alcoholism, *Q. J. Stud. Alcohol,* 13, 296, 1956.
7. Kalodner, C.R., Delucia, J.L., and Ursprung, A.W., An examination of the tension reduction hypothesis: the relationship between anxiety and alcohol in college students, *Addict. Behav.,* 14, 649, 1989.
8. Soyka, M., *Alkoholismus: Eine Krankheit und ihre Therapie,* Wissenschaftliche Verlagsgesellschaft, Stuttgart, 1997.
9. Merikangas, K.R., Leckman, J.F., Prusoff, B.A., Pauls, D.L., and Weissman, M.M., Familial transmission of depression and alcoholism, *Arch. Gen. Psychiatry,* 42, 367, 1985.
10. Merikangas, K.R., Risch, N.J., and Weissman, M.M., Comorbidity and co-transmission of alcoholism, anxiety and depression, *Psychol. Med.,* 24, 69, 1992.
11. Kessler, R.C., Crum, R.M., Warner, L.A., Nelson, C.B., Schulenberg, J., and Anthony, J.C., Lifetime co-occurrence of DSM–III-R alcohol abuse and dependence with other psychiatric disorders in the national comorbidity survey, *Arch. Gen. Psychiatry,* 54, 313, 1997.
12. Merikangas, K.R. and Gelernter, C.S., Comorbidity for alcoholism and depression, *Psychiatr. Clin. North. Am.,* 13, 613, 1990.
13. Maier, W., Lichtermann, D., Minges, J., Delmo, C., and Heun, R., The relationship between bipolar disorder and alcoholism: a controlled family study, *Psycholog. Med.,* 24, 787, 1995.
14. Cox, B.J., Norton, G.R., Swinson, R.P., and Endler, N.S., Substance abuse and panic related anxiety: a critical review, *Behav. Res. Ther.,* 28, 385, 1990.
15. Mullan, M.J., Gurling, H.M.D., Oppenheim, B.E., and Murray, R.M., The relationship between alcoholism and neurosis: evidence from a twin study, *Br. J. Psychiatry,* 148, 435, 1986.
16. Cowley, D.S., Alcohol abuse, substance abuse and panic disorders, *Am. J. Med.* (Suppl. 1A), 41, 1992.
17. Smail, P., Stockwell, T., Canter, S., and Hodgson, R., Alcohol dependence and phobic anxiety states I. A prevalence study, *Br. J. Psychiatry,* 144, 53, 1984.
18. Stockwell, T., Smail, P., Hodgson, R., and Canter, S., Alcohol dependence and phobic anxiety states. II. A retrospective study, *Br. J. Psychiatry,* 144, 58, 1984.
19. Merikangas, K.R., Risch, N.J., and Weissman, M.M., Comorbidity and co-transmission of alcoholism, anxiety and depression, *Psycholog. Med.,* 24, 69, 1994.
20. Boyd, J.H., Burke, J.D., Gruenberg, E., Holzer, C.E., Rae, D.S., George, L.K., Karno, M., Stolzman, R., McEvoy, L., and Nestadt, G., Exclusion criteria of DSM-III: a study of co-occurrence of hierarchy-free syndromes, *Arch. Gen. Psychiatry,* 41, 983, 1984.
21. Cadoret, R.J. and Winokur, G., Depression in alcoholism, *Ann. N.Y. Acad. Sci.,* 233, 34, 1974.
22. Schuckit, M.A., Alcoholic patients with secondary depression, *Am. J. Psychiatry,* 140, 711, 1983.
23. Murphy, G.E. and Wetzel, R.D., The lifetime risk of suicide in alcoholism, *Arch. Gen. Psychiatry,* 47, 383, 1990.

24. Guze, S.B., Cloninger, C.R., Martin, R., and Clayton, P.J., Alcoholism as a medical disorder, *Compr. Psychiatry*, 27, 501, 1986.

25. Yates, W., Petty, F., and Brown, K., Factors associated with depression among primary alcoholics, *Compr. Psychiatry*, 29, 28, 1988.

26. Hensel, B., Dunner, D.L., and Fieve, R.R., the relationship of family history of alcoholism to primary affective disorder, *J. Affect. Disord.*, 1, 105, 1990.

27. Merrill, J., Milner, G., Owens, J., and Vale, A., Alcohol and attempted suicide, *Br. J. Addict.*, 87, 83, 1992.

28. Winokur, G., The development and validity of familial subtypes in primary unipolar depression, *Pharmacopsychiatry*, 15, 142, 1982.

29. O'Sullivan, Whillans, P., Daly, M., Carroll, B., Clare, A., and Cooney, J., A comparison of alcoholics with and without coexisting affective disorder, *Br. J. Psychiatry*, 143, 133, 1983.

30. Penick, E.C., Powell, B.J., Othmer, E., Bingham, S.F., Rice, A.S., and Liese, B.S., Subtyping alcoholics by coexisting psychiatric syndromes: course, family history, outcome, *Long. Res. Alcoholism*, 167, 196, 1984.

31. Coryell, W., Winokur, G., Keller, M., Scheftner, W., and Endicott, J., Alcoholism and prime major depression: a family study approach to co-existing disorders, *J. Affect. Disorders*, 24, 93, 1992.

32. Freed, E.X., Alcoholism and schizophrenia: the search for perspectives, *J. Stud. Alcohol*, 36, 853, 1975.

33. Alterman, A.I., Ayre, F.R., and Williford, W.O., Diagnostic validation of conjoint schizophrenia and alcoholism, *J. Clin. Psychiatry*, 45, 300, 1984.

34. Chutuape, M.A.D. and DeWit, H., Preferences for ethanol and diazepam in anxious individuals: an evaluation of the self-medication hypothesis, *Psychopharmacology*, 121, 91, 1995.

35. Schuckit, M.A., Tipp, J.E., Bucholz, K.K., Nurnberger, J.I., Hesselborck, V.M., Crowe, R.R., and Kramer, J., The life-time rates of three major mood disorders and four major anxiety disorders in alcoholic and controls, *Addiction*, 92, 1289, 1997.

36. Kessler, R.C., McGonagle, K.A., Zhao, S., Nelson, C.B., Hughes, M., Eshleman, S., Wittchen, H.U., and Kendler, K.S., Lifetime and 12-month prevalence of DSM-III-R psychiatric disorders in the United States. Results from the National Comorbidity Survey, *Arch. Gen. Psychiatry*, 51, 8, 1994.

37. Kessler, R.C., Nelson, C.B., McGonagle, K.A., Edlund, M.J., Frank, R.G., and Leaf, P.J., The epidemiology of co-occurring addictive and mental disorders: implications from prevention and service utilization, *Am. J. Orthopsychiatry*, 66, 17, 1996.

38. Grant, B.F., Comorbidity between DSM IV alcohol use disorders and major depression: results of a national survey of adults, *J. Subst. Abuse*, 7, 481, 1995.

39. Winokur, G., Coryell, W., Akiskal, H.S., Maser, J.D., Keller, M.B., Endicott, J., and Mueller, T., Alcoholism in manic-depressive (bipolar) illness: familial illness, course of illness, and the primary-secondary distinction, *Am. J. Psychiatry*, 152(3), 365, 1995.

40. Powell, B.J., Penick, E.C., Othmer, E., Bingham, S.F., and Rice, A.S., Prevalence of additional psychiatric syndromes among male alcoholics, *J. Clin. Psychiatry*, 43, 404, 1982.

41. Galbaud Du Fort, G., Newman, S.C., and Bland, R.C., Psychiatric comorbidity and treatment seeking. Sources of selection bias in the study of clinical populations, *J. Nerv. Mental Dis.*, 181, 468, 1993.

42. Brown, S.A. and Schuckit, M.A., Changes in depression among abstinent alcoholics, *J. Stud. Alcohol*, 49, 412, 1988.

43. Schuckit, M.A., The clinical implications of primary diagnostic groups among alcoholics, *Arch. Gen. Psychiatry*, 42, 1043, 1985.

44. Hesselbrock, M.N., Hesselbrock, V.M., Tennen, H., Meyer, R.E., and Workman, K.L., Methodological considerations in the assessment of depression in alcoholics, *J. Cons. Clin. Psychol.*, 51, 399, 1983.

45. Hesselbrock, V.M., Family history of psychopathology in alcoholics: a review and issues, Meyer, R.E., Ed., *Psychopathology and Addictive Disorders*, Guilford Press, New York, 1986, 41.

46. Howed, M.J. and Hokanson, J.E., Conversational and social responses to depressive interpersonal behavior, *J. Abnorm. Psychol.*, 88, 625, 1979.

47. Hatsukami, D. and Pickens, R.W., Posttreatment depression in an alcohol and drug abuse population, *Am. J. Psychiatry*, 139, 1563, 1982.

48. Schuckit, M.A. and Monteiro, M.G., Alcoholism, anxiety and depression, *Br. J. Addict.*, 83, 1373, 1988.

49. Bland, R.C., Newman, S.C., and Orn, H., Schizophrenia: lifetime comorbidity in a community sample, *Acta Psychiatr. Scand.,* 75, 383, 1987.

50. Alling, C., Balldin, J., Bokstroem, K., Gottfries, C.G., Karlsson, I., and Langstrom, G., Studies on duration of a late recovery period after chronic abuse of ethanol, *Acta Psychiatr. Scand.,* 66, 384, 1982.

51. Bibb, J.L. and Chambliss, D.L., Alcohol use and abuse among diagnosed agoraphobics, *Behav. Res. Therapy,* 24, 49, 1986.

52. Schatzberg, A.F., Bipolar disorder: recent issues in diagnosis and classification, *J. Clin. Psychiatry,* 59 (Suppl. 6), 5, 1998.

53. Chilcoat, D.H. and Breslau, N., Posttraumatic stress disorder and drug disorder, *Arch. Gen. Psychiatry,* 55, 913, 1998.

54. Schuckit, M.A., Tipp, J.E., Anthenelli, R.M., Bucholz, K.K., Hesselbrock, V.M., and Nurnberger, J.I., Anorexia nervosa and bulimia nervosa in alcohol-dependent men and women and their relatives, *Am. J. Psychiatry,* 153, 74, 1996.

55. Bulik, C.M., Drug and alcohol abuse by bulimic women and their families, *Am. J. Psychiatry,* 144, 1604, 1987.

56. Newman, M.M. and Gold, M.S., Preliminary findings of patterns of substance abuse in eating disorder patients, *Am. J. Drug Alcohol Abuse,* 18, 207, 1992.

57. Henzel, H.A., Diagnosing alcoholism in patients with anorexia nervosa, *Am. J. Drug Alcohol Abuse,* 10, 461, 1984.

58. Eckert, E.D., Goldberg, S.C., Halmi, K.A., Casper, R.C., and Davis, J., Depression in anorexia nervosa, *Psychol. Med.,* 12, 115, 1982.

59. Hudson, J.I., Weiss, R.D., and Pope, H.G., Jr., Eating disorders in hospitalized substance abusers, *Am. J. Drug Alcohol Abuse,* 18, 75, 1992.

60. Maier, W. and Merikangas, K., Co-occurrence and cotransmission of affective disorders and alcoholism in families, *Br. J. Psychiatry,* 168 (Suppl. 30), 93, 1996.

61. Strakowski, S.M., Keck, P.E., McElroy, S.L., Lonczak, H.S., and West, S.A., Chronology of comorbid and principal syndromes in first-episode psychosis, *Compr. Psychiatry,* 36, 106, 1995.

62. Hambrecht, M. and Haefner, H., Fuehren Alkohol – oder Drogenmissbrauch zu Schizophrenie, *Nervenarzt* 67, 36, 1996.

63. Raskin, V.D. and Miller, N.S., The epidemiology of the comorbidity of psychiatric and addictive disorders: a critical review, *J. Addict. Dis.,* 12, 45, 1993.

64. Parker, J.B., Meiller, R.M., and Andrews, G.W., Major psychiatric disorders masquerading as alcoholism, *South. Med. J.,* 53, 560, 1960.

65. Mueser, K.T., Yarnold, P.R., Levinson, D.F., Singh, H., Bellack, A.S., Kee, K., Morrison, R.L., Yadalam, K.G., Prevalence of substance abuse in schizophrenia: demographic and clinical correlates, *Schizophrenia Bull.,* 166, 31, 1990.

66. Soyka, M., Albus, M., Finelli, A., Hofstetter, M., Holzbach, R., Immler, B., Kathmann, N., and Sand, P., Prevalence of alcohol and drug abuse in schizophrenic inpatients, *Eur. Arch. Psychiatry Clin. Neurosci.,* 242, 362, 1993.

67. Soyka, M., Albus, M., and Kathmann, N., Praevalenz von Suchterkrankungen bei schizophrenen Patienten – Erste Ergebnisse einer Studie an 447 stationaeren Patienten eines großstadtnahen psychiatrischen Bezirkskrankenhauses, Schon, D.R., Krausz, M., Eds., *Psychose und Sucht. Krankheitsmodelle, Verbreitung, therapeutische Ansaetze,* Lambertus, Freiburg, 1992, 59.

68. Sher, K.J. and Trull, T.J., Personality and disinhibitory psychopathology: alcoholism and antisocial personality disorder, *J. Abnorm. Psychol.,* 103, 92, 1994.

69. Bierut, L.J., Dinwiddie, S.H., Begleiter, H., Crowe, R.R., Hesselbrock, V.M., Nurnberger, J.I., Porjesz, B., Schuckit, M.A., and Reich, T., Familial transmission of substance dependence: alcohol, marijuana, cocaine and habitual smoking, *Arch. Gen. Psychiatry,* 55, 982, 1998.

70. Rounsaville, B.J., Kosten, T.R., Weissman, M.M., Prosoff, B., Puals, D., Anton, S.F., and Merikangas, K., Psychiatric disorders in relatives of probands with opiate addiction, *Arch. Gen. Psychiatry,* 48, 33, 1991.

71. Schuckit, M.A., Tipp, J.E., Bergman, M., Reich, T., Hesselbrock, V., and Smith, T.L., A comparison of induced and independent major depressive in 2,945 alcoholics, *Am. J. Psychiatry,* 154, 948, 1997.

72. World Health Organization, *Tobacco or Health: A Global Status Report,* WHO, Geneva, 1997.

73. Driessen, M., Veltrup, C., Wetterling, T., John, U., and Dilling, H., Axis I and axis II comorbidity in alcohol dependence and the two types of alcoholism, *Alcohol. Clin. Exp. Res.*, 22, 77, 1998.

74. Hesselbrock, M., Meyer, R.E., and Keener, J.J., Psychopathology in hospitalized alcoholics, *Arch. Gen. Psychiatry*, 42, 1050, 1985.

75. Cadoret, R.J., O'Gorman, T.W., Troughton, E., and Heywood, E., Alcoholism and antisocial personality disorder, *Arch. Gen. Psychiatry*, 42, 161, 1985.

76. Hesselbrock, M., Gender comparison of antisocial personality disorder and depression in alcoholism, *J. Subst. Abuse*, 3, 205, 1991.

77. Dinwiddie, S.H. and Reich, T., Genetic and family studies in psychiatric illness and alcohol and drug dependence, *J. Addict. Dis.*, 12, 17, 1993.

78. Cadoret, R.J., Troughton, E., and O'Gorman, T.W., Genetic and environmental factors in alcohol abuse and antisocial personality, *J. Stud. Alcohol*, 48, 1, 1987.

79. Cloninger, C.R., Bohman, M., and Sigvardsson, S., Inheritance of alcohol abuse: cross-fostering analysis of adopted men, *Arch. Gen. Psychiatry*, 38, 861, 1981.

80. Cloninger, C.R., Bohman, M., Sigvardsson, S., and von Knorring, A.L., Psychopathology in adopted-out children of alcoholics. The Stockholm adoption study, *Recent Developments in Alcoholism*, Galanter, M., Ed., 1985, 37.

81. Merikangas, K.R., Stevens, D.E., Fenton, M., Stolar, M., O'Malley, S., Woods, S.W., and Risch, N., Co-morbidity and familial aggregation of alcoholism and anxiety disorders, *Psych. Med.*, 28, 773, 1998.

82. Tsuang, M.T., Lyons, M.J., Meyer, J.M., Doyle, T., Eisen, S.A., Goldberg, J., True, W., Lin, N., Toomey, R., and Eaves, L., Co-occurrence of abuse of different drugs in men: the role of drug-specific and shared vulnerabilities, *Arch. Gen. Psychiatry*, 55, 967, 1998.

83. Lilenfeld, L.R., Kaye, W.H., Greeno, C.G., Merikangas, K.R., Plotnicov, K., Pollice, C., Rao, R., Strober, M., Bulik, C.M., and Nagy, L., Psychiatric disorders in women with bulimia nervosa and their first degree relatives: effects of comorbid substance dependence, *Int. J. Eat. Disord.*, 22, 253, 1997.

84. Kendler, K.S., Walters, E.E., Neale, M.C., Kessler, R.C., Health, A.C., and Eaves, L.J., The structure of the genetic and environmental risk factors for six major psychiatric disorders in women, *Arch. Gen. Psychiatry*, 52, 374, 1995.

85. Kaye, W.H., Lilenfeld, L.R., Plotnicov, K., Merikangas, K.R., Nagy, L., Strober, M., Bulik, C.M., Moss, H., and Greeno, C.G., Bulimia nervosa and substance dependence: association and family transmission, *Alcohol. Clin. Exp. Res.*, 20, 878, 1996.

86. Bartels, S.J., Drake, R.E., and Wallach, M.A., Long-term course of substance use disorders among patients with severe mental illness, *Psychiatr. Serv.*, 46, 248, 1995.

87. DeQuardo, J.R., Carpenter, C.F., and Tandon, R., Patterns of substance abuse in schizophrenia: nature and significance, *J. Psychiatr. Res.*, 28, 267, 1994.

88. Soyka, M., Sucht und Schizophrenie: nosologische klinische und therapeutische Fragestellungen. 1. Alkoholismus und Schizophrenie, *Fortschr. Neurol. Psychiat.*, 62, 71, 1994.

89. Lester, D., The association between alcohol consumption and suicide and homicide rates: a study of 13 nations, *Alcohol Alcohol.*, 30, 465, 1995.

90. Gruenewald, P.J., Ponici, W.R., and Mithell, P.R., Suicide rates and alcohol consumption in the United States, 1970–89, *Addiction*, 90, 1063, 1995.

91. Holderness, C.C., Brooks-Gunn, J., and Warren, M.P., Co-morbidity of eating disorders and substance abuse: review of the literature, *Int. J. Eating Disord.*, 16, 1, 1994.

92. Garner, D.M. and Garfinkel, P.E., Social-cultural factors in the development of anorexia nervosa, *Psych. Med.*, 10, 647, 1980.

93. Kendler, K.S., MacLen, C., Neale, M., Kessler, R., Heath, A., and Eyves, L., The genetic epidemiology of bulimia nervosa, *Am. J. Psychiatry*, 142, 1627, 1991.

94. Roy, A., Rylander, G., and Sarchiapone, M., Genetic studies of suicidal behavior, *Psychiatr. Clin. North. Am.*, 20(3), 595, 1997.

95. Kofoed, L., Friedman, M.J., and Peck, R., Alcoholism and drug abuse in patients with PTSD, *Psychiatric Q.*, 64, 151, 1993.

96. Rounsaville, B.J., Dolinsky, Z.S., Babor, T.F., and Meyer, R.E., Psychopathology as a predictor of treatment outcome in alcoholics, *Arch. Gen. Psychiatry*, 44, 505, 1987.

97. Davidson, J.R., Kudler, H.S., Saunders, W.B., and Smith, R.D., Symptom and comorbidity patterns in World War II and Vietnam veterans with posttraumatic stress disorder, *Compr. Psychiatry,* 31, 162, 1990.

98. Miller, N.S. and Gold, M.S., Comorbid cigarette and alcohol addiction: epidemiology and treatment, *J. Addict. Dis.,* 17, 55, 1993.

99. Hurt, R.D., Offord, K.P., Croghan, I.T., Gomez-Dahl, L., Kottke, T.E., Mores, R.M., and Melton, L.J., Mortality following inpatient addiction treatment: role of tobacco use in a community-based cohort, *JAMA,* 275(14), 1097, 1996.

100. Helzer, J.E. and Przybeck, T.R., The co-occurrence of alcoholism with other psychiatric disorders in the general population and its impact on treatment, *J. Stud. Alcohol,* 49, 219, 1988.

101. Fichter, M.M., Narrow, W.E., Roper, M.T., Rehm, J., Elton, E., Rae, D.S., Locke, B.Z., and Regier, D.A., Prevalence of mental illness in Germany and the United States, *J. Nerv. Ment. Dis.,* 184, 598, 1996.

102. Kendler, K.S., A twin study of individuals with both schizophrenia and alcoholism, *Br. J. Psychiatry,* 147, 48, 1985.

103. Moscicki, E.K., O'Carroll, P., Rae, D.S., Locke, B.Z., Roy, A., and Regier, D.A., Suicide attempts in the Epidemiologic Catchment Area Study, *Yale J. Biol. Med.,* 61, 259, 1988.

104. Jellinek, E.M., Alcoholism: a genus and some of its species, *Can. Med. Assoc. J.,* 93, 1341, 1960.

105. Del Boca, F.K., Sex gender and alcoholic typologies, *Types of alcoholics: Evidence from Clinical, Experimental and Genetic Research,* Babor, T.F., Hesselbrock, V., Meyer, R., and Shoemaker, W., Eds., Annals of the New York Academy of Sciences, New York, 1994.

106. Babor, T.F., Hofman, M., Del Boca, F., Hesselbrock, V., Meyer, R., Dolinsky, Z., and Rounsaville, B., Types of alcoholics. I: Evidencefor an empirically derived typology based on indicators of vulnerability and severity, *Arch. Gen. Psychiatry,* 49, 599, 1992.

107. Sigvardsson, S., Bohman, M., Cloninger, C.R., Replication of the Stockholm adoption study of alcoholism. Confirmatory cross-fostering analysis, *Arch. Gen. Psychiatry,* 53, 681, 1996.

108. Babor, T.F., The classification of alcoholics. *Alcohol Health Res. World,* 20, 6, 1996.

109. Glenn, S.W. and Nixon, S.J., Investigation of Cloninger's subtypes in a male alcoholic sample: applications and implications, *J. Clin. Psychol.,* 52, 219, 1996.

110. Penick, E.C., Powell, B.J., Nickel, E.J., Read, M.R., Gabrielli, W.F., Liskow, B.I., Examination of Cloninger's type I and type II alcoholism with a sample of men alcoholics in treatment, *Alcohol. Clin. Exp. Res.,* 14, 623, 1990.

111. Rubio, G., Leon, G., Pascual, F.F., Santo-Domingo, J., Clinical significance of Cloninger's classification in a sample of alcoholic Spanish men, *Addiction,* 93, 93, 1998.

112. Sannibale, C. and Hall, W., An evaluation of Cloninger's typology of alcohol abuse, *Addiction,* 93, 1241, 1998.

113. Schuckit, M.A. and Irwin, M., An analysis of the clinical relevance of type 1 and type 2 alcoholics, *Br. J. Addict.,* 84, 869, 1989.

114. Schuckit, M.A., Tipp, J.E., Smith, T.L., Shapiro, E., Hesselbrock, V.M., Bucholz, K.K., Reich, T., and Nurnberger, J.I., An evaluation of type A and B alcoholics, *Addiction,* 90, 1189, 1995.

115. Brown, J., Babor, T.F., Litt, M.D., and Kranzler, H.R., The type A/type B distinction: Subtyping alcoholics according to indicators of vulnerability and severity, *Types of Alcoholics: Evidence from Clinical, Experimental and Genetic Research,* Babor, T.F., Hesselbrock, V.M., Meyer, R., and Shoemaker, W., Eds., Annals of the New York Academy of Sciences, New York, 1994.

116. Litt, M.D., Babor, T.F., Del Boca, F.K., Kadden, R.M., Cooney, N.L., Types of alcoholics. II. Application of an empirically derived typology to treatment matching, *Arch. Gen. Psychiatry,* 49, 609, 1992.

117. Kranzler, H.R., Burleson, J.A., Brown, J., and Babor, T.F., Fluoxetine treatment seems to reduce the beneficial effects of cognitive-behavioral therapy in type B alcoholics, *Alcohol Clin. Exp. Res.* 20, 1534, 1996.

27 Heritability

Suchitra Krishnan-Sarin

OVERVIEW

Family and twin studies provide strong evidence to support genetic transmission of alcoholism, but also indicate an equally important role for shared environment. Further examination of the role of genetics and shared environment in mediating initiation, maintenance, and relapse to alcohol drinking suggests that while drinking patterns may be genetically determined, an individual's ability to quit may be mediated more by environmental factors. Evidence for familial transmission of alcoholism has prompted a number of investigations on physiological markers and specific genes that might mediate susceptibility to alcohol dependence and a number of candidates have been identified. However, alcoholism is a polygenic disease and confirming a role for these markers and genes in mediating vulnerability for alcoholism is a difficult task. Moreover, potential confounds produced by other disorders such as tobacco use and depression, which are highly comorbid with alcohol use, should not be disregarded. Nevertheless, the determination of specific genes and physiological correlates of alcoholism would significantly enhance our ability to develop improved treatments, and perhaps even prevent alcohol abuse/dependence disorders.

INTRODUCTION

Alcoholism is a genetically influenced disorder, the mode of inheritance of which involves multiple genes. Moreover, development of this disorder is believed to arise from a complex interplay of environmental and genetic factors. Over the past decade, a number of investigations have focused on identifying specific risk factors and genes involved in the development of alcohol abuse or dependence.

FAMILY AND TWIN/ADOPTION STUDIES

The idea that alcoholism may run in families was first suggested by a series of *family studies*.[1,2] A review of 39 family studies concluded that one in three alcoholics had at least one alcoholic parent and that rates of alcoholism were lower in non-alcoholic probands.[3] The degree of risk of developing alcoholism was found to be correlated with the frequency of (number of relatives), and the proximity (closeness of the relationship) of, relatives with the disorder. A more detailed review of only those family studies that had control subjects concluded a sevenfold higher risk of developing alcoholism in first-degree relatives of alcohol-dependent subjects.[4] While family studies suggest genetic transmission of alcoholism, they do not control for effects produced by shared environment or by cultural inheritance. A comparison of shared environment vs. genetic transmission is provided by adoption/twin studies.

Adoption studies examine alcohol abuse/dependence behavior in children who have been raised by unrelated adoptive parents and not by their biological parents. Adoption studies have the ability to separate genetic from environmental factors by examining behavior in biological parents, adoptive parents, as well as biologically unrelated siblings raised in the same environ-

0-8493-7801-X/00/$0.00+$.50
© 2000 by CRC Press LLC

ment and biologically related siblings raised in different environments. The far-reaching message from most adoption studies is that alcoholism is genetically transmitted. A number of studies have documented higher rates of alcoholism among adopted children born to alcoholic compared to non-alcoholic parents.[5-8] It has also been suggested that regardless of home environment, children whose biological parents have alcoholism have a 2.5-fold higher chance of becoming alcoholic.[4] Cloninger and colleagues analyzed data from a large Swedish adoptee sample and identified two separate types of inherited vulnerability to alcoholism: type I and type II.[7] Type I alcoholism, which has a stronger environmental influence, occurs in both men and women, develops after the age of 25, is associated with mild adult-onset alcoholism in a biological parent, and is often accompanied by feelings of guilt and fear about alcohol dependence. In contrast, type II alcoholism is more severe and influenced more by genetic rather than environmental factors, occurs primarily in males, develops early (before the age of 25), and is frequently characterized by aggression and spontaneous alcohol-seeking behavior. Additionally, Hill and colleagues have also proposed the existence of a third type of alcoholism that has a significant genetic component but which is without the antisocial behavior seen in Cloninger's type II alcoholics.[9]

Twin studies go a step beyond adoption studies and actually examine the parallelism of alcoholic behavior between pairs of genetically identical (monozygotic or MZ) vs. fraternal (dizygotic or DZ) twins. Twin studies are based on the premise that differences between DZ twins could be mediated either by genes or by environment, while differences between MZ twins are mediated only by environmental differences. This being the case, if a disorder is genetically mediated, then identical twins with shared environments should be more similar than fraternal twins with shared environments. Twin studies evaluate similarities between twin pairs using concordance rates, which are measures of the extent to which both members of a twin pair share a trait. For example, a concordance rate of 0.5 for a particular trait would indicate that in 50% of cases studied, both members of a twin pair expressed the trait.

To date, all the twin studies have emphasized a strong genetic component for this disorder.[10] Gender (male, female) and diagnosis (alcohol abuse vs. dependence) have also been shown to affect concordance rates, with twins meeting DSM-III criteria for either alcohol abuse, alcohol dependence, or both, evidencing slightly lower but not significantly different concordance rates for identical (0.76 for males and 0.36 for females) and fraternal (0.61 for males and 0.25 for females) pairs.[11] In contrast, meeting criteria for alcohol dependence only resulted in concordance rates that were significantly different between identical twins (0.59 for males and 0.25 for females) and fraternal twins (0.36 for males and 0.05 for females), indicating that genetic factors seem to play a more prominent role in the development of alcohol dependence. Significant heritability of alcoholism has also been found in an Australian female twin sample.[12]

Twin studies have also established a role for shared environment in vulnerability to alcoholism. A review of studies of alcohol use in the Finnish Twin Cohort, which controlled for gender differences by having same-sex adult twin pairs, found that while genetic factors significantly influenced alcohol use, twins in more frequent contact (i.e., with more shared environment) had greater similarities in alcohol use.[13] Clifford and colleagues also found a strong effect of shared environment (42%) and genetic factors (37%) in the development of this disorder.[14] An elegant analysis of data from adult Australian twins showed that factors that determined frequency and quantity of use were genetically based, while factors that mediated abstinence from alcohol were strongly influenced by shared environment.[15] Similar results were also reported in a U.S. sample of older twins such that lifetime abstinence from alcohol was influenced by both shared environmental factors (42%) and by genetic factors (40%), while frequency/quantity of alcohol use was primarily influenced by genetic factors.[16] A recent analysis of data from a sample of volunteer adult Australian twins, the majority of whom were mildly affected and did not meet DSM-IIIR criteria for alcohol dependence, reported that the ability of genetic vs. nonshared environmental factors to mediate the risk of becoming alcohol dependent was 2:1.[17]

More recently, Reed and coworkers compared and contrasted genetic vulnerability to alcoholism in MZ and DZ twins with susceptibility to two medical complications of alcoholism — liver cirrhosis and alcoholic psychosis — and found that shared factors accounted for almost 85% of the overall genetic risk to all three diseases.[18] The small amount of genetic risk not accounted for by shared factors was attributed to other genetic factors for cirrhosis and psychosis.

Twin/family designs have also examined the issue of cultural inheritance. Cultural transmission is when children learn behaviors from parents. Many investigators have documented evidence that suggests that parental alcohol use and parental attitudes toward alcohol significantly influence alcohol use in adolescents.[19-21] Twin/family designs augment twin data with information on family members. An examination of genetic vs. cultural reasons for familial aggregation of alcoholism in adult female twin pairs and their parents concluded that there was no evidence of cultural transmission.[22] Cultural transmission may be more important in the development of alcohol drinking behavior in younger adolescents, who are more likely to be influenced by parental behavior and by their peers.[23] However, most large-scale twin studies that have examined this issue have found very little support for cultural transmission of alcoholism.

The high comorbidity between alcohol and tobacco use has also prompted several recent twin studies that investigated shared genetic influences on alcohol and tobacco dependence. Shared environmental factors were found to be more important than genetic factors in mediating comorbid alcohol and tobacco use, in 12- to 16-year-olds from an adolescent and young-adult Dutch twin sample.[23] In contrast, for 17- to 25-year-olds from the same twin sample, alcohol and tobacco use was genetically determined and shared environmental factors played a smaller role. These data suggest that environmental factors may be more important in initiation of alcohol and tobacco use, while genetic factors may mediate maintenance of this behavior. A recent analysis of alcohol and tobacco use in adult MZ and DZ twin pairs found that a common genetic factor seemed to mediate correlations between both average and heavy patterns of alcohol and tobacco use.[25] Similarly, a common genetic factor was also found to mediate the relationship between smoking and perceived alcohol-induced intoxication in women from an Australian twin sample.[26] These studies suggest that history of smoking may influence tolerance to alcohol.

MARKERS OF VULNERABILITY TO ALCOHOLISM

The knowledge that alcoholism is genetically transmitted had prompted a number of investigations on the search for biochemical characteristics or trait markers that could be used to identify a predisposition for alcoholism. It has been suggested that the primary requirements for such a marker are reliability and ease of measurement, and the ability to be detected prior to the onset of alcoholism and during abstinence from alcohol, and not to be influenced by other coexisting disorders.[27] Additionally, such a trait should also be identified in an alcoholic subject's first-degree relatives and among relatives who are also alcohol dependent.[28] Such trait markers would not only help to identify individuals who are vulnerable to development of the disorder, but also could be used to identify candidate genes that may mediate development of this disorder.

In order to identify alcoholism traits, investigators have studied the existence of a number of markers in individuals with a positive family history of alcoholism (FHP) compared with individuals with a negative family history of alcoholism (FHN). Most of these studies have concentrated on three primary areas: (1) electrophysiological markers; (2) biochemical markers; and (3) physiological and neurochemical markers of reactions to alcohol.

ELECTROPHYSIOLOGICAL MARKERS

Electrical activity in the brain, as measured by electrophysiological techniques, has been examined as a marker of alcoholism. An early study found that sons of alcoholics, who had not consumed alcohol, had excess beta-activity and deficient delta-, alpha-, and theta-activity.[29] However, a later study found that while these differences were not detectable at baseline, significant differences in beta-activity could only be observed following consumption of alcohol in individuals with positive vs. those with negative family history of alcoholism.[30] Controversial differences have also been found in fast-frequency alpha-activity, with reports of greater activity at baseline followed by reduction in this energy after consumption of alcohol,[31] as well as reports of increases in alpha-energy in response to alcohol.[32] These disparities have been attributed to differences in the design of these studies, including differences in doses of alcohol used and differences in subtype of alcoholism.

A number of investigators have also examined differences in the ability of the alcoholic brain to respond to auditory, visual, and olfactory stimuli, as measured by event-related potentials, and have found an attenuation in the amplitude of a waveform that is seen 300 ms after exposure to a stimulus (P300 component) in alcoholics. The P300 waveform has been associated with a role in information processing, attention, decision-making, and memory. However, the use of this waveform as an indicator of vulnerability to alcoholism is controversial, with some investigators finding smaller P300 waves[33] in sons of alcoholics and others being unable to replicate these findings.[34] Moreover, prolonged P300 latencies have also been found in neuropsychiatrically ill patients (with or without polysubstance abuse).[35] More recent reports indicate that while alcoholics and non-alcoholics differ in P300 latencies, they do not differ in P300 amplitudes.[36] Moreover, neither amplitudes nor latencies of the P300 waveform were significantly altered by a family history of alcoholism. Therefore, the use of the P300 waveform as a marker of vulnerability to alcoholism remains to be established.

BIOCHEMICAL MARKERS

A number of enzymes that are influenced by alcohol use have also been examined as neurochemical markers of vulnerability to alcoholism. Monoamine oxidase (MAO) is an enzyme that mediates metabolism of monoamine neurotransmitters such as dopamine and norepinephrine, which have been associated with roles in mediating reinforcement from alcohol. MAO activity in blood platelets is believed to correlate well with similar activity in the brain. Many investigators have examined MAO activity in the platelets of alcoholics and have found both reductions[37,38] and no differences.[39,40] Several studies have also indicated that low platelet MAO activity may be a marker of type II or early-onset alcoholism.[40,41] Female alcoholics have also been found to exhibit lower platelet MAO levels.[42] One cautionary note regarding MAO is that decreased MAO activity has been associated with other psychiatric and medical illnesses, metabolic factors, personality traits, and cigarette smoking (to name a few), and therefore, the specificity of MAO activity as a specific marker for alcoholism remains to be established.[27,43] Morevoer, recent evidence from the Collaborative Study on the Genetics of Alcoholism data set suggests that cigarette smoking and male gender — and *not* alcohol dependence — determined decreases in platelet MAO activity, suggesting that MAO activity may be a state marker of cigarette smoking rather than a trait marker of alcohol dependence.[44]

Adenylate cyclase (AC) is an enzyme involved in the formation of a second messenger cAMP that mediates a number of cellular biochemical events. The adenylate cyclase/cyclic AMP pathway has been proposed to be important in mediating reinforcement from, and tolerance to, alcohol and a number of other drugs.[45] Activation of adenylate cylcase in platelets and lymphocytes by numerous non-alcohol-related stimuli has been reported to be lower in alcoholics when compared with controls.[45,46] Several studies have also documented that a family history of alcoholism is associated with lower stimulated AC activity.[42,47] It has been suggested that since low AC activity is seen in alcoholics even following long periods of abstinence from alcohol, that this may be a true trait marker of genetic predisposition to alcoholism. In support of this hypothesis, the transmission of AC activity in families has been reported to be mediated by a single gene.[48] However, many investigators have also suggested that, like other trait markers, low AC activity may increase the risk for alcoholism but not necessarily cause the disease.[48,49]

Some other neurochemical markers for which there is preliminary evidence include the opioids, gamma-aminobutyric acid (GABA), and serotonin. Both preclinical and clinical studies indicate that positive family history for alcoholism is associated with an enhanced sensitivity of the pituitary opioid peptide β-endorphin system to alcohol.[51,52] Moreover, a preliminary study by Froehlich and colleagues examined β-endorphin levels, both prior to and following a dose of alcohol, in a twin sample and found that the alcohol-induced β-endorphin response was significantly heritable.[53] GABA levels are also known to be altered during abstinence from alcohol, and sons of alcoholics (when compared with matched controls) have been shown to have significantly greater increases in plasma GABA-like activity in response to an alcoholic drink.[54] Similarly, alcoholics have also been shown to have low serotonin levels, with significantly higher rates of platelet serotonin uptake in subjects with alcoholic fathers.[55] However, all this evidence is preliminary and needs to be replicated in larger samples.

PHYSIOLOGICAL AND NEUROCHEMICAL MARKERS

MARKERS OF DIFFERENCES IN REACTION OF ALCOHOL

It has been proposed that individuals with a family history of alcoholism may find alcohol more reinforcing when compared with individuals with a negative family history of alcoholism. A number of investigations have been directed at characterizing this effect using both physiological and neuroendocrine tools. Men with a positive family history of male alcoholism have been shown to have significantly larger increases in heart rate following ingestion of a high dose of alcohol, and the alcohol-induced increases in heart rate have been found to correlate significantly with weekly rates of normal alcohol consumption.[56] A number of investigators have also reported that, compared with control subjects, sons of alcoholic fathers exhibit lower physiological reactivity (body sway, hormonal response, and brain activity) and self-reports of intoxication in response to low or moderate doses of alcohol,[57-59] but that this effect disappears when high doses of alcohol are administered.[60-62] A long-term follow-up study of family history positive (FHP) and family history negative (FHN) males who were initially tested for their responses to alcohol found that low levels of initial response to alcohol in both FHPs and FHNs was a good predictor for subsequent alcohol abuse or dependence.[63]

GENES INFLUENCING A PREDISPOSITION TO ALCOHOLISM

The knowledge that alcoholism is a complex, polygenic disease has also prompted a search for candidate genes that may be found specifically in individuals with a predisposition to alcoholism. Most genetic studies to date have used the "genetic association method," in which affected and unaffected individuals are compared for the occurrence of a particular allele of a gene that is thought to mediate predisposition to the disease. This method requires prior neurochemical or knowledge of a possible association between the disease and the gene.

GENES AFFECTING ALCOHOL METABOLISM

One of the first genes that was discovered and suggested to influence vulnerability to alcoholism was a defective allele of the gene encoding liver aldehyde dehydrogenase, which is involved in the breakdown of alcohol. The discovery of this gene was based on the observation of the alcohol flushing reaction commonly observed in some Asian populations (e.g., Chinese, Japanese, Koreans). Approximately 50% of Asians experience the alcohol-induced flushing response, which has been shown to be associated with an elevated level of acetaldehyde.[64] Elevations in acetaldehyde levels can be the result of either higher than normal conversion of alcohol to acetaldehyde by alcohol dehydrogenase (ADH), or slower than normal metabolism of acetaldehyde by aldehyde dehydrogenase (ALDH).

ALDH has four isozymes, of which ALDH2 is responsible for most of the acetaldehyde breakdown in the cell. Thus, a defect in ALDH2 is believed to mediate flushing and other alcohol sensitivity reactions. The gene for ALDH2 has two variants or alleles: ALDH2[1], which encodes a functional enzyme subunit, and ALDH2[2], which encodes a defective subunit. Since each individual inherits two copies of each gene, three combinations of ALDH2 alleles are possible: two ALDH2[1] alleles, one ALDH2[1] allele and one ALDH2[2] allele, and two ALDH2[2] alleles. Therefore, an individual with two ALDH2[2] alleles will have less enzyme activity than an individual with one of each allele, who will have less enzyme activity than an individual with two ALDH2[1] alleles. Interestingly, it has been shown that nearly all Caucasians and African Americans are homozygous for the ALDH2[1] allele; in comparison, 50% of Asians are homozygous for the ALDH2[1], 30 to 40% are heterozygous, and 5 to 10% are homozygous for the ALDH2[2] allele.[65] Similarly, Asians who have the ALDH2[2] allele drink very little alcohol.[66] Moreover, rates of alcohol drinking and alcohol dependence are significantly lower in Asians who are heterozygous, compared with those who are homozygous for the functional genotype (ALDH2[1]/2[1]). A review of a series of investigations conducted in Asians with different alleles suggests that individuals who are homozygous for the defective allele report more negative reactions (nausea, vomiting, tachycardia) to alcohol.[67] Interestingly, heterozygous individuals experience a more intense positive response to alcohol compared to those who were homozygous for the functional allele, suggesting that heterozygotes may have heightened sensitivity to alcohol and therefore may have to drink less to experience the effects of alcohol. In support of this hypothesis, alcohol consumption in heterozygous individuals has been shown to result in a greater magnitude of effects on the P300 wave (increased latency and decreased amplitude) when compared with those who were homozygous for the functional allele. However, despite all the above findings, the ALDH2[2] allele is found only in Asians and not in Caucasians, suggesting that this may not be a good genetic marker of differences in alcohol use patterns in Caucasian samples.

Alcohol dehydrogenase has six isozymes, of which two have been identified as being important in ethanol metabolism: ADH2 has been shown to have three alleles and ADH has two alleles. Asian alcoholics, when compared with non-alcoholics have significantly lower frequencies of ADH2[2] and ADH3[1].[68,69] Alcoholics who were homozygous for ADH2[1] also had higher ADH3[2] allele frequencies. It has been suggested that individuals with ADH2[2] and ADH3[1] alleles would rapidly convert alcohol to acetaldehyde and therefore have less tolerance to alcohol's effects and thus be less at risk for development of alcohol abuse. In contrast, Caucasians do not seem to have any differences in these genotypes of ADH, again suggesting that alcoholism in Caucasians may not be mediated by an inherited defect in alcohol metabolism.[70,71]

GENES FOR NEUROTRANSMITTERS AND ALCOHOLISM

Alcohol-induced reinforcement and behavior have been attributed to alterations in a number of neurotransmitter systems, including dopamine, serotonin, opioids, and GABA. Investigations into the roles of genes for these neurotransmitters and their receptors in determining vulnerability to alcoholism are currently underway. A few of these studies are described in detail below.

Dopamine is a neurotransmitter that has been associated with a central role in alcohol reinforcement and development of alcohol dependence.[72] The dopamine receptor, the site which binds the dopamine molecule, has been shown to have five subtypes. Initial investigations examined the population association of the A1 allele of the gene that regulates synthesis of the D2 receptor (also known as DRD2) with alcoholism and found high rates of this allele in alcoholics compared with non-alcoholics.[73] However, subsequent studies failed to replicate these findings and found either weaker associations[74,75] or failed to find any association.[76-78] It has been proposed that these controversial results could be due to a lack of adequate control of other factors that may influence genetic composition, such as ethnicity in the samples being studied. However, a recent study in an ethnically well-defined southwestern American Indian tribe with high rates of alcoholism, also found no association between the defective allele of the DRD2 receptor and alcoholism.[79] Interestingly, an association between a functional variant of a different dopamine receptor, the D4 receptor, and alcoholism has also been reported in a sample of severely affected Japanese alcoholics.[80] Moreover, dopamine transporter genes, which are responsible for removing dopamine from the synapse and terminating dopamine activity, have also been studied. A significantly high incidence of an allele of the dopamine transporter gene (DAT1) has been found in alcoholics who reported withdrawal seizures or delirium.[81] These results need to be replicated in a larger sample. Therefore, while dopamine is known to play an important role in brain reward circuits, the role of dopamine receptor and transporter genes in mediating vulnerability to alcoholism remains to be established.

The neurotransmitter serotonin has also been proposed to have a role in the development of alcohol dependence.[82] A number of investigators have proposed that deficiencies in serotonin levels may mediate increased risk of depression, suicide, and alcoholism.[83] Nielsen and colleagues examined the genes for the enzyme tryptophan hydroxylase, which is involved in the synthesis of serotonin, in alcoholics and found an allele of TPH to be associated with suicidal behavior.[84] The extensive evidence indicating a role for the endogenous opioids in alcohol reward, tolerance and withdrawal has also prompted investigations into the relationship between the genes for opioid receptors and alcohol dependence. The evidence to date is still controversial with some studies indicating a modest association between the mu receptor OPRM1 alleles and substance (cocaine, alcohol, or opioid) dependence,[85] and yet others indicating no associations,[86,87] and more recent evidence suggesting that genetic variations of the OPRM1 gene may mediate sensitivity of the dopaminergic system during alcohol withdrawal.[88]

Recently, the results of an NIAAA-supported multi-centered study called COGA (Collaborative Study on Genetics of Alcoholism) have been published. COGA investigators chose to use genetic linkage techniques to identify genes for alcoholism. Genetic linkage studies examine the inheritance of alcoholism in multigenerational families that have been affected by the disease. COGA investigators identified affected families and then conducted genome-wide scans to identify genes that may mediate susceptibility for alcohol dependence. Recent results of this investigation suggest that genes affecting vulnerability to alcoholism could be found on chromosomes 1 and 7.[89] The results also present modest evidence for a gene that could protect against alcoholism on chromosome 4. Similarly, genome scans conducted on alcohol-dependent subjects from a southwestern American Indian tribe also found evidence of a susceptibility gene on chromosome 11 and a protective gene on chromosome 4.[90] It is interesting to note that the alcohol dehydrogenase genes (ADH2 and ADH3), which have been proposed to have protective effects in Asian populations, are located near the protective chromosome 4 locus. Each one of these chromosomal regions consists of many genes, and further high-resolution mapping of each region could help determine the genes involved in mediating vulnerability to alcoholism. Determination of genes responsible for mediating susceptibility to alcoholism would contribute significantly to furthering our knowledge about this disease and also help in the treatment and possibly prevention of alcohol dependence.

REFERENCES

1. Amark, C.A., A study in alcoholism: clinical, socialpsychiatric and genetic investigations, *Acta Psychiatr. Neurol. Scand.,* 70, 1, 1951.
2. Bleuler, M., Familial and personal background of chronic alcoholism, *Etiology of Chronic Alcoholism,* Diethelm, O., Thomas, Springfield, IL, 1955, 110.
3. Cotton, N.S., The familial incidence of alcoholism: a review, *J. Stud. Alcohol.,* 40, 89, 1979.
4. Merikangas, K.R., The genetic epidemiology of alcoholism, *Psychol. Med.,* 20, 11, 1990.
5. Cadoret, R.J., Cain, C.A., and Grove, W.M., Development of alcoholism in adoptees raised apart from alcoholic biologic relatives, *Arch. Gen. Psychiatry,* 37, 561, 1980.
6. Bohman, M., Sigvardsson, S., and Cloninger, C.R., Maternal inheritance of alcohol abuse: Cross-fostering analysis of adopted women, *Arch. Gen. Psychiatry,* 38, 965, 1981.

7. Cloninger, C.R., Bohman, M., and Sigvardsson, S., Inheritance of alcohol abuse: cross-fostering analysis of adopted men, *Arch. Gen. Psychiatry,* 38, 861, 1981.

8. Goodwin, D.W., Schulsinger, F., Hermansen, L., Guze, S.B., and Winokur, G., Alcohol problems in adoptees raised apart from alcoholic biological parents, *Arch. Gen. Psychiatry,* 28, 238, 1973.

9. Hill, S.Y., Absence of paternal sociopathy in the etiology of severe alcoholism: is there a type III alcoholism? *J. Stud. Alcohol.,* 53, 161, 1992.

10. Cadoret, R.J., Genetics of alcoholism. In *Alcohol and the Family: Research and Clinical Perspectives,* R.L. Collins, K.E. Leonard, and J.S. Searles, Eds., Guilford Press, New York, 1990, 39.

11. Pickens, R.W., Svikis, D.S., McGue, M., Lykken, D.T., Heston, L.L., and Clayton, P.J., Heterogeneity in the inheritance of alcoholism: a study of male and female twins, *Arch. Gen. Psychiatry,* 48, 19, 1991.

12. Kendler, K.S., Heath, A.C., Neale, M.C., Kessler, R.C., and Eaves, L.J., A population-based twin study of alcoholism in women, *JAMA,* 268, 1877, 1992.

13. Kaprio, J., Rose, R.J., Romanov, K., and Koskenvuo, M., Genetic and environmental determinants of use and abuse of alcohol: the Finnish Twin Cohort studies, *Alcohol Alcohol.* (Suppl.), 131, 1991.

14. Clifford, C.A., Hopper, J.L., Fulker, D.W., and Murray, R.M., A genetic and environmental analysis of a twin family study of alcohol use, anxiety, and depression, *Genet. Epidemiol.,* 1, 63, 1984.

15. Heath, A.C., Meyer, J., Jardine, R., and Martin, N.G., The inheritance of alcohol consumption patterns in a general population twin sample: II. Determinants of consumption frequency and quantity consumed, *J. Stud. Alcohol.,* 52, 425, 1991.

16. Prescott, C.A., Hewitt, J.K., Heath, A.C., Truett, K.R., Neale, M.C., and Eaves, L.J., Environmental and genetic influences on alcohol use in a volunteer sample of older twins, *J. Stud. Alcohol.,* 55, 18, 1994.

17. Heath, A.C., Bucholz, K.K., Madden, P.A.F., Dinwiddie, S.H., Slutske, W.S., Bierut, L.J., Statham, D.J., Dunne, M.P., Whitfield, J.B., and Martin, N.G., Genetic and environmental contributions to alcohol dependence risk in a national twin sample: consistency of findings in women and men, *Psychol. Med.,* 27, 1381, 1997.

18. Reed, T., Page, W.F., Viken, R.J., and Christian, J.C., Genetic predisposition to organ-specific endpoints of alcoholism, *Alcohol. Clin. Exp. Res.,* 20, 1528, 1996.

19. Weinberg, N.Z., Dielman, T.E., Mandell, W., and Shope, J.T., Parental drinking and gender factors in the prediction of early adolescent alcohol use, *Int. J. Addictions,* 29, 89, 1994.

20. Duncan, T.E., Duncan, S.C., and Hops, H., The effects of family cohesiveness and peer encouragement on the development of adolescent alcohol use: a cohort-sequential approach to the analysis of longitudinal data, *J. Stud. Alcohol.,* 55, 588, 1994.

21. Ary, D.V., Tildesley, E., Hops, H., and Andrews, J., The influence of parent, sibling, and peer modeling and attitudes on adolescent use of alcohol, *Int. J. Addictions,* 28, 853, 1993.

22. Kendler, K.S., Neale, M.C., Heath, A.C., Kessler, R.C., and Eaves, L.J., A twin-family study of alcoholism in women, *Am. J. Psychiatry,* 151, 707, 1994.

23. Koopmans, J.R. and Boomsma, D.I., Familial resemblances in alcohol use: genetic or cultural transmission? *J. Stud. Alcohol.,* 57, 19, 1996.

24. Swan, G.E., Carmelli, D., and Cardon, L.R., The consumption of tobacco, alcohol, and coffee in caucasian male twins: a multivariate genetic analysis, *J. Stud. Alcohol.,* 8, 19, 1996.

25. Swan, G.E., Carmelli, D., and Cardon, L.R., Heavy consumption of cigarettes, alcohol and coffee in male twins, *J. Stud. Alcohol.,* 58, 182, 1997.

26. Madden, P.A.F., Heath, A.C., and Martin, N.G., Smoking and intoxication after alcohol challenge in women and men: genetic influences, *Alcohol. Clin. Exp. Res.,* 21, 1732, 1997.

27. Anthenelli, R.M. and Tabakoff, B., The search for biochemical markers, *Alcohol Health Res. World,* 19, 176, 1995.

28. Begleiter, H. and Porjesz, B., Potential biological markers in individuals at high risk for developing alcoholism, *Alcohol. Clin. Exp. Res.,* 12, 488, 1988.

29. Gabrielli, W.F., Mednick, S.A., Volavka, J., Pollock, V.E., Schulsinger, F., and Itil, T.M., Electroencephalograms in children of alcoholic fathers, *Psychphysiology,* 19, 404, 1982.

30. Ehlers, C.L. and Schuckit, M.A., EEG fast frequency activity in sons of alcoholics, *Biolog. Psychiatry,* 27, 631, 1990.

31. Ehlers, C.L. and Schuckit, M.A., Evaluation of EEG alpha activity in sons of alcoholics, *Neuropsychopharmacology,* 4, 199, 1991.

32. Pollock, V.E., Volavka, J., Goodwin, D.W., Mednick, S.A., Gabrielli, W.F., Knop, J., and Schulsinger, F., The EEG after alcohol administration in men at risk for alcoholism, *Arch. Gen. Psychiatry,* 40, 857, 1983.

33. Begleiter, H., Porjesz, B., and Tenner, M., Neuroradiological and neurophysiological evidence of brain deficits in chronic alcoholics, *Acta Psychiatr. Neurol. Scand.,* 286, 3, 1980.

34. Polich, J. and Bloom, F.E., Event-related brain potentials in indiviuals at high and low risk for developing alcoholism: failure to replicate, *Alcohol. Clin. Exp. Res.,* 12, 368, 1988.

35. Blum, K., Braverman, E.R., Dinardo, M.J., Wood, R.C., and Sheridan, P.J., Prolonged P300 latency in a neuropsychiatric population with the D2 dopamine receptor A1 allele, *Pharmacogenetics,* 4, 313, 1994.

36. Keenan, J.P., Freeman, P.R., and Harrell, R., The effects of family history, sobriety length, and drinking history in younger alcoholics on P300 auditory-evoked potentials, *Alcohol Alcohol.,* 32, 133, 1997.

37. Faraj, B.A., Lenton, J.D., Kutner, M., Camp, V.M., Stammers, T.W., Lee, S.R., Lolies, P.A., and Chandora, D., Prevalence of low monoamine oxidase function in alcoholism, *Alcohol. Clin. Exp. Res.,* 11, 464, 1987.

38. Pandey, G.N., Fawcett, J., Gibbons, R., Clark, D.C., and Davis, J.M., Platelet monoamine oxidase in alcoholism, *Biol. Psychiatry,* 24, 15, 1988.

39. Tabakoff, B., Hoffman, P.L., Lee, J.M., Saito, T., Willard, B., and de Leon-Jones, F., Differences in platelet enzyme activity between alcoholics and nonalcoholics, *N. Engl. J. Med.,* 318, 134, 1988.

40. von Knorring, A.L., Bohman, M., von Knorring, L., and Oreland, L., Platelet MAO activity as a biological marker in subgroups of alcoholism, *Acta Psychiatr. Neurol. Scand.,* 72, 51, 1985.

41. Tabakoff, B., Whelan, J.P., and Hoffman, P.L., Two biological markers of alcoholism, *Genetics and Biology of Alcoholism.* C.R. Cloninger and H. Begleiter, Eds., Cold Spring Harbor Laboratory Press, Cold Spring Harbor, 1990, 195.

42. Lex, B.W., Ellingboe, J., LaRosa, K., Teoh, S.K., and Mendelson, J.H., Platelet adenylate cyclase and monoamine oxidase in women with alcoholism or a family history of alcoholism, *Harvard Rev. Psychiatry,* 1, 229, 1993.

43. Sher, K.J., Bylund, D.B., Walitzer, K.S., Hartman, J., and Ray-Prenger, C., Platelet monoamine oxidase (MAO) activity: personality, substance use, and the stress-response dampening effect of alcohol, *Exp. Clin. Psychopharmacol.,* 2, 53, 1994.

44. Anthenelli, R.M., Tipp, J., Li, T.K., Magnes, L., Schuckit, M.A., Rice, J., Daw, W., and Nurnberger, J.I., Platelet monoamine oxidase activity in subgroups of alcoholics and controls: results from the Collaborative Study on the Genetics of Alcoholism, *Alcohol. Clin. Exp. Res.,* 22, 598, 1998.

45. Nestler, R.J., Molecular neurobiology of drug addiction, *Neuropsychopharmacology,* 11, 77, 1994.

46. Diamond, I., Wrubel, B., Estrin, W., and Gordon, A., Basal and adenosine receptor-stimulated levels of cAMP are reduced in lymphocytes in alcoholic patients, *Proc. Natl. Acad. Sci. U.S.A.,* 84, 1413, 1987.

47. Saito, T., Katamura, Y., Ozawa, H., Hatta, S., and Takahata, N., Platelet GTP-binding protein in long-term abstinent alcoholics with an alcoholic first-degree relative, *Biolog. Psychiatry,* 36, 495, 1994.

48. Devor, E.J., Cloninger, C.R., Hoffman, P.L., and Tabakoff, B., A genetic study of platelet adenylate cyclase activity: evidence for a single major locus effect in fluoride-stimulated activity, *Am. J. Hum. Genet.,* 49, 372, 1991.

49. Greenberg, D.A., Linkage analysis of "necessary" disease loci versus "susceptibility" loci, *Am. J. Hum. Genet.,* 52, 135, 1993.

50. Froehlich, J.C., and Li, T.-K., *Opioid Involvement in Alcohol Drinking,* Vol. 739, New York Academy of Science, New York, 1994.

51. Gianoulakis, C., Béliveau, D., Angelogianni, P., Meaney, M., Thavundayil, J., Tawar, V., and Dumas, M., Different pituitary β-endorphin and adrenal cortisol response to ethanol in individuals with high and low risk for future development of alcoholism, *Life Sci.,* 45, 1097, 1989.

52. Gianoulakis, C., Krishnan, B., and Thavundayil, J., Enhanced sensitivity of pituitary beta-endorphin to ethanol in subjects at high risk of alcoholism, *Arch. Gen. Psychiatry,* 53, 250, 1996.

53. Froehlich, J.C., Rhoades-Hall, C.E.R., Zink, R., Li, T.-K., and Christian, J.C. Heritability of plasma beta-endorphin following an alcohol challenge, *Alcohol. Clin. Exp. Res.,* 19(Suppl.) 72A, 1995.

54. Moss, H.B., Yao, J.K., Burns, M., Maddock, J., and Tarter, R.E., Plasma GABA-like activity in response to ethanol challenge in men at high risk for alcoholism, *Biolog. Psychiatry,* 27, 617, 1990.

55. Rausch, J.L., Monteiro, M.G., and Schuckit, M.A., Platelet serotonin uptake in men with family histories of alcoholism, *Neuropsychopharmacology*, 4, 83, 1991.

56. Pihl, R.O. and Peterson, J.B., Abiobehavioural model for the inherited predisposition to alcoholism, *Alcohol Alcohol.*, 1(Suppl.), 151, 1991.

57. Pollock, V.E., Teasdale, T.W., Gabrielli, W.F., and Knop, J., Subjective and objective measures of response to alcohol among young men at risk for alcoholism, *J. Stud. Alcohol.*, 47, 297, 1986.

58. O' Malley, S.S., and Maisto, S.A., Effects of family drinking history and expectancies on responses to alcohol in men, *J. Stud. Alcohol.*, 46, 289, 1985.

59. Schuckit, M.A., Low level of response to alcohol as a predictor of future alcoholism, *Am. J. Psychiatry*, 155, 184, 1994.

60. Finn, P.R., Zeitouni, N.C., and Pihl, R.O., Effects of alcohol on psychophysiological hyperactivity to nonaversive and aversive stimuli in men at high risk for alcoholism, *J. Abnorm. Psychol.*, 99, 79, 1990.

61. Peterson, J.B., Weiner, D., Pihl, R.O., Finn, P.R., and Earleywine, M., The tridimensional personality questionnaire and the inherited risk for alcoholism, *Addictive Behav.*, 16, 549, 1991.

62. Schuckit, M.A., Subjective responses to alcohol in sons of alcoholics and control subjects, *Arch. Gen. Psychiatry*, 41, 879, 1984.

63. Schuckit, M.A. and Smith, T.L., An 8-year follow-up of 450 sons of alcoholics and controls, *Arch. Gen. Psychiatry*, 53, 202, 1996.

64. Harada, S., Agarwal, D.P., and Goedde, H.W., Aldehyde dehydrogenase deficiency as cause of facial flushing reaction to alcohol in Japanese, *Lancet, II*, 982, 1981.

65. Goedde, H.W., Agarwal, D.P., Fritze, G., Meiertackmann, D., Singh, S., Beckmann, G., Bhatia, K., Chen, L.Z., Fang, B., Lisker, R., Paik, Y.K., Rothhammer, F., Saha, N., Segal, B., Srivastava, L.M., and Czeizel, A., Distribution of ADH2 and ALDH2 genotypes in different populations, *Human Genet.*, 88, 334, 1992.

66. Takeshita, T., Morimoto, K., Mao, X.Q., Hashimoto, T., and Furuyama, J.-I., Characterization of the three genotypes of low Km aldehyde dehydrogenase in a Japanese population, *Human Genet.*, 94, 217, 1994.

67. Wall, T.L. and Ehlers, C.L., Genetic influences affecting alcohol use among Asians, *Alcohol Health Res. World*, 19, 184, 1995.

68. Thomasson, H.R., Edenberg, H.J., Crabb, D.W., Mai, X.L., Jerome, R.E., Li, T.K., Wang, S.P., Lin, Y.T., Lu, R.B., and Yin, S.J., Alcohol and aldehyde dehydrogenase genotypes and alcoholism in Chinese men, *Am. J. Hum. Genet.*, 48, 667, 1991.

69. Thomasson, H.R., Crabb, D.W., Edenberg, H.J., and Li, T.K., Alcohol and aldehyde dehydrogenase polymorphisms and alcoholism, *Behav. Genet.*, 23, 131, 1993.

70. Gilder, F.J., Hodgkinson, S., and Murray, R.M., ADH and ALDH genotype profiles in Caucasians with alcohol-related problems, *Addiction*, 88, 383, 1993.

71. Couzigou, P., Fleury, B., Groppi, A., Cassaigne, A., Begueret, J., and Iron, A., Genotyping study of alcohol dehydrogenase class I polymorphism in French patients with alcoholic cirrhosis. The French Group for Research on Alcohol and Liver, *Alcohol Alcohol.*, 25, 623, 1990.

72. DiChiara, G., The role of dopamine in drug abuse viewed from the perspective of its role in motivation, *Drug Alcohol Depend.*, 38, 95, 1995.

73. Blum, K., Noble, E.P., Sheridan, P.J., Montgomery, A., Ritchie, T., Jagadeeswaran, P., Nogami, H., Briggs, A.H., Cohn, J.B., Allelic association of human dopamine D2 receptor gene in alcoholism, *JAMA*, 263, 2055, 1990.

74. Parsian, A., Todd, R.D., Devor, E.J., O' Malley, K.L., Suarez, B.K., Reich, T., and Cloninger, C.R., Alcoholism and alleles of the human D_2 dopamine receptor locus, *Arch. Gen. Psychiatry*, 48, 655, 1991.

75. Blum, K., Noble, E.P., Sheridan, P.J., Finley, O., Montgomery, A., Ritchie, T., Ozkaragoz, T., Fitch, R.J., Sadlack, F., Sheerfield, D., Dahlmann, T., Halbardier, S., and Nogami, H., Association of the A1 allele of the D_2 dopamine receptor gene, *Alcohol*, 8, 409, 1991.

76. Gelernter, J., Goldman, D., and Risch, N., The A1 allele at the D_2 dopamine receptor gene and alcoholism, *JAMA*, 269, 1673, 1993.

77. Goldman, D., Dean, M., Brown, G.L., Bolos, A.M., Tokola, R., Virkkunen, M., and Linnoila, M., D_2 dopamine receptor genotype and cerebrospinal fluid homovanillic acid, 5-hydroxyindoleacetic acid and 3-methoxy-4-hydroxyphenylglycol in alcoholics in Finland and the United States, *Acta Psychiatr. Scand.*, 86, 351, 1992.

78. Goldman, D., Brown, G.L., Albaugh, B., Robin, R., Goodson, S., Trunzo, M., Akhtar, L., Lucas-Derse, S., Long, J., Linnoila, M., and Dean, M., DRD2 dopamine receptor genotype, linkage disequilibrium, and alcoholism in American Indians and other populations, *Alcohol. Clin. Exp. Res.,* 17, 199, 1993.

79. Goldman, D., Urbanek, M., Guenther, D., Robin, R., and Long, J.C., Linkage and association of a functional DRD2 variant [Ser3 11 Cys] and DRD2 markers to alcoholism, substance abuse, and schizophrenia in Southwestern American Indians, *Am. J. Med. Genet. (Neuropsychiatr. Genet.,),* 74, 386, 1997.

80. Muramatsu, T., Higuchi, S., Murayama, M., Matsushita, S., and Hayashida, M., Association between alcoholism and the D4 receptor gene, *J. Med. Genet.,* 33, 113, 1996.

81. Sander, T., Harms, H., Podschus, J., Finckh, U., Nickel, B., Rolfs, A., Rommelspacher, H., and Schmidt, L.G., Allelic association of dopamine transporter gene polymorphism in alcohol dependence with withdrawal seizures or delirium, *Biolog. Psychiatry,* 41, 299, 1997.

82. Litten, R.Z. and Allen, J.P., Pharmacotherapies for alcoholism: promising agents and clinical issues, *Alcohol. Clin. Exp. Res.,* 15, 620, 1991.

83. Pihl, R.O., Peterson, J.B., and Lau, M.A., A biosocial model of the alcohol-aggression relationship, *J. Stud. Alcohol* (Suppl.) 11, 128, 1993.

84. Nielsen, D.A., Goldman, D., Virkkunen, M., Tokola, R., Rawlings, R., and Linnoila, M., Suicidality and 5-hydroxyindoleacetic acid concentration associated with a tryptophan hydroxylase polymorphism, *Arch. Gen. Psychiatry,* 51, 34, 1994.

85. Kranzler, H.R., Gelernter, J., O'Malley, S.S., Hernandez-Avila, C.A., and Kaufman, D., Association of alcohol or other drug dependence with alleles of the mu opioid receptor gene (OPRM1), *Alcohol. Clin. Exp. Res.,* 22, 1359, 1998.

86. Sander, R., Gscheidel, N., Wendel, B., Samochowiec, J., Smolka, M., Rommelspacher, H., Schmidt, L.G., and Hoeche, M.R., Human mu-opioid receptor variation and alcohol dependence, *Alcohol. Clin. Exp. Res.,* 22, 2108, 1998.

87. Bergen, A.W., Kokoszka, J., Peterson, R., Long, J.C., Virkkunen, M., Linniola, M., and Goldman, D., Mu opioid receptor gene variants: lack of association with alcohol dependence, *Mol. Psychiatry,* 2, 490, 1997.

88. Smolka, M., Sander, T., Schmidt, L.G., Samochowiec, J., Rommelspacher, H., Gscheidel, N., Wendel, B, and Hoehe, M.R., mu-opioid receptor variants and dopaminergic sensitivity in alcohol withdrawal, *Psychoneuroendocrinology,* 24, 629, 1999.

89. Reich, T., Edenberg, H.J., Goate, A., Williams, J.T., Rice, J.P., Eerdewegh, P.V., Foroud, T., Hesselbrock, V., Schuckit, M.A., Bucholz, K., Porjesz, B., Li, T.K., Conneally, P.M., Nurnberger, J.I., Tischfield, J.A., Crowe, R.R., Cloninger, C.R., Wu, W., Shears, S., Carr, K., Crose, C., Willig, C., and Begleiter, H., Genome-wide search for genes affecting the risk for alcohol dependence, *Am. J. Med. Genet. (Neuropsychiatr. Genet.),* 81, 207, 1998.

90. Long, J.C., Knowler, W.C., Hanson, R.L., Robin, R.W., Urbanek, M., Moore, E., Bennett, P.H., and Goldman, D., Evidence for genetic linkage to alcohol dependence on chromosomes 4 and 11 from an autosome-wide scan in an American Indian population, *Am. J. Med. Genet. (Neuropsychiatr. Genet.),* 81, 216, 1998.

28 Pathogenesis of Alcoholic Liver Disease

Peter Fickert and Kurt Zatloukal

OVERVIEW

Alcohol consumption of more than 40 g alcohol per day in women and more than 60 g alcohol per day in men significantly increases the risk for developing alcoholic liver disease (ALD). The pathogenesis of ALD is multifactorial. When alcohol is metabolized, oxygen is consumed, centrilobular hypoxia develops, and proinflammatory cytokines and toxic metabolites are produced. Additionally, cofactors such as gender, genetic predisposition, and nutrition play important roles in initiating and promoting ALD.

INTRODUCTION

Chronic alcohol abuse is the most important etiologic factor for liver cirrhosis in Western countries. Although prevention of alcoholism would be the best treatment, it is clear that we will have to continue to manage the medical problems. Successful therapy depends on our understanding of the pathogenetic mechanisms leading to ALD. It is important to bear in mind that **chronic alcohol abuse may lead to two different types of liver disease/damage**. Most drinkers develop **fatty liver** (Figure 28.1A), which by itself is reversible and unlikely to progress to liver cirrhosis (Figure 28.1C). Approximately 20% of heavy drinkers, however, develop a special type of ALD, namely, **alcoholic hepatitis** (AH) (Figure 28.1B), which rapidly progresses to liver cirrhosis in most cases.

At present, it is not known why the liver has this heterogeneous response to the consumption of alcohol and why only about 20% of alcoholics develop severe ALD. Answers to these questions can be found in the broad spectrum of pathogenetic factors, ranging from direct and indirect hepatotoxic effects of alcohol and its metabolites to genetic and environmental factors.

ALCOHOL OXIDATION

Ingested alcohol is mainly metabolized in the liver by the cytosolic enzyme **alcohol dehydrogenase (ADH)** and, in the pathological situation, after induction by the **microsomal ethanol oxidizing system (MEOS)**.[1] These pathways lead to production of acetaldehyde, which is oxidized in the liver by the mitochondrial aldehyde dehydrogenase (ALDH) to acetate. Acetate is mostly utilized by peripheral tissues (90%). The first metabolite, acetaldehyde, is a highly reactive electrophilic molecule that interacts with lipids and proteins. Interaction of acetaldehyde with lipids, particularly polyunsaturated fatty acids and cholesterol, initiates lipid peroxidation. This process structurally and functionally impairs the cellular and subcellular membranes and also generates free radicals. Furthermore, all these metabolic events require oxygen, thus possibly contributing to centrolobular hypoxia, a typical finding in ALD.

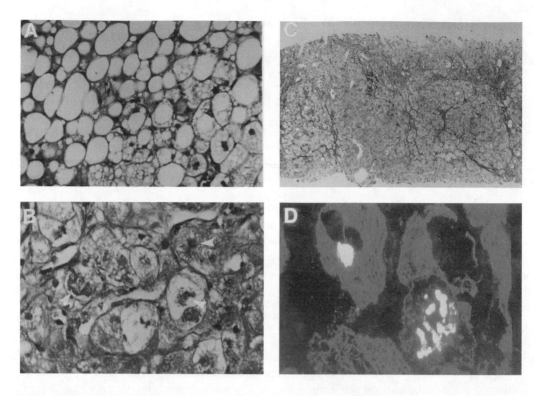

FIGURE 28.1 Morphologic alterations in alcoholic liver disease: A, alcoholic fatty liver with predominantly macrovesicular steatosis; B, alcoholic hepatitis with ballooned hepatocytes containing Mallory bodies (arrowheads); C, advanced stage of alcoholic hepatitis with development of liver cirrhosis; D, double-label immunofluorescence micrograph of a liver with alcoholic hepatitis using antibodies to cytokeratin (red) and a Mallory body specific antibody M_M120-1 (green). Mallory bodies appear in yellow because of colocalization of the non-cytokeratin component detected by M_M120-1 and cytokeratin. A-C, chromotrope aniline blue staining; Magnifications: A, × 224; B, × 224; C, × 36; D, × 360.

The electrophilic nature of acetaldehyde facilitates covalent binding of residues of proteins to form the so-called "acetaldehyde–protein adducts." Direct functional impairment of proteins and an immune response to these adducts are the two proposed pathogenetic mechanisms of the acetaldehyde–protein adducts.[6] Moreover, acetaldehyde adducts may affect inflammation and fibrosis in the liver.

FREE RADICAL GENERATION AND OXIDATIVE STRESS

The main candidates for oxidative stress generated in ALD include superoxide anion, hydrogen peroxide, hydroxyl radical, and alcohol-derived free radicals.[2] These highly reactive species arise from microsomal, mitochondrial, peroxisomal, and cytosolic sources. They are able to interact with several vital cellular molecules, leading to structural and metabolic modification and eventually cell death. Covalent binding of free radicals to proteins, including enzymes or receptors, leads to oxidative destruction of amino acids, cross-linking, or aggregation, and thus impairment of cell function. These interactions also initiate DNA damage, particularly affecting the mitochondria, thus leading to impairment of mitochondrial function. There is also considerable evidence that oxidative stress and/or lipid peroxidation are major factors in the initiation and promotion of liver fibrogenesis.

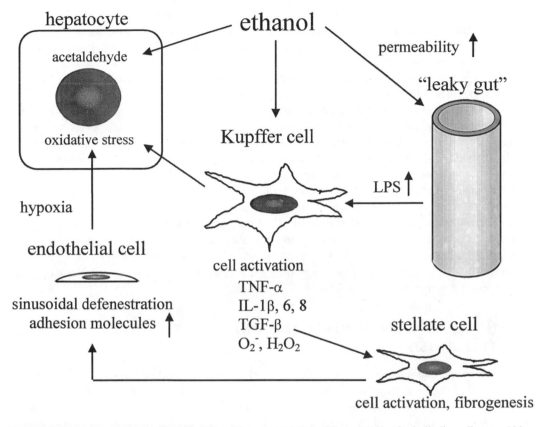

FIGURE 28.2   Interactions of hepatocytes and non-parenchymal liver cells in alcoholic liver disease. Abbreviations: TNF-α, tumor necrosis factor-alpha; Il-1β, 6,8, Interleukin-1-beta, 6,8; TGF-β, Transforming growth factor-beta; O_2^-, superoxide anion; H_2O_2, hydrogen peroxide.

Reactive oxygen species stimulate production of collagen in hepatic stellate cells. Furthermore, inflammation is a consequence of reactive oxygen species action. It is becoming increasingly apparent that they amplify and initiate inflammation through the up-regulation of several different genes involved in inflammatory processes — for example, via induction of the nuclear factor-kappa-B (NF-κB).

EFFECTS OF ALCOHOL ON NONPARENCHYMAL CELLS

For many years, the major interest of ALD research focused on the effects of alcohol and its metabolites on hepatocytes. Recently, there has been an information explosion on cytokine-mediated inflammation and how, in addition to fibrogenesis, these mediators may be involved in ALD (Figure 28.2). Kupffer cells (KC) (hepatic macrophages), endothelial cells, hepatic stellate cells (lipocytes), and pit cells (natural killer cells), constitute the so-called nonparenchymal liver cells, contributing 5% of the liver volume. These cells play a major role in liver homeostasis through uptake of soluble waste molecules and defense against bacteria and viruses. Of special interest in ALD is the ability of KCs to respond to and clear bacterial lipopolysacharides (endotoxin). Plasma levels of endotoxin are increased in patients with ALD.[3,4] Activated KCs are the main source of cytokines, eicosanoids, and reactive oxygen species in the liver. Proinflammatory cytokines play an important role in the pathogenesis of ALD, especially in the case of AH. Induction and increased serum levels of several proinflammatory cytokines such as tumor necrosis factor alpha (TNF-α), interleukin 8 (IL-8), interleukin 6 (IL-6), and interleukin-1-beta (IL-1β), have been reported in

AH.[5] The transcription factor **NF-κB** is a key player in stimulating gene expression of these proinflammatory cytokines. NF-κB is bound to an inhibitor located in the cytoplasm. Upon activation (e.g., by stimuli such as oxidative stress and endotoxin), NF-κB is uncoupled from its inhibitor and is translocated into the nucleus, inducing gene expression.

Some typical symptoms in ALD can be attributed to the action of various cytokines.[5] TNF-α and IL-1β, together with endotoxin, enhance the gene expression of leptin with subsequent anorexia. Anorexia is a regular feature of ALD, and it increases with disease severity. Cholestasis/jaundice is a frequent complication of ALD. Lipopolysaccharides (LPS)-stimulated monocytes and proinflammatory cytokines are known to cause cholestasis and decreased bile flow in experimental animal models. Increased bioactivity of IL-1β, TNF-α, and IL-8 help explain fever and neutrophilia that frequently complicate AH. IL-6, also known as hepatocyte stimulating factor, is important in mediating many of the hepatic aspects of the acute-phase response. Hepatocytes have the ability to proliferate in response to IL-6, which provides a protective mechanism by which the liver is able to recover from toxin-mediated damage. IL-8 mediates hepatic neutrophil infiltration, and plasma levels correlate with disease severity and mortality in AH. Today, there is much interest in anticytokine strategies to treat AH. However, it is important to bear in mind that cytokines such as TNF-α and IL-6 can be important in liver regeneration. It could be of vital interest to block negative and to attempt positive effects of cytokines.

MORPHOLOGIC ALTERATIONS IN ALD AND THEIR RELATION TO PATHOGENESIS

Differences in the pathogenesis of fatty liver and AH are clearly evident from their morphologic appearance. In fatty liver, hepatocytes contain huge amounts of fat in their cytoplasma, but this fat has no major effects on liver function. The accumulation of fat in hepatocytes is well explained by the metabolism of ethanol and the metabolic situation of the patients. In contrast, little is known about the pathogenesis of AH[6]; here, hepatocytes balloon to two or three times their original diameter and contain cytoplasmic inclusions, termed "Mallory bodies" (MBs) (Figure 28.1B). In AH, apoptosis, necrosis, steatosis, a chicken-wire-like fibrosis, inflammation with predominantly polymorphnuclear granulocytes, activation of Kupffer cells, and cholestasis are also seen.

One of the major hepatocytic structures affected in AH is the cytokeratin (CK) intermediate filament cytoskeleton. The CK cytoskeleton of MB-containing hepatocytes is severely deranged, and there are even some hepatocytes that appear to be completely devoid of CK filaments. CK becomes hyperphosphorylated at multiple sites, and hyperphosphorylated CK preferentially accumulates in MBs. Hyperphosphorylation of CK is accompanied by marked overexpression of CK mRNA, which is most pronounced in MB-containing hepatocytes, implying a possible relationship between CK overexpression and MB formation. Biochemical and immunological analyses of MBs revealed that, besides CKs, non-CK components (namely, the stress-inducible M_M 120-1 antigen, a 62-kDa MB component recognized by the antibody SMI 31, and ubiquitin, which is a common constituent of a variety of cytoplasmic inclusions occurring in different chronic degenerative diseases) are present in MB.

The role of these different components in MB formation, as well as the relevance of MBs and the cytoskeletal alterations in the course of AH, was, at least in part, elucidated with the help of CK gene knockout mice. Experiments with these clearly showed that CK8 is the nucleating MB component and that the other non-CK MB components either bind to or coassemble with CK8 in the course of MB formation. It was further shown that MBs by themselves are not detrimental to hepatocytes but can be considered as a product of a defense response involving CK8, and that overexpression of CK enables hepatocytes to better tolerate toxic damage, which is a novel non-structural function of CK. The importance of these findings was underlined by our observation of impressive overexpression of CK8 in human AH.[7]

GENETIC FACTORS

Only a small subpopulation of alcoholics develop severe ALD, and there is no clear relationship between the consumed alcohol dose and the severity of AH. This fact raises the question of whether there is a genetic predisposition for ALD. Modern molecular biologic techniques have allowed identification of genetic polymorphisms for ADH, ALDH, Cytochrome P450, and the TNF-α-promotor.[8,9] Genetic variants of ADH may predispose to higher levels of acetaldehyde after alcohol consumption, which predisposes individuals to ALD. ALDH-polymorphism as found in Asians does protect individuals from heavy drinking because of unpleasant side effects like flushing and such symptoms as headache and nausea that result from accumulation of aceltaldehyde. TNF-α-promotor-polymorphism could make individuals more sensitive to stimuli like LPS because of increased TNF-α production. All of these genetic differences may be important factors influencing the course of ALD, but up to now, we are far away from satisfying answers. Further studies in this direction are warranted, and physicians should put more emphasis on family history in patients suffering from ALD to elucidate the role of genetic risk factors.

GENDER

Women are more susceptible to the toxic effects of alcohol than men and thus more likely to develop AH and cirrhosis at a younger age. Gender-related differences are multifactorial. These differences may be due to different pharmacokinetics of ethanol, which in turn could be a function of the sensitivity of ADH activity to sex hormones. In recent years, data have accumulated on differences in endotoxin sensitivity between female and male animals.[10,11] Endotoxinemia is a common observation in ALD, as mentioned above. Animal models of toxic liver injury have shown a greater susceptibility of female animals with regard to liver damage and mortality. Similarly, application of estrogen in male animals has been shown to enhance toxic effects of LPS. Clinical studies are warranted to confirm these findings in humans.

NUTRITION

Until recently, ALD was believed to be only a consequence of malnutrition. Not all alcoholics are malnourished, nor do all alcoholics develop liver disease.[12] Nevertheless, there is evidence in the literature showing that most alcoholics with ALD are malnourished and nutrition in fact plays a critical role in the pathogenesis of ALD. There are numerous nutritional deficiencies in ALD including: (1) protein-caloric deficiencies via decreased cellular homeostasis and antioxidant defense, (2) lipotropic factors, including deficiencies in choline and methionine, vitamins (B6, B12, E, thiamine, folate), zinc, and selenium. Dietary fat is of special interest in the pathogenensis of ALD. Not only the amount but rather the source and type of fat consumed is critical for the potentiation of the toxic effects of alcohol. Studies have shown a positive correlation between the intake of unsaturated fatty acids and the incidence of cirrhosis. Pathogenetic mechanisms underlying the effect of polyunsaturated fatty acids are currently unknown and the subject of intense research. One can speculate on the role of fatty acids in the induction of the MEOS resulting in enhanced oxidative stress. Another attractive point is the ability of these fatty acids to activate KCs, the important liver macrophage population and main production site of proinflammatory cytokines.

IRON OVERLOAD

The consumption of alcohol affects human iron homeostasis, and hepatic iron overload is a typical finding in ALD. In fact, mild to moderate iron overload is found in 50 to 60% of alcoholic patients.[13] Moreover, consumption of red wine, which contains high levels of iron, is associated with a higher risk of developing ALD. In addition, studies in hereditary hemochromatosis have shown an additive hepatotoxic effect of alcohol resulting in significantly reduced long-term survival.[14] Iron absorption occurs primarily in the proximal small intestine and appears to regulate total body iron balance. Both major proteins of iron metabolism — ferritin and transferrin — are affected by alcohol. The cause of iron overload in alcoholics is unknown but also may be related to ineffective erythropoiesis associated with alcohol-related folate deficiency and sideroblastic abnormalities, or alcohol-related increase in iron absorption with preferential hepatic deposition. The possible cell toxicity of iron is believed to result from its ability to participate in oxidation-reduction reactions. Catalytically active iron may damage and affect multiple cellular substrates such as lipids, proteins, and nucleic acids. Currently, exact mechanisms of iron-induced cellular injury and fibrogenesis are under investigation. Studies regarding the role of heterozygous mutations of the HFE gene, which is responsible for hemochromatosis, in the so-called secondary iron overload in ALD are warranted.

VIRAL HEPATITIS

Concomitant viral infections with hepatitis B and hepatits C (HCV) viruses are known risk factors for development of severe ALD. Alcoholics have an increased incidence of these infections; this may be due to their generally low socioeconomic status or impairment of the immune system function in ALD. Little is known about interactions between viral hepatitis and progression of ALD. Patients infected with HCV and concomitant significant alcohol intake (>40 g alcohol per day in women and >60 g alcohol per day in men for >5 years) have a two- to threefold greater risk of liver cirrhosis and decompensated liver disease.[15] Moreover, patients with ALD and chronic HCV infection have a markedly increased risk to develop hepatocellular carcinoma. Currently, there is great interest regarding the influence of the different HCV genotypes on ALD.

REFERENCES

1. Nanji, A.A. and Zakim, D., Alcoholic liver disease, in *Hepatology: A Textbook of Medicine*, 3rd ed., Zakim, D. and Boyer, T.D, Eds., W.B. Saunders, New York, 1996, 891-940.
2. Lieber, C.S. and De Carli, L.M., Hepatotoxicity of ethanol, *J. Hepatol.*, 12, 394, 1991.
3. Bode, C., Kugler, V., and Bode, J.C., Endotoxemia in patients with alcoholic and non-alcoholic cirrhosis and in subjects with no evidence of chronic liver disease following acute ethanol excess, *J. Hepatol.*, 4, 8, 1987.
4. Bjarson, I., Ward, K., and Peters, T.J., The leaky gut of alcoholism: possible route of entry for toxic compounds, *Lancet*, 1, 179, 1984.
5. McClain, C.J., Hill, D., Schmidt, J., and Diehl, A.M., Cytokines and alcoholic liver disease, *Semin. Liver. Dis.*, 13, 170, 1993.
6. Denk, H., Stumptner, C., and Zatloukal, K., Mallory bodies revisited, *J. Hepatol.*, in press, 2000.
7. Kenner, L., Trauner, M., Fickert, P., Stauber, R.E., Eferl, R., Denk, H., and Zatloukal, K., Overexpression of keratin-8 and -18 RNA is associated with mallory body formation in patients with alcoholic hepatitis, *Hepatology*, 28, Abs. 564, 1998.
8. Crabb, D.W., Biological markers for increased risk of alcoholism and for quantitation of alcohol consumption, *J. Clin. Invest.*, 853, 11, 1990.
9. Grove, J., Daly, A.K., Bassendine, M.F., and Day, C.P., Association of a tumor necrosis factor promotor polymorphism with susceptibility to alcoholic steatohepatitis, *Hepatology*, 26, 143, 1997.
10. Iimuro, Y., Frankenberg, M.V., and Arteel, G.E., Female rats exhibit greater susceptibility to early alcohol-induced induced liver injury than males, *Am. J. Phys.*, 272, 1186, 1997.
11. Ikejima, K., Enomoto, N., Iimuro, Y., et al., Estrogen increases sensitivity of hepatic Kupffer cells to endotoxin, *Am. J. Phys.*, 274, 669, 1998.
12. Carithers, R.L., Alcoholic hepatitis and cirrhosis, *Liver and Biliary Diseases*, 2nd ed., Kaplowitz N., Ed.,Williams & Wilkins, Baltimore, 1996, 377.
13. Bacon, B.R. and Brown, K.E., Iron metabolism and Disorders of Iron Overload, *Liver and Biliary Diseases*, 2nd ed., Kaplowitz N., Ed.,Williams & Wilkins, Baltimore, 1996, 349.

14. Adams, P.C. and Agnew, S., Alcoholism in heriditary hemochromatosis revisited: prevalences and clinical consequences among homocygous siblings, *Hepatology,* 23, 724, 1996.

15. Wiley, T.E., McCarthy, M., Breidi, L., McCathy, M., and Layden, T., Impact of alcohol on the histological and clinical progression of hepatitis C infection, *Hepatology,* 28, 805, 1998.

29 Harmful Alcohol Consumption

Linda Baier Manwell and Michael Fleming

OVERVIEW

A clear dose–response relationship between the level of alcohol use and strokes, liver disease, cancer, and heart disease has been demonstrated in a number of studies. For example, Figure 29.1 summarizes the findings from six studies on the relationship between alcohol use and liver cirrhosis. Persons who drank more than 40 to 60 g per day (three to four standard drinks per day) had a two- to twelve-fold increased risk of liver disease. Overall mortality (including traffic accidents, violent deaths, and cancer) in many epidemiological studies suggests a cut-off of two to four standard drinks per day (i.e., 30 to 60 g per day) for men. Risks for women and older adults appear greater and are reflected in the lower limits of alcohol use recommended for these populations.

RISK AND THE NEW PUBLIC HEALTH PARADIGM

The alcohol field is moving toward a public health harm reduction paradigm and away from an exclusive focus on the identification and treatment of alcoholism and abstinence-based endpoints. The harm reduction paradigm focuses on reducing alcohol use to low-risk levels. This shift is based on three observations. First, most problems related to alcohol use occur in persons who are not alcohol dependent. It is estimated that the ratio of problem drinkers to those severely affected by alcohol is about 3:1 to 4:1.[1] Most people who experience alcohol-related accidents, health problems, or family difficulties do not meet criteria for alcoholism; rather, they simply drink too much, often in high-risk situations.[2-4]

The second observation is that the natural history of recovery is very complicated and does not fit a single model. The classic Jellinek model of progressive disease does not represent the natural history of most persons who drink too much. It is also becoming increasingly clear that many problem drinkers who quit or reduce their use do so without specialized treatment. This is illustrated by a Canadian study to assess the frequency of recovery from alcohol problems with and without treatment.[4] The study included whether recovery involved abstinence or moderate drinking. Investigators examined data from two national studies: the National Alcohol and Drug Survey (n = 11,634) and the Ontario Alcohol and Drug Opinion Survey (n = 1034). Both studies were conducted by random sample telephone interview. They found that 78% of the problem drinkers in sample 1 and 78% in sample 2 reported recovery for at least 1 year with no treatment. They also found that 38% of the problem drinkers in sample 1 and 63% in sample 2 were able to resume drinking at low-risk levels.

Other studies suggest that just asking a problem drinker about alcohol consumption can reduce use.[5,6] These findings parallel a large body of research showing that 80 to 90% of smokers who quit do so on their own with minimal professional intervention.[7]

A third observation is the use of a new term, "at-risk drinking," which has emerged in place of the terms "hazardous" or "heavy" drinking. The term "risk" is intended to place heavy alcohol use in the context of other health risks such as high blood pressure, elevated cholesterol, or high blood sugar levels. Not all patients with elevated blood pressure or cholesterol or blood sugar will develop a stroke, ischemic heart disease, or kidney failure, but they are clearly at greater risk than

0-8493-7801-X/00/$0.00+$.50
© 2000 by CRC Press LLC

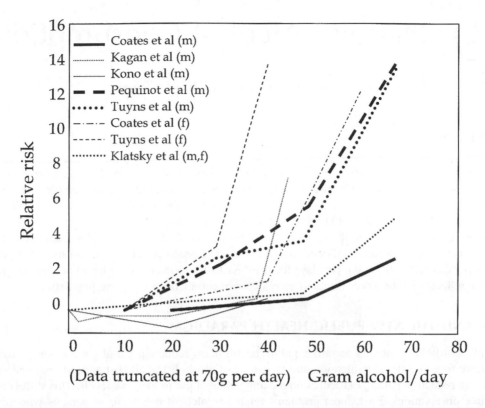

FIGURE 29.1   Relationship between alcohol use and liver cirrhosis: a summary of the findings from six studies. (From Anderson, P., Cremona, A., Paton, A., Turner, C., and Wallace, P., *Addiction,* 88, 1493, 1993. With permission.)

persons with a normal blood pressure or cholesterol level or blood sugar. Similarly, we know that many persons who drink alcohol above recommended limits do not develop liver disease or other medical problems related to their alcohol use, but they are at greater risk than people with lower consumption levels. By utilizing terms such as "risk," we place heavy drinking in the context of a health risk that can be identified and treated by primary health care providers.

The definition of "at-risk" use is based on the dose-response relationship discussed in the beginning of this chapter. As stated before, Figure 29.1 illustrates a dose-response relationship between alcohol use and liver cirrhosis. Figure 29.2 depicts the association between alcohol consumption and mortality in young men, mostly aged 18–19. The relative risk of death among men with a high consumption of alcohol (>250 g/wk) was 3.0 compared with those who had moderate consumption (1-100 g/wk). After adjustment for social background variables, the relative risk was reduced to 2.1.

DEFINITION OF "AT-RISK," "HARMFUL," AND "DEPENDENT" ALCOHOL USE

The terms "heavy" drinkers, "hazardous" drinkers, and "at-risk" drinkers are often used interchangeably. The term "at-risk" is preferred as it fits in the context of other health concerns such as elevated blood pressure, cholesterol, or blood sugar. For the purpose of this chapter, "at-risk" drinkers are defined as men who drink more than 14 standard drinks per week (12 g alcohol per drink or >168 g per week), or more than four drinks per occasion one or more times per week; and women who drink more than seven drinks per week (>98 g alcohol per week), or more than three drinks per

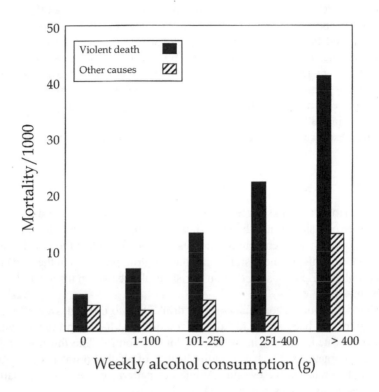

FIGURE 29.2 Association between alcohol consumption and 15-year mortality among young men. (From Andreasson, S., Allebeck, P., and Romelsjo, A., Alcohol and mortality among young men: longitudinal study of Swedish conscripts, *Br. Med. J.,* 296, 1021, 1988. With permission.)

occasion one or more times per week. These criteria are recommended by the U.S. National Institute on Alcohol Abuse and Alcoholism (NIAAA).[10] Persons who drink less than these limits are considered "low-risk" drinkers unless they are drinking during pregnancy, in the presence of certain medical problems such as diabetes, or in high-risk situations such as when operating machinery or driving a motorized vehicle.

The limits described above are based on conservative estimates of alcohol and risk.[8] There is no widespread agreement on a definition of "at-risk alcohol use." The NIAAA uses lower limits than many other countries. Most research in the United Kingdom uses higher consumption limits: greater than 21 drinks per week for men, greater than 14 drinks per week for women, and greater than 5 drinks per occasion for either men or women. The grams of alcohol per standard drink also vary widely by country, ranging from 8 to 14 grams. For example, England has 8 g alcohol per glass of beer and North America has up to 14 g alcohol per standard drink.

"Harmful" alcohol use is defined using ICD-10 criteria, which specifies a "pattern of alcohol use that is causing both physical or mental damage to health." The criteria requires that actual damage has occurred to the physical or mental health of the user. Other terms that are used interchangeably include "alcohol abuse" or "problem drinking." "Harmful" drinking is preferred over "alcohol abuse" due to the moralistic connotation of the word "abuse" and the need to focus on a harm reduction model. The definition of "alcohol abuse" using DSM-IV criteria[11] is broader and less specific than ICD-10 criteria. To meet a definition of alcohol abuse, the patient needs to meet at least one of the following four criteria in the previous 12 months: (1) continued alcohol use despite recurring problems; (2) recurrent use in hazardous situations; (3) drinking resulting in failure to fulfill major role obligations; or (4) recurrent legal problems. Persons who do not meet these criteria, but who drink above recommended limits, are considered at-risk drinkers.

Persons who meet ICD-10 criteria for dependent alcohol use must meet three of the following seven criteria: (1) tolerance; (2) withdrawal; (3) loss of control; (4) progressive neglect of alternative activities; (5) increased time spent on obtaining alcohol or recovering from use; (6) persistent drinking despite evidence of harm; (7) a compulsion to drink. While there are some minor differences between ICD-10 and DSM-IV criteria for alcohol dependence, for the purposes of this chapter, we will consider them to be the same.[12] Other terms for alcohol dependence include "alcoholism" and "addiction." These terms should be used carefully due to the moral, social, and employment implications of such labels.

The following case examples illustrate persons who meet criteria for at-risk, harmful, and dependent drinking.

AT-RISK DRINKERS

Michael is a physician who drinks three to four times per week with friends. He usually drinks five to six drinks per occasion. While he sometimes becomes intoxicated, he rarely drives his car until the alcohol is out of his system. He has no health problems related to his alcohol use and has no risk factors (no family history, no history of alcohol or drug problems in the past) for developing alcohol-related problems. He is classified as an at-risk drinker based on his level of use and absence of alcohol problems.

Christina is a 45-year-old school teacher who drinks two to three glasses of wine with dinner daily. Her use pattern has been stable for about 10 years. She has no problems with her level of use, never gets intoxicated, and has no history of loss of control. She did use alcohol, however, during both of her pregnancies. She has a family history of alcohol problems. She says she drinks to relieve stress and to relax in the evening. While her pattern of use is stable, daily alcohol use above recommended limits places her in the at-risk category.

HARMFUL ALCOHOL USE

Karl is a 35-year-old farmer who drinks three to six beers every day when he has finished his farm chores. He has a history of high blood pressure and chronic epigastric pain that responded to ranitidine. While he does not get visibly drunk, his family has been complaining about his heavy alcohol use and has asked him to stop. His blood pressure measurements over a 3-month period ranged from 160/110 to 140/98. A laboratory exam revealed an elevated GGT. He remains abstinent 6 months after his physician and family confronted him. His blood pressure problems and epigastric pain have resolved. Karl is considered a former harmful drinker based on his history of high blood pressure, epigastric pain, and heavy use.

Maria is a 25-year-old unmarried graduate student who drinks four to five beers two or three times per week. She was recently treated in the emergency room for a head injury. She reportedly slipped on a patch of ice outside her apartment. She gets drunk about once per week and occasionally drives herself home while intoxicated. The emergency department physician has told her to limit her alcohol use to one or two drinks per occasion and to see her regular health care provider if she has any problems reducing her drinking. Maria is considered a harmful drinker based on her history of injury, driving while drunk, and heavy use.

ALCOHOL DEPENDENT

John is a 32-year-old unmarried lawyer. In the past 2 years, he has had two serious motor vehicle accidents while drinking. He drinks three to four times per week and usually stops at five to six drinks. He is a hard-working district attorney who was recently nominated to serve as an appellate court judge. He always drives himself home, even when drunk. While he sometimes drinks alone, he usually drinks with colleagues after work and at parties on weekends. He has a history of depression and two hospitalizations for fractures occurring in alcohol-related car accidents. He does not have a personal physician; the orthopedic surgeon who set his fractures confronted him. John denied any problems related to his drinking and refused to abstain or get help. The next year, while intoxicated, John was involved in an accident involving a fatality. John meets criteria for alcohol dependence based on multiple accidents, heavy use, denial, and lack of control.

REFERENCES

1. Institute of Medicine, Division of Mental Health and Behavioral Medicine, *Broadening the Base of Treatment for Alcohol Problems,* National Academy Press, Washington, D.C., 1990.
2. Fuchs, C.S., Stampfer, M.J., Colditz, G.A., et al. Alcohol consumption and mortality among women. *N. Engl. J. Med.,* 332, 1245, 1995.
3. Gentilello, L.M., Cobean, R.A., Walker, A.P., Moore, E.E., Wertz, M.J., and Dellinger, E.P., Acute ethanol intoxication increases the risk of infection following penetrating abdominal trauma, *J. Trauma,* 34, 669, 1993.
4. Sobell, L.C., Cunningham, J.A., and Sobell, M.B., Recovery from alcohol problems with and without treatment: prevalence in two populations surveys, *Am. J. Public Health,* 86, 966, 1996.
5. Bien, T.H., Miller, W.R., and Tonigan, J.S., Brief interventions for alcohol problems: a review, *Addiction,* 88, 315, 1993.
6. Fleming, M.F., Barry, K.L., Manwell, L.B., Johnson, K., and London, R., Brief physician advice for problem alcohol drinkers: a randomized controlled trial in community-based primary care practices, *JAMA,* 277, 1039, 1997.
7. Fiore, M.C., Ed., *Smoking Cessation. Clinical Practice Guideline Number 18.* U.S. Department of Health and Human Services, Agency for Health Care Policy and Research, Centers for Disease Control and Prevention, AHCPR Publication No. 96-0692, 1996.
8. Anderson, P., Cremona, A., Paton, A., Turner, C., and Wallace, P., The risk of alcohol, *Addiction,* 88, 1493, 1993.
9. Andreasson, S., Allbeck, P., and Romelsjo, A., Alcohol and mortality among young men: longitudinal study of Swedish conscripts, *Br. Med. J.,* 296, 1021, 1988.
10. National Institute on Alcohol Abuse and Alcoholism, *The Physicians' Guide to Helping Patients with Alcohol Problems,* U.S. Department of Health and Human Services, Public Health Service, National Institutes of Health, 1995, NIH publication no. 95-3769. http://silk.nih.gov/silk/niaaa1/publication/physicn.htm.
11. American Psychiatric Association, *Diagnostic and Statistical Manual of Mental Disorders,* 4th ed., Washington, D.C., APA, 1994. *J. Trauma,* 34, 669, 1993.
12. Grant, B.F., DSM-IV, DSM-III-R, and ICD-10 alcohol and drug abuse/harmful use and dependence, United States, 1992: a nosological comparison, *Alcohol. Clin. Exp. Res.,* 20, 1481, 1996.

30 Psychometric Instruments to Evaluate Outcome in Alcoholism Treatment

Andrea C. King, Peter A. Vanable, and Harriet de Wit

OVERVIEW

What precisely determines treatment success is still an open question in the field of addiction research. Alcohol dependence has been defined largely as a chronic relapsing disorder. Developments have been made in the last 20 years in treatment options for alcohol-dependent patients, providing a range of treatment goals and therapeutic modalities. The continued refinement of psychometric instruments to reliably assess alcoholism treatment outcome is crucial to these efforts to enhance treatment effectiveness. In contrast to more traditional procedures to define success as 100% continuous abstinence, newer and more innovative measures are available to determine psychosocial consequences and alcohol-related diagnoses, precise drinking patterns, and other important constructs such as post-treatment alcohol craving and stage of change. This chapter highlights various psychometric instruments used in large-scale clinical trials with the focus on practical applications for use in various clinic settings. Most of these psychometric instruments can be found in an alphabetical list in Chapter 44.

INTRODUCTION

One of the most difficult aspects of evaluating the effectiveness of treatment for substance use disorders is how one defines outcome. Comparisons across distinct treatment modalities can be largely a product of when, how, and by what method a researcher uses to assess outcome. Although advances have been made in the past 10 to 20 years in developing sensitive and standard assessment tools for alcoholism treatment, there is currently no single gold-standard instrument or questionnaire to evaluate treatment effectiveness. Historically, treatment outcome in alcoholism trials was largely defined in narrow terms, such as evaluating self-reports of 100% continuous abstinence. Treatment success rates using this restrictive definition were relatively low and did not take into account the relapsing nature of this disorder and/or gains made in other areas of functioning. In addition, the emergence of newer treatment modalities using a harm reduction model (i.e., in which the goal is a reduction in drinking and/or hazardous consequences rather than strict abstinence) underscored the importance of employing outcome measures more consistent with the goals of treatment.

The development of more comprehensive and flexible outcome measures has aided clinical researchers in determining a variety of clinically relevant endpoint measures. Objective measures and biomarkers of chronic and recent alcohol drinking, such as liver enzyme levels, mean corpuscular volume, and carbohydrate-deficient transferrin tests, have been used with some success as a measure of outcome. However, the specificity of such laboratory results is relatively low, as other medical conditions can elevate these biological indicators.[1] Urine toxicology and/or breathalyzer recordings have occasionally been used in conjunction with outcome assessment instruments.

However, these are rarely used alone because they only detect recent use and do not provide information on overall trends in use, psychosocial impairment, and consequences of drinking.

The psychometric tools currently used in published alcoholism treatment studies include interviews (diagnostic or comprehensive evaluation of alcohol and other relevant areas of functioning) and questionnaires (assessing alcohol drinking parameters, symptoms of the alcohol dependence syndrome, and subjective alcohol craving). This chapter describes and compares features of the most commonly used psychometric instruments to assess alcohol treatment. This information can guide clinicians and researchers in evaluating the literature on clinical trials outcome research and can also inform practitioners as to which instruments might be most useful for evaluating the success of their own treatment programs.

STRUCTURED CLINICAL INTERVIEW
FOR DSM-IV DISORDERS (SCID)

The Structured Clinical Interview for DSM-IV Disorders (SCID)[2] is a semi-structured clinical interview that assesses clinical disorders listed in the American Psychiatric Association's Diagnostic and Statistical Manual for Mental Disorders, or DSM-IV.[3] The SCID is a clinical interview to determine current and lifetime prevalence of the major mental disorders in the DSM, including a comprehensive module on alcohol and drug use disorders. The SCID is typically administered by a master's or Ph.D. level clinician and can be used in both research and clinical settings to establish diagnoses at the outset of treatment and at follow-up. The SCID has been shown to be a reliable and valid instrument in substance abuse populations.[4]

The substance use disorders section of the SCID, or "Module E," takes approximately 15 minutes to administer. If time does not permit administering the full SCID, Module E can be administered as a stand-alone assessment tool. One drawback to administering only Module E is that related lifetime comorbid psychiatric diagnoses, which are estimated to occur in approximately one third of alcoholics,[5,6] cannot be determined.

The interview format for the SCID Module E includes an initial screen for evidence of any lifetime excessive drinking, followed by items for specific diagnoses of Alcohol Abuse and Dependence, and course specifiers (i.e., partial vs. full remission; early vs. sustained). Each item is scored 1 (not present), 2 (mildly present or unclear), or 3 (present). A rating of "3" on three or more of the seven listed criteria for alcohol dependence indicates a positive diagnosis. Again, the SCID also contains items to establish diagnosis of alcohol abuse if dependence is not warranted.

The advantages to using either the full SCID or SCID Module E include achieving definitive DSM-related diagnoses at baseline and during various treatment intervals. With the SCID, a clinician or researcher has carefully assessed core clinical features and widely used, standardized diagnoses, without the unnecessary burden of using secondary measures or questionnaires with which to infer diagnoses. One of the main disadvantages of the SCID in practical terms is that it should be administered by a trained clinician, and is therefore more costly than self-report, questionnaire outcome measures in terms of the time and cost needed to conduct the interview. In addition, the SCID does not provide detailed information on the absolute amount, frequency, patterns of use, or situational factors related to alcohol drinking.

ADDICTION SEVERITY INDEX (ASI)

The Addiction Severity Index (ASI)[7,8] is perhaps the most comprehensive outcome assessment instrument and has been widely used for the evaluation of large-scale clinical trials for alcohol and drug dependence. The ASI has been in use for nearly 20 years and is currently in its fifth edition. It is a 45- to 60-minute semi-structured interview delivered by a trained technician at baseline (i.e., before treatment) and at follow-up intervals. The ASI assesses recent (last 30 days) and lifetime problems in seven substance use-related areas. The ASI has been shown to be a reliable and valid instrument (for review, see Reference 8) and has been used in a variety of treatment contexts and patient subpopulations. In addition, the ASI has been translated into 14 languages, making it suitable for use with a variety of non-English-speaking patient populations.

A trained technician typically administers the ASI to the patient in an individual interview format. The ASI assesses seven areas of functioning, including alcohol use, drug use, family/social, psychiatric, employment, medical, and legal status. Scoring for the ASI includes an overall severity index as well as composite scores for each of the separate areas of functioning. This instrument provides a broad range of clinical information, including information about alcohol and drug use and about employment and family functioning. This breadth of information permits the clinician or researcher to evaluate treatment success therefore in a variety of substance and nonsubstance areas of functioning.

The primary disadvantage of the ASI, like the SCID, is that it must be administered by a trained person, and is therefore more costly than self-report outcome measures. Moreover, ASI interviewers must undergo specific training. Potential interviewers must have the ability to establish rapport with the patient and to adequately probe or restate questions. ASI interviewers may be trained using the Instruction Manual and Fifth Edition of the ASI[8] or attend an on-site training seminar (University of Pennsylvania, Philadelphia, PA). Another potential disadvantage of the ASI (also like the SCID) is that it measures frequency, but not quantity, of alcohol and drug use, and therefore might provide inadequate information for treatments designed to target drinking moderation or reduction in harmful use.

ALCOHOL DEPENDENCE SCALE (ADS)

The Alcohol Dependence Scale (ADS)[9,10] is a 25-item questionnaire assessing severity of alcohol-related symptomatology. It can be administered in approximately 5 minutes by either self-report (paper-and-pencil or computer testing) or interview with a technician. The items comprising the ADS were derived from the 147-item Alcohol Use Inventory[11] and encompass four key aspects of the dependence syndrome, including loss of behavioral control (e.g., gulping drinks), psychoperceptual disturbance during withdrawal (e.g., hallucinations), physiological withdrawal symptoms (e.g., hangover, delirium tremens), and compulsive drinking patterns (e.g., sneaking drinks).

The philosophy of the ADS is based on the *alcohol dependence syndrome* originally proposed by Edwards and Gross,[12] conceiving alcoholism as existing along a severity continuum rather than as a unitary categorical diagnosis. The item format reflects this distinction: questions are worded with choice responses along a dichotomous, three-, or four-choice range with individual item scores ranging from 0 to 4. The total ADS score ranges from 0 to 47, with a total score greater than 9 being highly predictive of a DSM diagnosis of alcohol dependence.[13]

Advantages of the ADS include its theoretical base and relative ease of use. The ADS can also allow the practitioner to measure symptoms of alcohol dependence at baseline and follow-up by altering the instructions to include symptoms present in the 12 months preceding treatment and at 6-month intervals during and after treatment cessation. The disadvantages of the ADS mainly include that it is strictly focused on measuring alcohol-related disability and symptoms of withdrawal, which diverge slightly from the most recent focus on DSM-IV criteria of alcohol dependence, defined less by the physiological and more by psychosocial consequences of use.

OBSESSIVE-COMPULSIVE DRINKING SCALE (OCDS)

The 14-item Obsessive-Compulsive Drinking Scale (OCDS) is a recently developed self-report inventory of cognitive and behavioral dimensions of alcohol craving.[14,15] Although a precise definition of what constitutes "craving" has yet to be determined, most clinical researchers acknowledge that recurrent alcohol-related urges and thoughts are important features of the disorder and are likely to be related to outcome.[14] The ICD-10, i.e., the most recent version of the International Classification of Diseases, includes craving in its conceptualization of alcohol dependence, while the DSM-IV lists the "inability to cut down or control alcohol consumption" as a core feature, with craving described as a common related phenomenon. The importance of the craving concept has been recently underscored with the advent of potentially useful pharmacological adjuncts, such as opioid antagonists, which are speculated to attenuate alcohol craving as part of their therapeutic effect. Historically, craving has been measured by unitary visual-analog scales, leaving the burden of what is meant by craving up to the patient.

The key components of alcohol craving (i.e., compulsive drive to consume alcohol, recurrent and persistent thoughts, and attempts to control this condition) have been suggested to be similar to the core features of obsessive-compulsive illness.[12,16,17] This concept led researchers to develop the OCDS, which was derived from the Yale-Brown Obsessive-Compulsive Scale and its related version for heavy drinkers.[16-19] Each of the 14 items on the scale are scored from 0 to 4, with the inclusion of four split items with only the higher of the two scored items to be used in the total score. The OCDS total score ranges from 0 to 40. Test-retest reliability and validity (i.e., strong correlation to the ADS and ASI alcohol scale) for the OCDS have been established.[14,15] In addition, the OCDS appears to represent an independent domain of alcohol dependence, given its low shared variance with the ASI and ADS, and is also sensitive to treatment response.[14] Scores on the OCDS are lower during early stages of abstinence (75% reduction in total score during first 2 weeks of sobriety), with the highest scores remaining in those who relapse to drinking.

The advantages of the OCDS include that it is an easily obtained (~5 min) self-report measure of an independent domain of alcohol dependence and can be given at baseline and at different treatment intervals to assess improvement during the clinical treatment process. One disadvantage of the OCDS is that there are no established threshold or cut-off scores to indicate clinically significant changes. Also, patients who exhibit largely concrete thought patterns or who are particularly defensive about their alcohol use may not endorse items reflecting recurrent preoccupation with drinking, despite continued alcohol dependence.

TIMELINE FOLLOW-BACK (TLFB) AND QUANTITY-FREQUENCY (QF) MEASURES

Simply stated, one of the principal goals of alcohol treatment is to modify drinking behavior. Therefore, careful assessment of alcohol consumption pre- and post-treatment is important. Two general types of primary drinking measures have been developed for these purposes:[20] the Time-Line Follow-Back (TLFB)[21,22] and Quantity-Frequency (QF)[23,24] methods. Both scales have been used extensively in outcome trials, and can be used in an interview format or by self-administration. These direct alcohol consumption instruments take into consideration the complexities of the amount, type, frequency, and associated patterns of alcohol consumption. Although beyond the scope of this chapter, the Form-90[25] is an extensive instrument combining the techniques of TLFB and QF and developed specifically for use in a recent large multi-site alcoholism treatment trial called Project MATCH.[26]

The Alcohol TLFB is a reliable and valid calendar assessment of drinking estimates over a specified time course (i.e., 1 month, 3 months, 1 year, etc.). Unlike the previously discussed scales, which comprise listed items to derive either a diagnosis or a severity score, the TLFB is a retrospective calendar-based technique where numerous outcome measures can be extracted. These include calculating the percent days abstinent, number of drinks consumed per drinking occasion, and number or percent days of alcohol withdrawal. Typically, the TLFB is conducted with an interviewer to help patients use anchor points (holidays, important life events, etc.) and other memory aids for enhancing recall of drinking and sober days. This method is especially relevant in evaluating treatment outcome and comparisons across treatments, where precise estimates of alcohol consumption pre- and post-treatment are needed.

The advantages of the TLFB method are its relative flexibility, ease of use, and low-to-moderate training required. The TLFB can be a particularly useful method for assessing drinkers with variable alcohol use patterns, such as binge drinkers, because alterations in drinking pattern can be estimated and identified. Although the TLFB can provide various precise drinking outcome measures, its shortcomings include that other related drinking factors, such as consequences and psychosocial effects, and information related to diagnoses, are not measured.

The QF instruments usually derive estimates of *typical* alcohol drinking and are among the earliest developed techniques to assess alcoholism treatment outcome. Currently, there are over six versions of the QF measurement, which can create confusion for the clinical researcher. The major differences among these QF scales are their emphasis on *usual* vs. *variable* alcohol consumption patterns and the ranges employed to define "very heavy" alcohol drinking occurrences. In general, QF scales determine recent typical patterns for each alcohol beverage type, and then employ calculations to derive an aggregate alcohol consumption index. As with TLFB, the time period of interest is flexible, depending on the desired pre- and post-treatment interval (i.e., 1 month, 3 months, 1 year, etc.).

The largest criticism of QF scales is that although they provide reliable information about total consumption and number of drinking days, they are usually not sensitive to occasional high and low consumption days. Sporadic or binge drinkers, therefore, are often underreported by QF measures. Some QF scales have attempted to overcome this limitation by adding additional items to discern maximum drinking days and frequency. By adding items to inquire about such occurrences, however, the instrument may lose two of its advantages, its brevity and ease of use. Another limitation of QF measures is that physical and psychosocial consequences of drinking cannot be ascertained. These limitations notwithstanding, QF measures are commonly used in clinical studies, and are particularly useful in assessing quantity and frequency of alcohol use in severely alcohol-dependent persons, since variability of drinking pattern is potentially less of an issue with this subgroup than with alcohol abusers or problematic users.

READINESS TO CHANGE MEASURES

For patients who misuse alcohol but are not severely dependent, treatment may consist of modalities other than the traditional abstinence-based methods. For example, in recent years, there has been increasing interest in the use of harm reduction, alcohol drinking moderation, and stages of change-based treatment for individuals not ready to consider a goal of sobriety. There is growing recognition that briefer and flexible interventions are needed to suit this population of patients. The previously mentioned consumption, diagnostic, and severity inventories may be of limited value in ascertaining treatment effectiveness and/or outcome in these patients.

Several useful instruments have been recently developed for applications to motivation-based and brief interventions. These scales assess a client's stage of change, based on the model proposed by Prochaska and DiClemente,[27,28] which posits that individuals go through sequential stages when considering changing a target behavior. Two of these scales are The Stages of Change Readiness and Treatment Eagerness Scale (SOCRATES)[29] and the University of Rhode Island Change Assessment Scale (URICA).[30,31] However, the shortest and perhaps most convenient of the change assessment scales is the Readiness to Change Questionnaire (RTCQ).[32,33] This brief 12-item questionnaire can be self-administered in approximately 5 minutes and, because of its ease of use and breadth of applications, has been used in a variety of clinical settings, including general medical practice.

The RTCQ identifies three stages of change: *precontemplation* = no plans to change behavior; *contemplation* = consider making a change; and *action* = taking necessary steps and implementing change. The highest score indicates the current stage for the patient. Thus, in contrast to the traditional treatment outcome instruments, the RTCQ does not yield information on consumption patterns or consequences of use, or severity of dependence. Rather, this instrument is used strictly to identify the patient's current stage of change. Obtaining such a measure is particularly important for motivationally based interventions, which aim to help move a patient along the stages of change in order to effectively alter drinking behavior. In practical terms, this is an easily attained instrument and can be given at treatment onset and at regular post-treatment follow-ups.

This scale is frequently used as an outcome measure to help discern whether a particular intervention has helped to move a patient along this continuum of change (e.g., precontemplation to contemplation or action stage). Some studies suggest that the longer a patient remains in a particular stage, the more unlikely he/she is to progress to making the necessary behavioral change.[28] Additionally, stage of change has been shown to have significant predictive validity for outcome, as indicated by significant positive correlation with alcohol consumption behavior at follow-up.[34] The RTCQ and its related measures are rarely used alone, but rather, in concert with other drinking-related measures to help clinicians and researchers determine other outcome determinants that more closely match the purposes of the intervention.

CONCLUSIONS

In determining whether a particular intervention for any disorder is efficacious, it is first important to understand the common features associated with the disorder. For alcohol use disorders, continued clinical research will help yield more effective, targeted, and clinically validated treatments to match a particular patient's needs. Along with these efforts, it is vital for clinical researchers to apply sensitive and comprehensive assessments in order to determine a variety of treatment outcome dimensions.

This chapter reviewed treatment instruments in four distinct categories of outcome: diagnoses, severity of dependence, primary drinking measures, and newer conceptual areas, such as intensity of alcohol craving and readiness to change. At present, it is recommended that a combination of several of these measures be utilized to determine outcome for a particular program or clinic. Selection of instruments can be determined by both treatment goals and philosophy as well as by practical factors, such as time availability, staff training, and financial issues. As with most areas of mental health treatment, demonstrating treatment efficacy will be necessary for program viability. For the allied health practitioner, consideration of outcome will also aid in assessing effectiveness and/or meeting the particular needs of any patient population in alcohol and drug use disorders. Awareness of the multidimensional nature of alcohol treatment "outcome" and various techniques to measure outcome is the first step in developing more effective, targeted treatments and ongoing evaluation of these treatments.

ACKNOWLEDGMENTS

This work was supported by NIAAA (#AA11133-02) and the Alcohol Beverage Medical Research Foundation.

REFERENCES

1. Salaspuro, M., Biological state markers of alcohol abuse, *Alcohol Health Res. World,* 18, 131, 1994.
2. First, M.B., Spitzer, R.L., Gibbon, M., and Williams, J.B.W., Structured Clinical Interview for DSM-IV Axis I Disorders — Patient Edition (SCID-I/P, Version 2.0), Biometrics Research Department, New York, 1995.

3. American Psychiatric Association, *Diagnostic and Statistical Manual of Mental Disorders*, 4th ed., American Psychiatric Association, Washington, D.C., 1994.

4. Kranzler, H.R., Kadden, R.M., Babor, T.F., and Rounsaville, B.J., Validity of the SCID in substance abuse patients, *Addiction*, 91, 859, 1996.

5. Penick, E.C., Powell, B.J., Nickel, E.J., Bingham, S.E., Riesenmy, K.R., Read, M.R., and Campbell, J., Co-morbidity of lifetime psychiatric disorder among male alcoholic patients, *Alcohol. Clin. Exp. Res.*, 18, 1289, 1994.

6. Regier, D.A., Farmer, M.E., Rae, D.S., Locke, B.Z., Keith, S.J., Judd, L.L., and Goodwin, F.K., Comorbidity of mental disorders with alcohol and other drug abuse: results from the Epidemiologic Catchment Area (ECA) Study, *JAMA*, 264, 2511, 1990.

7. McLellan, A.T., Luborsky, L., O'Brien, C.P., and Woody, G.E., An improved diagnostic instrument for substance abuse patients: the Addiction Severity Index, *J. Nerv. Ment. Dis.*, 168, 26, 1980.

8. McLellan, A.T., Kushner, H., Metzger, D., Peters, R., Smith, I., Grisson, G., Pettinati, H., and Argeriou, M., The fifth edition of the Addiction Severity Index, *J. Subst. Abuse Treatment*, 9, 199, 1992.

9. Skinner, H.A. and Allen, B.A., Alcohol dependence syndrome: measurement and validation, *J. Abnorm. Psychol.*, 91, 199, 1982.

10. Skinner, H.A. and Horn, J.L., *Alcohol Dependence Scale: Users Guide*, Addiction Research Foundation, Toronto, 1984.

11. Horn, J.L., Wanberg, K.W., and Foster, F.M., *The Alcohol Use Inventory*, Center for Alcohol Abuse Research and Evaluation, Denver, CO, 1974.

12. Edwards, G. and Gross, M.M., Alcohol dependence: provisional description of a clinical syndrome, *Br. Med. J.*, 1, 1058, 1976.

13. Ross, H.E., Gavin, D.R., and Skinner, H.A., Diagnostic validity of the MAST and Alcohol Dependence Scale in the assessment of DSM-III alcohol disorders, *J. Stud. Alcohol*, 51, 506, 1990.

14. Anton, R.F, Moak, D.H., and Latham, P.K., The Obsessive Compulsive Drinking Scale: a new method of assessing outcome in alcoholism treatment, *Arch. Gen. Psychiatry*, 53, 225, 1996.

15. Moak, D.H., Anton, R.F., and Latham, P.K., Further validation of the Obsessive-Compulsive Drinking Scale (OCDS): relationship to alcoholism severity, *Am. J. Addictions*, 7, 14, 1998.

16. Modell, J.G., Glaser, F.B., Mountz, J.M., Schmaltz, S., and Cyr, L., Obsessive and compulsive characteristics of alcohol abuse and dependence: quantification by a newly developed questionnaire, *Alcohol. Clin. Exp. Res.*, 16, 266, 1992.

17. Modell, J.G., Glaser, F.B., Cyr, L., and Mountz, J.M., Obsessive and compulsive characteristics of craving for alcohol in alcohol abuse and dependence, *Alcohol. Clin. Exp. Res.*, 16, 272, 1992.

18. Goodman, W.K., Price, L.H., Rasmussen, S.A., Mazure, C. Delgado, P., Heninger, G.R., and Charney, D.S., The Yale-Brown Obsessive Compulsive Scale I: development, use, and reliability, *Arch. Gen. Psychiatry*, 46, 1006, 1989.

19. Goodman, W.K., Price, L.H., Rasmussen, S.A., Mazure, C. Delgado, P., Heninger, G.R., and Charney, D.S., The Yale-Brown Obsessive Compulsive Scale II: validity, *Arch. Gen. Psychiatry*, 46, 1012, 1989.

20. Sobell, L.C. and Sobell, M.B., Alcohol consumption measures, *Assessing Alcohol Problems: A Guide for Clinicians and Researchers*, NIAAA Treatment Handbook Series 4, USDHHS, Bethesda, MD, 1995.

21. Sobell, L.C. and Sobell, M.B., *Alcohol Timeline Follow-Back Users' Manual*, Addiction Research Foundation, Toronto, 1995.

22. Sobell, L.C., Maisto, S.A., Sobell, M.B., and Cooper, A.M., Reliability of alcohol abusers' self-reports of drinking behavior, *Behav. Res. Ther.*, 17, 157, 1979.

23. Cahalan, V., Cisin, I., and Crossley, H.M., *American Drinking Practices*, Rutgers Center for Alcohol Studies, New Brunswick, NJ, 1969.

24. Straus, R. and Bacon, S.D., *Drinking in College*, Yale University Press, New Haven, CT, 1953.

25. Miller, W.R., Form 90: a structured assessment interview for drinking and related behaviors test manual, Project MATCH Monograph Series Vol. 5, USDHHS, Bethesda, MD, 1996.

26. Miller, W.R. and Del Boca, F. K., Measurement of drinking behavior using the Form 90 family of instruments, *J. Stud. Alcohol*, Suppl. 12, 112, 1994.

27. Prochaska, J.O. and DiClemente, C.D., Toward a comprehensive model of change, Miller, W.R. and Heather, N., Eds., *Treating Addictive Behaviors: Processes of Change*, Plenum, New York, 3, 1986.

28. Prochaska, J.O., DiClemente, C., and Norcross, J.C., In search of how people change: applications to addictive behaviors, *Am. Psychologist,* 47, 1102, 1992.

29. Miller, W.R. and Tonigan J.S., Assessing drinkers' motivation for change: The Stages of Change Readiness and Treatment Eagerness Scale (SOCRATES), unpublished manuscript, Center on Alcoholism, Substance Abuse, and Addictions, University of New Mexico, Albuquerque, NM, 1994.

30. DiClemente, C.C. and Hughes, S.O., Stages of change profiles in outpatient alcoholism treatment, *J. Subst. Abuse,* 2, 217, 1990.

31. McConnaughy, E.A., Prochaska, J.O., and Velicer, W.F., Stages of change in psychotherapy: measurement and sample profiles, *Psychother. Theory Res. Pract.,* 20, 368, 1983.

32. Heather, N., Gold, R., and Rollnick, S., Readiness to Change Questionnaire: User's Manual, Technical Report 15, National Drug and Alcohol Research Centre, University of New South Wales, Kensington, Australia, 1991.

33. Rollnick, S., Heather, N., Gold, R., and Hall, W., Development of a short "Readiness to Change" questionnaire for use in brief opportunistic interventions, *Br. J. Addict.,* 87, 743, 1992.

34. Heather, N., Rollnick, S., and Bell, A., Predicitive validity of the Readiness to Change Questionnaire, *Addiction*, 88, 1667, 1993.

31 Meta-Analysis of Pharmacotherapeutic Trials

Claudia Schoechlin and Rolf R. Engel

OVERVIEW

During the last years, developments in relapse prevention in alcoholism were presented mainly in the field of pharmacological treatment. A meta-analysis of 18 placebo-controlled, randomized clinical trials was performed; this analysis included 2658 patients with a minimum duration of 3 months on drugs tested for their effectiveness in decreasing alcohol consumption or preventing relapse in alcohol-dependent patients (acamprosate, atenolol, bromocriptine, buspirone, citalopram, fenfluramine, γ-hydroxybutyrate (GHB), nalmefene, naltrexone, and tiapride). Effect sizes ranged between r = –0.09 and 0.65, corresponding to drug-placebo response rate differences of about 10% in favor of placebo and 65% in favor of drugs. Studies including non-detoxified patients showed higher effect sizes than studies with detoxified patients. Higher efficacy was found with controlled drinking as response criterion and for quantitative measures (e.g., drinking days) compared to abstinence and qualitative measures (relapse), respectively. The number of patients treated with the individual substances differs; therefore, comparison of substances concerning efficacy must be interpreted with caution. The largest data pool came from studies with acamprosate (1785 of 2658 patients). Compounds, in general, revealed to be superior to placebo in the relapse prevention in alcohol dependence, which means that they are effective. The available data are not sufficient to permit definitive conclusions on differences between the substances. Study design variables may influence the results; studies on detoxified patients, for example, yield lower effect sizes than studies on nondetoxified patients.

INTRODUCTION: CONCEPTS OF RELAPSE PREVENTION IN ALCOHOLISM

The long-term treatment of alcohol dependence has been the domain of sociotherapeutic and psychotherapeutic interventions. There are, however, a large number of patients for whom such strategies have not been very helpful, and alternative possibilities of treatment are necessary.[1] Several pharmacological strategies were developed and tested in the past. They are discussed on the bases of biological processes in alcoholism as suggested by animal research.[2,3] Currently, three approaches can be distinguished. (1) By means of a pharmacological agent, aversive consequences following alcohol consumption are induced; a prototype of this strategy is the long-term administration of disulfiram. (2) Coexisting psychiatric disorders or symptoms are treated in order to replace alcohol, which is considered to be "self-medication" for psychiatric or psychological problems. This is useful only for certain subgroups of patients. Merikangas et al.,[4] for example, found a causal relationship between anxiety and alcohol consumption in alcoholics, but only for social phobia, not for panic disorder. A critical discussion of the so-called self-medication hypothesis is furnished in this handbook (see Chapters 7 and 26). Several antidepressant and anxiolytic drugs — including tricyclic antidepressants, selective serotonin reuptake inhibitors (SSRIs), and lithium — have been tested in this indication. (3) A drug is given with the aim of blocking (at least some of) the psychoactive effects of alcohol and thereby reducing drug self-administration, that is, acting as an agent that inhibits craving for alcohol, which is supposed to be responsible for alcohol intake. In this indication, several drugs have been used and tested, including serotonin re-uptake inhibitors, GABAergic drugs, opiate antagonists, dopamine agonists and beta-adrenergic blocking agents. These "anti-craving" substances are supposed to biologically influence central systems responsible for the "reward" following alcohol consumption. Their pharmacological actions are different and currently not fully understood, nor is there a consensus on either the meaning or the measurement of "craving."[5,6] Spanagel and Hoelter, for example, discuss in Chapter 36 their findings concerning the role of dopamine in alcohol reward, as well as problems related to the concept of craving. Despite the controversial discussion that accompanies clinical research concerning craving, we focus on this concept, for three reasons. (1) This chapter gives a statistical presentation of existing studies. It describes the logic that can be seen beyond strategies and does not promote any logic. (2) Craving is a weak concept, but psychological concepts in psychiatry often are not "strong," and a central concept in alcoholism. Psychological dimensions are much more difficult to operationalize in humans than in rats. (3) We are dealing with clinical research, not primarily with basic research. To our knowledge, there are few drugs whose development is due only to profound research based on non-controversial theoretical concepts, at least in psychiatry. Craving, in our view, is a hypothetical construct, and ultimately a question of definition. If substances reduce alcohol intake, they must reduce craving; as, for example, why do people drink if they do not crave alcohol?

Nevertheless, from a clinical point of view, these compounds present new and interesting pharmacotherapeutical approaches to relapse prevention in alcoholism. The aim of the present chapter is to review published placebo-controlled clinical studies with pharmacological agents in the treatment of alcohol dependence by means of a quantitative meta-analysis of results. Not only clinical but also methodological aspects are considered. We want to answer the following questions:

1. Are drugs superior to placebo in the prevention of alcoholic relapse?
2. If there are differences in the magnitude of active drug vs. placebo differences between studies, which study- or patient-related factors can account for them? (The first and most obvious factor might be the *substance* investigated; a second one, *study duration*; and the third one, *pretreatment*.
3. Are there systematic differences between the various outcome criteria that have been used in the studies?

Although our main strategy was to average effect sizes over all measures used by the authors of a given paper, we nevertheless decided to compare the measures in a second step across studies.

METHODS OF META-ANALYSIS

STUDIES

English-, German-, and French-language literatures were searched for studies of drug treatment of alcoholism, using *Medline*, *Current Contents*, and manual cross-referencing in existing reviews. Included in the meta-analysis were randomized placebo-controlled clinical trials with a treatment duration of at least 3 months, including patients with severe substance abuse and investigating a substance whose clinical efficacy may be supposed to be based on its "anti-craving" effect. Studies were not included if a second psychiatric diagnosis was an inclusion criterion in the trial. Studies were included if they were accessible before mid-1997; studies published later are mentioned in the discussion.

OUTCOME MEASURES

Despite the number of assessment instruments that have been developed for the use in alcoholism (see Chapter 4 on psychometric screening instruments), there is no generally accepted outcome measure in alcoholism research that meets all clinical and statistical requirements (see Reference 7, page 54; for an overview on outcome criteria, see also Chapter 30), a problem often met in meta-analysis. Effect sizes were therefore calculated for all available clinical outcome variables that were presented in sufficient detail to allow a statistical comparison between the subjects in the drug and placebo groups. Not included were laboratory data. Thus, efficacy was calculated for frequency data such as responder rates, as well as for quantitative measures, such as drinking days or craving ratings.

DROPOUTS

In long-term studies with substance-dependent patients, it is a conservative approach to assume that virtually all patients lost in the course of the study have a relapse, that is, they are to be treated as drug non-responders.[8-10] Responder rates used in this meta-analysis were therefore referenced to the number of patients intended to treat (N_{itt}), and not to a smaller denominator as would have been the number of patients not violating the protocol rules or the number of patients completing the study. Our rates may therefore be different from those given in the original papers. This is a conservative way of analysis that, in turn, better reflects the situation in clinical practice. Regrettably, a similar conservative approach was not possible in the analysis of quantitative measures. Here, the analysis depends completely on the data given in the papers. These refer often to the completers, without any correction for patients lost during the study (like the last-observation-carried-forward method).

EFFECT SIZE CALCULATION

As a common value of effect size, the correlation coefficient r was calculated as proposed by Rosenthal[11] and others. When used as a measure of effect size, r denotes the association between treatment and response. Possible values range from $r = 1$ (indicating a perfect association between treatment and response) through $r = 0$ (indicating no effect of treatment) to $r = -1$ (for a perfect negative relationship). Response rates effect sizes were calculated as fourfold correlation coefficients between treatment group membership (drug vs. placebo) and outcome group membership (positive outcome vs. no positive outcome). For quantitative data, r was calculated from the statistics given in the paper (e.g., means, t-, or F-values, exact probabilities) by methods given as given in Rosenthal.[11] When several measures were given (and interpreted) in a paper, effect sizes were calculated for all of them and then averaged (via z-transformation, to account for statistical characteristics of effect sizes). A thorough explanation of the statistical concepts involved is beyond the scope of this review. The reader is referred to the literature.[11] Homogeneity of study effect sizes was assessed by the usual chi-square test for homogeneity of correlation coefficients, weighted for the sample size of the studies.[11,12] Explorative comparisons of specific effect sizes were performed by means of contrasts (for details, see Reference 11), a method that compares to t-testing in usual statistics. Given p values are two-tailed.

RESULTS OF THE ANALYSIS OF DRUG STUDIES

STUDIES AND PATIENTS INCLUDED

Eighteen studies with 2658 patients could be located that fulfilled the inclusion criteria. The studies are listed in Table 31.1, which also shows the main study characteristics. All patients, except those

TABLE 31.1
Characteristics of the Trials and Patients Included in Meta-Analysis

Source, Year (Ref.)	Substance[a]	Dose	Duration[b]	Diagnosis	Detoxification[c]	N[d]	Drop-outs[e]
Lhuintre, 1985 (56)	Aca.	250 mg/10 kg/d	3	Severe alcoholics; >200 g/d alc. or 2 previous detoxific.; gamma-GT	Yes	85	18%
Lhuintre, 1990 (21)	Aca.	1,3 g/d	3	Alcohol withdrawal syndrome, gamma-GT increase	Yes	569	37%
Ladewig, 1993 (15)	Aca.	1,3 /2 g/d	6	DSM-III (1 year), chron./episodic type, gamma-GT increase, CAGE, MAST (dep.)	Yes	61	36%
Paille, 1995 (57)	Aca.	2.0 g	12	DSM-III-R dependence	Yes	350	57%
Sass, 1995 (16)	Aca.	0.6–2 g/d	12	5 DSM-III-R criteria for alc. dependence, MALT (dependence)	Yes	272	51%
Withworth, 1996 (58)	Aca.	1,3 /3 g/d	12	DSM-III crit. for chronic/episodic alc. dependence, min. 12 months	Yes	448	61%
Gottlieb, 1995 (19)	Atenolol	0, 50, or 100 mg/d	12	Chronic alcoholism, SADQ (moderate degree), regular employment	Yes	100	85%
Borg, 1983 (24)	Bromoc.	7.5–15 mg/d	6	Motivated gamma-alcoholics (Jellinek)	No	50	16%
Malec, 1996 (59)	Buspir.	40 mg/d	12	DSM-III-R alcohol dep. >3 months, 25–60 y, socially stable	No	57	37%
Naranjo, 1995 (22)	Citalop.	40 mg/d	3	Mildly to moderately dependent drinkers (>27 drinks/week), socially stable	No	99	27%
Tiihohen, 1996 (60)	Citalop.	40 mg/d	3	DSM-III-R alcohol dependence	Yes	62	45%
Krasner, 1976 (13)	Fenflur.	120 mg/d	12	WHO 1952: chronic alcoholics	Yes	34	47%
Kranzler, 1995 (23)	Fluoxet.	47 mg/d	3	DSM-III-R alcohol dependence	Yes	101	6%
Gallimberti, 1992 (17)	GHB	50 mg/kg	3	DSM-III-R alcoholism, at least 5 years, last 2 years: 150 g alcohol per day	No	82	13%
Mason, 1994 (20)	Nalme.	40 mg/d	3	DSM-III-R dependence, ADS (mild-to-severe)	No	14	64%
Volpicelli, 1992 (25)	Naltre.	50 mg/d	3	5 DSM-III-R crit. for alcohol dependence, MAST (> 5) (male veterans)	Yes	70	14%
O'Malley, 1992 (14)	Naltre.	50 mg/d	3	DSM-R-III dependence (SCID)	Yes	104	35%
Shaw, 1994 (18)	Tiapride	300 mg/d	3	Chemically dependent alcoholics	Yes	100	46%
Total						2658	40%[f]

[a] Aca. = acamprosate; Bromoc.= bromocriptine; Buspir. = buspirone; Citalop. = citalopram; Fenflur. = fenfluramine; fluoxet. = fluoxetine; GHB = γ-hydroxybutyric acid; Nalme. = nalmefene; Naltre. = naltrexone. [b] Duration of treatment period in months. [c] Detoxification: yes, if detoxification was a requirement for inclusion into the study; no otherwise. [d] No. of patients included in the study with the intention to treat. [e] Drop-outs, according to the authors, refers to patients who did not complete the study, independent of the reason of premature termination. [f] Weighted average.

of Krasner et al.,[13] fulfilled the criteria for alcohol dependence according to DSM-III or DSM-III-R. In 15 of the studies, patients with other psychiatric diagnoses or those in need of treatment with other psychotropic drugs were excluded. If duration of illness was specified in the paper, it was between 7 and 20 years (mean: 12.5 y, median: 11 y). Patients' mean age was 42 years (median: 42; range: 37–47); an average of 24% of the patients were female (median: 25; range: 0–44). The nature of recruitment, as far as it was indicated, differed between the studies: six studies recruited patients during detoxification, four were conducted in special centers for treatment of alcohol-dependent patients, and four recruited patients by public announcement. Thirteen of the papers required patients to be detoxified; a minority accepted those still drinking. Wash-out phase was between 0 and 30 days.

The drugs tested were acamprosate (6 studies; $N_{ITT} = 1785$), atenolol (1; 100), bromocriptine (1; 50), buspirone (1; 57), citalopram (2; 161), fenfluramine (1; 34), fluoxetine (1; 101) γ-hydroxy-butyric acid (GHB, 1; 82), naltrexone (2; 174), nalmefene (1; 14) and tiapride (1; 100). Studies with acamprosate contribute 67% of all patients in this meta-analysis, naltrexone 7%, citalopram 6%, and all others less than 5%. Ten of the 18 studies had treatment periods of 3 months; six of the studies lasted 1 year. One study[14] also examined the effect of psychosocial interventions; most of the others accepted or offered concomitant or supportive interventions. In only five of the studies, no concomitant psychological or psychosocial treatment was mentioned.[13,15-18]

Patients drop-out rates ranged from 6 to 85%. This large variation may result from differences in efficacy or side effect profile, but also from differences in protocols. In Gottlieb et al.'s publication,[19] for example, patients were terminated from treatment if criteria for relapse were met. Mason,[20] in contrast, regards a relapse as a common aspect of early recovery and did not exclude patients when they relapsed. In the present meta-analysis of response rates, all drop-outs were counted as treatment failures.

With the exception of Lhuintre et al.[21] and Naranjo et al.,[22] all studies reported responder rates as one (and usually the pivotal) outcome measure (be it for the criterion of abstinence or for a criterion of "controlled drinking" or for both), and most studies reported in addition one or more quantitative measures (amount of alcohol consumption, days of drinking, amount of craving, time until first relapse, gamma-glutamyltransferase activity).

OUTCOME

Table 31.2 shows effect sizes for the various outcome measures reported in the individual studies. The table differentiates between "quantitative" and "qualitative" criteria; for example, dichotomous (i.e., response yes/no) variables. In the last three columns, the weighted averaged effect sizes for the individual studies and the confidence intervals of the study effect sizes are presented. Study effect sizes ranged between –0.09 (Reference 23) and 0.65 (Reference 24). Confidence intervals indicate the significance of the difference between drug and placebo treatment: in 7 of the 18 studies, confidence intervals do not include zero; this indicates a significant difference between drug and placebo, with a superiority of drug. In nine studies, drug patients did slightly better than placebo patients. Two studies — on atenolol and fluoxetine — yielded negative effect sizes, indicating a (nonsignificant) superiority of placebo.

Studies differ markedly in their results, and the chi-square-test for heterogeneity was highly significant (chi-square (17) = 44, $p < 0.001$). When all studies are pooled, a significant superiority of anti-craving substances compared to placebo ($r_{total} = 0.16$; 95% confidence interval of 0.12 to 0.19, $p < 0.001$) results. Given the clear heterogeneity of the studies, it is not appropriate to interpret the mean value of all studies. Instead, one must look for moderator variables that might have influenced study results.

An obvious variable of influence should be the type of medication. Table 31.3 shows effect sizes for the different substances. At first glance, compounds seem to influence the outcome of the studies — atenolol showing the worst, GHB and bromocriptine showing the best results. There are,

TABLE 31.2
Effect Sizes r for Different Outcome Criteria

Source, Year (Ref.)	Substance	N_{ITT}	Quantitative Outcome Criteria[n]				Qualitative Criteria		Weighted Mean r Basis = n_{itt}	Confidence Interval	
			Drink. Days	Alc. Consumption	Craving	Clinical Rating	Contr. Drinking	Abstinence		Lower Limit	Upper Limit
Lhuintre, 1985 (56)	Aca.	85						0.16	0.16	-0.06	0.36
Lhuintre, 1990 (21)	Aca.	569				0.10			0.10	0.02	0.18
Ladewig, 1993 (15)	Aca.	61	0.25[a]				0.18[f]		0.22	-0.03	0.45
Paille, 1995 (57)	Aca.	350	0.19,[b] 0.13[c]					0.10	0.14	0.04	0.24
Sass, 1995 (16)	Aca.	272	0.23[b]					0.22	0.23	0.11	0.34
Withworth, 1996 (58)	Aca.	448	0.14[b]					0.16	0.15	0.06	0.24
Gottlieb, 1995 (19)	Atenolol	100						-0.03	-0.03	-0.23	0.17
Borg, 1983 (24)	Bromoc.	50				0.81		0.40	0.65	0.45	0.79
Malec, 1996 (59)	Buspir.	57		0.14[d]	0.11			0.06	0.08	-0.27	0.41
Naranjo, 1995 (22)	Citalop.	99	0.10[a]	-0.10[d]	0.02				0.07	-0.13	0.26
Tiihonen, 1996 ( )	Citalop.	62				0.22		0.09	0.15	-0.10	0.39
Krasner, 1976 (13)	Fenflur.	34	0.37[a]					0.00	0.10	-0.25	0.42
Kranzler, 1995 (23)	Fluoxet.	101	-0.14	-0.16[d]–0.05[e]			0.08[g]	0.00	-0.09	-0.28	0.11
Gallimberti, 1992 (17)	GHB	82	0.52[a]	0.57[d]	0.63		0.43[h]	0.27	0.49	0.31	0.64
Mason, 1994 (20)	Nalme.	14					0.14[i]		0.14	-0.42	0.62
Volpicelli, 1992 (25)	Naltre.	70	0.29[a]		0.33		0.23[k]	0.03	0.22	-0.02	0.43
O'Malley, 1992 (14)	Naltre.	104	0.29[a]		0.09		0.25[l]	0.19	0.21	0.02	0.39
Shaw, 1994 (18)	Tiapride	100	0.58[a]	0.42[e]			0.07[m]	0.03	0.22	0.03	0.40

[a] Abstinence in % of days. [b] Cumulative abstinence duration. [c] Time until first relapse. [d] Daily drinks. [e] Daily intake on (heavy) drinking day. [f] No relapse. [g] <3 lapses (alcohol consumption) within a 4-week interval. [h] Alcohol consumption <40 mg/d. [i] <5 drinks/day or [j] <5 drink. days/week. [k] <5 days alc. consumption within 1 week or <4 drinks per drinking occasion or <100 mg/l blood alcohol concentration. [l] <60 mg/d alc (<5 drinks/occasion), 40 mg/d (<4 drinks/occasion). [m] <4 occasions in any 1 week, <5 units/occasion. [n] Quantitative outcome criteria were based on ITT population, if possible. If for one criterion two effect sizes were calculated for one study, these were averaged.

TABLE 31.3
Pooled Results (Effect Sizes ES, *r*) for Different Substances and Design Variables, Ranked by Effect Size

Substance	No. of Studies	No. of Patients	ES *r*, weighted	Design Variables: Duration (months)	Detoxification
Atenolol	1	100	−0.03	12	Yes
Buspirone	1	57	0.08	3	No
Citalopram	2	161	0.10	3, 3	Yes, no
Fenfluramine	1	34	0.10	12	Yes
Acamprosate	6	1816	0.15	3, 3, 6, 12, 12, 12	Yes
Nalmefene	1	14	0.14	3	No
Naltrexone	2	174	0.21	3	Yes
Tiapride	1	100	0.22	3	Yes
GHB	1	82	0.49	3	No
Bromocriptine	1	50	0.65	6	No

Note: Calculation of *r* is based on the averaged effect sizes of the studies, which take into account all outcome criteria.

however, other potential moderator variables that are also displayed in Table 31.3, which may be confounded with the influence of medication. One of them, study duration, did not correlate with effect size ($r = 0.14$ vs. $r = 0.17$; weighted contrast between effect sizes: $z = 0.81$, $p > 0.05$, for duration = 3 months vs. duration >3 months). Another inclusion criterion, detoxification, did correlate with effect size, better results being obtained in studies with non-detoxified patients. The difference in effect sizes of these five studies combined ($r = 0.33$) vs. those including detoxified patients ($r = 0.13$) was statistically significant ($z = 3.12$, $p = 0.002$). This could mean that the tested drugs can better demonstrate their potential effect in the presence rather than in the absence of alcohol. This hypothesis could be further tested by contrasting outcome measures derived in the presence and absence of alcohol. Five studies[13,14,17,18,25] gave responder rates for both abstinence and controlled drinking as a criterion. In three of the five studies, the drug effect compared to placebo was stronger under the criterion of controlled drinking (mean effect size for abstinence $r = 0.12$; for controlled drinking $r = 0.22$; $z = 1.4$; $p = 0.15$. This difference misses statistical significance. Shaw et al.,[18] however, present two definitions of controlled drinking; the more conservative one was chosen for this meta-analysis for reasons of comparability with the other studies. The less conservative definition yields an effect size of 0.25; including this one into the comparison, the difference between controlled drinking and abstinence effect sizes reaches statistical significance.

In a further analysis of outcome measures, all quantitative data presented in Table 31.2, such as drinking days or amount of alcohol consumption, were compared with response rate data. In this comparison, only studies were included that presented quantitative and qualitative data. The weighted mean effect size of all quantitative variables of all studies ($r = 0.27$; 21 effect sizes) was significantly higher than that of the qualitative variables ($r = 0.16$; 18 effect sizes; $z = 3.77$; $p < 0.001$).

Table 31.4 shows response rates and their differences for abstinence and controlled drinking, all drop-outs being considered as treatment failures (ITT). Response rates vary between 6 and 75% under drug and between 0 and 52% under placebo, with drug placebo differences varying between −3 and 44%. It was mentioned above that the magnitude of the difference between active drug and placebo is correlated with the definition of response (controlled drinking obtaining larger differences than abstinence). Single response rates indicate that this is due to an increase of responders in the active drug group when controlled drinking serves as response criterion, and not, for example, to a decrease of responder in the placebo group. The difference between abstinence and controlled

TABLE 31.4
Response Rates (ITT)

Source, Year (Ref.)	Substance	N_{ITT}	Abstinence			Controlled Drinking		
			Drug	Placebo	Diff.	Drug	Placebo	Diff.
Lhuintre, 1985 (56)	Aca.	85	47%	29%	18%			
Ladewig, 1993 (15)	Aca.	61				41%	22%	20%
Paille, 1995 (57)	Aca.	350	19%	11%	8%			
Sass, 1995 (16)	Aca.	272	43%	21%	22%			
Withworth, 1996 (58)	Aca.	448	18%	7%	11%			
Gottlieb, 1995 (19)	Atenolol	100	14%	16%	02%			
Borg, 1983 (24)	Bromoc.	50	75%	31%	44%			
Malec, 1996 (59)	Buspirone	57	7%	10%	−3%			
Tiihonen, 1996 (60)	Citalop.	62	19%	10%	9%			
Krazner, 1976 (13)	Fenflur.	34	6%	0%	6%	18%	12%	6%
Kranzler, 1995 (23)	Fluoxet.	62	53%	53%	0%			
Gallimberti, 1992 (17)	GHB	82	27%	5%	22%	63%	20%	43%
Volpicelli, 1992 (25)	Naltre.	70	37%	31%	06%	60%	34%	26%
O'Malley, 1992 (14)	Naltre.	104	38%	19%	19%	56%	29%	27%
Mason, 1994 (20)	Nalme.	14				57%	29%	29%
Shaw, 1994 (18)	Tiapride	100	20%	18%	2%	26%	18%	8%

drinking responder rate differences seems to be caused, in particular, by an increase of responder in the drug group in the controlled drinking data.

DISCUSSION OF THE RESULTS

The present meta-analysis of placebo-controlled clinical trials of drug treatment for alcohol dependence focuses on currently tested drugs, which are discussed to influence alcohol intake by influencing the "craving" for alcohol. The surveyed clinical trials do not represent a specific pharmacological class of drugs, but rather a heterogeneous sample of agents with GABAergic, dopaminergic, opiate antagonistic, and beta-adrenergic-blocking activity. The sample represents the state of affairs today: the theory behind the concept of craving is still *in statu nascendi*, and most agents have only been tested in one or two clinical trials with small samples of subjects. An exception to this is acamprosate, an NMDA-receptor-blocking agent, which has recently been tested in a number of clinical trials across Europe.[16] Most of these studies were not yet published in sufficient detail to be included in this meta-analysis. Even so, the 1785 patients of the six acamprosate trials included make up two thirds of the meta-analysis sample. We could have collected a larger sample of studies and patients if we had included trials with a shorter treatment duration. In particular, some studies on serotonergic substances were not included in the meta-analysis, as their treatment duration was too short,[22,26] the design was experimental,[27] or patient sample was more heterogeneous.[28] We focused on a minimal treatment duration of 3 months because we wanted to include only trials with a clinical view on relapse prevention, and not a primarily experimental view.

As could be expected from the heterogeneous sample of drugs, effect sizes of the individual studies ranged from lower zero to $r = 0.65$. The large heterogeneity does not make it easy to draw conclusions on the effect of "anticraving" drugs in general. There seem to be large differences between the effects of the individual drugs, but these are confounded with other methodological factors, which will be discussed below. Most of the drugs were represented with one study only and sample sizes were generally small. In such situations, one should be aware of the "file-drawer problem":[29] as there is no international registry of clinical trials (and their results), we cannot control the selection effects leading to the publication or non-publication of a clinical trial (although many authors have thought and commented on the problem, see, e.g., References 12, 29, and 30). Chances are high that positive trials have a greater probability to appear in print.

Acamprosate was investigated in six trials published before mid-1997. It showed a homogeneous (chi square = 3.7, p = 0.6) positive effect size with a weighted mean value of r = 0.15, which is based on 1785 patients and beyond any doubt better than placebo ($p < 10^{-10}$). Results from the other ten placebo-controlled studies across Europe seem to show a similar, if not better, effect size, although at the time of writing, the results are only available in the form of a general review.[16] An effect size of 0.15 is comparable to a responder rate difference between drug and placebo of 15 percentage points. If we assume the mean placebo response under the criterion of abstinence to be 20%, the drug would have produced a mean increase of the responder rate to 35% — or 15 patients more from every 100 included. This is a considerable effect given the usually low responder rates in long-term trials with alcohol-dependent patients. It can be compared with other long-term treatments in psychiatry, for example, the maintenance treatment of unipolar depression with antidepressant drugs. In a meta-analytic review using a similar method as in this paper, Dang and Engel[31] have come to a mean effect size of r = 0.35. Reviewing the same question, Davis et al.[32] reported a mean relapse rate of 23% under drug and 50% under placebo, giving a drug-placebo-difference of 27% points. Compared to these figures, the long-term treatment of alcohol-dependent patients with acamprosate seems to be less effective, but — again — it is significantly better than placebo. Naltrexone, a compound approved in a number countries for the treatment of alcoholism, especially in the U.S., was investigated in only two of the studies that were published in sufficient detail to be included in meta-analysis. With an effect size of 0.21 and 174 patients included, it shows a relatively stable superiority to placebo. This database, however, is markedly smaller than the acamprosate database. Numerically, the effect sizes of some of the other agents included in the present meta-analysis were higher, but they are less reliable due to the small base of studies. The more studies that exist on a compound, and the more patients that are included in trials on a certain compound, the more probable it is that the mean result (the difference between active drug and placebo) is not due to chance. A numerically correct way to take the different sample sizes of the acamprosate and naltrexone trials into account would be to give confidence intervals for the pooled effect sizes. However, due to differences among studies (e.g., detoxified vs. non-detoxified patients, different outcome criteria), giving the confidence intervals for the pooled effect sizes would suggest a level of statistical accuracy that, in reality, cannot be obtained. There are, however, a number of studies underway, especially on opioid antagonists such as naltrexone, serotonergic substances such as ritanserin, and dopaminergic substances such as tiapride, lisuride, or flupentixol decanoate. The ritanserin study published by Johnson and colleagues (in 1996) was not included in our work, as its double-blind treatment phase was only 11 weeks. The authors found a significant reduction in drinking measures but no differences between treatment groups. A discussion of the studies on dopaminergic substances, on which sufficient data for meta-analysis are missing, is provided in Chapter 36.

In addition to the possible differences between drugs, we have described explorative analyses of the influence of methodological procedures (detoxification at inclusion?) and measures (e.g., numerous vs. dichotomous data). Several sources of information indicate that anti-craving drugs may be more effective in the presence of alcohol than in its absence:

1. The combined effect size of studies including patients still drinking alcohol was significantly larger than that of studies accepting detoxified patients only. Naturally, this effect is assessed across studies and therefore it is confounded with drug and other factors and may only be taken as a hypothesis.
2. Combining the four studies measuring relapse rates for "controlled drinking" as well as for complete abstinence, the response rate difference between drug and placebo (i.e., the effect size) was significantly higher for the former. This outcome is measured **within**

studies and, consequently, confounding with other factors is ruled out. The effect seems to be independent of the individual medication, as was demonstrated in studies investigating GHB, naltrexone and, depending on the definition of controlled drinking, also tiapride.

3. These different effect sizes are predominantly due to an increase of the responders in the drug group for the criterion of controlled drinking.

Within the framework of a meta-analysis, the question must stay unanswered as to whether alcohol-dependent subjects may profit more from an anticraving drug under less restrictive abstinence conditions. The issue is also discussed controversially in the literature.[33] Naranjo et al.[35] report data of a controlled study on bromocriptine, including 366 alcoholics (this study was not included in meta-analysis, as is was published after inclusion was terminated). They found, in contrast to Borg[24] and Dongier,[36] no superiority of bromocriptine over placebo. They discuss that one of the differences between the study protocols was their inclusion of abstinent alcoholics, compared to non-detoxified patients in the study of Borg. It certainly would be worthwhile to design and run controlled experiments to answer this question.

We have included in this meta-analysis all available measures of the individual papers that have been presented in sufficient detail to allow the computation of between-group effect sizes and that have been interpreted as a relevant criterion for clinical purposes. This is a very liberal strategy that makes sense only in the context of this rather new research paradigm with "anti-craving" substances. Long-term drug trials in other fields of clinical pharmacopsychiatry have more or less standardized on reporting response (or relapse) rates only complemented by one or the other quantitative measure. The effect of drop-outs can be described much better and handled more systematically using rate measures instead of quantitative data. Quantitative data, on the other hand, give more information, but only under the condition of complete data sets that never exist in long-term clinical trials. Within the 18 studies analyzed in this chapter, qualitative data showed in their sum an effect size significantly lower than quantitative data, a finding which was also reported by Huges et al.[37] in a review on disulfiram treatment. Two possible explanations for this finding can be formulated. The first one is a methodological one: quantitative data refer either to the last-planned or to the last-observed values of a patient. When a patient stays sober for some time and then does not show up anymore for unknown reason, then his or her last value is sometimes used in the analysis. In our intent-to-treat analysis, he or she is counted as a non-responder. In addition to this methodological bias, there might exist a substantial difference in the sense that alcohol consumption is a more sensitive measure for therapeutic efficacy, be it for statistical reasons or because anti-craving drugs are better able to reduce alcohol consumption than to reduce relapses.

Ratings of "craving" were positively influenced by some of the drugs analyzed. The relationship between craving and relapse, up to now, is not definitively elucidated.[38-41] Nevertheless, it would be worthwhile to examine whether "anti-craving" drugs do what their name implies. This question, up to now, remains open, as only in five publications was it dealt with in such detail that a statistical meta-analysis was possible; and in three of the five, no clear effect on craving, measured usually with visual analog scales, was found — according to our criteria.

Moncrieff and Drummond[42] published a comprehensive review on clinical trials in relapse prevention of alcoholism. They discuss a number of methodological flaws that may have introduced bias and therefore may have invalidated the studies' results. In fact, there are some special problems in alcoholism research such as very high drop-out rates, but most of the methodological problems discussed by the authors concern all clinical studies in psychiatry. Nonetheless, clinical trials, such as those included in this meta-analysis, are at present the only way to create knowledge upon which decisions on further research and therapy can be based.

No comparable meta-analytic data exist on relapse prevention by aversive effects (disulfiram) and by treatment of (coexisting) mood disorders. Reviews, indeed, report questionable general efficacy of aversive treatment with disulfiram.[43-47] Treatment of comorbid psychiatric symptoms with, for example, lithium[48,49] or classical antidepressants,[50,51] also shows limited success; for an overview, see also Reference 52. For psychosocial interventions, a meta-analysis of controlled studies[53] found a significant superiority over control (placebo) procedures in only 3 among 15 studies, the types of successful psychotherapeutic interventions not being mentioned in enough detail in the publication for accurate description. Only very few controlled studies investigate a possible interaction between pharmacotherapy and psychotherapy. Given the diverse methodological problems jeopardizing the field of alcoholism research and psychotherapy research, it is necessary to design studies that address these questions directly, instead of integrating literature results. There is, however, some evidence that psychotherapy may reinforce the effects of medication.[54,55] The pharmacological treatment seems to be an important strategy among the current concepts of relapse prevention, although the empirical database is still small and questions of clinical research methodology must be addressed in empirical studies.

REFERENCES

1. Soyka, M., Pharmacotherapy and psychotherapy for the treatment of alcoholism in Germany, *Drug Alcohol Depend*, 39, 9, 1995.
2. Litten, R.Z., Allen, J., and Fertig, J., Pharmacotherapies for alcohol problems: a review of research with focus on developments since 1991, *Alcohol. Clin. Exp. Res.*, 20, 853, 1996.
3. Myers, R.D., New drugs for the treatment of experimental alcoholism, *Alcoholism*, 11, 439, 1994.
4. Merikangas, K.R., Stevens, D.E., Fenton, B., Stolar, M., O'Malley, S., Woods, S.W., and Risch, N., Comorbidity and familial aggregation of alcoholism and anxiety disorders, *Psychol. Med.*, 28, 773, 1998.
5. Pickens, R.W. and Johanson, C.E., Craving: consensus of status and agenda for future research, *Drug Alcohol Depend.*, 30, 127, 1992.
6. Sitharthan, T., McGrath, D., Sitharthan, G., and Saunders, J.B., Meaning of craving in research on addiction, *Psychol. Rep.*, 71, 823, 1992.
7. The Plinius Maior Society, Guidelines on evaluation of treatment of alcohol dependence, *Alcoholism*, 30, 1994.
8. Ogborne, A. and Annis, H., The reactive effect of follow-up assessment procedures: an experimental study, *Addict. Behav.*, 13, 123, 1988.
9. Sobell, L.C., Sobell, M.B., Frequent follow-up as data gathering and continued care with alcoholics, *Int. J. Addict.*, 16, 1077, 1980.
10. Mackenzie, A., Funderburk, F., Allen, P., and Stefan, R., The characteristics of alcoholics frequently lost to follow-up, *J. Stud. Alcohol*, 48, 119, 1987.
11. Rosenthal, R., *Meta-analytic Procedures for Social Research*, Sage, Beverly Hills, 1991.
12. Mantel, N. and Haenszel, W., Statistical aspects of the analysis of data from retrospective studies of disease, *J. Natl. Cancer. Inst.*, 22, 719, 1959.
13. Krasner, N., Moore, M.R., Goldberg, A., Booth, J.C.D., Frame, A.H., and McLaren, A.D., A trial of fenfluramine in the treatment of the chronic alcoholic patient, *Br. J. Psychiatry*, 128, 346, 1976.
14. O'Malley, S.S., Jaffe, A.J., Chang, G., Richard, S., Schottenfeld, M.D., Meyer, E., and Rounsaville, B., Naltrexone and coping skills therapy for alcohol dependence, *Arch. Gen. Psychiatry*, 49, 881, 1992.
15. Ladewig, D., Knecht, T., Leher, P., and Fendl, A., Acamprosat — ein Stabilisierungsfaktor in der Langzeitentwoehnung von Alkoholabhaengigen, *Ther. Rundschau*, 50, 182, 1993.
16. Sass, H., Results from a pooled analysis of 11 European trials comparing acamprosate and placebo on the treatment of alcohol dependence, *Alcohol Alcohol.*, 30, 484, 1995.
17. Gallimberti, L., Ferri, M., Ferrara, S.D., Fadda, F., and Gessa, G.L., Gamma-hydroxybutric acid in the treatment of alcohol dependence: a double-blind study, *Alcohol. Clin. Exp. Res.*, 16, 673, 1992.
18. Shaw, G.K., Waller, S., Majumdar, S.K., Alberts, J.L., Latham, C.J., and Dunn, G., Tiapride in the prevention of relapse in recently detoxified alcoholics, *Br. J. Psychiatry*, 165, 515, 1994.
19. Gottlieb, L.D., Horwith, R.I., Kraus, M.L., Segal, S.R., and Viscoli, C.M., Randomized controlled trial in alcohol relapse prevention: role of atenolol, alcohol craving, and treatment adherence, *J. Subst. Abuse. Treatm.*, 11, 253, 1994.

20. Mason, B.J., Ritvo, E.C., Morgan, R.O., Salvato, F.R., Goldberg, G., Welch, B., and Mantero-Atienza, E., A double-blind, placebo-controlled pilot study to evaluate the efficacy and safety of oral nalmefene HCL for alcohol dependence, *Alcohol. Clin. Exp. Res.*, 18, 1162, 1994.

21. Lhuintre, J.P., Moore, N., Tran, G., Steru, L., Langrenon, S., Daoust, M., Parot, P., Ladure, P., Libert, C., Boismare, F., and Hillemands, B., Acamprosate appears to decrease alcohol intake in weaned alcoholics, *Alcohol Alcohol.*, 25, 613, 1990.

22. Naranjo, C.A., Bremner, K.E., and Lactôt, K.L., Effects of citalopram and a brief psycho-social intervention on alcohol intake, dependence and problems, *Addiction*, 90, 87, 1995.

23. Kranzler H.R., Burleson, JA., Korner, P., Del-Boca, F.K., Brown, M.J., and Liebowitz, N., Placebo-controlled trial of fluoxetine as an adjunct to relapse prevention in alcoholics, *Am. J. Psychiatry,* 153, 391, 1995.

24. Borg, V., Bromocriptine in the prevention of alcohol abuse, *Acta. Psychiatr. Scand.*, 68, 100, 1983.

25. Volpicelli, J.R., Alterman, A.I., Hayashida, M., and O'Brien, C.P., Naltrexone in the treatment of alcohol dependence, *Arch. Gen. Psychiatry,* 49, 876, 1992.

26. Naranjo, C.A., Poulos, C.X., Bremner, K.E., and Lanctot, K.L., Citalopram decreases desirability, liking, and consumption of alcohol in alcohol-dependent drinkers, *Clin. Pharmacol. Ther.,* 51, 729, 1992.

27. Gorelick, D.A. and Paredes, A., Effect of fluoxetine on alcohol consumption in male alcoholics, *Alcohol. Clin. Exp. Res.,* 16, 261, 1992.

28. Cornelius, J.R., Salloum, I.M., Cornelius, M.D., Perel, J.M., Thase, M.E., Ehler, J.G., and Mann, J.J., Fluoxetine trial in suicidal depressed alcoholics, *Psychopharmacol. Bull.,* 29, 195, 1993.

29. Rosenthal, R., The "file drawer problem" and tolerance for null results, *Psychol. Bull.,* 86, 638, 1979.

30. Gilbody, S. and House, A., Publication bias and meta-analysis, *Br. J. Psychiatry,* 167, 266, 1995.

31. Dang, T. and Engel, R.R., Long-term drug treatment of bipolar and depressive disorders: meta-analysis of controlled clinical trials with Lithium, Carbamazepin and antidepressant agents, *Pharmacopsychiatry,* 28, 170, 1995.

32. Davis, J.M., Wang, Z., and Janicak, P.G., A quantitative analysis of clinical drug trials for the treatment of affective disorders, *Psychopharmacol. Bull.,* 29, 175, 1993.

33. Levy, M.S., The disease controversy and psychotherapy with alcoholics, *J. Psychoactive Drugs,* 24, 251, 1992.

34. Naranjo, C.A., Poulos, C.X., Lanctot, K.L., Bremner, K.E., Kwok, M., Umana, M., and Ritanserin, A central 5-HT2 antagonist, in heavy social drinkers: desire to drink, alcohol intake and related effects, *Addiction,* 90, 893, 1995.

35. Naranjo, C.A., Dongier, M., and Bremner, K.E., Long-acting injectable bromocriptine does not reduce relapse in alcoholics, *Addiction,* 92, 969, 1997.

36. Dongier, M., Vachon, L., and Schwartz, G., Bromocriptine in the treatment of alcohol dependence, *Alcohol. Clin. Exp. Res.,* 15, 970, 1991.

37. Huges, J.G. and Cook, C.C., The efficacy of disulfiram: a review of outcome studies, *Addiction,* 92, 381, 1997.

38. Kuefner, H., Denis, A., Roch, I., Arzt, J., and Rug, U., *Stationaere Krisenintervention bei Drogenab-haengigen. Ergebnisse der wissenschaftlichen Begleitung des Modellprogramms,* Nomos Verlagsge-sellschaft, Baden-Baden, 1994.

39. Lucki, I., Volpicelli, J.R., and Schweizer, E., Differential craving between recovering abstinent alco-holic-dependent subjects and therapeutic users of benzodiazepines, *NIDA Res. Monogr.,* 105, 322, 1991.

40. Velleman, R., *Counselling for Alcohol Problems,* Sage, Beverly Hills, 1994.

41. Veltrup, C., Eine empirische Analyse des Rueckfallgeschehens bei entzugsbehandelten Alkoholab-haengigen, Koerkel, J., Lauer, R., and Scheller, R., Eds., *Brennpunkte der Rueckfallforschung,* Springer-Verlag, Berlin, 1993.

42. Moncrieff, J. and Drummond, C.D., New drug treatments for alcohol problems: a critical appraisal, *Addiction,* 92, 939, 1997.

43. Brewer, C., Controlled trials of Antabuse in alcoholism: the importance of supervision and adequate dosage, *Acta. Psychiatr. Scand.,* 369, 51, 1992.

44. Chick, J., Gough, K., Falkowski, W., Kershaw, P., Hore, B., Mehta, B., Rison, B., Ropner, R., and Torley, D., Disulfiram treatment of alcoholism, *Br. J. Psychiatry,* 161, 84, 1992.

45. Critchfild, G.C. and Eddy, D.M., A confidence profile analysis of the effectiveness of disulfiram in the treatment of chronic alcoholism, *Med. Care,* 25, 66, 1987.

46. Fuller, R.K., Branchey, L., Brightwell, D.R., Derman, R.M., Emrick, C.D., Iber, F.L., James, K.E., Lacoursiere, R.B., Lee, K.K., Lowenstramm, I., Manny, I., Neiderhisre, D., Nocks, S., and Shaw, J.J., Disulfiram treatment of alcoholism: a veterans administration cooperative study, *JAMA,* 256, 1449, 1986.

47. Kristenson, H., Long-term antabuse treatment of alcohol-dependent patients, *Acta Psychiatr. Scand. Suppl.,* 369, 41, 1992.

48. Lejoyeux, M. and Ades, J., Evaluation of lithium treatment in alcoholism, *Alcohol Alcohol.,* 28 273, 1993.

49. Fawcett, J., Clark, D.C., Gibbons, R.D., Aagesen, C.A., Pisani, V.D., Tilkin, J.M., Sellers, D., and Stutzman, D., Evaluation of lithium therapy for alcoholism, *J. Clin. Psychiatry,* 45 494, 1984.

50. Mason B.J. and Kocsis, J.H., Desimipramine treatment of alcoholism, *Psychopharmacol. Bull.,* 27, 155, 1991.

51. Nunes, E.V., McGrath, P.J., Quitkin, F.M., Stewart, J.P., Tricamo, H.W., and Ocepek-Welikson, K., Imipramine treatment of alcoholism with comorbid depression, *Am. J. Psychiatry,* 150, 963, 1993.

52. Gorelick, D.A., Overview of pharmacologic treatment approaches for alcohol and other drug addiction, *Psychiatr. Clin. North. Am.,* 16, 141, 1993.

53. Agosti V., The efficacy of controlled trials of alcohol misuse treatment in maintaining abstinence: a meta-analysis, *Int. J. Addict.,* 29, 759, 1994.

54. O'Malley, S.S. and Carroll, K.M., Psychotherapeutic considerations in pharmacological trials, *Alcohol. Clin. Exp. Res.,* 20(Suppl. 7), 17A, 1996.

55. Carroll, K.M., Integrating psychotherapy and pharmacotherapy to improve drug abuse outcomes, *Addict. Behav.,* 22, 233, 1997.

56. Lhuintre, J.P., Moore, N.D., Saligaut, C., Boismare, F., Daoust, M., Chretien, P., Tran, G., and Hillemand, B., Ability of calcium bis acetyl homotaurine, a gaba antagonist, to prevent relapse in weaned alcoholics, *Lancet,* 4, 1010, 1985.

57. Paille, F.M., Guelfi, J.D., Perkins, A.C., Royer, R.J., Steru, L., and Parot, P., Double-blind randomized multicentre trial of acamprosate in maintaining abstinence from alcohol, *Alcohol Alcohol.,* 20, 239, 1995.

58. Withworth, A.B., Fischer, F., Lesch, O.M., Nimmerrichter, A., Oberbauer, H., Platz, T., Potgieter, A., Walter, H., and Fleischhacker, W., Comparison of acamprosate and placebo in long-term treatment of alcohol dependence, *Lancet,* 347, 1438, 1996.

59. Malec, E., Malec, M.A., Gagné, M.A., and Dongier, M., Buspirone in the treatment of alcohol dependence: a placebo-controlled trial, *Alcohol. Clin. Exp. Res.,* 20, 307, 1996.

60. Tiihohen, J., Ryynaenen, O.P., Kauhanen, J., Hakola, H.P.A., and Salaspuro, M., Citalopram in the treatment of alcoholism: a double-blind placebo-controlled study, *Pharmacopsychiatry,* 29, 27, 1996.

32 Meta-analysis Without Tears: a Step-by-Step Introduction

Georg Kemmler

OVERVIEW

This chapter provides an introduction to meta-analysis for medical research workers, which requires little prior knowledge in statistics. First, some important aspects for planning meta-analyses are discussed, in particular the issue of *study selection*. Then the concept of *effect size* is introduced, and two common effect size measures are discussed (standardized treatment difference and odds ratio). The actual analysis procedure is then described in some detail for two important cases (continuous and dichotomous outcome variable). They are illustrated by a worked example. Finally, some common problems and caveats when dealing with meta-analyses are outlined and suggestions for further reading are given.

INTRODUCTION

Meta-analyses have become very popular in recent years.[1] Despite its name, there is no magic behind this procedure. It is simply a statistically founded synopsis of the results of a *series* of trials studying the same scientific question, e.g, if a certain compound XYZ is efficacious for the pharmacotherapy of alcohol dependence. When comparing such studies, one usually finds remarkable differences between them. Thus, different studies may use different outcome criteria (e.g., percent continuously abstinent patients, percent drinking days, amount of alcohol consumed, rating on a scale of social functioning, etc.). In addition, results obtained under one and the same outcome criterion might vary considerably across trials. Meta-analysis is a scientifically sound way to take these differences into account, whereas ad hoc methods, such as counting those trials favoring *one* treatment against those favoring the other treatment, must be dismissed as unscientific because they do not distinguish between, for example, large and small studies, large and small treatment effects, and many other aspects in which studies can differ from one another.

Although the issue of meta-analysis is methodologically quite demanding, its basic ideas are simple and can be explained without using more than elementary statistics. For certain types of data, this also applies for the computations. This chapter concentrates on such cases. However, meta-analysis is not just a matter of statistical analysis, but includes several other issues of importance. Some of these will be addressed in this contribution, in particular the issue of study selection (cf. next subsection) and that of heterogeneity of studies and some related topics (to be addressed in the last two sections).

This chapter pursues two aims. The first is to provide the reader with a basic knowledge for understanding publications dealing with meta-analyses. The second is to enable the reader to do his or her *own* meta-analyses, at least in simple cases. Readers interested in a more detailed account of the topic will find a good presentation of the material in the monograph by Petitti[2] and, mathematically more elaborate, in the "classic" by Hedges and Olkin.[3]

0-8493-7801-X/00/$0.00+$.50
© 2000 by CRC Press LLC

SELECTION OF STUDIES

When starting a meta-analysis, the first question is how to find all the trials relevant for the issue under study. This requires, to start with, that the issue be clearly defined, for example, comparison of two treatments, an active drug (A) vs. placebo (B), for the treatment of alcohol dependence with respect to efficacy, measured by a specified outcome variable (e.g., percent continuously abstinent patients). An extensive literature search should follow to obtain the complete set of studies from which the ones to be used in the meta-analysis can be selected. Usually, not all published trials on an issue are suitable for a meta-analysis (e.g., because a trial was performed in a group of patients with a somewhat different diagnosis, or simply because it appeared in Japanese and is thus incomprehensible for the conductor of the meta-analysis). Therefore, in a next step, criteria regarding eligibility have to be set up. This will include year of publication, language, study design, originality (if the same data have been published twice, only one of the two publications can be considered), sample characteristics (diagnosis, age, etc.), similarity of treatment modalities, similarity of outcome criteria, and completeness of information (e.g., regarding outcome criteria). These criteria must be defined in advance, that is, *before* inspecting study results. In a final step, *all* studies meeting the eligibility criteria are selected for the meta-analysis. More about the selection of studies for meta-analysis can be found in the literature.[2,4] It should be noted that study selection may be subject to considerable bias. In particular, one should take into consideration the possibility of a publication bias: trials with a nonsignificant outcome are usually less likely to be accepted for publication than trials with a statistically significant outcome.[5] We will come back to this problem at the end of the chapter.

THE CONCEPT OF EFFECT SIZE AND SOME COMMON EFFECT SIZE MEASURES

Once the studies eligible for meta-analysis have been selected, one can start with the main task, namely the quantitative "synopsis" of the studies. In order to do so, one needs a suitable measure of the treatment effect (effect size) for an individual study. Suppose, for example, that in a certain study, two drugs for the treatment of alcohol dependence, A and B, are compared and that under A a proportion of 40% of the patients remain abstinent while the corresponding proportion for therapy B (possibly placebo) is only 20%. What one is looking for is a measure to express the superiority of A over B (40 vs. 20% responders) in a single number, allowing comparisons across several studies. Such measures are referred to as *effect size* measures. Consider the two cases below.

Case 1: Dichotomous Outcome Variable

Suppose that the outcome criterion for an individual patient is a variable with only two possible values, for example, "continuous abstinence during 1 year: yes/no." For a group of patients, this gives rise to a percentage (or rate), namely, in the present example, "percent of patients continuously abstinent." For illustration, take the numbers from above, 40% continuously abstinent patients under drug A ($p_A = 40\% = 0.4$) vs. 20% under drug B ($p_B = 20\% = 0.2$). Obviously, the chance of being continuously abstinent during 1 year is two times higher under drug A compared with drug B, since 40%/20% (or 0.4/0.2) = 2. This ratio is *one* useful measure to quantify the superiority of therapy A over B. It measures the relative advantage when using drug A rather than B. (As it is often used in the assessment of risks rather than positive events, it is usually called the *relative risk*.)

A more versatile effect size measure is the so-called *odds ratio*, which is closely related to the relative risk. Taking the same abstinence rates as above, $p_A = 0.4$ (= 40%) and $p_B = 0.2$ (= 20%), the odds ratio is given by:

$$\{p_A : (1 - p_A)\}/\{p_B : (1 - p_B)\}$$

$$= (0.4 : 0.6)/(0.2 : 0.8) = 0.667/0.25 = 2.667$$

The odds ratio is always somewhat higher than the relative risk; but if p_A and p_B are fairly low (up to about 0.2 = 20%), both measures are quite similar in size. The odds ratio is equal to 1 if A and B perform equally well with respect to the outcome criterion ($p_A = p_B$); it is greater if A performs better than B, and lower if B performs better than A. There is no universal rule for interpreting the size of an odds ratio, in terms of "large" or "small." However, as a rule of thumb, odds ratios between about 1 and 1.5 usually indicate rather small treatment effects; odds ratios between 1.5 and 2.5 describe moderate effects; and those greater than 2.5 to 3 generally indicate fairly large effects.

Case 2: Continuous Outcome Variable

Now suppose that the outcome of an individual patient is measured on a (continuous) numerical scale. An example would be "number of abstinent days within 1 year." For a study comparing two drugs A and B, one can summarize the outcome by taking the mean number of abstinent days under drug A (y_A = 120 days) together with the standard deviation (s_A = 55 days) and the same under drug B ($y_B \pm s_B$, 80 days (±45 days). A possible effect size measure would simply be the difference between the two means (120 – 80 = 40 days). However, to facilitate comparisons across studies, a more useful measure of effect size is the *standardized difference* between the outcome means. It is given by

$$d = (y_A - y_B)/s$$

where s is the pooled estimate of the standard deviation of the outcome variable in the two groups. In many cases, a good approximation of s is given by ($s_A + s_B$)/2 (i.e., the average of s_A and s_B). The exact formula is $s = \sqrt{\{((n_A - 1) s_A^2 + (n_B - 1) s_B^2)/(n_A + n_B - 2)\}}$, where n_A and n_B denote the sample sizes of the two groups. In this case, $s \approx (55 + 45)/2 = 50$, and thus

$$d \approx (120 - 80)/50 = 40/50 = 0.8.$$

The standardized difference of means, d, is 0 if therapy A and B perform equally well; it is greater than 0 if A performs better; and lower than 0 otherwise. Although no universal guidelines can be given for the interpretation of the size of standardized differences (since this depends on the context), one will in most cases find that values of d between 0 and 0.3 indicate rather small effects; values between 0.3 and 1 describe moderate effect sizes; and values greater than 1 point to fairly large effect sizes.

The two measures of effect size just introduced — the odds ratio and the standardized difference of means — are probably those most commonly used in meta-analyses of clinical trials. However, in the literature, several further effect size measures are found. They are summarized in Table 32.1.

EFFECT SIZE OF A SERIES OF STUDIES

Assume now that there is a *series* of k studies comparing treatments A and B, each giving rise to an effect size d_i (i = 1, ..., k) (the d_i's may be either standardized differences or odds ratios or some different effect size measure.). What one is looking for in a meta-analysis is a "joint" (or pooled) effect size d summarizing the effect sizes d_i in a statistically sound manner. A simple, straightforward

TABLE 32.1
Some Common Measures of Effect Size

Effect Size Measure	Applicable for Following Type(s) of Outcome Variable	Equality of Treatments ("no effect") Indicated By	Range (theoretical)	Range Usually Met in Real-Life Examples
Standardized difference of means, d	Continuous (numerical)	$d = 0$	$-\infty$ to $+\infty$	≈ -3 to $+3$
Odds ratio, OR	Dichotomous	$OR = 1$	0 to $+\infty$	≈ 0.1 to 10
Relative risk, RR	Dichotomous	$RR = 1$	0 to $+\infty$	≈ 0.1 to 10
Correlation coefficient, r	Continuous, ordinal, dichotomous (also a combination of these)	$r = 0$	-1 to $+1$	≈ -0.8 to $+0.8$

approach to this problem is taken in the so-called *fixed-effects model*. This is the approach most commonly used in applications. The underlying assumption is that *all* of the d_i, despite their different values, are estimates of the *same* unknown "true" effect size δ. One can then use the combined information of the k studies to obtain a more precise estimate d of δ than any of the d_i's would be. The task in the following will be to work out how to determine the joint effect size d. There are cases where the homogeneity assumption does not hold. We shall come back to this problem at the end of the chapter.

META-ANALYSIS FOR STUDIES WITH A CONTINUOUS OUTCOME VARIABLE

Start with the case of a series of studies comparing two treatments, A and B, with respect to a *continuous* outcome variable. To allow the reader to follow the computations step by step, we use an example of six studies comparing acamprosate (A) with placebo (B) using the outcome criterion "number of abstinent days within observation period" (observation period was usually 12 months; in two cases, 6 months). For each study, means and standard deviations of the outcome variable under acamprosate ($y_A \pm s_A$) and placebo ($y_B \pm s_B$) as well as the sample sizes n_A and n_B are displayed in Table 32.2. The computations necessary for the meta-analysis can be split into four steps. A mathematical derivation of the formulae can be found in the book by Hedges and Olkin.[3]

TABLE 32.2
Example Data for Meta-analysis with a Continuous Outcome Measure: Comparison of Acamprosate (A) and Placebo (B) with respect to Total Number of Abstinent Days During 1 Year

Study Number	Drug A (Acamprosate)		Drug B (Placebo)		Total Sample Size ($N = n_A + n_B$)	Standard Deviation[b] ($s_0 = (s_A + s_B)/2$)	Effect Size ($d = (y_A - y_B)/s_0$)	Weight	Ref.
	n_A	Abstinent Days $y_A \pm s_A$ (mean ± SD)	n_B	Abstinent Days $y_B \pm s_B$ (mean ± SD)					
1[a]	29	121.8 ± 139.1	32	77.5 ± 99.3	61	119.2	0.372	15.0	6
2	361	210.0 ± 133.5	177	173.0 ± 126.0	538	129.8	0.285	117.7	7
3	136	224.6 ± 136.6	136	162.0 ± 132.2	272	134.4	0.466	66.2	8
4	224	138.8 ± 137.5	224	103.8 ± 119.0	448	128.2	0.273	111.0	9
5[a]	128	61.0 ± 70.0	134	43.0 ± 58.0	262	64.0	0.281	64.9	10
6	55	136.9 ± 147.5	55	74.7 ± 107.9	110	127.7	0.487	26.7	11

[a] Observation period was only 180 days. [b] Approximation of the exact formula.

Step 1: Calculate the effect sizes (standardized mean differences) for the individual studies

These are worked out as shown above. To distinguish individual studies use subscript i for the i-th study: the effect size of the i-th study will be denoted by d_i, the sample sizes by $n_{i,A}$ and $n_{i,B}$, etc. Then,

$$d_i = \left(y_{i,A} - y_{i,B}\right)/s_i,$$

where s_i denotes the pooled standard deviation of the two samples, which can here always be approximated by the average of the two standard deviations ($s_i = (s_{i,A} + s_{i,B})/2$).

For the first study, we obtain $s_1 \approx (139.1 + 99.3)/2 = 119.2$ and, thus,

$$d_1 = \left(121.8 - 77.5\right)/119.2 = 44.3/119.2 = 0.372;$$

for the others, the computations run accordingly (cf. Table 32.2).

Step 2: Obtain weights (w_i) for the individual studies

The rationale behind the idea of weighting is basically that studies with a large sample size (giving rise to a rather precise estimate of the effect size) should be given a higher impact than studies with a small sample size (giving rise to a fairly inaccurate estimate of the effect size). A good approximation to the optimal weight value is given by

$$w_i = 2\,N_i/\left(8 + d_i^2\right),$$

where w_i is the weight for the i-th study and N_i the total sample size in the i-th study. For very unequal sample sizes in the two groups (e.g., if one sample exceeds the other by more than 50%), N_i has to be replaced by $4\,(n_{i,A} * n_{i,B})/(n_{i,A} + n_{i,B})$. For the first study, one obtains

$$w_1 = 2*61/\left(8 + 0.372^2\right) = 122/8.138 = 14.99 \left(\approx 15.0\right).$$

Note that in the second study, the two sample sizes are very different from each other, and thus N_i should be replaced by $4\,(n_{i,A} * n_{i,B})/(n_{i,A} + n_{i,B})$. Here it amounts to $4 * (361 * 177)/(361 + 177) = 475.07$, which is considerably smaller than $N = 538$.

Step 3: Calculate the joint effect size

This is simply the weighted mean of the individual effect sizes d_i:

$$d = \left\{\Sigma\, w_i\, d_i\right\}/\Sigma\, w_i,$$

where Σ means summation over all studies (i = 1, ..., k). In this example,

$$d = \left\{0.372*15.0 + 0.285*117.7 + ...\right\}/\left\{15.0 + 117.7 + ...\right\} = 131.5/401.4 = 0.328.$$

Using the rule of thumb of the last section, this has to be considered a small to moderate effect size.

Step 4: Calculate the 95% confidence interval for the joint effect size

The formulae for the 95% confidence interval are

$$\text{Lower bound: } d_{lower} = d - 1.96 * \sqrt{\left\{1/\left(\Sigma\ w_i\right)\right\}},$$

$$\text{Upper bound: } d_{upper} = d + 1.96 * \sqrt{\left\{1/\left(\Sigma\ w_i\right)\right\}}.$$

In this example, one obtains

$$d_{lower} = 0.328 - 1.96 * \sqrt{\left\{1/401.4\right\}} = 0.328 - 1.96 * 0.0499 = 0.230,$$

$$d_{upper} = 0.328 + 1.96 * \sqrt{\left\{1/401.4\right\}} = 0.328 + 1.96 * 0.0499 = 0.426.$$

The 95% confidence interval contains only positive values (excluding 0). Therefore, the joint effect size is significantly greater than zero on the 5% level ($p < 0.05$). Expressed verbally, overall, acamprosate performed significantly better than placebo with respect to the outcome criterion "time without relapse."

The exact p-value can be determined by computing

$$z = d/\sqrt{\left\{1/\left(\Sigma\ w_i\right)\right\}} = 0.328/0.0499 = 6.57$$

and looking up this value in a table of the standardized normal distribution (this yields the one-sided p-value). Here, z exceeds all the tabulated values. For example, a one-sided p of 0.00005 would correspond to z = 3.89. Therefore, the two-sided p in our case is lower than $2 * 0.0005 = 0.0001$.

META-ANALYSIS FOR STUDIES WITH A DICHOTOMOUS OUTCOME VARIABLE

If the outcome variable for an individual patient is dichotomous, the techniques used above are not directly applicable. However, the general approach is similar. One can demonstrate the procedure using the same studies as above and the outcome variable "continuous abstinence during one year: yes/no." The numbers required for the computations (sample sizes n_A and n_B, response rates p_A and p_B) are displayed in Table 32.3.

Step 1: Calculate effect size for individual studies

As noted before, the effect size for the comparison of studies with a dichotomous outcome variable is usually expressed as the *odds ratio* of the two proportions p_A and p_B (in the following formulae, they are expressed as numbers between 0 and 1 rather than percentages):

$$\textit{Odds ratio, } OR = \frac{p_A/\left(1 - p_A\right)}{p_B/\left(1 - p_B\right)}$$

For example, for the first study, one obtains

$$OR_1 = \left(0.379 : 0.621\right)/\left(0.156 : 0.844\right) = 0.610/0.185 = 3.30.$$

TABLE 32.3

Example Data for Meta-analysis with a Dichotomous Outcome Measure: Comparison of Acamprosate (A) and Placebo (B) with Respect to Continous Abstinence During 1 Year

Study Number	Drug A (Acamprosate)		Drug B (Placebo)		Total Sample Size $(N = n_A + n_B)$	Odds Ratio (A vs. B) $\left(OR = \dfrac{p_A/(1-p_A)}{p_B/(1-p_B)}\right)$	ln (OR)	Weight	Ref.
	n_A	% continuously abstinent patients: p_A	n_B	% continuously abstinent patients: p_B					
1[a]	29	37.9	32	15.6	61	3.30	1.19	2.61	6
2	361	18.6	177	11.3	538	1.79	0.58	13.39	7
3	136	42.6	136	20.6	272	2.86	1.05	13.33	8
4	224	18.3	224	7.1	448	2.93	1.08	10.25	9
5[a]	128	19.5	134	9.7	262	2.26	0.81	7.41	10
6	55	25.5	55	14.5	110	2.02	0.70	4.13	11

[a] Observation period was only 180 days.

Step 2: Obtain weights for individual studies

Similar to the case of a continuous outcome variable, the odds ratio of the series is basically a weighted sum of the individual odds ratios. The somewhat complicated-looking formula is given by

$$w = \frac{n_A \, p_A \left(1-p_A\right) * n_B \, p_B \left(1-p_B\right)}{n_A \, p_A \left(1-p_A\right) + n_B \, p_B \left(1-p_B\right)}.$$

These weights must be calculated in turn for each study (w_i, i = 1, ..., k). For the first study, one obtains

$$w_1 = \frac{29 * 0.379 * 0.621 * 32 * 0.156 * 0.844}{29 * 0.379 * 0.621 + 32 * 0.156 * 0.844} = 28.757/11.038 = 2.61.$$

Step 3: Calculate joint odds ratio for series of studies

The formula is somewhat more complicated than for a continuous outcome variable. First calculate the natural logarithm (ln) of all the odds ratios (second last column in Table 33.3). One obtains the logarithm of the joint odds ratio as the weighted mean of the individual values:

$$\ln\left(OR_{series}\right) = \left\{\Sigma \, w_i \, \ln\left(OR_i\right)\right\} / \Sigma \, w_i,$$

where subscript i indicates the i-th study.

In the example,

$$\ln\left(OR_{series}\right) = \left\{2.61 * 1.19 + 13.39 * 0.58 + ...\right\} / \left\{2.61 + 13.39 + ...\right\} = 44.9/51.1 = 0.878.$$

The joint odds ratio, OR_{series}, is obtained by exponentiation:

$$OR_{series} = e^{\left\{\text{expression on r.h.s. of formula}\right\}} = e^{0.878} = 2.406.$$

Step 4: Calculate 95% confidence interval

An approximate 95% confidence interval for the odds ratio of the series of studies can be calculated using the following formulae:

$$OR_{series,lower} = OR_{series} * \exp\left\{-1.96 * \sqrt{\left(1/\Sigma\ w_i\right)}\right\},$$

$$OR_{series,upper} = OR_{series} * \exp\left\{1.96 * \sqrt{\left\{1/\Sigma\ w_i\right\}}\right\},$$

where "exp" denotes exponentiation $[\exp(x) = e^x]$. In this example, one obtains

$$1.96\ \sqrt{\left\{1/\left(\Sigma\ w_i\right)\right\}} = 1.96 * \sqrt{\left\{1/51.1\right\}} = 0.2741$$

and, hence,

$$OR_{series,lower} = 2.406 * e^{-0.2741} = 1.829$$

$$OR_{series,upper} = 2.406 * e^{0.2741} = 3.165$$

The joint odds ratio, OR_{series}, is significantly greater than 1 ($OR = 1$ would correspond to equality of treatments A and B) with $p < 0.05$, since the 95%-confidence interval contains only values greater than 1. Again, as in the case of a continuous outcome variable, the exact p-value can be found via the z-value $z = \ln (OR_{series})/\sqrt{\{1/(\Sigma w_i)\}}$. We skip the computations here (in the example, $z = 6.28$, giving rise to a p-value < 0.0001).

According to the above-mentioned criteria, the odds ratio of 2.406 is moderate in size, but fairly close to the upper end of the region termed "moderate." Together with the high level of statistical significance ($p < 0.0001$), this shows a clear superiority of treatment A (acamprosate) over treatment B (placebo) with respect to the variable "continuous abstinence."

A FEW CAVEATS

Caution should be exercised when performing a meta-analysis or studying the results of published meta-analyses. In particular, the following should be kept in mind:

1. The results of a meta-analysis may be flawed by a *publication bias*, that is, by the fact that some studies on the issue investigated have never been published. Various methods to check for this have been developed and the reader is referred to the literature.[2,12,13]
2. The methods described here are based on the assumption of a *homogeneous* series of studies; that is, it is assumed that the observed differences in effect size between studies are only due to sampling error in random sampling and not to any other sources of error. A statistical test for homogeneity of a series of studies can be easily performed and methods to deal with heterogeneous series are available.[2,14,15]
3. Heterogeneity of a series of studies may, among other reasons, be due to *differences in important patient characteristics* between studies. For example, the patients in the individual studies may differ with respect to age or severity of symptomatology. Alternatively, there may be differences regarding *study characteristics* (e.g., year of study conduct).[16] There are special ways to deal with this particular type of heterogeneity.[1,3,17]

CONCLUDING REMARKS

This chapter provided an introduction to the topic of meta-analysis. While it attempted to keep things fairly simple, the reader should be reminded that meta-analysis as such is a complex subject matter. Complexity is not primarily entered by statistical difficulties but rather by issues lying beyond the scope of statistics. In doing a meta-analysis, we subsume a number of studies differing in many respects, both quantitative (e.g., mean age of study participants) and qualitative (e.g., quality of study conduct). The former, quantitative aspects, can be dealt with by appropriate statistical methods. However, this is much less clear for the latter (i.e., qualitative aspects). Here, some method of operationalization must be found first, before statistical handling is possible. It is mainly because of such qualitative aspects that meta-analyses continue to be an issue of considerable controversy in the scientific literature.[17-20] This should be borne in mind when studying published meta-analyses or when embarking on one's own meta-analysis.

For further reading, the above-mentioned monograph by Petitti[1] is recommended; it also contains a large number of cross-references. An excellent review of meta-analysis methodology is given by Friedenreich which, despite its title, concerns both clinical as well as epidemiologic studies.[21] Some important aspects of the state of the art in meta-analysis are also dealt with by Lau et al.,[1] Pogue et al.,[20] and Moher and Olkin,[22] among others.

REFERENCES

1. Lau, J., Ioannidis, J.P.A., and Schmid, C.H., Summing up evidence: one answer is not always enough, *Lancet*, 351, 123, 1998.
2. Petitti, D.B., *Meta-Analysis, Decision Analysis, and Cost-Effectiveness Analysis*, Oxford University Press, New York, 1994.
3. Hedges, L.V. and Olkin, I., *Statistical Methods for Meta-Analysis*, Academic Press, Orlando, 1985.
4. Sacks, H.S., Berrier, J., Reitman, D., Ancona-Berk, V.A., and Chalmers, T.C., Meta-analyses of randomized controlled trials, *N. Eng. J. Med.*, 316, 450, 1987.
5. Easterbrook, P.J., Berlin, J.A., Gopalan, R., and Matthews, D.R., Publication bias in research, *Lancet*, 337, 867, 1991.
6. Ladewig, D., Knecht, T., Leher, P., and Fendl, A., Acamprosat — ein Stabilisierungsfaktor in der Langzeitentwoehnung von Alkoholabhaengigen, *Ther. Umschau*, 50, 182, 1993.
7. Paille, F.M., Guelfi, J.D., Perkins, A.C., Royer, R.J., Stern, L., and Parot, P., Double-blind randomized multicentre trial of acamprosate in maintaining abstinence from alcohol, *Alcohol Alcohol.*, 30, 239, 1995.
8. Sass, H., Soyka, M., Mann, K., and Zieglgaensberger, W., Relapse prevention by acamprosate. Results from a placebo-controlled study on alcohol dependence, *Arch. Gen. Psychiatry*, 49, 673, 1996.
9. Whitworth, A.B., Fischer, F., Lesch, O.M., Nimmerrichter, A., Oberbauer, H., Platz, H., Potgieter, A., Walter, H., and Fleischhacker, W.W., Comparison of acamprosate and placebo in long-term treatment of alcohol dependence, *Lancet*, 347, 1438, 1996.
10. Geerlings, P.J., Ansoms, C., and Van den Brink, W., Acamprosate and prevention of relapse in alcoholics. Results of a randomized placebo-controlled, double-blind study in out-patient alcoholics in the Netherlands, Belgium and Luxembourg, *Eur. Addiction Res.*, 3, 129, 1997.
11. Besson, J., Aeby, F., Kasas, A., Lehert, P., and Potgieter, A., Combined efficacy of acamprosate and disulfiram in the treatment of alcoholism: a controlled study, *Alcohol. Clin. Exp. Res.*, 22, 573, 1998.
12. Chalmers, T.C., Frank, C.S., and Reitman, D., Minimizing the three stages of publication bias, *JAMA*, 263, 1392, 1990.
13. Berlin, J.A., Begg, C.B., and Louis, T.A., An assessment of publication bias using a sample of published clinical trials, *J. Am. Stat. Assoc.*, 84, 381, 1989.
14. DerSimonian, R. and Laird, N., Meta-analysis in clinical trials, *Controlled Clin. Trials*, 7, 177, 1986.
15. Thompson, S.G. and Pocock, S.J., Can meta-analyses be trusted? *Lancet*, 338, 1127, 1991.
16. Rothwell, P.M. and Robertson, G., Meta-analyses of randomised controlled trials, *Lancet*, 350, 1181, 1997.

17. Davey Smith, G. and Egger, M., Meta-analysis of randomised controlled trials, *Lancet*, 350, 1182, 1997.

18. Editorial, Meta-analysis under scrutiny, *Lancet*, 350, 675, 1997.

19. LeLorier, J., Gregoire, G., Benhaddad, A., Lapierre, J., and Derderian, F., Discrepancies between meta-analyses and subsequent large randomized, controlled trials, *N. Engl. J. Med.*, 337, 536, 1997.

20. Pogue, J. and Yusuf, S., Overcoming the limitations of current meta-analysis of randomised controlled trials, *Lancet*, 351, 47, 1998.

21. Friedenreich, C.M., Methods for pooled analyses of epidemiologic studies, *Epidemiology*, 4, 295, 1993.

22. Moher, D. and Olkin, I., Meta-analysis of randomized clinical trials: a concern for standards, *JAMA*, 274, 1962, 1995.

33 Patient-to-Treatment Matching

Richard K. Fuller and John P. Allen

OVERVIEW

Matching treatments according to the specific needs of alcoholic patients has evoked considerable interest among researchers, practitioners, and policy-makers. Scientific literature on "patient-treatment matching" is reviewed in this chapter. The primary emphasis is on the results of Project MATCH, a multisite U.S. trial of patient-treatment matching comparing three different psychotherapeutic treatments: Twelve-Step Facilitation (TSF), Cognitive-Behavioral Therapy (CBT), and Motivational Enhancement Therapy (MET). Project MATCH tested 21 predicted matches. Only four were verified — three in the outpatient cohort arm and one in the aftercare group (i.e., those who had a period of inpatient, residential, or day hospital treatment just prior to being treated with one of the MATCH therapies). Among the outpatients, those high in anger had better outcomes when treated with MET, and those with a social network permissive of drinking or who were low in psychiatric severity benefited more from TSF. The match between patients low in psychiatric severity and TSF treatment did not persist 1 year after treatment. Those patients initially treated as inpatients and who were higher in severity of dependence benefited more from TSF. While these results only weakly support the patient-treatment matching hypothesis, they do suggest that there will be some incremental improvement in treatment outcome if outpatients are screened for anger, type of social network, and psychiatric severity and aftercare patients for severity of alcohol dependence.

INTRODUCTION

The excessive use of alcohol can result in a wide array of physical, emotional, family, and social problems. Some of the more common alcohol-related problems seen in physician offices are hypertension, insomnia, abdominal pain, frequent trauma, and depression.[1] It is not surprising, therefore, that up to 20% of the patients seeking care in primary care settings meet criteria for alcohol abuse or dependence. Primary care physicians are thus in a pivotal position to identify these patients and provide care for both the immediate presenting complaints as well as the misuse of alcohol that may cause or exacerbate these problems.

PATIENT–TREATMENT MATCHING

Assigning patients to different treatments as a function of the clinical features of the illness or particular personal characteristics is commonly done in medicine. For example, a man with prostate cancer may receive surgery or radiation based on extent of the disease (clinical feature) or age (patient attribute). Matching individuals to treatment by patient attributes has been studied in psychotherapy and education as well as in medicine.[2] For many years, matching has also been advocated for alcoholism treatment. Because many alcoholics benefit from treatment and no single treatment is effective for all, the concept of matching patients to specific treatments rather than the traditional treatment strategy of "one size fits all" holds great promise for improving alcoholism treatment outcomes.

0-8493-7801-X/00/$0.00+$.50
© 2000 by CRC Press LLC

Prior to the initiation of Project MATCH, a large, multisite clinical trial designed to evaluate alcoholism patient-treatment interactions, at least 28 studies on the topic had been previously reported.[3] Most of these projects focused on the role of personality features and alcohol-related variables. Earlier matching studies generally involved secondary analysis of data sets rather than being specifically designed and conducted prospectively to evaluate matching effects. Few of the projects involved replication in settings or sites beyond the original study location. Thus, it is difficult to determine how robust or generalizable their findings might be and the advantages that might derive from incorporating patient-treatment matching strategies into applied treatment settings. Finally, these studies, with apparently only four exceptions, were conducted in the context of alcoholism treatment or psychiatric programs. Hence, the degree to which findings might extend to primary care or other settings remains unclear.

These limitations notwithstanding, some conclusions can be drawn from this corpus of literature:

1. Matching effects typically occurred for only one of the two or more treatments under investigation and often only for individuals at one level (usually at the high or low end) of the patient attribute. For example, those low in conceptual level, or high in sociopathy, or more dependent on alcohol were reported to respond better to one of two treatments offered, whereas those at the other extreme of these dimensions did equally well in either of the two treatments.

2. On the positive side, results across studies were not contradictory, and in no instance did observed matching effects reverse themselves within studies. None of the studies suggested, for example, that while one treatment would be most beneficial in terms of improved drinking status at early follow-up, an alternative treatment would be more beneficial at a later point in time.

3. From the existing evidence, it appears that patients with more severe problems, whether in terms of their alcohol dependence, cooccurring psychiatric problems, or deficiencies in personal resources, tended to achieve more favorable outcomes when assigned to more intense interventions (e.g., inpatient rather than outpatient). Patients without these significant liabilities typically did equally as well in both less intense and more intense treatments.

4. Sociopathy seemed to be an especially potent matching variable. Patients higher in sociopathy or related problems in general typically gained more from behavioral therapies stressing the acquisition of coping skills. On the other hand, those low in sociopathy appeared to do as well in treatments that reinforced improvements of interpersonal relationships as they did in interventions that were intended to develop more effective coping skills.

PROJECT MATCH: RATIONALE AND DESIGN

Despite the small scale of most of the previous studies on patient-alcoholism treatment interactions, as well as their frequent methodologic limitations, the "matching hypothesis" attracted considerable interest from treatment providers and researchers in the field. An expert panel assembled by the Institute of Medicine strongly urged that systematic and definitive studies of patient-treatment matching be done.[4]

The rationale and protocol of Project MATCH have been described in more detail elsewhere.[5] Therefore, only the basic design of the study will be briefly summarized here. Project MATCH was conducted at nine clinical sites and included two separate arms. Patients in the "aftercare" arm had received a course of inpatient or day hospital treatment beyond detoxification before receiving the MATCH treatments. They were usually enrolled in Project MATCH within a week of discharge. Those in the "outpatient" arm were recruited at outpatient clinics rather than hospital, residential, or day hospital facilities.

A total of 1726 patients were randomly assigned to three treatments. The three interventions were Twelve-Step Facilitation (TSF), Cognitive-Behavioral Therapy (CBT), and Motivational Enhancement Therapy (MET). The objective of TSF was to facilitate not only attendance but involvement in Alcoholics Anonymous (AA). Patients were actively encouraged to attend AA meetings, obtain a sponsor, read the AA literature, and complete the first few steps of the 12 steps. Cognitive Behavioral Therapy was based on social learning theory. It was designed to overcome coping skills deficits and increase the ability to constructively deal with events, either intrapersonal (e.g., depression) or external (e.g., social pressure to drink), that commonly precipitate relapse. Motivational Enhancement Therapy was based on principles of motivational psychology. It focused on strengthening commitment and motivation to resolve drinking problem and employed strategies to mobilize the individual's own resources.

These treatments were selected based on their potential for matching, distinctiveness from each other, practicability of being implemented in community treatment settings, and previous evidence of efficacy.[6] TSF and CBT consisted of 12 weekly 1-hour sessions. MET entailed four hourly sessions during the 12-week period. Treatments were administered in a one-on-one format and each session was guided by a standardized manual. Manuals for the three treatments employed in Project MATCH can be obtained from the National Clearinghouse for Alcohol and Drug Information, P.O. Box 2345, Rockville, MD 20847-2345; (http://www.health.org/pubs/catalog/ordering.htm).

Of the 21 *a priori* hypotheses that predicted a variety of matches to the three treatments, 10 were considered primary and 11 secondary. Although the secondary hypotheses were also formulated before analysis of the data, either the literature that prompted them appeared less compelling than that leading to the selection of the primary hypotheses, or the patient characteristic included in a secondary hypothesis was somewhat overlapping with one in a primary hypothesis. The primary and secondary hypotheses were based on previous alcohol research findings as well as on reflection about matching effects observed in the broad psychotherapy literature. The hypotheses were tested separately in the two arms. Matching effects were evaluated across time on two primary dependent variables: percentage of days abstinent and the average number of drinks on those days when the patient drank.

Follow-up assessments were done at 3-month intervals from the point of randomization to 15 months later (1 year after the 3-month treatment period concluded). Additionally, patients in the outpatient sites had an additional assessment at 39 months (3 years after treatment).

Only one of the ten primary hypotheses was validated.[6] As predicted, *outpatients* low in psychiatric severity assigned to TSF drank on fewer days than did those assigned to CBT. The matching effect was most pronounced at 6 months after treatment, with the low psychiatric severity patients assigned to TSF drinking on only 13% of the days, but low psychiatric severity patients assigned to CBT consuming alcohol on 27% of the days. This matching effect persisted for 8 months but was no longer present 1 year after treatment ended.

Three matches were also seen in tests of the secondary hypotheses. In the *outpatient* arm of the trial, the degree of patient anger at baseline interacted with treatment. Subjects higher in anger achieved better outcomes on both dependent variables if assigned to MET than if assigned to TSF and CBT ($p < 0.014$ and $p < 0.011$ for percent days abstinent and drinks per drinking day, respectively.)[7] The finding that MET produced more abstinent days and fewer drinks per drinking day for those higher in anger at baseline was also found at the 3-year follow-up.[8]

In the *aftercare* arm, patients with more severe alcohol dependence experienced a higher percent of alcohol-free days ($p < 0.006$) and consumed fewer drinks on those days in which they did drink ($p < 0.010$) if treated with TSF than if treated with CBT. Conversely, those individuals lower in alcohol dependence did better with CBT.[7]

Finally, an interesting matching effect was found in the 3-year follow-up of *outpatient* subjects.[8] Patients having pre-treatment social networks (peers, coworkers, and family) more supportive of drinking had more abstinent days if assigned to TSF than if treated in MET. Those with social support networks supportive of drinking and who were assigned to TSF drank on only 23% of the days, whereas patients with social support networks supportive of drinking and assigned to MET drank on 39% of the days. Similarly, "matched" patients averaged only 4.5 drinks per drinking day vs. 6.0 drinks per drinking day if they were "mismatched" to treatment. For patients whose social networks did not encourage drinking, MET, TSF and CBT resulted in approximately equivalent outcomes.[9] In a series of secondary analyses, Longabaugh et al.[9] determined that at least part of the reason for the favorable matching effect was due to the fact that TSF participation was associated with greater involvement in Alcoholics Anonymous.

In summary, only 4 of 21 predicted matches were found: 3 in the outpatient arm and 1 in the aftercare arm. One match (the one in which patients scoring low in psychiatric severity had a better outcome when treated with TSF) did not persist for the entire 1 year following treatment. These results, at best, support the broad patient-treatment matching hypothesis only weakly, but they still have some relevance for alcoholism treatment programs. They suggest that patients be screened for degree of anger, severity of dependence, type of social network, and psychiatric severity. In Project MATCH, the Spiegelberger State-Trait Anxiety Scale, Edinburgh Dependence Scale, the Important Persons and Activities Interview, and the psychiatric severity subscale of the Addiction Severity Index were used to assess for these patient attributes. This assessment takes approximately 1 hour. The small investment of time could ensure more appropriate treatment. For those patients whose networks are supportive of drinking, it would be important to facilitate involvement in Twelve-Step programs.

Several reasons have been suggested for why the patient-treatment interaction effects observed in Project MATCH were not greater in number. Clearly, one possibility is that, despite previous findings and the attractiveness of the matching hypotheses, matching does not substantially augment treatment outcome.[6] Were the treatments more radically different, such as contrasting a verbal therapy with a medication, perhaps matching effects might have been greater. Also, Project MATCH did not study assigning patients to treatment settings differing in intensity (e.g., residential vs. outpatient).

Second, the three treatments achieved similar main effects on the two primary outcome measures, percent days abstinent, and drinks per drinking day (Table 33.1). However, Twelve-Step Facilitation resulted in significantly longer sustained abstinence (1 year continuous abstinence) in the *outpatients* than CBT or MET (24 vs. 15 and 14%, respectively). This was not the case for the aftercare arm; there, the three treatments were equivalent in achieving 35% 1-year continuous abstinence.

Third, patients stayed in treatment longer than is generally the experience in outpatient alcoholism treatment and as a group did remarkably well (Table 33.2). Overall, there was a marked reduction in drinking frequency and quantity after entry into treatment, a reduction in alcohol-related problems as well as drinking for at least 1 year, and a reduction in drinking that persisted for 3 years. It may well be that some type of treatment "ceiling" effect occurred, suppressing the

---

TABLE 33.1
Effects of CBT, MET, and TSF on Two Indices of Drinking

	3 Months Prior to Treatment		15-Month Follow-up	
	% Days Abstinent	Drinks per Drinking Day	% Days Abstinent	Drinks per Drinking Day
Aftercare arm				
CBT	23	15	89	2
MET	19	15	88	2
TSF	24	15	88	2
Outpatient arm				
CBT	27	11	79	3
MET	27	11	79	3
TSF	30	11	83	2

TABLE 33.2
Long-Term Effects of MATCH Treatments

Variables	Baseline Prior 3 Months	39 Months Prior 3 Months
Median days abstinent (all Ss)	28%	86%
Median drinks per drinking day (all Ss)	11.54	4.21
Median days abstinent (excluding abstainers at follow-up)	27%	68%
Median drinks per drinking day (excluding abstainers at follow-up)	10.88	6.24

potential benefits of matching. This latter possibility may well have been the case since other features of treatment such as counselor characteristics, patient characteristics, and type of treatment accounted for much smaller percentages of outcome variance than is generally found in alcoholism treatment efficacy studies.

MATCH IMPLICATIONS FOR PRIMARY CARE

While Project MATCH was not conducted in primary care settings, its findings seem to have implications for family practice physicians treating alcoholics. Given its somewhat lower cost, lower intensity, and near-equal effects with CBT and TSF, primary care physicians might well use features of MET in their practices. At the same time, they should encourage participation in AA or in some other peer support group. This would seem particularly advisable for patients who have social networks that support drinking and for patients who do not suffer significant psychopathology.

Procedures for conducting MET are described in detail in the Project MATCH MET treatment manual.[10] This document is available from the National Clearinghouse for Alcohol and Drug Information, P.O. Box 2345, Rockville, MD 20847-2345; (http://www.health.org/pubs/catalog/ordering.htm). MET can be modified to meet the constraints imposed by the practice setting (e.g., time limitations, fiscal resources).

MET begins with an assessment battery that inquires about the patient's usual quantity and frequency of drinking, as well as periods of high consumption. Also evaluated is the nature of problems related to alcohol use. DrInC, a measure of such consequences, can be employed in this regard.[11] (This instrument and its documentation are also available from the National Clearinghouse for Alcohol and Drug Information.) Additionally, measures of the severity of alcohol dependence as well as biochemical measures of heavy drinking (e.g., gamma-glutamyl transpeptidase) should be employed. Other factors that should be assessed include neuropsychological functioning; individual risk factors, such as positive family history of alcohol problems; and the level of patient motivation. Results of these tests are provided to the patient in the form of a personalized feedback report. This extensive assessment is beyond the capabilities of a typical primary care practice, and referral to outside resources may be necessary. A practice employing a nurse or health education specialist with sufficient time may find it feasible to implement MET.

MET is based on principles of the psychology of motivation. It attempts to utilize the client's own resources for effecting change. MET incorporates the "FRAMES" model. FRAMES is a mnemonic referring to six elements found to enhance brief interventions for alcohol problems:[12]

*F*eedback on personal risk of alcohol abuse or excessive consumption
Emphasis on the patient's own *R*esponsibility for changing drinking behavior
Clear *A*dvice to the patient to diminish or cease consumption
A *M*enu of options for the patient on how to reduce drinking
*E*mpathetic rather than confrontational style of counseling
Enhancement of *S*elf-efficacy or -optimism in the patient that he or she is able to make changes

The spouse or some other person who is significant to the patient typically participates in the first two MET sessions.

While it may not be practical to implement MET as developed for Project MATCH, certain elements appear important and feasible for the primary care setting. Feedback specific to the patient appears to motivate change.[12] Because patients may fail to acknowledge that drinking is a cause of their problems, possibly because of embarrassment or simply failing to appreciate the adverse effects of drinking on their health or well-being, it is important that the physician discuss the problem with the patient in a non-judgmental manner. It is also important that the physician be encouraging that the problem can be treated. Advice should be given in a direct, albeit supportive, manner.

Outside of the family and the workplace, the physician's office may be the only place that the alcohol problem comes to light. Thus, it is important not to miss an opportunity to treat the underlying alcohol abuse or dependence as well as to diagnose and treat the presenting problem.

REFERENCES

1. Barry, K.L. and Fleming, M.F., The family physician, *Alcohol Health Res. World*, 18, 105, 1994.
2. Mattson, M.E., Allen, J.P., Longabaugh, R., Nickless, C.J., Connors, G.J., and Kadden, R.M., A chronological review of empirical studies matching alcoholic clients to treatment, *J. Stud. Alcohol*, Suppl. 12, 16, 1994.
3. Allen, J.P. and Kadden, R.M. Matching clients to alcohol treatments, R.K. Hester and W.R. Miller, Eds., *Handbook of Alcoholism Treatment Approaches*, 2nd ed., Allyn and Bacon, Boston, 1995, 278.
4. Institute of Medicine, *Broadening the Base of Treatment for Alcohol Problems*, National Academy Press, Washington, D.C., 1990.
5. Project MATCH Research Group, Project MATCH: rationale and methods for a multisite clinical trial matching patients to alcoholism treatment, *Alcohol. Clin. Exp. Res.*, 17, 1130, 1993.
6. Project MATCH Research Group, Matching alcoholism treatments to client heterogeneity: Project MATCH posttreatment drinking outcomes, *J. Stud. Alcohol*, 58, 7, 1997.
7. Project MATCH Research Group, Project MATCH secondary a priori hypotheses, *Addiction*, 92, 1671, 1997.
8. Project MATCH Research Group, Matching alcoholism treatments to client heterogenity: Project MATCH three-year drinking outcomes, *Alcohol. Clin. Exp. Res.*, 22, 1300, 1998.
9. Longabaugh, R., Wirtz, P.W., Zweben, A., and Stout, R.L., Network support for drinking, Alcoholics Anonymous and long-term matching effects, *Addiction*, 93, 1313, 1998.
10. Miller, W.R., Zweben, A., DiClemente, C.C., and Rychtarik, R.G., *Motivational Enhancement Therapy Manual*, National Institute on Alcohol Abuse and Alcoholism, Rockville, MD, 1992.
11. Miller, W.R., Tonigan, J.S., and Longabaugh, R. *The Drinker Inventory of Consequences (DrInC): An Instrument for Assessing Adverse Consequences of Alcohol Abuse*, Test Manual. NIAAA Project MATCH Monograph Series, Vol. 4, NIH Pub. No. 95-3911, U.S. Government Printing Office, Washington, D.C., 1995.
12. Bien, T.H., Miller, W.R., and Tonigan, J.S., Brief interventions for alcohol problems: a review, *Addiction*, 88, 315, 1993.

34 Molecular Pharmacology and Neuroanatomy

Elio Acquas

OVERVIEW

Until recently, the psychiatric and somatic effects of alcohol were considered to result from "non-specific" membrane fluidizing properties. However, the discovery that alcohol acts on receptor-gated ion channels ($GABA_A$, NMDA, and $5HT_3$) in a saturable and specific manner has now led to the belief that the behavioral and neurochemical properties of alcohol are the consequence of a number of specific receptor interactions of this chemical in the brain. Besides its interactions with $GABA_A$, NMDA, and $5HT_3$ receptors, alcohol has also been found to specifically interact with the dopaminergic, opioidergic, as well as adenosine receptors. Overall, the investigation into alcohol's specific receptor interactions is still evolving; thus, the following brief overview should be taken only as snapshot of a rapidly evolving field of research. Alcohol's actions on such a multitude of target systems may be due to the convergence of more than just one mechanism of this simple chemical. Such a high degree of redundancy in the molecular and functional effects of alcohol still awaits a clarification.

ALCOHOL AND GABA

The advancement of knowledge about alcohol's actions at molecular level has progressively transformed its pharmacology from a unified hypothesis (mostly referring to "nonselective" effects on neuronal membranes) to the description of its discrete molecular mechanisms. The basis for the progress toward the identification of the molecular basis of alcohol mechanisms in the brain was the observation that a positive relationship exists between blood alcohol concentrations (<50 mmol l^{-1}) and the appearance of alcohol behavioral effects. Allan and Harris described that the GABA-benzodiazepine receptor complex is sensitive to low (5 to 15 mmol l^{-1}) alcohol concentrations.[5] Indeed, alcohol shares, with other compounds known to act at the $GABA_A$ receptor complex (i.e., benzodiazepines and barbiturates), a number of pharmacological effects such as sedation, ability to reduce anxiety, loss of righting reflex (defined in rats as deep sedation with inability to move from the upside-down position), and hypnosis.

The $GABA_A$ receptor is an oligomeric protein complex associated with a receptor-gated ion channel and contains specific allosteric binding sites for benzodiazepines and barbiturates.[100,123] $GABA_A$ receptors are embedded in the membrane of neurons and consist of five protein subunits to form a channel. Thus, when GABA or GABA-like compounds bind to the receptor and activate it, the channel opens and allows the passage of chloride ions (from outside to inside the neuron), therefore decreasing neuronal excitability. Each subunit of the $GABA_A$ receptor complex consists of a large extracellular region of four segments spanning the cell membrane and of several intracellular regions (Figure 34.1). The phosphorylation of specific intracellular regions of these segments by protein kinase C (PKC) may regulate the function of these receptors and it was suggested that subunit phosphorylation might be the requirement for alcohol's action taking place at the $GABA_A$ receptor complex. A recent study on transgenic mice, in which the gene for the γ-isoform

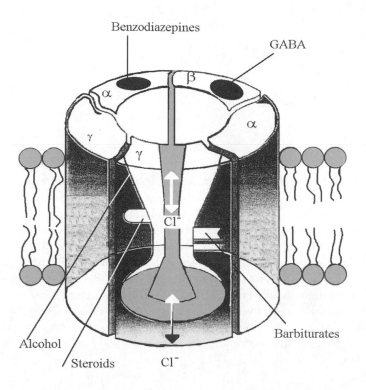

FIGURE 34.1 Schematic three-dimensional representation of the GABA$_A$ receptor complex with the recognition sites for GABA, benzodiazepines, alcohol, steroids, and barbiturates.

of PKC was knocked out, showed that some of the behavioral effects of alcohol (loss of the righting reflex and hypothermia) were abolished, thus suggesting that genetic differences in PKC isozymes might be responsible for differences in sensitivity to alcohol.[62] GABA$_A$ receptor subunits fall into four main categories — α, β, γ, and δ — and each of these categories can exist in different subunits (i.e., γ$_1$ ... γ$_2$) that are differentially distributed within the brain. Although the exact molecular composition of the GABA$_A$ receptors is not known, it is widely accepted that the stoichiometry of these macromolecular complexes is formed by two α, one β, and two γ subunits.

The specificity of compounds such as GABA itself, benzodiazepines, or barbiturates might refer to the specific subunit composition in terms of their binding properties to the GABA$_A$ receptor complex[90,100] and, overall, the pharmacological properties mediated by ligands at GABA$_A$ receptors may differ as a function of their subunit composition.[90,127] Thus, while alcohol's actions at the GABA$_A$ receptors appear mediated by the presence of the γ$_2$ subunit in its long variation (γ$_{2L}$), which carries a site for phosphorylation by PKC, the same does not apply for the action of drugs such as benzodiazepines or barbiturates whose sedative, anxiolytic, and hypnotic effects are also mediated by a potentiation of GABA actions onto these receptors.[81]

Behavioral studies indeed showed a large number of interactions between alcohol and drugs known to act at the GABA$_A$ receptor complex, and also that signs of alcohol withdrawal are efficaciously reversed by GABA agonists, benzodiazepines, and barbiturates. The behavioral effects of alcohol with respect to its actions onto GABA$_A$ receptors have been pharmacologically characterized by drug discrimination studies. This procedure involves training animals to make an operant response to obtain a reward when treated with a specific drug and to make an alternative response when treated with an alternative drug or placebo. Animals can discriminate reliably between a wide range of drugs. Thus, when the training drug is substituted by compounds with similar discriminative properties and subjective effects, the animals show appropriate dose-related and drug-appropriate responses if the discriminative drug has a similar profile of action. Alcohol's discrimination effects have been shown to substitute for a number of GABA agonists.[120] Animals generalize to compounds known to potentiate GABA function rather than to direct GABA agonists. Thus, it has been reported that the direct GABA agonist muscimol failed to substitute for alcohol,[120] as it also failed to substitute for barbiturates[61] or for benzodiazepines.[8,9] These behavioral data suggest that alcohol's actions are due to a stimulation of GABA activity at the $GABA_A$ receptor complex, rather than to a direct GABA-mimetic action. However, similar drug discrimination studies indicated subtle differences between alcohol and some benzodiazepines or barbiturates, which lends further support to the view that differences in the subunit composition of the receptor complex or in the actions mediated by isozymes of PKC might be responsible for differences between alcohol and other compounds in terms of their pharmacological effects mediated by the $GABA_A$ receptor complex.[60,128]

ALCOHOL AND GLUTAMATE

The NMDA receptor complex is one of the receptor subtypes for glutamate and is widely distributed throughout the brain. Drug discrimination studies indicated that alcohol might be interfering with glutamatergic neurotransmission at the NMDA receptor, since noncompetitive NMDA antagonists substitute for alcohol.[55,56,120] Accordingly, signs of alcohol withdrawal are extinguished by NMDA antagonists as well. Such behavioral evidence is supported by *in vitro* data showing that alcohol inhibits NMDA-induced ion currents in a concentration-dependent manner within a range of concentrations (5 to 50 mmol l^{-1}) that is considered to be relevant for its pharmacological effects.[85] Alcohol also decreases NMDA-mediated Ca^{2+} influx[42,65] and reduces excitatory electrical signals evoked by NMDA.[133] Long-sleep (LS) and short-sleep (SS) mice are selectively bred to differ for their sensitivities to the anesthetic effects of alcohol, while slow and fast mice are selectively bred for differences in their sensitivities to the locomotor stimulant effects of alcohol. Using microsacs (cell-free membrane preparations) from cortices and hippocampi from SS and LS mice, Daniell and Phillips[25,26] demonstrated that alcohol dose-dependent decreases L-glutamate-stimulated Ca^{2+} influx from slow but not from fast mice, and that high alcohol concentrations (200 mmol l^{-1}) reduced the NMDA-mediated responses in hippocampal microsacs from LS mice, suggesting that genetic differences might be at the basis for different sensitivity to alcohol. A reduction of this neurochemical measure of glutamatergic neurotransmission through the NMDA receptor complex is one of the primary targets for the molecular mechanism(s) of alcohol in the brain,[57,60,128] and as in the case of $GABA_A$ receptors, alcohol's actions on the NMDA receptor complex seem to depend on its subunit composition,[128] which is not completely known, although functional NMDA receptors appear to have NR_1 and NR_2 proteic subunits.[93]

Given that NMDA antagonists (dizocilpine [MK-801], ketamine, and phencyclidine) show sedative, anaesthetic, and motor performance impairing effects[24,126,138] similar to alcohol, it is very likely that they also share the same molecular target. Alcohol withdrawal symptoms seem to be mediated — at least in part — through NMDA receptors. Thus, increases of the NR_1 protein in the hippocampus,[101,131] of NR_{2A} in hippocampus and cortex from mice chronically treated with alcohol were reported.[124] Also, *in vivo* glutamate neurotransmission in the striatum of freely moving rats made dependent on alcohol was reported to be profoundly increased by withdrawal from chronic alcohol.[111]

To summarize, the following evidence suggests that alcohol and NMDA agonists share a common neurochemical basis with drugs of abuse: dopamine neurotransmission in the nucleus accumbens is increased by NMDA antagonists;[70,87,129] chronic alcohol consumption causes profound decreases of dopamine neuronal activity,[32,34,35] and dopamine release in the nucleus accumbens,[33,110] and administration of the NMDA receptor antagonist dizocilpine, reverse these changes.[44,110]

ALCOHOL AND SEROTONIN

Alcohol's actions in the brain also involve changes in the central serotonergic system. Acute alcohol administration has been shown to increase brain serotonin (5HT) concentrations[82] and reductions of serotonin levels were pointed as a causal factor for promoting alcohol-taking behavior.[97,115] Low doses of $5HT_{1A}$ agonist, 8-OH-DPAT, which reduces serotonin availability at the synapses by its action onto presynaptic receptors on dorsal raphe neurons, also preferentially increases alcohol intake in rats.[115,130] With respect to genetic differences among alcohol preferring and alcohol non-preferring rats, lower levels of forebrain serotonin (and its main metabolite 5-HIAA) were described in rats selectively bred as alcohol preferring than in their non-preferring counterparts;[53,102] decreased serotonin turnover rate[94] and reduced number of serotonin fibers[143] were also reported. This evidence can be extended to serotonin receptor studies. Thus, preferential increases in the binding of $5HT_{1A}$ receptors[88,139] were reported in high alcohol drinker rats. On the other hand, comparative studies with genetically selected high and low alcohol drinkers provided no clear-cut results on the role of the $5HT_{2A}$ serotonin receptor subtypes.[88,89] In contrast, both animal and human studies suggested that serotonin, acting on $5HT_3$ receptors, is involved in the regulation of behavioral and neurochemical effects of alcohol.[59,119] Thus, $5HT_3$ receptor antagonists have been involved in the regulation of alcohol consumption in alcohol preferring rats[43] and in non-severely alcohol-dependent patients.[119] $5HT_3$ receptor antagonists also regulate the discriminative stimulus effects of alcohol,[54] attenuate its locomotor stimulant effects,[106] and block the stimulation of dopamine release in the rat nucleus accumbens[18,21] (Figure 34.2). All together, these findings indicate that serotonin, by acting on $5HT_3$ receptors, modulates neurochemically based motivational properties of alcohol[37] and therefore might control alcohol-taking behaviors.

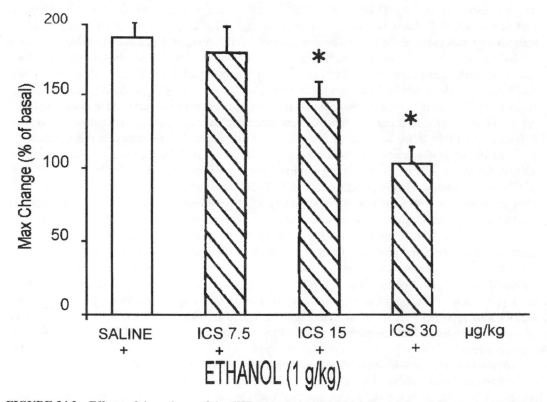

FIGURE 34.2 Effects of three doses of the $5HT_3$ antagonist ICS 205-930, on ethanol (1 g/kg i.p.)-induced stimulation of dopamine release in the nucleus accumbens. Values are expressed as maximal change (%) from baseline. (Modified from Carboni, E., Acquas, E., Frau, R., and Di Chiara, G., Differential inhibitory effects of a 5-HT$_3$ antagonist on drug-induced stimulation of dopamine release, *Eur. J. Pharmacol.*, 164, 515, 1989. With permission.)

$5HT_3$ receptors, in contrast to all other 5HT receptors in the brain, are associated with ion channels that regulate the flow of Na^+ and K^+ cations[28] and are mainly distributed in limbic and cortical areas.[74,134] Recent reports demonstrated that alcohol potentiates $5HT_3$-mediated ion currents in neuroblastoma cells[83] and in isolated preparations of adult rat neurons.[84] $5HT_3$ receptors are found in the ventral tegmental area (VTA)[15,19,91,92,107,132] and in the nucleus accumbens.[18,21] Local application of alcohol in the VTA of Sprague-Dawley rats elevates both dopamine and serotonin concentrations in this region.[19,141] Therefore, alcohol-induced elevations of extracellular concentrations of dopamine, both in the VTA[141] and in the nucleus accumbens[18,69] (see Figure 34.6), might be directly related to its reinforcing properties. Furthermore, alcohol was shown to excite dopaminergic neurons in the VTA[14,15,50] (see Figure 34.5). An elevation of serotonin concentrations in the VTA increases firing activity of dopaminergic neurons via $5HT_{1D}$ serotonin receptors.[17]

$5HT_3$ receptor antagonists displace ^3H-flunitrazepam binding,[75] and it was postulated that the $5HT_3$ antagonist MDL 72222 might also have inverse agonist properties at the $GABA_A$ receptor complex. The finding that this $5HT_3$ receptor antagonist exacerbates the severity of alcohol withdrawal-induced seizures[58] may reflect some anxiogenic-like properties of this compound, which might also account for differential mechanisms through which compounds of this class block alcohol-related behaviors.[43,54]

ALCOHOL AND OPIOID PEPTIDES

Endogenous opioids are critically involved in alcohol addiction as well as in acute alcohol effects. The experimental evidence available for the involvement of endogenous opioid systems on alcohol's actions is supported by the use of the non-selective opioid receptor antagonist naltrexone in clinical practice for the treatment of alcoholism.[99,135] The endogenous opioid peptides are identified as β-endorphins (β-EP), Met- and Leu-enkephalins (ENK), and Dynorphins (DYN) as they derive, respectively, from the precursors pro-opiomelanocortin (POMC), pro-enkephalin (PENK), and pro-dynorphin (PDYN). The β-EP system (which is relevant for the reinforcing effects of alcohol) originates in the nucleus arcuatus paraventricularis of the mediobasal hypothalamus and projects its long axons to a number of structures, among which are the VTA and the nucleus accumbens.[86] Similarly, although ENK-containing elements have mostly short axons, endings of the enkephalinergic neurons have been found in a number of structures of the forebrain and in particular in the nucleus accumbens,[114] where their actions are mediated (Figure 34.3). The functional receptors for β-EP and ENK are, respectively, indicated as μ- and δ-opioid receptors, and μ- and δ-receptor-mediated functions may be relevant for the rewarding/motivational properties of alcohol.[64] A compelling body of evidence, in addition, has shown that key anatomical structures for the mediation of rewarding effects of β-EP and ENK are the VTA, also indicated as A10 area, and the nucleus accumbens, a component of the extended amygdala,[63] the origin and target areas of dopaminergic neurons of the mesolimbic system, respectively. Rats self-administer μ-opioid receptor agonists.[13] Also, systemic administration of the prototypical agonists of μ-opioid receptors, morphine and heroin,[95,125] or local administration of μ- and δ-opioid receptor agonists produces place preference conditioning.[10,121,122] Thus, while these effects of opioid agonists are due to primary actions on opioid receptors, their motivational properties appear mediated by activation of the dopaminergic mesolimbic system (VTA — nucleus accumbens).[38,64] However, dopamine-independent mechanisms might also be involved in opioid reinforcement,[49] this latter possibility being interpreted as somehow linked to the mesolimbic dopamine system as well, since these actions can be viewed as located post-synaptically in the nucleus accumbens.[119]

Three lines of evidence point to the β-EP and ENK opioid systems as being involved in alcohol's actions. The first line of evidence is supported by studies showing that blockade of μ- and/or δ-opioid receptors reduce alcohol consumption in animals selectively bred for high alcohol drinking.[45,46,52,66,78–80,112] The second line of evidence, which refers to the opioid deficiency hypothesis of

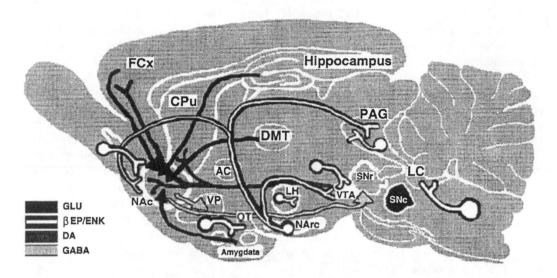

FIGURE 34.3   Schematic representation of some of the reward pathways in the rat brain. Abbreviations: AC: anterior commisure; CPu: caudate putamen; DA: dopamine; DMT: dorsal medial thalamus; FCx: frontal cortex; GLU; glutamate; LC: locus coeruleus; LH: lateral hipothalamus; NAc: nucleus accumbens septi; NArc: nucleus arcuatus paraventricularis; SNc: substantia nigra pars compacta; SNr: substantia nigra pars reticulata; PAG: periacqueductal gray; VP: ventral palidum; VTA: ventral tegmental area.

alcoholism,[108] originates from the observation that there appears to exist an inverse correlation between alcohol consumption and brain concentrations of β-EP, ENK,[51] and mRNA content for the β-EP precursor, POMC.[6,116] The third line of evidence is supported by *in vivo* microdialysis studies that demonstrate that the acute effects of alcohol on dopamine transmission[69] in the nucleus accumbens are antagonized by naloxone (μ/δ-opioid antagonist)[11] and by the δ-opioid antagonist naltrindole[2] (Figure 34.4).

The exact molecular mechanism(s) through which alcohol generates its actions involving the β-EP and ENK systems is(are) not presently known. Genetic differences, however, seem to be the discriminative element for an increased sensitivity to some of the alcohol's actions on opioid peptides functions[29,30] and receptors.[31] Thus, high alcohol drinkers (Alko Alcohol, AA) consistently show increased propensity to higher rates of opioid self-administration[68] and intake[67] than their low drinker counterparts (Alko non-Alcohol, ANA). Furthermore, the acquisition and expression of motivational effects of alcohol need an intact dopaminergic mesolimbic system,[38,40,64] and it is conceivable to speculate that the activation of the mesolimbic dopaminergic system, as expressed by increased release of dopamine in the nucleus accumbens[36,69] or by increased firing activity of dopamine neurons in the VTA[50] (Figure 34.5), is secondary to the interaction of alcohol with the opioidergic pathways relevant for its rewarding effects. Aversive states can be obtained by blockade of μ-opioid receptors,[3,122] thus suggesting that the opioid system can be viewed as a reward system independent from mesolimbic dopamine and that alcohol rewarding effects might therefore have a component that does not involve increases of dopamine release in the mesolimbic system.[49,117] In any case, it is noteworthy that dopamine receptor antagonists for the D_1 subtype have been shown to block the aversive effects caused by μ-opioid receptor antagonists.[3,122]

Recent studies suggest that the molecular mechanism by which morphine increases dopamine release in the nucleus accumbens,[36] as well as somatodendritic release in the VTA, is mediated by the stimulation of inhibitory μ-opioid receptors on inhibitory GABA interneurons in this structure.[38,71,72,76] Moreover, these effects were shown to be potentiated by the $GABA_A$ agonist muscimol.[76] Thus, at least as far as the actions of alcohol on dopaminergic neurons in the VTA (and the release of dopamine in the nucleus accumbens) are concerned, it might be speculated that a

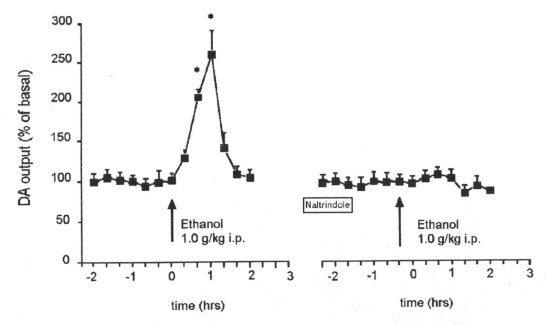

FIGURE 34.4   Effect of local application, by reverse dialysis, of the δ-opioid receptor antagonist, naltrindole (1 µmol l⁻¹), on ethanol (1 g/kg i.p.) -stimulated dopamine release in the nucleus accumbens. (Modified from Acquas, E., Meloni, M., and Di Chiara, G., Blockade of δ-opioid receptors in the nucleus accumbens prevents ethanol-induced stimulation of dopamine release, *Eur. J. Pharmacol.* 230, 239, 1993, and Di Chiara, G., Acquas, E., Tanda, G., and Cadoni, C., Drugs of abuse: biochemical surrogates of specific aspects of natural reward?, *Biochem. Soc. Symp.*, 59, 65, 1993, with permission.)

mechanism through which alcohol increases firing activity of dopaminergic neurons in the VTA[14,50] and dopamine release in the nucleus accumbens[69] is through an increase in β-EP levels[52] and therefore by a potentiation of the actions of GABA onto GABA$_A$ receptors.

ALCOHOL AND ADENOSINE

Alcohol shares with the neuromodulator adenosine some functional characteristics, such as the ability to cause sedation and motor performance impairment. Animal studies demonstrated that alcohol-induced sedation and ataxia are potentiated by adenosine as well as by the adenosine reuptake inhibitor, dilazep; conversely, adenosine antagonists may reduce the intensity of these alcohol actions.[27] Cross-sensitivity between alcohol and adenosine is segregated in genetically selected mice for differential responses to alcohol (Long-sleep and Short-sleep).[105] Thus, alcohol might act on central adenosine neurotransmission by increasing adenosine concentrations as a consequence of selective blockade of a nucleoside transporter, thereby indirectly modulating adenosine's actions of other neurotransmitters. Finally, it was suggested that some of the pharmacological effects of alcohol (ataxia) might stem from acetate, the peripherally obtained alcohol metabolite.[23,103]

It has been reported that acute administration of alcohol increases adenosine concentrations in the medium of mutant S49 and NG 108-15 cell preparations and it was suggested that alcohol acts by selectively blocking a subtype of facilitative transporter for adenosine.[77] These alcohol-induced increases of adenosine are paralleled by increases of cyclic AMP (cAMP) and may cause, after chronic alcohol exposure, (heterologous) desensitization of the transporter. This desensitization results in the loss of ability of alcohol to block the transporter[96,113] and it was suggested to depend on reduced cAMP production and on reduced protein kinase A (PKA)-mediated phosphorylation. Furthermore, chronic alcohol may cause a reduction in cAMP production, also as a consequence

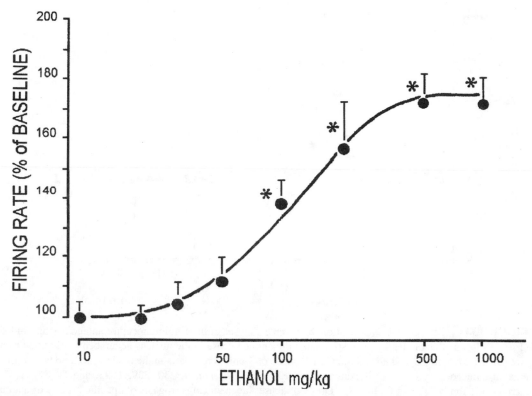

FIGURE 34.5   Dose-response curve of the effect of intravenous ethanol on the firing rate of dopaminergic neurons in the VTA. (Modified from Gessa, G.L., Muntoni, F., Collu, M., Vargiu, L., and Mereu, G., Low doses of ethanol activate dopaminergic neurons in the ventral tegmental area, *Brain Res.*, 348, 201, 1985.. With permission.)

of the activation of receptor-mediated actions due to different neurotransmitters which act through G_S proteins.

Given that adenosine interferes with a number of neurochemical systems, either facilitating and inhibiting neurotransmitter release, it is not surprising that some of the pharmacological actions of alcohol might be modulated (at least in part) by adenosine.

Thus, for example, although the molecular mechanism(s) is still unknown, a recent study showed that alcohol increases β-EP levels in a number of brain areas, and that the combined administration of alcohol and adenosine receptor agonists or antagonists potentiates or reduces, respectively, these effects of alcohol on β-EP levels.[7] Also, K+-stimulated glutamate release from hippocampal slices was reported to be inhibited by alcohol, and pretreatment with an adenosine A_1 receptor antagonist was shown to block this alcohol-induced inhibition.[109]

Alcohol is not metabolized in the brain and it has been claimed that its liver biotransformation product, acetate, may have some central effects in common with alcohol and adenosine as well.[23,103] This increased bioavailability of acetate, following alcohol consumption, as a consequence of its transformation to acetyl CoA, causes increased ATP utilization, which ultimately increases blood adenosine concentrations and, therefore, also brain adenosine. Interestingly, acetate was also reported to lower the requirement of a number of general anaesthetics needed to induce anaesthesia.[20] However, although acetate also causes some behavioral effects similar to those of alcohol,[23] the hypothesis of the role of acetate in the mediation of alcohol's actions was recently questioned on the basis of failure to obtain alterations of physiological responses by acetate on a hippocampal slice preparation.[16]

ALCOHOL AND DOPAMINE

Electrophysiological, neurochemical, and behavioral evidence indicates that the mesolimbic dopaminergic system plays a key role in the motivational responses triggered by alcohol consumption. This evidence, supported by extensive literature, was prompted by early clinical and experimental observations that dopaminergic mechanisms could mediate the stimulant and euphorigenic properties of alcohol in rats and humans.[4,22] Acute administration of alcohol was originally reported[50] to excite dopaminergic neurons in the VTA (Figure 34.5). These authors showed that low doses of alcohol in unanesthetized rats increased their firing rate, a finding also confirmed in identified dopaminergic neurons in a VTA slice preparation.[14] More recently, a series of experiments demonstrated that the firing activity of VTA neurons, measured *in vivo*, in rats withdrawn from chronic alcohol is long-lastingly reduced.[32-35] These authors also showed that the reduction of neuronal activity caused by abrupt discontinuation of alcohol intake could be rapidly reversed by alcohol itself or by γ-hydroxybutyric acid (GHB),[35] a compound suggested to be of potential usefulness for the treatment of alcoholism.[47,48] Neurochemical evidence for the actions of alcohol on mesolimbic dopamine transmission *in vivo* were originally provided by Imperato and Di Chiara,[36,69] who reported the preferential stimulation of dopamine release in the rat nucleus accumbens as compared to the dorsal striatum, thus pointing to site-specific actions of alcohol on this dopaminergic system (Figure 34.6). Following these original investigations, a large number of studies unequivocally confirmed these neurochemical actions of acute alcohol.[2,12,18,21,140,142]

Changes in the activity of the mesolimbic dopaminergic system after either acute or chronic alcohol consumption are considered to be relevant in terms of the motivational properties of this chemical (and of a number or other drugs of abuse as well as of natural rewards).[38,40] Thus, while positive reinforcing effects of alcohol (and of other drugs of abuse) are suggested to be directly related to increases of dopamine transmission in the nucleus accumbens (and more recently in its shell subdivision),[104] negative, dysphoric effects of alcohol withdrawal may be related to the depression of VTA firing activity[34] as well as to the dramatic decreases of dopamine transmission in the nucleus accumbens.[110] In this regard, reductions of basal dopamine extracellular concentrations in the nucleus accumbens might be viewed as a common feature of withdrawal not only from alcohol, but also from a number of other drugs of abuse.[1,110]

With respect to the current hypothesis on the role of dopamine in the motivational effects of alcohol,[41] it is noteworthy that alcohol self-administering rats similarly show decreased dopamine release in the nucleus accumbens[137] when withdrawn from alcohol. In addition, when allowed to drink alcohol again, this voluntary intake quickly reinstates dopamine extracellular concentrations at the pre-withdrawal levels.[137] Quantitatively different increases of dopamine release in the nucleus accumbens of self-administering genetically selected rats as high alcohol drinkers vs. genetically heterogeneous Wistar rats were described.[136] This latter study further differentiated between the pharmacological effects of comparable blood alcohol levels on dopamine release and the effects of operant responding per se among genetically selected and genetically heterogeneous rats: when asked to respond for oral self-administration of saccharin, both groups showed identical responses in terms of changes of dopamine transmission in the nucleus accumbens during either the pre-saccharin or the saccharin consumption periods,[136] thus suggesting that preferentially higher increases of dopamine release in genetically selected animals might represent a neurochemical measure of discrimination for propensity to alcohol consumption. However, this hypothesis is far from being conclusive because the above evidence, obtained in P rats vs. heterogeneous Wistars,[136,137] contrasts with other studies showing that systemic administration[73] or orally self-administered[98] alcohol fails to produce significantly higher increases of nucleus accumbens dopamine release in AA as compared with ANA rats.[73,98]

As in the case of alcohol's actions at the opioid peptide systems, the molecular mechanism(s) responsible for the pharmacological actions of alcohol that involve the mesolimbic dopaminergic system remains to be fully elucidated. However, given the role that dopamine plays in goal-directed

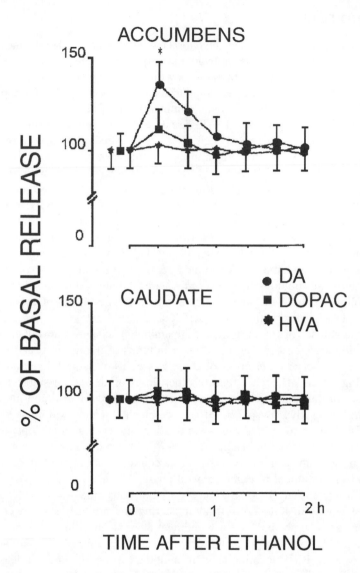

FIGURE 34.6   Effect of ethanol (0.25 g/kg i.p.) on dopamine (DA), dihydroxyphenylacetic acid (DOPAC), and homovanillic acid (HVA) output in the nucleus accumbens (upper) and caudate (lower). (Modified from Imperato, A. and Di Chiara, G., Preferential stimulation of dopamine release in the nucleus accumbens of freely moving rats by ethanol, *J. Pharmacol. Exp. Ther.,* 239, 219, 1986, with permission.)

behavior and in motivational learning,[41] it is intriguing to suggest that some of the alcohol's pharmacological actions, primarily exerted on neurochemical systems other than the dopaminergic one, may nonetheless converge on the VTA-nucleus accumbens dopaminergic system to cause its characteristic emotional, motivational, and drug-seeking behaviors.[40,128]

ACKNOWLEDGMENTS

This work is dedicated to Niccolo'. I wish to express my gratitude to Dr. Gerald Zernig, who provided helpful discussions throughout the preparation of the manuscript and always had a funny and sweet way to hold out for some views expressed in it.

REFERENCES

1. Acquas, E. and Di Chiara, G., Depression of mesolimbic dopamine transmission and sensitization to morphine during opiate abstinence, *J. Neurochem.*, 58, 1620, 1992.

2. Acquas, E., Meloni, M., and Di Chiara, G., Blockade of δ-opioid receptors in the nucleus accumbens prevents ethanol-induced stimulation of dopamine release, *Eur. J. Pharmacol.* 230, 239, 1993.

3. Acquas, E. and Di Chiara, G., D_1 receptor blockade stereospecifically impairs the acquisition of drug conditioned place preference and place aversion, *Behav. Pharmacol.*, 5, 555, 1994.

4. Alhenius, S., Carlsson, A., Engel, J., Svensson T.H., and Sodersten, P., Antagonism by α-methyl-tyrosine of the ethanol-induced stimulation and euphoria in man, *Clin. Pharm. Ther.*, 14, 586, 1973.

5. Allan, A.M. and Harris, R. A., Acute and chronic ethanol treatments alter GABA receptor-operated chloride channels, *Pharmacol. Biochem. Behav.,* 27, 665, 1987.

6. Angelogianni, P. and Gianoulakis, C., Chronic ethanol exposure increases proopiomelanocortin gene expression in the rat hypothalamus, *Neuroendocrinology*, 57, 106, 1993.

7. Anwer, J. and Soliman, M.R., Ethanol-induced alterations in beta-endorphin levels in specific rat brain regions: modulation by adenosine agonist and antagonist, *Pharmacology*, 51, 364, 1995.

8. Ator, N.A. and Griffits, R.R., Discriminative stimulus effects of atypical anxiolytics in baboons and rats, *J. Pharmacol. Exp. Ther.,* 237, 393, 1986.

9. Ator, N.A., Drug discrimination and drug stimulus generalization with anxiolytics, *Drug Dev. Res.*, 20, 189, 1990.

10. Bals-Kubik, R., Shippeberg, T.S., and Herz, A., Involvement of central μ and δ opioid receptors in mediating the reinforcing effects of β-endorphin in the rat, *Eur. J. Pharmacol.*, 175, 63, 1990.

11. Benjamin, D., Grant, E.R., and Pohorecky, L.A., Naltrexone reverses ethanol-induced dopamine release in the nucleus accumbens in awake, freely moving rats, *Brain Res.*, 621, 137, 1993.

12. Blomqvist, O., Ericson, M., Engel, J.A., and Soderpal, B., Accumbal dopamine overflow after ethanol: localization of the antagonizing affect of mecamylamine, *Eur. J. Pharmacol.*, 334, 149, 1997.

13. Bozarth, M.A. and Wise, R.A., Heroin reward is dependent on a dopaminergic substrate, *Life Sci.*, 29, 1881, 1986.

14. Brodie, M.S., Shefner, S.A., and Dunwiddie, T.V., Ethanol increases the firing rate of dopamine neurons in the rat ventral tegmental area *in vitro, Brain Res.*, 508, 65, 1990.

15. Brodie, M.S., Trifunovic, R.R., and Shefner, S.A., Serotonin potentiates ethanol-induced excitation of ventral tegmental area neurons in brain slices from three different rat strains, *J. Pharmacol. Exp. Ther.,* 273, 1139, 1995.

16. Brundege, J.M. and Dunwiddie, T.V., The role of acetate as a potential mediator of the effects of ethanol in the brain, *Neurosci. Lett.*, 186, 214, 1995.

17. Cameron, D.L. and Williams, J.T., Cocaine inhibits GABA release in the VTA through endogenous 5-HT, *J. Neurosci.*, 14, 6763, 1994.

18. Campbell, A.D. and McBride, W.J., Serotonin-3 receptor and ethanol-stimulated dopamine release in the nucleus accumbens, *Pharmacol. Biochem. Behav.*, 51, 835, 1995.

19. Campbell, A.D., Kohhl, R.R., and McBride, W.J., Serotonin-3 receptor and ethanol-stimulated soma-todentritic dopamine release, *Alcohol*, 13, 569, 1996.

20. Campisi, P., Carmichael, F.J.L., Crawford, M., Orrego, H., and Khanna, J.M., Role of adenosine in the ethanol-induced potentiation of the effects of general anesthetics in rats, *Eur. J. Pharmacol.*, 325, 165, 1997.

21. Carboni, E., Acquas, E., Frau, R., and Di Chiara, G., Differential inhibitory effects of a 5-HT_3 antagonist on drug-induced stimulation of dopamine release, *Eur. J. Pharmacol.*, 164, 515, 1989.

22. Carlsson, A., Engel, J., Strombom, U., Svensson, T.H., and Waldeck, B., Suppression by dopamine agonists of the ethanol-induced stimulation of locomotor activity and brain dopamine synthesis, *Naunyn-Schmiedeberg's Arch. Pharmacol.*, 283, 117, 1974.

23. Carmichael, F.J., Israel, Y., Crawford, M., Minhas, K., Saldivia, V., Sandrin, S., Campisi, P., and Orrego, H., Central nervous system effects of acetate: contribution to the central effects of ethanol, *J. Pharmacol. Exp. Ther.,* 259, 403, 1991.

24. Daniell, L.C. and Harris, R.A., Neuronal intracellular calcium concentrations are altered by anesthe-tics: relationship to membrane fluidization, *J. Pharmacol. Exp. Ther.,* 245, 1, 1988.

25. Daniell, L.C. and Phillips, T.J., Ethanol sensitivity of brain NMDA receptors in mice selectively bred for differences in response to the low-dose locomotor stimulant effects of ethanol, *Alcohol. Clin. Exp. Res.*, 18, 1474, 1994.

26. Daniell, L.C. and Phillips, T.J., Differences in ethanol sensitivity of brain NMDA receptors of long-sleep and short-sleep mice, *Alcohol. Clin. Exp. Res.*, 18, 1482, 1994.

27. Dar, M.S., Central adenosinergic system involvement in ethanol-induced motor incoordination in mice, *J. Pharmacol. Exp. Ther.,* 255, 1202, 1990.

28. Derkach, V., Surprenant, A., and North, R.A., 5-HT$_3$ receptors are membrane ion channels, *Nature*, 339, 706, 1989.

29. De Waele, J.P., Papachristou, D.N., and Gianoulakis, C., The alcohol-preferring C57BL/6 mice present an enhanced sensitivity to the hypothalamic β-endorphin system to ethanol than alcohol-avoiding BDA/2 mice, *J. Pharmacol. Exp. Ther.,* 261, 788, 1992.

30. De Waele, J.P., Kiianmaa, K., and Gianoulakis, C., Spontaneous and ethanol-stimulated *in vitro* release of β-endorphin by the hypothalamus of AA and ANA rats, *Alchol. Clin. Exp. Res.*, 18, 1468, 1994.

31. De Waele, J.P., Kiianmaa, K., and Gianoulakis, C., Distribution of the mu and delta opioid binding sites in the brain of the alcohol-preferring AA and alcohol-avoiding ANA lines of rats, *J. Pharmacol. Exp. Ther.,* 275, 518, 1995.

32. Diana, M., Pistis, M., Muntoni, A., Rossetti, Z.L., and Gessa, G., Marked decrease of A10 dopamine neuronal firing during ethanol withdrawal syndrome in rats, *Eur. J. Pharmacol.*, 221, 403, 1992.

33. Diana, M., Pistis, Carboni, S., Gessa, G., and Rossetti, Z.L., Profound decrement of mesolimbic dopaminergic neuronal activity during ethanol withdrawal syndrome in rats: electrophysiological and biochemical evidence, *Proc. Natl. Acad. Sci. U.S.A.,* 90, 7966, 1993.

34. Diana, M., Pistis, M., Muntoni, A., and Gessa, G., Ethanol withdrawal does not induce a reduction in the number of spontaneously active dopaminergic neurons in the mesolimbic system, *Brain Res.*, 682, 29, 1995.

35. Diana, M., Pistis, M., Muntoni, A., and Gessa, G., Mesolimbic dopaminergic reductions outlasts ethanol withdrawal syndrome: evidence of protracted abstinence, *Neuroscience*, 71, 41, 1996.

36. Di Chiara, G. and Imperato, A., Drugs abused by humans preferentially increase synaptic dopamine concentrations in the mesolimbic system of freely moving rats, *Proc. Natl. Acad. Sci. U.S.A.,* 85, 5274, 1988.

37. Di Chiara, G., Acquas, E., and Carboni, E., Role of mesolimbic dopamine in the motivational effects of drugs: brain dialysis and place preference studies, *The Mesolimbic Dopamine System: From Motivation to Action,* Willner, P. and Scheel-Kruger, J., Eds., J. Wiley & Sons, Chichester, 1991, 367.

38. Di Chiara, G. and North, R.A., Neurobiology of opiate abuse, *TiPS*, 13, 185, 1992.

39. Di Chiara, G., Acquas, E., Tanda, G., and Cadoni, C., Drugs of abuse: biochemical surrogates of specific aspects of natural reward?, *Biochem. Soc. Symp.*, 59, 65, 1993.

40. Di Chiara, G., Acquas, E., and Tanda, G., Ethanol as a neurochemical surrogate of conventional reinforcers: the dopamine-opioid link, *Alcohol*, 13, 13, 1996.

41. Di Chiara, G., A motivational learning hypothesis of the role of mesolimbic dopamine in compulsive drug use, *J. Psychopharmacol.*, 12, 54, 1998.

42. Dildy, J.E. and Leslie, S.W., Ethanol inhibits NMDA-induced increases in free intracellular Ca^{2+} in dissociated brain cells, *Brain Res.*, 499, 383, 1989.

43. Fadda, F., Garau, B., Marchei, F., Colombo, G., and Gessa, G.L., MDL 72222, a selective 5-HT$_3$ receptor antagonist, suppresses voluntary ethanol consumption in alcohol preferring rats, *Alcohol Alcohol.*, 26, 107, 1991.

44. Fadda F. and Rossetti, Z.L., Chronic ethanol consumption from neuroadaptation to neurodegeneration, *Progr. Neurobiol.*, 56, 385, 1998.

45. Froehlich, J.C., Harts, J., Lumeng, L., and Li, T.-K., Naloxone attenuates voluntary ethanol intake in rats selectively bred for high ethanol preference, *Pharmacol. Biochem. Behav.*, 35, 385, 1990.

46. Froehlich, J.C., Zweifel, M., Harts, J., Lumeng, L., and Li, T.-K., Importance of delta opioid receptors in maintaining high alcohol drinking, *Psychopharmacology*, 103, 467, 1991.

47. Gallimberti, L., Gentile, N., Cibin, M., Fadda. F., Canton, G., Ferri, M., Ferrara, S. D., and Gessa, G.L., Gamma-hydroxybutyric acid for treatment of alcohol withdrawal syndrome, *Lancet*, 30, 787, 1989.

48. Gallimberti, L., Ferri, M., Ferrara, S.D., Fadda, F., and Gessa, G.L., Gamma-hydroxybutyric acid in the treatment of alcohol dependence: a double-blind study, *Alcohol. Clin. Exp. Res.*, 16, 673, 1992.

49. Gerrits, M., Ramsey, N.F., Wolterink, G., and Van Ree, J.M., Lack of evidence for an involvement of nucleus accumbens D1 receptors in the initiation of heroin self-administration in the rat, *Psychopharmacology*, 114, 486, 1994.

50. Gessa, G.L., Muntoni, F., Collu, M., Vargiu, L., and Mereu, G., Low doses of ethanol activate dopaminergic neurons in the ventral tegmental area, *Brain Res.*, 348, 201, 1985.

51. Gianoulakis, C., De Waele, J.P., and Kiianmaa, K., Differences in the brain and pituitary β-endorphin system between the alcohol-preferring AA and alcohol-avoiding ANA rats, *Alcohol. Clin. Exp. Res.*, 16, 453, 1992.

52. Gianoulakis, C., De Waele, J.-P., and Thavundyil, J., Implication of the endogenous opioid system in excessive ethanol consumption, *Alcohol*, 13, 19, 1996.

53. Gongwer, M.A., Murphy, J.M., McBride, W.J., Lumeng, L., and Li, T.-K., Regional brain contents of serotonin, dopamine and their metabolites in the selectively bred high- and low-alcohol drinking lines of rats, *Alcohol*, 6, 317, 1989.

54. Grant, K.A. and Barrett, J.E., Blockade of the discriminative stimulus effects of ethanol with 5HT$_3$ receptor antagonists, *Psychopharmacology*, 104, 451, 1991.

55. Grant, K.A., Colombo, G., and Tabakoff, B., Competitive and noncompetitive antagonists of the NMDA receptors complex have ethanol-like discriminative stimulus effects in rats, *Alcohol. Clin. Exp. Res.*,15, 321, 1991.

56. Grant, K.A. and Colombo, G., Discriminative stimulus effect of ethanol: effect of training dose on the substitution of N-methyl-D-aspartate antagonists, *J. Pharmacol. Exp. Ther.*, 264, 1241, 1993.

57. Grant, K.A., Emerging neurochemical concepts in the actions of ethanol at ligand-gated ion channels, *Behav. Pharmacol.*, 5, 383, 1994.

58. Grant, K.A., Hellevuo, K., and Tabakoff, B., The 5HT$_3$ antagonist MDL 72222 exacerbates ethanol withdrawal seizures in mice, *Alcohol Clin. Exp. Res.*, 18, 410, 1994.

59. Grant, K.A., The role of 5-HT$_3$ receptors in drug dependence, *Drug Alcohol Dep.*, 38, 155, 1995.

60. Grant, K.A. and Lovinger, D.M., Cellular and behavioral neurobiology of alcohol: receptor mediated neuronal processes, *Clin. Neurosci.*, 3, 155, 1995.

61. Grech, D.M. and Balster, R.L., Pentobarbital-like discriminative stimulus effects of direct GABA agonists in rats, *Psychopharmacology*, 110, 295, 1993.

62. Harris, R.A., McQuilkin, S.J., Paylor, R., Abeliovich, A., Tonegawa, S., and Wehner, M.E., Mutant mice lacking the γ isoform of protein kinase C show decreased behavioral actions of ethanol and altered function of γ-aminobutyrate type A receptors, *Proc. Natl. Acad. Sci. U.S.A.*, 92, 3658, 1995.

63. Heimer, L., Zham, D.S., Churchill, L., Kalivas, P.W., and Wohltmann, C., Specificity in the projection patterns of accumbal core and shell in the rat, *Neuroscience*, 41, 89, 1991.

64. Herz, A., Endogenous opioid systems and alcohol addiction, *Psychopharmacology*, 129, 99, 1997.

65. Hoffman, P.L., Rabe, C.S., Moses, F., and Tabakoff, B., *N*-Methyl-*D*-aspartate receptors and ethanol inhibition of calcium flux and cyclic GMP production, *J. Neurochem.*, 52, 1937, 1989.

66. Hyytia, P., Involvement of μ-opioid receptors in alcohol drinking by alcohol-preferring AA rats, *Pharmacol. Biochem. Behav.*, 45, 697, 1993.

67. Hyytia, P. and Sinclair, J.D., Oral etonitazene and cocaine consumption by AA, ANA and Wistar rats, *Psychopharmacology*, 111, 409, 1993.

68. Hyytia, P., Schulteis, G., and Koob, G.F., Intravenous heroin and ethanol self-administration by alcohol preferring AA and ANA alcohol avoiding ANA rats, *Psychopharmacology*, 125, 2448, 1996.

69. Imperato, A. and Di Chiara, G., Preferential stimulation of dopamine release in the nucleus accumbens of freely moving rats by ethanol, *J. Pharmacol. Exp. Ther.*, 239, 219, 1986.

70. Imperato, A., Scrocco, M.G., Bacchi, S., and Angelucci, L., NMDA receptors and *in vivo* dopamine release in the nucleus accumbens and caudatus, *Eur. J. Pharmacol.*, 187, 555, 1990.

71. Johnson, S.W. and North, R.A., Opioids excite dopamine neurons by hyperpolarization of local interneurons, *J. Neurosci.*, 12, 483, 1992.

72. Kalivas, P.W., Duffy, P., and Eberhardt, H., Modulation of A10 dopamine neurons by γ-aminobutyric acid agents, *J. Pharmacol. Exp. Ther.*, 253, 858, 1990.

73. Kiinmaa, K., Nurmi, M., Nykaenen, I., and Sinclair, J.D., Effect of ethanol on extracellular dopamine in the nucleus accumbens of alcohol-preferring AA and alcohol-avoiding ANA rats, *Pharmacol. Biochem. Behav.*, 52, 29, 1995.

74. Kilpatrick, G.J., Jones, B.J., and Tyers, M.B., Identification and distribution of 5HT3 receptors in rat brain using radioligand binding, *Nature*, 330, 746, 1987.

75. Klein, R.L., Sanna, E., McQuilkin, S.J., Whiting, P.J., and Harris, R.A., Effects of 5-HT$_3$ receptor antagonists on binding and function of mouse and human GABA$_A$ receptors, *Eur. J. Pharmacol.*, 268, 237, 1994.

76. Klitenick, M.A., DeWitte, P., and Kalivas, P.W., Regulation of somatodentric dopamine release in the ventral tegmental area by opioids and GABA: an *in vivo* microdialysis study, *J. Neurosci.* 12, 2623, 1992.

77. Krauss, S.W., Ghirnikar, R.B., Diamond, I., and Gordon, A.S., Inhibition of adenosine uptake by ethanol is specific for one class of nucleoside transporters, *Mol. Pharmacol.*, 44, 1024, 1993.

78. Krishnan-Sarin, S., Jing, S.-L., Kurz, D.L., Zweifel, M., Portoghese, P.S., Li, T.-K., and Froehlich, J.C., The delta opioid receptor antagonist naltrindole attenuates both alcohol and saccharin intake in rats selectively bred for alcohol preference, *Psychopharmacology*, 120, 177, 1995.

79. Krishnan-Sarin, S., Portoghese, P.S., Li, T.-K., and Froehlich, J.C., The delta$_2$-opioid receptor antagonist naltriben selectively attenuates alcohol intake in rats bred for alcohol preference, *Pharmacol. Biochem Behav.*, 52, 153, 1995.

80. Lê, A.D., Poulos, C.X., Quan, B., and Chow, S., The effects of selective blockade of delta and mu opioid receptors on ethanol consumption by C57BL/6 mice in a restricted access paradigm, *Brain Res.*, 630, 330, 1993.

81. Leidenheimer, N.J., Whiting, P.J., and Harris, R.A., Activation of calcium-phospholipid-dependent protein kinase enhances benzodiazepine and barbiturate potentiation of the GABA$_A$ receptor, *J. Neurochem.*, 60, 1972, 1993.

82. LeMarquand, D., Pihl, R.O., and Benkelfat, C., Serotonin and alcohol intake, abuse and dependence: clinical evidence, *Biol. Psychiatry*, 36, 326, 1994.

83. Lovinger, D.M., Ethanol potentiation of 5-HT$_3$ receptor-mediated ion current in NCB-20 neuroblastoma cells, *Neurosci. Lett.*, 122, 57, 1991.

84. Lovinger, D.M. and White, G., Ethanol potentiation of 5-hydroxytryptamine$_3$ receptor-mediated ion current in neuroblastoma cells and isolated adult mammalian neurons, *Mol. Pharmacol.*, 40, 263, 1991.

85. Lovinger, D.M., White, G., and Weight, F.F., Ethanol inhibits NMDA-activated ion current in hippocampal neurons, *Science*, 243, 1721, 1989.

86. Mansour, A., Khachaturian, H., Lewis, M.E., Akil, H., and Watson, S.J., Anatomy of CNS opioid receptors, *TiNS*, 1, 308, 1988.

87. Mathé, J.M., Nomikos, G.G., Hildebrand, B.E., Hertel, P., and Svensson, T.H., Prazosin inhibits MK-801-induced hyperlocomotion and dopamine release in the nucleus accumbens, *Eur. J. Pharmacol.*, 309, 1, 1996.

88. McBride, W.J., Murphy, J.M., Lumeng, L., and Li, T.-K., Serotonin, dopamine and GABA involvement in alcohol drinking of selectively bred rats, *Alcohol*, 7, 199, 1990.

89. McBride, W.J., Chernet, E., Rabold, J.A., Lumeng, L., and Li, T.-K., Serotonin-2 receptors in the CNS of alcohol-preferring and non-preferring rats, *Pharmacol. Biochem. Behav.*, 46, 631, 1993.

90. McKernan, R.M. and Whiting, P.J., Which GABA$_A$-receptor subtypes really occur in the brain?, *TiNS*, 19, 139, 1996.

91. Minabe, Y., Ashby, C.R. Jr., Schwartz, J.E., and Wang, R.Y., The 5-HT$_3$ receptor antagonist LY 277359 and granisetron potentiate the suppressant action of apomorphine on the basal firing rate of ventral tegmental dopamine cells, *Eur. J. Pharmacol.*, 209, 143, 1991.

92. Minabe, Y., Ashby, C.R. Jr., and Wang, R.Y., The effect of acute and chronic LY 277359, a selective 5-HT$_3$ receptor antagonist, on the number of spontaneously active midbrain dopamine neurons, *Eur. J. Pharmacol.*, 209, 151, 1991.

93. Monyer, H., Sprengel, R., Schoepfer, R., Herb, A., Highuchi, M., Lomeli, H., Burnashev, N., Shakman, B., and Seeburg, P., Heteromeric NMDA receptors: molecular and functional distinction of subtypes, *Science*, 256, 1217, 1992.

94. Morinan, A., Reduction in striatal 5-hydroxytryptamine turnover following chronic administration of ethanol to rats, *Alcohol Alcohol.*, 22, 53, 1987.

95. Mucha, R.F. and Iversen, S.D., Reinforcing properties of morphine and naloxone revealed by conditioned place-preferences: a procedural examination, *Psychopharmacology*, 82, 241, 1984.

96. Nagy, L.E., Diamond, I., Collier, K., Lopez, L., Ullman, B., and Gordon, A.S., Adenosine is required for ethanol-induced heterologous desensitization, *Mol. Pharmacol.*, 36, 744, 1989.

97. Naranjo, C.A. and Sellers, E.M., Serotonin uptake inhibitors attenuate ethanol intake in problem drinkers, *Rec. Dev. Alcohol.*, 7, 255, 1989.

98. Nurmi, M., Ashizawa, T., Sinclair, J.D., and Kiinmaa, K., Effect of prior ethanol experience on dopamine overflow in accumbens of AA and ANA rats, *Eur. J. Pharmacol.*, 315, 277, 1996.

99. O'Brien, C.P., Volpicelli, L.A., and Volpicelli, J.R., Naltrexone in the treatment of alcoholism: a clinical review, *Alcohol*, 13, 35, 1996.

100. Olsen, R.W. and Tobin, A.J., Molecular biology of GABA$_A$ receptors, *FASEB J.*, 4, 1469, 1990.

101. Ortiz, J., Fitzgerald, L.W., Charlton, M., Lane, S., Trevisan, L., Guitart, X., Shoemaker, W., Duman, R.S., and Nestler, E.J., Biochemical actions of chronic ethanol exposure in the mesolimbic dopamine system, *Synapse*, 21, 289, 1995.

102. Overstreet, D.H., Rezvani, A.H., and Janowsky, D.S., Genetic animal models of depression and ethanol preference provide support for cholinergic and serotonergic involvement in depression and alcoholism, *Biol. Psychiatry*, 31, 919, 1992.

103. Phillis, J.W., O'Regan, M.H., and Perkins, L.M., Actions of ethanol and acetate on rat cortical neurons: ethanol/adenosine interactions, *Alcohol*, 9, 541, 1992.

104. Pontieri, F.E., Tanda, G., and Di Chiara, G., Intravenous cocaine, morphine, and amphetamine preferentially increase extracellular dopamine in the "shell" as compared to the "core" of the rat nucleus accumbens, *Proc. Natl. Acad. Sci. U.S.A.*, 92, 12304, 1995.

105. Proctor, W.R. and Dunwiddie, T.V., Behavioral sensitivity to purinergic drugs parallels ethanol sensitivity in selectively bred mice, *Science*, 224, 519, 1984.

106. Rajachandran, L., Spear, N.E., and Spear, L.P., Effects of the combined administration of the 5HT$_3$ antagonist MDL 72222 and ethanol on conditioning in the periadolescent and adult rat, *Pharmacol. Biochem. Behav.*, 46, 535, 1993.

107. Rasmussen, K., Stockton, M.E., and Czachura, J.F., The 5-HT$_3$ receptor antagonist zatosetron decreases the number of spontaneously active A10 dopamine neurons, *Eur. J. Pharmacol.*, 205, 113, 1991.

108. Reid, L.D., Endogenous opioids and alcohol dependence: opioid alkaloids and the propensity to drink alcoholic beverages, *Alcohol*, 13, 5, 1996.

109. Reynolds, J.D. and Brien, J.F., The role of adenosine A$_1$ receptor activation in ethanol-induced inhibition of stimulated glutamate release in the hippocampus of the fetal and adult guinea pig, *Alcohol*, 12, 151, 1995.

110. Rossetti, Z.L., Hmaidan, Y., and Gessa, G.L., Marked inhibition of mesolimbic dopamine release: a common feature of ethanol, morphine, cocaine, and amphetamine abstinence in rats, *Eur. J. Pharmacol.*, 221, 227, 1992.

111. Rossetti, Z.L. and Carboni, S., Ethanol withdrawal is associated with increased extracellular glutamate in the rat striatum, *Eur. J. Pharmacol.*, 283, 177, 1995.

112. Samson, H.H. and Doyle, T.F., Oral ethanol self-administration in the rat: effect of naloxone, *Pharmacol. Biochem. Behav.*, 22, 91, 1985.

113. Sapru, M.K., Diamond, I., and Gordon, A.S., Adenosine receptors mediate cellular adaptation to ethanol in NG 108-15 cells, *J. Pharmacol. Exp. Ther.*, 271, 542, 1994.

114. Sar, M., Stumpf, W.E., Miller, R.J., Chang, K.-J., and Cuatrecasas, P., Immunohistochemical localization of enkephalin in rat brain and spinal cord, *J. Comp. Neurol.*, 182, 17, 1978.

115. Schreiber, R., Opitz, K., Glaser, T., and De Vry, J., Ipsapirone and 8-OH-DPAT reduce ethanol preference in rats: involvement of presynaptic 5-HT$_{1A}$ receptors, *Psychopharmacology*, 112, 100, 1993.

116. Seizinger, B.R., Hollt, V., and Herz, A., Effects of chronic ethanol treatment on the *in vitro* biosynthesis of pro-opiomelanocortin and its postranslational processing to beta-endorphin in the intermediate lobe of the rat pituitary, *J. Neurochem.*, 43, 607, 1984.

117. Self, D.W. and Nestler, E.J., Molecular mechanisms of drug reinforcement and addiction, *Annu. Rev. Neurosci.*, 18, 463, 1995.

118. Sellers, E.M., Higgins, G.A., and Sobell, M.B., 5-HT and alcohol abuse, *TiPS*, 13, 69, 1992.

119. Sellers, E.M., Toneatto, T., Romach, M.K., Somer, G.R., Sobell, L.C., and Sobell, M.B., Clinical efficacy of the 5-HT$_3$ antagonist odansetron in alcohol abuse and dependence, *Alcohol. Clin. Exp. Res.*, 18, 879, 1994.

120. Shelton, K.L. and Balster, R.L., Ethanol drug discrimination in rats: substitution with GABA agonists and NMDA antagonists, *Behav. Pharmacol.*, 5, 441, 1994.

121. Shippenberg, T.S., Bals-Kubik, R., and Herz, A., Motivational properties of opioids: evidence that an activation of δ-receptors mediates reinforcement processes, *Brain Res.*, 436, 234, 1987.

122. Shippenberg, T.S., Bals-Kubuk, R., and Herz, A., Examination of the neurochemical substrates mediating the motivational effects of opioids: role of the mesolimbic dopamine system and D-1 vs. D-2 dopamine receptors, *J. Pharmacol. Exp. Ther.*, 265, 53, 1993.

123. Smith, G.B. and Olsen, R.W., Functional domains of GABA$_A$ receptors, *Trends Physiol. Sci.*, 16, 162, 1995.

124. Snell, L.D., Nunley, K.R., Lickteig, R.L., Browning, M.D., Tabakoff, B., and Hoffman, P.L., Regional and subunit specific changes in NMDA receptor mRNA and immunoreactivity in mouse brain following chronic ethanol ingestion, *Mol. Brain Res.*, 40, 71, 1996.

125. Spiraki, C., Fibiger, H.C., and Phillips, A.G., Attenuation of heroin reward in rats by disruption of the mesolimbic dopamine system, *Psychopharmacology*, 79, 278, 1983.

126. Stone, C.J. and Forney, R.B., The effects of phencyclidine on ethanol and sodium hexobarbital in mice, *Toxicol. Appl. Pharmacol.*, 40, 177, 1977.

127. Tabakoff, B., Current literature reviewed and critiqued, *Alcohol. Clin. Exp. Res.*, 19, 1597, 1995.

128. Tabakoff, B. and Hoffman, P.L., Alcohol addiction: an enigma among us, *Neuron*, 16, 909, 1996.

129. Taber, M.T. and Fibiger, H.C., Electrical stimulation of the prefrontal cortex increases dopamine release in the nucleus accumbens of the rat: modulation by metabotropic glutamate receptors, *J. Neurosci.*, 15, 3896, 1995.

130. Tomkins, D.M., Higgins, G.A., and Sellers, E.M., Low doses of the 5-HT$_{1A}$ agonist 8-hydroxy-2-(di-*n*-propylamino)-tetralin (8-OH DPAT) increase ethanol intake, *Psychopharmacology*, 115, 173, 1994.

131. Trevisan, L., Lawrence, W.F., Brose, N., Gasic, G.P., Heinemann, S.F., Duman, R.S., and Nestler, E.J., Chronic ingestion of ethanol up-regulates NMDAR1 receptor subunit immunoreactivity in rat hippocampus, *J. Neurochem.*, 62, 1635, 1994.

132. Trifunovic, P.D. and Brodie, M.S., The effects of clomipramine on the excitatory action of ethanol on dopaminergic neurons of the ventral tegmental area *in vitro*, *J. Pharmacol. Exp. Ther.*, 276, 34, 1996.

133. Tsai, G., Gastfriend, D.R., and Coyle, J.T., The glutamatergic basis of human alcoholism, *Am. J. Psychiatry*, 152, 332, 1995.

134. Van Bockstaele, E.J., Cestari, D.M., and Pickel, V.M., Synaptic structure and connectivity of serotonin terminals in the ventral tegmental area: potential sites for modulation of mesolimbic dopamine neurons, *Brain Res.*, 647, 307, 1994.

135. Volpicelli, J.R., Alterman, A.I., Hayashida, M., and O'Brien, C.P., Naltrexone in the treatment of alcohol dependence, *Arch. Gen. Psychiatry*, 49, 8786, 1992.

136. Weiss, F., Lorang, M.T., Bloom, F.E., and Koob, G.F., Oral alcohol self-administration stimulates dopamine release in the rat nucleus accumbens: genetic and motivational determinants, *J. Pharmacol. Exp. Ther.*, 267, 250, 1993.

137. Weiss, F., Parson, L.H., Schulteis, G., Hyytia, P., Lorang, M.T., Bloom, F.E., and Koob, G.F., Ethanol self-administration restores withdrawal-associated deficiencies in accumbal dopamine and 5-hydroxytryptamine release in dependent rats, *J. Neurosci.*, 16, 3474, 1996.

138. Wessinger, W.D. and Balster, R.L., Interactions between phencyclidine and central nervous system depressants evaluated in mice and rats, *Pharmacol. Biochem. Behav.*, 27, 323, 1987.

139. Wong, D.T., Threlkeld, P.G., Lumeng, L., and Li, T.-K., Higher density of serotonin$_{1A}$ receptors in the hippocampus and cerebral cortex of alcohol-preferring P rats, *Life Sci.*, 46, 231, 1990.

140. Wozniak, K.M., Pert, A., Mele, A., and Linnoila, M., Focal application of alcohols elevates extracellular dopamine in rat brain: a microdialysis study, *Brain Res.*, 540, 31, 1991.

141. Yan, Q.-S., Reith, M.E.A., Jobe, P.C., and Dailey, J.W., Focal ethanol elevates extracellular dopamine and serotonin concentrations in the rat ventral tegmental area, *Eur. J. Pharmacol.*, 301, 49, 1996.

142. Yoshimoto, K., McBride, W.J., Lumeng, L., and Li, T.-K., Alcohol stimulates the release of dopamine and serotonin in the nucleus accumbens, *Alcohol*, 9, 17, 1991.

143. Zhou, F.C., Bledsoe, S., Lumeng, L., and Li, T.-K, Immunostained serotonergic fibers are decreased in selected brain regions of alcohol preferring rats, *Alcohol*, 8, 425, 1991.

35 Behavioral Pharmacology

Gail Winger

OVERVIEW

This is a selected review of oral and intravenous models of the reinforcing effects of ethanol in non-human primates and rodents. The point of view is that studies of the reinforcing effects of ethanol in experimental animals must include demonstrations of high, sustained, voluntary ethanol intake of 8 to 12 g kg^{-1} d^{-1} and blood levels in the range of 200 to 300 mg% with clear behavioral intoxication in order to substantiate claims to measure an aspect of the reinforcing effects of ethanol relevant to the human condition of alcoholism. These criteria have clearly been met when non-human primates are trained to respond and receive intravenous ethanol. Thus far, however, using an oral route of administration, no rodent preparation and few primate preparations have provided these data. Although animals drink ethanol in patterns that closely resemble those shown with intravenous administration and demonstrate a reinforcing effect of ethanol, they do not drink as much, they do not develop marked intoxication, and, when access is continuous, they do not show sustained intakes. It is not clear why there is a marked difference in the amount of ethanol consumed under oral as compared with intravenous administration, but limits on fluid ingestion, delayed feedback effects, and different behavioral requirements are suggested as possible avenues to explore. The possibility that alcoholism in animals as in humans tends to be a slowly developing process, with a number of environmental as well as genetic constraints that limit the rapid establishment of symptomatic behavior, must be entertained.

INTRODUCTION

The prevalence of ethanol use is greater than the prevalence of use of any other psychoactive, nontherapeutic drug in the U.S., with the possible exception of nicotine. More than 64% of U.S. residents are current users of ethanol.[1] Given these levels of exposure to ethanol, it is not surprising that ethanol abuse and alcoholism are the major drug abuse problems in this country. Some 8% of the population can be classified as heavy drinkers or alcoholics.[1] Studies of the behavioral pharmacology of ethanol, particularly as it relates to abuse of this substance and treatment of such abuse, are therefore of considerable importance for medical and public health considerations.

Ethanol has many behavioral effects. For example, it stimulates some behavior at small doses, and produces a general retardation of behavior at larger doses.[2] It can disinhibit some behavior in a manner similar to that shown by anxiolytic drugs.[3] It has stimulus effects that can be mimicked by a variety of other depressant drugs.[4] At relatively small doses, it can impair behavior on selective attention tasks,[5] and this impairment might be responsible for the problems that occur when people drink and drive. With chronic administration, physical dependence on ethanol develops with a characteristic withdrawal syndrome.[2] There is really a single behavioral effect of ethanol, however, that is of overriding relevance to the condition of alcoholism. That is the reinforcing effect of ethanol, based on the stimulus provided by ethanol's neuropharmacological effects. A reinforcing effect of ethanol in this case means simply that these neuropharmacological effects of ethanol cause an increase in the behavior (drinking ethanol) that produces these effects. It is the reinforcing effect of ethanol that leads some people to return to this drug more and more frequently until it impairs their ability to function appropriately as individuals and in society.

It is possible to study ethanol as a reinforcer in laboratory animals by measuring the behavior that produces ethanol availability and/or ingestion; many investigators have invested considerable time and effort in this type of study. Much of this work has been reviewed earlier,[6,7] but before summarizing and updating these reviews, it is important to point out the problems that must be considered in evaluating animal research on ethanol as a reinforcer. Whenever animals are used to measure certain aspects of a condition that occurs in humans, it is important to know whether or not what the animals are telling us is relevant to the human condition. When the condition is a behavioral disorder rather than a physical disorder such as cancer, infection, or a physical disease, "relevance" can be fairly difficult to establish. The issue here is whether the reinforcing effects of ethanol as measured in animals are relevant to the reinforcing effects of ethanol in humans. Because so little is known about ethanol as a reinforcer in humans, it is difficult to make this assessment in many cases. It is probably safe to assume that humans find ethanol to be reinforcing because of its pharmacological effects as opposed to its taste, caloric value, or other nonpharmacological effects. This makes it important to demonstrate in animals that the measured reinforcing effect is related to ethanol's pharmacological effect, and specifically, that consumption by the animal is sufficient to produce a pharmacological effect. Unfortunately, there are no experimental studies in humans that answer the question of how much ethanol must be consumed to produce a pharmacologically based reinforcing effect. Neither is it known whether this amount differs among social drinkers, heavy drinkers, and alcoholics. A good animal model of human ethanol consumption should demonstrate ethanol consumption in rates and patterns that mimic those of the human counterpart; but again, there is very little documentation of how humans drink ethanol, particularly how they overconsume ethanol. Thus, our ignorance about ethanol drinking and alcoholism as it occurs in humans severely impairs our ability to establish credible animal models for this disorder.

The reinforcing effect of ethanol may, at its behavioral base, be no different from the reinforcing effects produced by other drugs of abuse, such as cocaine or heroin, or from the reinforcing effects produced by food, water, or personal contact. Certainly, the manner in which the reinforcing effects of these and other stimuli is frequently studied is quite similar, and under these conditions, ethanol as a reinforcer is difficult to distinguish from other reinforcers. If there is a distinction to be made between reinforcers that increase our quality of life and those that decrease it, it may not be in the stimuli themselves, but in the amount of time spent in acquiring and consuming them. Eating food is necessary for life; eating too much food can result in early death. Gambling is occasional entertainment for some and a major and detrimental preoccupation for others. Social drinking can provide needed relaxation and improve important interpersonal interactions. When carried to extremes, drinking isolates individuals, increases their anxiety, and severely decreases the quality of their lives.

The phenomenon of "overconsumption" of some reinforcers by some individuals is rarely studied when some drugs or other events are evaluated as reinforcing stimuli. More frequently, restrictions are in place in the experimental paradigm to prevent excessive intake and the undesired consequences of such excess such as morbidity or behavioral variability. It is perhaps these restrictions that prevent distinctions from being made among the various reinforcers that have been evaluated, and they may as well reduce the likelihood that animals will provide unambiguous models of the human condition. In the case of modeling human ethanol consumption in animals, however, at least by the oral route, the issue is not that overconsumption is prevented by restriction of access, it is that overconsumption is difficult to observe under any circumstances, and the reasons for this are puzzling.

In reviewing studies of animal models of the reinforcing effects of ethanol, it is useful to state the criteria for overconsumption that should be met to establish an animal model as relevant to the human condition of alcoholism. As might be guessed from the above discussion, this is not easy to do because there is no relevant standard for defining alcoholism in humans in terms of amount of ethanol consumed over long periods of time. The risk of decompensated cirrhosis increases with ethanol intakes over 150 gm per day,[8] suggesting that physical harm from ethanol can result in humans at these intake levels. But measures of behavioral harm from ethanol ingestion, in terms of increases in the amount of control it exercises over an individual's life, have not been related to the amount of ethanol consumed.

To ensure that pharmacological effects of ethanol are responsible for the reinforcing effects observed, relevant criteria are that ethanol is consumed in amounts that produce gross signs of intoxication, or in amounts that result consistently in blood ethanol levels in the range of 200 to 300 mg% in primates and perhaps higher in less-sensitive rodents. Blood levels in humans above 100 mg% are considered incompatible with safe driving in some parts of the U.S. In addition, this blood level should be observed, perhaps in a cyclic manner, over substantial periods of time. The development of physiological dependence on ethanol is *prima facie* evidence of sustained high levels of ethanol intake. A number of caveats need to be applied to the use of dependence as a criterion for an animal model, however, primarily in comparison with other drugs of abuse. Dependence on potent drugs can develop in the absence of a reinforcing effect, and a clearly relevant pharmacological effect can be obtained in the absence of physiological dependence, particularly using an intravenous route of administration with limited access conditions. Therefore, although it is important to note when physiological dependence has been shown to occur, and when it has not, this is only as an indicator of sustained, high intakes, and not as a hard-and-fast criterion for an animal model of alcoholism. Physiological dependence on ethanol in non-human primates has been demonstrated with consumption of approximately 8 g kg^{-1} d^{-1} for less than 1 week,[9] and in rats with an average consumption of 13 g kg^{-1} d^{-1} for 3 months;[10] these values can be set as approximations of the amount of ethanol that these respective animals need to consume in order to model the human condition of severe alcoholism. Dependence in humans has been determined by self-report to occur with approximately 10 years of consumption of approximately 4 g kg^{-1} d^{-1}.[15]

ORAL ROUTE OF ADMINISTRATION: PRIMATES

Most investigators interested in ethanol as a reinforcer in animals have used the oral route of administration. This is appropriate because people consume ethanol orally, and because route of administration is an important variable in drug self-administration and should be modeled as closely as possible. Because it is non-invasive, the oral route is also the one that will be most useful in long-term studies of the development of alcoholism, and studies of the social influences on ethanol consumption. However, it has been difficult to establish ethanol as a reinforcer by the oral route in a fashion that suggests human alcoholism. Animals do not readily come to drink ethanol in the quantities and in the compulsive patterns that are associated with human alcoholism.

Meisch and Stewart[6] have recently reviewed some of the literature on ethanol as a reinforcer in non-human primates. They note that early studies, including those in which monkeys drank ethanol in concentrations ranging from 5 to 20% in order to avoid electric shock presentation, in order to present food, or those using schedule-induced polydipsia procedures,[11-14] were generally unsuccessful in producing significant oral ethanol consumption in non-human primates. Simply making these concentrations of ethanol available as an alternative to water also did not lead to consumption of more than moderate amounts of ethanol, and resulted in consistent preference for water.

A breakthrough of sorts in producing a reinforcing effect of ethanol came with the discovery that monkeys would prefer lower concentrations of ethanol (2%) to water.[16,17] Subsequent studies have used various techniques to establish ethanol as a reinforcer, starting with these low concentrations. Food deprivation is an important element in establishing ethanol as a reinforcer according to some investigators,[6,18] but plays little role according to others.[19] Schedule-induced polydipsia, in which small pieces of food are given to primates spaced in time with ethanol solutions available,[20] and food-induced drinking, in which ethanol is made available during the time that the daily food ration is given,[21,22] have been notably successful in producing initial high ethanol consumption. However, others have found that simply making 2% ethanol available along with water will yield a preference for ethanol in some monkeys, in the absence of strong inducing conditions.[6,19,23] Once drinking of low concentrations of ethanol is occurring, the concentration can be increased, and the inducing conditions can be discontinued. Some[19] or most[6] of the monkeys under study can be induced to drink substantial amounts of ethanol under these conditions.

Once oral ethanol has been established as a reinforcer, it has been fairly common to alter the concentration of ethanol in a systematic manner. Henningfield and Meisch evaluated a wide range of ethanol concentrations in three monkeys and found that the animals drank less total volume of ethanol as the concentration increased, but maintained similar total ethanol intake (2.56 to 3 g kg^{-1} per 3-hour session) across the various concentrations.[24] After-session blood levels were between 200 and 265 mg%. These are impressive amounts of ethanol consumption, less than those obtained with intravenous self-administration (see below) but indicative of a pharmacologically relevant amount of ethanol ingestion. Interestingly, however, in a subsequent study, the investigators made two changes. They made water available concurrently with the ethanol, and they decreased the amount of food deprivation from 80 to 85% of free feeding weight. The three monkeys in this study drank significantly less ethanol (0.84 to 1.03 g kg^{-1} per 3-hour session), and showed lower blood ethanol levels (24 to 171 mg%).[25] Importantly, when the monkeys were allowed 23-h-per-day access to ethanol, they took only slightly more ethanol than under the 3-hour condition, and intake was variable across days. The authors attributed the decreased ethanol intake in the second study to the decreased amount of food deprivation.[25] Although this does not necessarily indicate that the primates were consuming ethanol for its caloric value, it does raise the issue of relevance to the human condition, where food deprivation is not thought to contribute to the development of alcoholism or the maintenance of large amounts of ethanol intake.

Baboons have also been used in experiments in oral ethanol consumption. Two baboons were given 3-hour access to ethanol once drinking was established using a food-induced drinking procedure. Concentrations were increased from 8 to 32%. The total ethanol intake remained relatively constant across these concentration increases, at approximately 1.5 g kg^{-1} (maximum blood levels of 157 mg%) for one baboon, and approximately 2.8 g kg^{-1} (maximum blood levels of 273 mg%) for the other. When water was made available along with ethanol solutions, the baboons showed a clear preference for the ethanol.[22] Although there have been a few additional demonstrations that ethanol serves as a reinforcer in baboons under limited access conditions,[26,27] demonstrations of overconsumption of ethanol in the context of long-term availability of ethanol, with the consequent development of physiological dependence, have not been published.

Although it is clear that significant progress has been made in inducing oral ethanol consumption in non-human primates, it is not yet clear that these preparations are relevant to human alcoholism. Under conditions of strong food deprivation, monkeys will drink amounts of ethanol that lead to blood levels indicative of an intoxicating effect. Yet, attempts to produce physical dependence on ethanol in non-human primates using an oral route of ethanol availability have not been successful.[25,28,29] Under conditions of continuous or frequent daily access, intakes by monkeys are fairly low relative to those necessary to produce and maintain intoxication and dependence. The reasons why monkeys drink substantial amounts of ethanol when access is limited, yet fail to continue to drink to excess when access is less limited, is puzzling, but evidence of a reason to be concerned about the validity of the oral model of ethanol consumption in primates.

Non-human primates will ingest intoxicating amounts of ethanol when sweetener or flavor is added to the ethanol solution.[30,31] Addition of sweeteners, however, makes it more difficult to ascertain that the fluid is being consumed for the pharmacological effects of ethanol rather than for the taste. Nevertheless, some very interesting studies of ethanol consumption have been done in monkeys using sweetened solutions of ethanol. Marku Linnoila and colleagues at the National

Institute on Alcohol Abuse and Alcoholism (NIAAA) have evaluated in monkeys some of the hypotheses put forward by Cloninger regarding types of alcoholism in humans.[32]

According to Cloninger, there are two types of alcoholics: type I is characterized by high anxiety and excessive avoidance of harm or novelty; type II is characterized by episodes of impulsive aggression. Both genetic and environmental factors influence these traits, and type II alcoholics in particular have decreased central nervous system serotonin function.

In attempting to develop animal models for these types of alcoholics, Higley et al.[33] evaluated consumption of aspartame-sweetened ethanol in two groups of young adult (50 months of age) rhesus monkeys. Individuals in one group had been raised by their mothers until they were 6 months old (maternally raised or MR). Those in the other group had been raised without their mothers but with other monkeys of a similar age (peer-raised or PR). After 6 months of age, all monkeys were placed in identical social environments. Sweetened 7% ethanol solutions were made available to the monkeys in their home cages for 1 hour each day under conditions that reduced the opportunity for one monkey to interfere with another monkey's consumption of ethanol. A similarly sweet, non-ethanol solution was available as well. The animals were then separated from their peer groups and placed in individual cages for four consecutive 4-day periods with 3 days of group housing between the periods of isolation. Sweetened ethanol was also available in the individual cages for 1 hour per day.

All monkeys drank sufficient amounts of the sweetened ethanol solution to produce signs of intoxication. They drank in patterns that resembled those described for monkeys drinking unsweetened ethanol solutions: intake was rapid when the solutions were initially available (60% of the total intake was consumed in the first 15 minutes), and then maintained at slower rates throughout the remaining exposure time. There were large individual differences in the amount of ethanol consumed; and when each animal was later given, by intragastric tube, the amount of ethanol it had consumed in the experiment, blood ethanol levels ranged between 25 and 380 mg%, with an average of 375 mg%. Of most interest was the finding that the PR monkeys in the group housing condition drank significantly more ethanol and showed higher levels of anxiety than did the MR monkeys. The MR monkeys, on the other hand, showed marked increases in ethanol ingestion when placed in the isolated living conditions. Earlier studies had indicated that intermittent social separation produced increases in intake of sweetened ethanol solutions,[34] extending the generality of these findings.

This experiment was repeated (using 8.4% ethanol in aspartame) in a second study with similar behavioral results.[35] The PR monkeys drank more ethanol than the MR monkeys during group housing conditions, and the MR monkeys increased their ethanol intake to match that of the PR monkeys during social isolation. Most monkeys drank more than 1.4 g kg^{-1} ethanol during the access hour on one or more occasions, and some drank as much as 5 g kg^{-1}. Blood levels of 270 mg% were measured in the monkeys later, when they received by gastric tube the amount of ethanol they had drunk in the study. In this study, measures of CSF levels of a metabolite of serotonin (5-HIAA) were taken over the monkeys' lives. The PR monkeys were found to have lower levels of 5-HIAA as both infants and adults than the MR monkeys. Independent of the rearing conditions, there was a negative correlation between rates of ethanol consumption during the isolated condition and levels of CSF HIAA during isolation. Monkeys with infrequent social interactions and reduced impulse control were also found to drink more ethanol.[35]

Interestingly, when animals had both ethanol-aspartame solutions and ethanol-free aspartame solutions to drink, they drank more of the ethanol-free fluid, although they drank intoxicating amounts of ethanol and generated high blood ethanol levels. Thus, although intoxicating amounts of ethanol were consumed, and interesting correlations were made between ethanol consumption, early life experience, and measures of central serotonin turnover, a reinforcing effect of ethanol in the form of preference was not demonstrated in these animals. A group of 12 monkeys from the NIAAA who consumed the most sweetened ethanol solutions under the conditions described by

Higley et al. were made available to investigators, who evaluated the reinforcing effects of ethanol in these monkeys and compared them with effects in a group of 12 age-matched controls. These monkeys were given unflavored and unsweetened ethanol to drink concurrently with water during 2-hour daily sessions in which four contacts on one of the two spouts were required to produce fluid delivery. The concentration of ethanol was varied from 0.25 to 16%. The monkeys selected for their high intakes of sweetened ethanol drank significantly more ethanol than water under these conditions, indicating that ethanol had a reinforcing effect in these animals. The maximum fluid intakes developed at 1 or 2% ethanol, and the maximum ethanol consumption occurred at 8% ethanol. At this concentration, the NIAAA monkeys drank an average of 1.5 g kg^{-1} and the control monkeys that had not been selected for ethanol consumption drank an average of 0.9 g kg^{-1}. In addition, there was a negative correlation between CSF levels of 5-HIAA and ethanol preference, regardless of the group from which the animals came.[28]

It remained puzzling and frustrating to find that monkeys with substantial exposure to sweetened ethanol solutions, which they consumed to the point of intoxication, did not drink unsweetened ethanol solutions to the point of intoxication although they demonstrated a reinforcing effect of the unsweetened ethanol. Thus, the role of ethanol remains unclear in situations in which its taste is masked, large amounts are consumed, and clear relations, which parallel those in humans, can be drawn between ethanol consumption and early life experiences, neurotransmitter levels, and behavioral signs of anxiety and aggressions.

INTRAVENOUS ROUTE OF ADMINISTRATION: PRIMATES

In contrast to the difficulties shown in inducing non-human primates to drink significant amounts of ethanol, ethanol appears to serve readily as an intravenous reinforcer in monkeys. In some monkeys, experience with self-administration of other drugs such as cocaine or methohexital was necessary before ethanol came to maintain responding;[9] but in other monkeys, intravenous ethanol was able to initiate as well as maintain responding.[9,36] When made available under continuous access conditions, intravenous ethanol was self-administered in amounts that led to profound intoxication (as much as 8.6 g kg^{-1} d^{-1}), and rather quickly to physical dependence and withdrawal signs. Binge patterns of spontaneous ethanol self-administration were observed much like those that have been described in human alcoholics.[37] When access to ethanol was restricted to 3 hours per day, ethanol-controlled responding became regular from day to day, and closely resembled responding controlled by other drug reinforcers. There was an inverted-U-shaped relationship between rates of responding and dose per injection;[38] presession administration of ethanol produced a compensatory decrease in the amounts of ethanol taken in a daily session; intake was in the range of 4 g kg^{-1}; and blood levels of ethanol reached values of 400 mg% during 3-hour sessions, and were maintained at the peak levels during 6-hour sessions.[36]

ORAL ROUTE OF ADMINISTRATION: RODENTS

The issues and problems involved in establishing an appropriate model of oral ethanol self-administration in non-human primates are present in studies in rodents as well. As with non-human primate studies, two different procedures have been used in rodents to indicate a reinforcing effect of ethanol. One is to present the rats with water and a solution of ethanol in a two-bottle, home-cage preference evaluation. If the rats drink more ethanol than water during the day, they are considered to be demonstrating a reinforcing effect of the ethanol solution. As with non-human primates, rats prefer low concentrations of ethanol to water, but they consistently refuse higher concentrations of ethanol if water is concurrently available. A number of strategies have been used to induce ethanol consumption in rodents, and just a few of these are considered in detail below.

One of the early procedures made ethanol available concurrently with intermittent food presentation. This induces overconsumption of any available fluid; and when the fluid was ethanol, the rats drank sufficient quantities to produce physical dependence.[10] Although this model satisfies the requirement of overconsumption (13 g kg^{-1} d^{-1}) and physical dependence, it was not clear that the consumption was due to the pharmacological effects of ethanol, as opposed to the fluid qualities of ethanol, because any available fluid is consumed in prodigious quantities under these feeding conditions.

Wolffgramm and Heyne[40] describe a model of ethanol addiction in which rats had several different concentrations of ethanol available along with water for as long as 50 weeks. The ethanol solutions were removed for 4 to 9 months and then returned. Animals greatly increased their ethanol consumption for a week when the ethanol solutions were again available. Intake in these animals was not markedly reduced by adding quinine to the ethanol solutions, although quinine typically decreased ethanol intake in rats not exposed to the inducing conditions. Social isolation, which normally produced increases in ethanol consumption of previously group-housed rats, no longer had an effect on ethanol intake in the induced animals. These data led the investigators to claim to have observed a "loss of control" of ethanol consumption in this situation. The primary drawback of this model of ethanol consumption is that the rats drank only 4 g kg^{-1} d^{-1} of ethanol when they were showing maximal intake. The investigators did not indicate the pattern of ethanol consumption, but it can be assumed that this amount is taken primarily during the dark part of the diurnal cycle, presumably a 12-hour period. This amount of ethanol consumed over this time period is not sufficient to produce the profound intoxication necessary to claim a model of human alcoholism. Although the investigators claim to see both intoxication and withdrawal signs in these rats, their measure of intoxication and withdrawal were much too sensitive to be considered relevant because intoxication was reported following 0.2 to 0.3 g kg^{-1} ethanol intake, and withdrawal signs were observed in rats given access to ethanol only once per week for 32 weeks.

Several groups of investigators have bred rats for their tendency to drink or to refuse to drink relatively high concentrations of ethanol.[41-44] The ethanol preferring (P) and non-ethanol preferring (NP) lines developed by Li and colleagues have been studied more intensively than the other strains; Li and McBride state that these animals meet all the criteria for a animal model of alcoholism and have been accepted by the ethanol research community as such.[45] Among the criteria that the P animals are said to have met are demonstrated consumption of large amounts of ethanol, with consequent high blood levels, for the pharmacological effects of ethanol, and to the point of physiological dependence. These are excellent criteria for the establishment of a rodent model of alcoholism, but it is arguable that the P rats meet these criteria.

Li et al.[46] indicated that P rats would eventually consume as much as 12 g kg^{-1} d^{-1} of ethanol when given a choice between 10% ethanol and water for a period of 10 weeks. Although this is a substantial amount of ethanol, indicative of a pharmacological basis of consumption, measures of blood ethanol levels at times when ethanol intake was high showed that the intakes were not reflected in blood ethanol levels, which were typically below 100 mg%. The authors suggested that metabolic tolerance could account for this discrepancy, but the development of such tolerance would only increase the intake requirements to confirm a pharmacological basis of the ethanol consumption. Spillage and evaporation were not directly assessed as alternative explanations for the discrepancy between consumption and blood levels. In a study of the development of metabolic tolerance to ethanol in P rats, Lumeng and Li[47] observed an increase in ethanol metabolism of 16 to 20% in rats that were given long-term access to 10% ethanol and water. The typical ethanol intakes were between 7.2 and 9.3 g kg^{-1} d^{-1}, although levels as high as 11.5 g kg^{-1} d^{-1} were recorded in the 7th week of the study. Blood ethanol levels in one or two of the ten rats were recorded at 130 mg% at the estimated time of peak ethanol intake, but the average of the group was approximately 50 mg%.[45] In another study,[48] P rats were given access to ethanol (10%) for 24 hours per day, for

4 consecutive hours per day, or for 1 hour of every four around the clock. Ethanol intake per hour of availability was highest at 1.1 g kg^{-1}/hr when ethanol was available discontinuously (4.4 g kg^{-1} d^{-1} compared with 6.9 g kg^{-1} d^{-1} for the 24-hour access condition), but blood ethanol levels were nearly the same in each group at approximately 60 mg%. Thus, the claim to high blood ethanol levels in the P line of rats is difficult to substantiate, and the finding of high daily intakes has not been replicated in more recent evaluations.

There have been at least two purported demonstrations of physiological dependence on ethanol in the P rats. In one,[46] the animals were food deprived and given ethanol in a saccharin, and NaCl solution. These animals drank 12 g kg^{-1} d^{-1} of ethanol, and many of them developed seizures when the ethanol solution was withdrawn. Although this is clear evidence of physiological dependence, it did not develop as a consequence of voluntary consumption of ethanol; a reinforcing function of ethanol in this situation was not demonstrated. In another study,[49] physiological dependence was indicated by scoring behaviors that ranged from tail stiffening to audiogenic seizures. P rats given access to ethanol solutions and water for 20 weeks demonstrated withdrawal signs, frequently in the form of teeth chatter and wet dog shakes, when the ethanol was discontinued. However, the animals in this experiment were drinking only 4.5 g kg^{-1} d^{-1} at the time ethanol was withdrawn, and it is unlikely that this small intake was responsible for the behavioral changes observed. The fact that no withdrawal signs were observed during the day when ethanol intake was low supports the notion that the behavioral changes may have been due to factors other than ethanol withdrawal.

The first method of demonstrating a reinforcing effect of ethanol was described as a home-cage, two-bottle preference measure. The second was to train the rats to respond on a lever to gain access to a solution of ethanol. The number of presses required for each delivery of ethanol can be altered, sessions of ethanol availability can be long or short, water and/or food can be available concurrently, or ethanol alone can be in the situation during a test session. If ethanol solutions maintain lever-pressing behavior in rats that are not otherwise deprived of food or fluid, it is demonstrated to be a reinforcer. The mechanism of its reinforcing function and whether that involves a pharmacological effect of ethanol are not often easy to demonstrate. Samson and colleagues have used a couple of procedures to induce ethanol-reinforced responding in rats. In one procedure, the animals were first trained to make an operant response during 30-min sessions and receive a dipper of 20% sucrose solution. The concentration of sucrose was then gradually reduced and ethanol was added to the fluid in gradually increasing concentrations until the animals were making responses to gain access to 10% ethanol. When responses on a second lever presented water, the rats made the majority of their responses on the lever that resulted in presentation of 10% ethanol. When responses on the second lever resulted in presentation of concentrations of sucrose as low as 1%, the rats chose both levers equally. With higher concentrations of sucrose, the lever selection became nearly exclusively on the one that presented sucrose. The maximum amount of ethanol that was consumed in rats that had experience with the sucrose-fading procedure was 0.94 g kg^{-1} in a 30-min period.[50] A second inducing procedure involved training rats to lick a spout containing 10% ethanol in order to gain access to a dipper of 20% sucrose.[51] Animals exposed to ethanol under these inducing conditions eventually responded on levers to gain access to 10% ethanol and consumed amounts comparable to animals exposed to the sucrose-inducing conditions.[52] Interestingly, rats that had not been induced to drink ethanol also came to drink these substantial quantities of ethanol, either initially or over a period of several weeks,[51] suggesting that the inducing conditions may play little role in the development of ethanol-reinforced responding.

These studies were designed primarily to demonstrate a reinforcing effect of ethanol in these rats. Although they accomplish this goal, the use of a very short session time (30 min) precludes any demonstration of overconsumption of ethanol in these animals, and reduces the potential relevance of this procedure to human alcoholism. These investigators have studied ethanol intake in situations where the animals remain in the operant chamber throughout the day, with food and water available (continuous access operant). They have also evaluated the effects of the inducing conditions on preference for ethanol solutions in a home cage two-bottle preference procedure. Thus, prior to exposure to one of the inducing procedures, Long-Evans rats showed a 25% preference (2 g kg^{-1} d^{-1} intake) for 10% ethanol paired with water in the home cage. Following the inducing procedure, home-cage preference increased to 55% (3 g kg^{-1} d^{-1}).[51] Similar tests in Alko alcohol preferring animals[54] and in the P line of preferring animals[55] indicated an increase in alcohol preference following the sucrose-substitution procedure to initiate ethanol drinking.

Samson and colleagues[51] observed a lack of correlation between the amount of ethanol rats drink in a home-cage, two-bottle preference procedure and the amount they consume when ethanol is contingent on lever-press responses under continuous access conditions. For example, rats exposed to one of the initiation procedures consumed significantly less ethanol when it was contingent on an operant response than when it was consumed in the home-cage, two-bottle situation. On the other hand, rats that were not exposed to the initiation procedure drank more ethanol in the continuous access operant situation than in the home-cage, two-bottle procedure.[51] This demonstration of a lack of correlation between the two most frequently used measures of ethanol's reinforcing effects is in need of much replication and consideration.

The ability of ethanol to reinforce behavior in the P rat line, bred for their willingness to consume 10% ethanol, has been studied with interesting results. In the 30-min sessions of ethanol availability, the P rats acted very much like outbred, initiated Long-Evans rats. They demonstrated a reinforcing effect of ethanol up to concentrations of 40%; but, as with the outbred strain, the P rats decreased their intake of ethanol when another lever was available that presented solutions of 5% sucrose.[52] Similar data were obtained with the Alko ethanol accepting rats that did not show reinforced ethanol drinking that was different from that of Wistar rats.[53-54] However, in the continuous access operant situation, the P rats consumed nearly twice as much ethanol as the outbred rats (4.4 g kg^{-1} d^{-1}).[55] Because pattern of drinking could be easily measured in this situation, the investigators compared these patterns in the two lines of rats. The P rats consumed most of their ethanol in bouts of responding and drinking, and had more bouts per day than the outbred rats. The size of each bout was nearly the same in the two lines. Following initiation procedures, in a home-cage, two-bottle preference procedure, P rats increased their ethanol preference from 50% (3.6 g kg^{-1} d^{-1}) to 90% (4 g kg^{-1} d^{-1}), a greater preference than shown by the Long-Evans strain, but with less total ethanol consumption than shown by the P rats in previous studies.[52]

The conclusion that can be drawn about oral ethanol consumption in rats is that there has been a tremendous research effort devoted to developing rats that drink large amounts of ethanol. Despite this effort, even under the best of conditions, and with clear demonstrations of a reinforcing effect of oral ethanol, daily ethanol consumption by these rats does not approximate the levels suggested as necessary to represent relevant overconsumption of ethanol.

Mice have also been studied for their oral ethanol consumption, frequently in the context of genetic contributions to ethanol ingestion. Ethanol drinking has been established in two strains of mice — C57BL/6J and BALB/cJ — by depriving the mice of food and making ethanol available along with their daily food rations. The food was then moved to after the 30-min daily session in which ethanol was available for responses on an FR1 schedule of reinforcement. Both the fixed ratio value and the concentration of ethanol was varied in both strains. The C57BL/6j mice responded more and drank more ethanol than BALB/cJ mice, and the former showed increased rates of responding as fixed ratio values increased. The greatest amount of ethanol was consumed when the concentration was 8%, and the FR was set at 1. Under these conditions, mice drank 2.2 to 2.4 g kg^{-1} per 30-min session, and had blood ethanol concentrations of approximately 140 mg%. Indeed, most of the ethanol consumption occurred in the initial 10 minutes of each session, during which high rates of responding were shown, and after which responding nearly stopped. A concentration-related reinforcing effect of ethanol was clearly present in this study in the C57BL/6J mice, and it is possible that the mice were intoxicated at these blood levels.[56] This pattern and amount of ethanol consumption is much like that observed in primates in studies.[24,25] Studies of ethanol consumption under less-limited access conditions have apparently not been published, so the critical question of whether these mice continue to consume intoxicating amounts of ethanol throughout a 24-hour period, for several days, to the point of physiological dependence has not been asked.

The importance of serotonin in the initiation and maintenance of ethanol drinking has been suggested in both humans and non-human primates. It was therefore interesting to measure ethanol intake in mice that were lacking the serotonin 1B receptor. These mice were more aggressive than normal mice, and consumed twice as much ethanol as normal mice, drinking an average of 10 g kg^{-1} d^{-1} of solutions of 20% ethanol available with water.[57] No withdrawal signs were observed following 12 days of access to this concentration of ethanol. Although these knockout mice did not differ from normal mice in their total fluid intake, preference for sweet or bitter solutions, rate of metabolism of ethanol, or intensity of ethanol withdrawal signs when they were exposed to ethanol vapor for 72 hours, they did show less ataxia following administration of 2 g kg^{-1} of ethanol, indicating a reduced sensitivity to ethanol. These studies are provocative and encourage further evaluation of the role of serotonin in the development of ethanol drinking and alcoholism.

INTRAVENOUS ROUTE OF ADMINISTRATION: RODENTS

There have been relatively few studies of intravenous ethanol-reinforced responding in rats. Of these, several indicated that ethanol did not serve as a reinforcer in this species.[55-61] In most of the remainder, ethanol was declared to be a reinforcer when delivered intravenously, but the doses of ethanol used were extremely small; and although it is not clear why the behavior was maintained, it is unlikely that the pharmacological effect of ethanol was responsible. Smith and Davis,[62] for example, demonstrated that 0.00012 g kg^{-1} inj^{-1} ethanol (keep in mind that 0.1 g kg^{-1} inj^{-1} is a typical intravenous dose for a monkey, and rats are very likely to be an order of magnitude less sensitive to ethanol than primates) produced a marked increase in responses in 8 of 11 rats exposed to this dose on an FR 1 schedule in 12-h d^{-1} sessions. Behavior returned to pre-ethanol levels when saline was made response-contingent. Sinden and LeMagnen[63] found that 0.001 g kg^{-1} inj^{-1}, but not 0.0005 or 0.005 g kg^{-1} inj^{-1}, available on an FR 1 schedule 24-h d^{-1}, produced increases in responses over a 5-day period to an average of 63 injections or 0.0063 g kg^{-1} d^{-1}. Hyytia et al. made 0.001 g kg^{-1} inj^{-1} ethanol available on an FR 1 TO 10s schedule of reinforcement in 3-hour daily sessions to AA and ANA rat strains whose behavior had been maintained by heroin. There was a dramatic increase in the number of responses made by the AA rats on the first day of ethanol availability, and this quickly returned to the level maintained by heroin and was not modified by increases in the dose to 0.002 and 0.004 g kg^{-1} inj^{-1}. The ANA rats only showed decreases in behavior when ethanol replaced heroin.[64]

In only one study[65] was a reinforcing effect of reasonable doses of ethanol described. In this study, one group of rats was made dependent on ethanol by frequent intravenous infusions to the point of anesthesia (9 to 16 g kg^{-1} d^{-1}) for 4 to 6 days prior to exposure to the self-administration conditions. If the rats did not respond (FR 1) and receive at least 5 g kg^{-1} d^{-1} ethanol during a 24-hour period, they were returned to another 4 to 6-day cycle of ethanol administration. Under these conditions, rats self-administered over 10 g kg^{-1} d^{-1} ethanol following three to eight cycles of ethanol exposure. Increasing the FR to 2 and 3 led to increased responses and maintenance of ethanol intakes. A second group of rats was given a similar opportunity to self-administer ethanol, but in the absence of chronic ethanol exposure; these rats did not self-administer ethanol.

It thus appears that rats do not typically develop rates of intravenous ethanol-maintained responding in a manner similar to that of monkeys. There is one study that indicates that intravenous ethanol can serve a reinforcing function in mice. Grahame and Cunningham[66] evaluated the reinforcing effects of 0.06 to 0.09 g kg^{-1} inj^{-1} intravenous ethanol in two strains of mice using a nose-poke response. Both strains, an oral ethanol preferring strain and a non-preferring strain, showed equal rates of i.v. ethanol-reinforced responding. Rates of nose-poke decreased when the dose of ethanol was either increased or decreased, but remained above that shown when saline was response contingent. The greatest amount of ethanol was taken by mice of the ethanol-preferring strain (2.37 g kg^{-1} per session) during daily 2-hour sessions when 0.09 g kg^{-1} inj^{-1} was available.

PHARMACOTHERAPY OF ALCOHOLISM IN ANIMAL MODELS

Two pharmacotherapies for alcoholism have recently been approved for the treatment of alcoholism. Naltrexone, a pure opioid antagonist, is currently used in the U.S. and has been shown to reduce ethanol drinking in controlled clinical trials.[67,68] Naltrexone, or the shorter-acting opioid antagonist naloxone, also reduced ethanol intake in a variety of animal models.[69] In rodents drinking ethanol (see, for example, References 70 and 71), in primates drinking ethanol,[23] and in primates self-administering ethanol by the intravenous route,[23] the opioid antagonists consistently reduced selection of, or rates of responding maintained by, ethanol. The mechanism for this effect is unclear. It is commonly thought that, because naltrexone is an opioid antagonist, its ability to block ethanol's reinforcing effects must be through this mechanism, and that opioids therefore mediate the reinforcing effects of ethanol.[72] This is not necessarily the case, although it has proven difficult to provide a clear alternative explanation. Studies using other opioid antagonists indicate that those selective for either mu-, kappa-, or delta-receptors may be unable to replicate the depressant effects of naltrexone on ethanol consumption.[73] The effects of naltrexone appeared limited to opioid antagonists with a chemical structure like that of naltrexone, such as nalmefene and naloxone.[29] The interaction between naltrexone and ethanol is not specific. Naltrexone reduced intake of any preferred solution. It reduced consumption of sucrose when sucrose was preferred to water, and it reduced consumption of water when water was preferred to high concentrations of ethanol.[74] Naltrexone therefore appeared to be blocking certain nonspecific appetitive factors, although its ability to suppress consumption of preferred solutions did not appear to be explained entirely by its ability to produce conditioned taste avoidance.[75]

The second pharmacotherapy for ethanol abuse is acamprosate, which has been approved for the treatment of alcoholism in some European countries. Acamprosate was shown in several clinical trials to produce an increase in abstinence in alcoholic patients.[76-78] Acamprosate is a depressant, but its mechanism of action is not entirely clear. It does not appear to act at GABA receptors, but may decrease the effects of glutamate acting through the NMDA receptors; it may also block calcium ion flux.[72] Acamprosate has not been evaluated as thoroughly as naltrexone in animal models of ethanol drinking, and not at all in intravenous models of ethanol's reinforcing effects. In studies in which ethanol drinking increased as a result of short-term removal of ethanol availability, acamprosate prevented these deprivation-induced increases.[79,80] In some studies, it decreased baseline ethanol consumption as well, and in others, it modified only the increases in ethanol consumption produced by ethanol deprivation.[81] More thorough evaluation of acamprosate's ability to decrease ethanol-induced drinking as well as to decrease the reinforcing effects of ethanol in intravenous models will give us more information about the relevance of the models and the usefulness and mechanism of action of acamprosate.

CONCLUSIONS

One conclusion from this chapter is that animal preparations of oral ethanol consumption succeed, at best, in increasing the concentration of ethanol that animals will select over water. This is accomplished by long-term exposure to low concentrations of ethanol, with or without one of a variety of inducing conditions, or with selective breeding. Although ethanol is clearly established as a reinforcer under some of these circumstances, the mechanism responsible for the reinforcing effect of ethanol, and the relevance to the human condition of alcoholism, have yet to be established.

This is because voluntary, pharmacologically induced overcomsumption of ethanol to the point of physical dependence has never been shown unambiguously in the oral models, and clear demonstrations of intoxication are rare. Although it is not necessary for physical dependence to be shown in order to establish a relevant reinforcing effect of orally presented drugs, in the case of ethanol drinking, dependence and intoxication are probably important to ensure that pharmacologically relevant amounts of ethanol have been consumed.

The issue of why animals do not consume greater amounts of oral ethanol is an interesting one. In many studies of oral ethanol intake, animals take smaller volumes of higher concentrations of ethanol, maintaining a fairly constant total ethanol intake.[6] This suggests that ethanol intake is being regulated at a certain value, and this regulation in turn indicates that the pharmacological properties of ethanol are important in maintaining ethanol ingestion. Similar regulation of intravenous ethanol intake has been used to support the notion of relevant ethanol control of this behavior as well.[39] However, the level at which ethanol intake is regulated is much higher for the intravenous than the oral route, with the intravenous route maintaining blood levels at least twice as high (and usually considerably higher) as those maintained under oral access conditions. Although there are fewer studies of oral administration of other drugs of abuse, the findings are similar: animals drink solutions of some stimulants, depressants, and opioids and indicate a reinforcing effect of these drugs, but the role of the drugs' pharmacological properties in this effect are difficult to ascertain because much less drug is consumed orally than is taken by the intravenous route, where profound intoxication is typically observed. The question of why the blood levels of ethanol and other drugs should be regulated at different values when the two routes of administration are used is an interesting and important one that has yet to be answered.

Comparisons between the oral and the intravenous routes with respect to patterns of intake raise similar questions. The pattern of oral ethanol consumption is largely invariant across individuals and across species, and is very similar to the pattern of i.v. ethanol intake where dramatically intoxicating amounts of ethanol are taken. The majority of responding and ethanol ingestion occurs at the beginning of the period of ethanol availability, and ethanol consumption occurs at much lower rates as the duration of ethanol availability is extended. It might be assumed that intoxication or satiation is responsible for the abrupt cessation of ethanol self-administration under both oral and intravenous conditions. The difference between the oral and intravenous patterns is that rates of ethanol intake decrease or stop after much smaller amounts of ethanol have been ingested in the oral situation. If intoxication or satiation is responsible for cessation consumption in both cases, why does it occur at much lower doses of ethanol in the oral case? It seems unlikely that the pharmacological effects of ethanol stop consumption in the relatively brief (10 minutes in some situations) periods sometimes observed, when absorption is probably incomplete. When the concentration of ethanol is low, it could be that fluid ingestion rather than intoxication is limiting oral intake. When ethanol concentration is high, greater than the 15% concentration used in most intravenous studies, the animals can receive the same amount of ethanol with less fluid ingestion by the oral as compared with the intravenous route. Thus, total fluid intake should not be limiting intake in these cases. It may be that the responses of drinking and swallowing are more susceptible to the rate-decreasing effects of ethanol than is the lever press response used in intravenous studies, and that the lack of a required drinking and swallowing response with the intravenous route accounts for larger intakes under these conditions. It may be that the faster feedback effects of intoxication by the intravenous route in some way encourage larger intake; oral ingestion may be maintained by the association between the taste of ethanol and the delayed pharmacological effects, and this conditioned reinforcing effect of oral ethanol may be more susceptible to the rate-decreasing effects of ethanol. It may be that oral ethanol is simply less reinforcing than intravenous ethanol, and behavior maintained by reinforcers of lower magnitude might be more susceptible to the rate-decreasing effects of drugs.

A large number of experiments appear to make it clear that animals do not drink ethanol for the calories it provides; there is little evidence that the taste of ethanol is responsible for ethanol consumption. Yet, the pharmacological effects of ethanol have not been clearly established as the mechanism behind its oral reinforcing effects in experimental animals. This is a mysterious circumstance that will probably not be soon resolved, in part because the investigators involved in studies of oral ethanol as a reinforcer have either convinced themselves that they have a relevant model of alcoholism, or they accept their demonstration of the reinforcing effects of ethanol as sufficient, and are therefore not continuing to try to determine why these preparations fail to attain the levels of overconsumption that are requisite in such a model.

The second conclusion from this review is that, with the possible exception of two studies in rodents, only in non-human primates has the intravenous route of ethanol delivery successfully demonstrated a reinforcing effect of pharmacologically relevant amounts of ethanol with accompanying severe intoxication, binge patterns of intake, and physiological dependence. Thus, intravenous ethanol self-administration in monkeys is the least ambiguous measure of the reinforcing effects of ethanol as they are relevant to the human condition of alcoholism. It is unfortunate that research using this procedure is so limited. It could be argued that humans do not demonstrate intoxication and dependence as readily as the monkey in studies of intravenous self-administration, and that this preparation is therefore also not homologous to the human condition. If a preparation was developed in which animals with orally available ethanol demonstrated increasing intake of ethanol over their life course, with periods of greater intake associated with particular environmental conditions, but culminating in frequent bouts of intoxication and physiological dependence in some genetically predisposed individuals, an entirely satisfactory model of alcoholism would be at hand, and its contribution to the understanding of this disease process would be profound.

REFERENCES

1. National Center for Health Statistics, Thornberry, O.T., Wilson, R.W., and Golden, P.M., Advance Data from Vital and Health Statistics, No. 1265, DHHS Publ. No. PHS 82-1250, Hyattsville, MD, Public Health Service, 1986.
2. Hobbs, W.R., Rall, T.W. and Verdoorn, T.A., Hypnotics and sedatives; ethanol, *Goodman and Gilman's The Pharmacological Basis of Therapeutics,* 9th ed., Hardman, J.G., Limbird, L.E., Molinoff, P.B., Ruddon, R.W., and Gilman, A.G., Eds., McGraw-Hill, New York, 1996, 361.
3. Koob, G.F. and Britton, K.T., Neurobiological substrates for the anti-anxiety effects of ethanol, *The Pharmacology of Alcohol and Alcohol Dependence,* Begleiter, H. and Kissen, B., Eds., Oxford University Press, New York, 1996, 477.
4. Grant, K.A., Colombo, G., and Gatto, G.J., Characterization of the ethanol-like discriminative stimulus effects of 5-HT receptor agonists as a function of ethanol training dose, *Psychopharmacology,* 133, 133, 1997.
5. Moskowitz, H., Effects of alcohol on peripheral vision as a function of attention, *Hum. Factors,* 16, 174, 1974.
6. Meisch, R.A. and Stewart, R.B., Ethanol as a reinforcer: a review of laboratory studies of non-human primates, *Behav. Pharmacol.,* 5, 425, 1994.
7. Stewart, R.B. and Grupp, L.A., Models of alcohol consumption using the laboratory rat, *Neuromethods: Animal Models of Drug Addiction,* Boulton, A.A., Baker, C.B., and Wu, P.H., Eds., Humana Press, Totowa, NJ, 1992, 1.
8. Arico, S. Galatola, G., Tabone, M., Corrao, G., Torchio, P., Valenti, M., and De la Pierre, M., The measure of life-time alcohol consumption in patients with cirrhosis: reproducibility and clinical relevance, *Liver,* 15, 202, 1995.
9. Winger, G.D. and Woods, J.H., The reinforcing property of ethanol in the rhesus monkey: I. Initiation, maintenance, and termination of intravenous ethanol reinforced responding, *Ann. N.Y. Acad. Sci.,* 215, 162, 1973.

10. Falk, J.L., Samson, H., and Winger, G., Behavioral maintenance of high concentrations of blood ethanol and physical dependence in the rat, *Science,* 177, 811, 1972.
11. Kamback, M.C., Drinking as an avoidance response by the pigtail monkey (*Macaca nemestrina*), *Q. J. Stud. Alc.,* 34, 331, 1973.
12. Mello, N.K. and Mendelson, J.H., Factors affecting alcohol consumption in primates, *Psychosomatic Med.,* 28, 529, 1966.
13. Mello, N.K. and Mendelson, J.H., Evaluation of a polydipsia technique to induce alcohol consumption in monkeys, *Physiol Behav.,* 7, 827, 1971a.
14. Mello, N.K. and Mendelson, J.H., The effects of drinking to avoid shock on alcohol intake in primates, *Biological Aspects of Alcohol,* Roach, M.K., McIsaac, M.K., and Creaven, P.J., Eds., University of Texas Press, Austin, 1971, 313.
15. Stuppaeck, C.H., Pycha, R., Miller, C., Whitworth, A.B., Oberbauer, H., and Fleishchacker, W.W., Carbamazepine versus oxazepam in the treatment of alcohol withdrawal: a double-blind study, *Alcohol Alcohol.,* 27, 153, 1992.
16. Kornet, M., Goosen, C., Ribbens, L.G., and Van Ree, J.M., Analysis of spontaneous alcohol drinking in rhesus monkeys, *Physiol Behav.,* 47, 679, 1990.
17. Macenski, M.J. and Meisch, R.A., Ethanol-reinforced responding of naive rhesus monkeys: acquisition without induction procedures, *Alcohol,* 9, 547, 1992.
18. Carroll, M.E. and Meisch, R.A., Enhanced drug-reinforced behavior due to food deprivation, *Advances in Behavioral Pharmacology,* Vol. 4, Thompson, T., Dews, P.B., and Barrett, J.E., Eds., Academic Press, New York, 1987, 47.
19. Pakarinen, E.D., Williams, K., and Woods, J.H., Food restriction and sex differences on concurrent, oral ethanol and water reinforcers in juvenile rhesus monkeys, *Alcohol,* 17, 35, 1999.
20. Meisch, R.A., The function of schedule-induced polydipsia in establishing ethanol as a positive reinforcer, *Pharmacolog. Rev.,* 27, 465, 1975.
21. Meisch, R.A. and Henningfield, J.E., Drinking of ethanol by rhesus monkeys: experimental strategies for establishing ethanol as a reinforcer, *Adv. Exp Med Biol.,* 85B, 443, 1977.
22. Henningfield, J.E., Ator, N.A., and Griffiths, R.R., Establishment and maintenance of oral ethanol self-administration in the baboon, *Drug Alc. Depend.,* 7, 113, 1981.
23. Williams, K.L., Winger, G., Pakarinen, E.D., and Woods, J.H. Naltrexone reduces ethanol- and sucrose-reinforced responding in rhesus monkeys, *Psychopharmacology,* 61, 53, 1998.
24. Henningfield, J.E. and Meisch, R.A., Ethanol drinking by rhesus monkeys, *Psychopharmacology,* 57, 133, 1978.
25. Henningfield, J.E. and Meisch, R.A., Ethanol drinking by rhesus monkeys with concurrent access to water, *Pharmacol. Biochem. Behav.,* 10, 777, 1979.
26. Ator, N.A. and Griffiths, R.R., Oral self-administration of triazolam, diazepam and ethanol in the baboon: drug reinforcement and benzodiazepine physiological dependence, *Psychopharmacology,* 108, 301, 1992.
27. Ator, N.A. and Griffiths, R.R., Oral self-administration of methohexital in baboons, *Psychopharmacology,* 79, 120, 1983.
28. Vivian, J.V., Higley, J.D., Linnoila, M., and Woods, J.H., Ethanol oral self-administration in rhesus monkeys: behavioral and neurochemical correlates, unpublished data, 1998.
29. Williams, K., personal communication, 1998.
30. Crowley, T.J. and Andrews, A.E., Alcoholic-like drinking in simian social groups, *Psychopharmacology,* 92, 196, 1987.
31. Fincham, J.E., Jooste, P.L., Seier, J.V., Taljaard, J.J., Weight, M.J., and Tichelaar, H.Y., Ethanol drinking by vervet monkeys (*cercopitheus pygerethrus*): individual responses of juvenile and adult males, *J. Med. Primat.,* 15, 183, 1986.
32. Cloninger, C.R., Bohman, M., Sigvardsson, S., Inheritance of alcohol abuse. Cross-fostering analysis of adopted men, *Arch. Gen. Psychiatry,* 38, 861, 1981.
33. Higley, J.D., Hasert, M.F., Suomi, S.L., and Linnoila, M., Nonhuman primate model of alcohol abuse: effects of early experience, personality, and stress on alcohol consumption, *Proc. Natl. Acad. Sci.,* 88, 7261, 1991.
34. Kraemer, G.W. and McKinney, W.T., Social separation increases alcohol consumption in rhesus monkeys, *Psychopharmacology,* 86, 182, 1985.

35. Higley, J.D., Suomi, S.L., and Linnoila, M., A nonhuman primate model of type II alcoholism? 1. Low cerebrospinal fluid 5-hydroxyindolacetic acid concentrations and dimished social competence correlate with excessive alcohol consumption, *Alcohol. Clin. Exp. Res.*, 20, 629, 1996.

36. Deneau, G., Yanagita, T. and Seevers, M.H., Self-administration of psychoactive substances by the monkey, *Psychopharmacologia*, 16, 30, 1969.

37. Nathan, P.E., Goldman, M.S., Lisman, S.A., and Augustus Taylor, H., Alcohol and alcoholics: a behavioral approach, *Trans. N.Y. Acad. Sci.*, 34, 602, 1972.

38. Carney, J.M., Lewellyn, M.E., and Woods, J.H, Variable interval responding maintained by intravenous codeine and ethanol injections in the rhesus monkey, *Pharmacol. Biochem. Behav.*, 5, 577, 1976.

39. Karoly, A.J., Winger, G., Ikomi, F., and Woods, J.H., The reinforcing property of ethanol in the rhesus monkey. II. Some variables related to the maintenance of intravenous ethanol-reinforced responding, *Psychopharmacology*, 58, 19, 1978.

40. Wolffgramm, J. and Heyne, A., From controlled drug intake to loss of control: the irreversible development of drug addiction in the rat, *Behav. Brain Res.*, 70, 77, 1995.

41. Mardones, J. and Segovia-Riquelme, N., Thirty two years of selection of rats for ethanol preference: UChA and UChB strains, *Neurobehav. Toxicol. Teratol.*, 5, 171, 1983.

42. Eriksson, K., The estimation of heritability for the self-selection of alcohol in the albino rat, *Ann. Med. Exp. Biol. Fenn.*, 47, 172, 1969.

43. Li, T.-K., Lumeng, L., McBride, W.J., and Waller, M.B., Indiana selection studies on alcohol-related behavior, *Development of Animal Models as Pharmacogenetic Tools*, McCreary, G.E., Deitrich, R.A, and Erwin, V.G., Eds., NIAAA Research Monograph 6, Department of Health and Human Services, 1981, 171.

44. Fadda, F., Mosca E., Colombo, G., and Gessa, G.L., Alcohol-preferring rats: genetic sensitivity to alcohol-induced stimulation, *Physiol. Behav.*, 47, 727, 1990.

45. Li, T.-K. and McBride, W.J., Pharmacogenetic models of alcoholism, *Clin. Neurosci.*, 3, 182, 1995.

46. Li, T-K., Lumeng, L., McBride, W.J., and Waller, M.B., Progress toward a voluntary oral consumption model of alcoholism, *Drug Alc. Depend.*, 4, 45, 1979.

47. Lumeng, L. and Li, T.-K., The development of metabolic tolerance in the alcohol-preferring P rats: comparison of forced and free-choice drinking of ethanol, *Pharmacol. Biochem. Behav.*, 25, 1013, 1986.

48. Murphy, J.M., Gatto, G.J., Waller, M.B., McBride, W.J., Lumeng, L., and Ti, T.-K., Effects of scheduled access on ethanol intake in alcohol-preferring (P) line of rats, *Alcohol*, 3, 331, 1986.

49. Waller, M.B., McBride, W.J., Lumeng, L., and Li, T.-K., Induction of dependence on ethanol by free-choice drinking in alcohol preferring rats, *Pharmacol. Biochem. Behav.*, 16, 501, 1982.

50. Samson, H., Initiation of ethanol reinforcement using a sucrose-substitution procedure in food- and water-sated rats, *Alcohol. Clin. Exp. Res.*, 10, 436, 1986.

51. Samson, H.H., Tolliver, G.A., and Schwartz-Stevens, K., Ethanol self-administration in a non restricted access situation: effect of ethanol initiation, *Alcohol*, 8, 45, 1991.

52. Schwartz-Stevens, K., Samson, H.H., Tolliver, G.A., Lument, L., and Li, T-K., The effects of ethanol initiation procedures on ethanol-reinforced behavior in the alcohol-preferring rat, *Alcohol. Clin. Exp. Res.*, 15, 277, 1991.

53. Files, F.J., Denning, C.E., Hyytia, R., Kiianmaa, K., and Samson, H.H., Ethanol-reinforced responding by AA and ANA rats following the sucrose-initiation procedure, *Alcohol. Clin. Exp. Res.*, 21, 749, 1997.

54. Ritz, M.C., George, F.R., and Meisch, R.A., Ethanol self-administration in ALKO rats. II. Effects of selection and fixed ratio size, *Alcohol*, 6, 235, 1989.

55. Files, F.J., Andrews, C.M., Samson, H.H., Lumeng, L., and Li, T.-K., Alcohol self-administration in a nonrestricted access situation with alcohol-preferring (P) rats, *Alcohol. Clin. Exp. Res.*, 16, 751, 1992.

56. Elmer, G.I., Meisch, R.A., Goldberg, S.R., and George, F.R., Fixed ratio schedules of oral ethanol self-administration in inbred mouse strains, *Psychopharmacology*, 96, 431, 1988.

57. Crabbe, J.C., Phillips, T.J., Feller, D.J., Hen, R., Wenger, C.D., Lessov, C.N., and Schafer, G.L., Elevated alcohol consumption in null mutant mice lacking 5-HT1B serotonin receptors, *Nature Genetics*, 14, 98, 1996.

58. Collins, R.J., Weeks, J.R., Cooper, M.M., Good, P.I. and Russell, R.R., Prediction of abuse liability of drugs using IV self-administration by rats, *Psychopharmacology*, 82, 6, 1984.

59. Numan, R., Naparzewska, A.M., and Adler, C.M., Absence of reinforcement with low dose intravenous ethanol self-administration in rats, *Pharmacol. Biochem. Behav.,* 21, 609, 1984.

60. DeNoble, V.J., Mele, P.C., and Porter, J.H., Intravenous self-administration of pentobarbital and ethanol in rats, *Pharmacol. Biochem. Behav.,* 23, 759, 1985.

61. Naruse, T. and Asami, T., Cross-dependence on ethanol and pentobarbital in rats reinforced on diazepam, *Arch. Int. Pharmacodynam. Ther.,* 304, 147, 1990.

62. Smith, S.G. and Davis, W.M., Intravenous alcohol self-administration in the rat, *Pharmacol. Res. Commun.,* 6, 397, 1974.

63. Sinden, J.D. and LeMagnen, J., Parameters of low-dose ethanol intravenous self-administration, *Pharmacol. Biochem. Behav.,* 16, 181, 1982.

64. Hyytia, P., Schulteis, G., and Koob, G.F., Intravenous heroin and ethanol self-administration by alcohol preferring AA and alcohol-avoiding ANA rats, *Psychopharmacology,* 125, 248, 1996.

65. Numan, R., Multiple exposures to ethanol facilitate intravenous self-administration of ethanol by rats, *Pharmacol. Biochem. Behav.,* 15, 101, 1981.

66. Grahame, N.J. and Cunningham, C.L., Intravenous ethanol self-administration in C57BL/6J and DBA/2J mice, *Alcohol. Clin. Exp. Res.,* 21, 56, 1997.

67. O'Malley, S., Jaffe, A., Chang, G., Shottenfeld, R. M., Meyer, R., and Rounsaville, B., Naltrexone and coping skills therapy for alcohol dependence, *Arch. Gen. Psychiatry,* 49, 881, 1992.

68. Volpicelli, J.R., Alterman, A.I., Hayashida, M., and O'Brien, C.P., Naltrexone in treatment of alcohol dependence, *Arch. Gen. Psychiatry,* 49, 876, 1992.

69. Ulm, R.R., Volpicelli, J.R., and Volpicelli, L.A., Opiates and alcohol self-administration in animals, *J. Clin. Psychiatry,* 56 (Suppl. 7), 5, 1995.

70. Berman, R.F., Lee, J.A., Olson, K.L., and Goldman, M.S., Effects of naloxone on ethanol dependence in rats, *Drug Alc. Depend.,* 13, 245, 1984

71. Froehlich, J.C., Harts, J., Lumeng, L., and Li, T.K., Naloxone attenuates voluntary ethanol intake in rats selectively bred for high ethanol preference, *Pharmacol. Biochem. Behav.,* 35, 385, 1990.

72. Spanagel, R. and Zieglgansberger, W., Anti-craving compounds for ethanol: new pharmacological tools to study addictive processes, *Trends Pharmacol. Sci.,* 18, 54, 1997.

73. Williams, K.L. and Woods, J.H., Oral ethanol-reinforced responding in rhesus monkeys: effects of opioid antagonists selective for the mu-, kappa-, or delta-receptor. *Alcohol. Clin. Exp. Res.,* 22, 1634, 1998

74. Williams, K.L. and Woods, J.H., Naltrexone reduces ethanol- and/or water-reinforced responding in rhesus monkeys: effect depends upon ethanol concentration, submitted manuscript.

75. Williams, K.L. and Woods, J.H. Conditioned effects produced by naltrexone doses that reduce ethanol-reinforced responding in rhesus monkeys, *Alcohol. Clin. Exp. Res.,* in press.

76. Pelc, I., Verbanck, P., Le Bon, O., Gavrilovic, M., Lion, K., and Lehert, P., Efficacy and safety of acamprosate in the treatment of detoxified alcohol-dependent patients. A 90-day placebo-controlled dose-finding study, *Br. J. Psychiatry,* 171, 73, 1997.

77. Poldrugo, F., Acamprosate treatment in a long-term community-based alcohol rehabilitation programme, *Addiction,* 92, 1537, 1997.

78. Sass, H., Soyka, M., Mann, K., and Zieglgansberger, W., Relapse prevention by acamprosate: results from a placebo-controlled study on alcohol dependence, *Arch. Gen. Psychiatry,* 53, 673, 1996.

79. Holter, S.M., Landgraf, R., Zieglgansberger, W., and Spanagel, R., Time course of acamprosate action on operant ethanol self-administration after ethanol deprivation, *Alcohol. Clin. Exp. Res.,* 21, 862, 1997.

80. Spanagel, R., Holter, S.M., Allingham, K., Landgraf, R., and Zieglgansberger, W. Acamprosate and alcohol: I. Effects on alcohol intake following alcohol deprivation in the rat, *Eur. J. Pharmacol.,* 305, 39, 1996.

81. Heyser, C.J., Schulteis, G., Durbin, P., and Koob, G.F., Chronic acamprosate eliminates the alcohol deprivation effect while having limited effects on baseline responding for ethanol in rats, *Neuropsychopharmacology,* 18, 125, 1998.

36   Controversial Research Areas

Rainer Spanagel and Sabine M. Hoelter

OVERVIEW

Research data in the biomedical field are controversial per se. There are many reasons for this, however; it is the living organism who offers such a heterogenity and sometimes it is the researcher by him/herself who is driven by expectations fitting into dogmatic and mainstream thinking and thus accepts false negative or false positive results. Our scientific apparatus and framework lead to dogmas and mainstream thinking in the biomedical field. This chapter presents some examples that demonstrate that dogmatism also takes place in biomedical research on alcohol and alcoholism. For example, a close link between dopamine and alcohol reward, craving and relapse, or anxiety and alcoholism has been postulated; however, a closer analysis of recent studies reveals controversial findings that imply that these hypotheses should be modified.

THE DOPAMINE HYPOTHESIS OF ALCOHOL REWARD: DOES DOPAMINE PLAY A ROLE IN ALCOHOL REWARD AND RELAPSE?

In 1954, it became clear from electrical brain stimulation experiments performed by Olds and Milner[1] that the brain must have some specialized sites for reward functions. In these experiments, brain sites were identified where electrical stimulation was rewarding in the sense that a rat will stimulate itself in these places frequently and regularly for long periods of time if permitted to do so. In particular, the midbrain dopamine system is sensitive to electrical self-stimulation and has been characterized as a neurochemical substrate of reward.[2] Midbrain dopamine neurons involved in reward processes originate in the ventral tegmental area and project to structures closely associated with the limbic system, most prominently the nucleus accumbens shell region. Not only natural rewards (such as food, water, and sex) but also a variety of drugs abused by humans (including alcohol) preferentially increase synaptic dopamine transmission in the nucleus accumbens shell region.[3-5] The following chapter sections describe animal and human studies that examined the relationship between alcohol and midbrain dopamine.

When alcohol is administered to rats, various techniques have indicated that the mesolimbic dopaminergic system is activated. The ventral tegmental area in particular has been implicated in the effects of alcohol. Thus, alcohol has an acute effect on these neurons in increasing cell firing when applied to isolated slices of the ventral tegmental area.[6] Alcohol injected intravenously also increases firing of dopamine cell bodies in this brain region.[7] Using microdialysis, it was found that acute administration of alcohol results in preferential release of dopamine from the nucleus accumbens shell region.[4] It is suggested that the manner by which acute alcohol administration increases extracellular dopamine within the nucleus accumbens is via changes in GABA interneurons, in the ventral tegmental area. Alcohol might decrease the activity of these GABAergic interneurons, which leads subsequently to a disinhibition of mesolimbic dopamine neurons. The observation that dopamine levels within the nucleus accumbens remained elevated after systemic alcohol administration, whereas somatodendritic release in the ventral tegmental area had already declined, suggests that alcohol has also some local effects in the nucleus acccumbens.[8] Since local infusion of GBR12909, a dopamine reuptake inhibitor, through the dialysis probe into the nucleus accumbens elevated dopamine levels therein and in parallel decreased dopamine levels in the ventral tegmental area,[8] it is suggested that elevating dopamine levels in the nucleus accumbens activates a long-loop negative GABAergic feedback system to the ventral tegmental area, which regulates dopamine cell body neuronal activity.[8,9] In summary, systemic alcohol probably has multiple actions affecting the ventral tegmental area and its afferents, and the nucleus accumbens and its afferents.

The activation of mesolimbic A10 neurons by alcohol seems to be associated with the reinforcing properties of the drug since rats will directly self-administer alcohol into the ventral tegmental area.[10] Numerous pharmacological studies have further investigated the role of midbrain dopamine in alcohol reinforcement, but the results have been contradictory. Although 6-hydroxy-dopamine-induced lesions do not affect the maintenance of alcohol self-administration,[11,12] acquisition of alcohol drinking is substantially reduced by this manipulation.[12] These findings demonstrate that different neuronal mechanisms mediate acquisition and maintenance of alcohol drinking and that functionality of midbrain dopamine neurons is not required to maintain alcohol self-administration. In contrast to these lesion studies, dopamine antagonists administered either systemically or locally into the nucleus accumbens decrease home-cage drinking and operant responding for alcohol.[13,14] These observations are underlined by a recent study showing that alcohol consumption and preference is markedly reduced in dopamine D_2-receptor-deficient mice.[15] Moreover, quantitative trait locus (QTL) analysis using recombinant mice inbred strains localized a QTL for alcohol preference at the location of the dopamine D_2-receptor on mouse chromosome 9.[16] Interestingly, the gene encoding the dopamine D_2-receptor on human chromosome 11 was also linked to alcohol consumption in humans. In particular, a positive relationship between the *Taq*I-A1 allele of the dopamine D_2-receptor and an increased vulnerability to alcohol drinking-related disorders was reported.[17] However, numerous further association and linkage studies in humans produced controversial results. To clarify the relationship between the dopamine D_2-receptor locus and alcohol drinking-related disorders, a large sample of families containing multiple alcoholics, collected by the Collaborative Study on the Genetics of Alcoholism (COGA),[18] was recently examined. Despite extensive analysis of two different polymorphisms in the dopamine D_2-receptor gene, no evidence for association or linkage of this gene with alcohol drinking-related disorders could be detected.[19]

Dopamine measurements in alcohol-preferring rat strains received by selective breeding have also produced conflicting results. Alcohol self-administration has been shown to produce a considerably greater relative stimulation of mesolimbic dopamine release in alcohol-preferring P rats than in control Wistar rats.[20] Moreover the expectancy of alcohol intake enhanced dopamine release in P rats but not in Wistar rats,[21] demonstrating that the mere anticipation of alcohol availability can mimic the pharmacological effects of alcohol in P rats. In contrast to these findings, a dose-dependent increase in mesolimbic dopamine release in another alcohol-preferring rat strain (AA rats), as well as in alcohol-avoiding rats (ANA rats), was reported,[22] indicating that alcohol reinforcement is not related to the amount of dopamine released by alcohol in these animals. Furthermore, prior alcohol experience by repeated alcohol injections had no influence on the dopaminergic response. Thus, the magnitude of dopamine release induced by alcohol was still similar in AA and ANA rats.[23] However, dopamine release in AA rats that had prior experience of several days of alcohol self-administration was completely blunted,[23] demonstrating that midbrain dopamine is not correlated with alcohol reinforcement in AA rats. Similar findings were obtained in yet another strain of alcohol-preferring rats. In alcohol-naive high-alcohol-drinking (HAD) and low-alcohol-drinking (LAD) lines of rats, alcohol dose-response curves for dopamine release showed no difference in the sensitivity to alcohol between the lines.[24] With regard to the apparent lack of congruity among the aforementioned studies of dopamine release, one must take into consideration that most of these experiments were done with experimenter-administered alcohol, and this is why one may not see differences between the preferring and non-preferring AA/ANA and HAD/LAD lines. So, clearly, further studies are warranted in these rat lines where dopamine measurements are performed during operant self-administration. However, since the non-preferring lines barely respond for ethanol, the appropriate controls for those experiments are missing.

Repeated administration of alcohol can lead either to a decrease (tolerance) or an increase (sensitization) in its behavioral effects. Behavioral sensitization occurs following repeated intermittent administration of a drug. In the search for the neurobiological basis of drug-induced behavioral sensitization, research has focused on the mesolimbic dopaminergic system. Although most drugs of abuse given under an intermittent injection schedule lead to a more pronounced increase in dopamine release as compared to the acute administration of these drugs,[25,26] it remains unclear whether or to what extent alcohol-induced behavioral sensitization has a dopaminergic basis. Thus, a lack of tolerance to alcohol-induced dopamine release in the nucleus accumbens following its repeated intermittent injection was demonstrated but not an augmented sensitized response.[27] On the other hand, a recent report demonstrated long-lasting hyperreactivity of mesolimbic dopamine neurons and cross-sensitization to psychostimulants and morphine following repeated treatment of rats with alcohol.[28] Clearly, further studies are needed, in particular microdialysis studies in mice since rats usually do not show alcohol-induced behavioral sensitization, in order to clarify the role of dopamine in this phenomenon. It has been hypothesized that alcohol-induced sensitization processes within the nucleus accumbens play a crucial role in the development of compulsive alcohol-seeking behavior, craving, and relapse.[29] However, since a dopaminergic basis of alcohol-induced behavioral sensitization has not explicitly been demonstrated and no animal studies on relapse behavior and midbrain dopamine have been performed thus far (but see Reference 30), it is not justified at the moment to make any conclusions about the role of dopamine in addictive behavior to alcohol.

Nevertheless, a number of dopaminergic compounds have already been tested in weaned alcoholics for relapse prevention and as possible anti-craving compounds. However, neither the dopamine receptor agonist bromocriptine nor the dopamine receptor antagonist tiapride were useful in this respect.[31,32] Interestingly, lisuride, which was tested in two placebo-controlled double-blind studies, even increased relapse rates in detoxified alcoholics.[33,30] Similar results were obtained recently with flupenthixol in a large clinical study. Thus, flupenthixol-treated patients relapsed significantly earlier than placebo-treated patients.[34] On the other hand, alcohol abuse patients show impairments in the function of central dopamine receptors that depend on the amount of prolonged alcohol consumption, and retardation in the recovery of dopamine function is associated with early relapse in alcoholics.[35] Although these results of clinical efficacy of dopaminergic compounds for relapse prevention is discouraging at the moment, one should emphasize that at least five different subtypes of dopamine receptors were found in the brain.[36] Due to its distribution in the brain, in particular in the midbrain dopamine system,[37,38] the dopamine D_3-receptor may be an appropriate target in the treatment of psychiatric disorders such as schizophrenia and drug addiction.[39] Recently, it was shown that long-term voluntary alcohol consumption, but not forced alcohol administration, led to specific changes in the dopamine D_3-receptor gene expression, whereas alcohol drinking did not alter the mRNA expression of any other dopamine receptor subtype.[40] Further elucidation of the functional role of the dopamine D_3-receptor in the mediation of reinforcing effects induced by alcohol and relapse behavior is warranted, but the appropriate studies are still severely hampered by the lack of selective dopamine D_3-receptor agonists and antagonists.

In summary, there is now little doubt that midbrain dopamine plays an essential role in the acquisition of an alcohol-seeking behavior. But changes in dopamine activity do not mediate emotional hedonic or anhedonic components of reinforcement processes; it seems rather likely that an enhanced dopamine signal highlights important stimuli and functions as a learning signal.[41,42] However, midbrain dopamine neurons do not seem to play a critical role in the maintenance of alcohol-reinforced behavior. Indeed, no consistent link has been established between the maintenance of alcohol self-administration and dopamine activity thus far. It was claimed that failure to observe a clear association between self-administration and dopamine release is due to the heterogenity of the nucleus accumbens.[5] Thus, dopamine responses to drugs of abuse differ in the core and shell region[5,43] as well as in the anteroposterior axis of the nucleus accumbens.[43] Clearly, further accurate microdialysis or voltammetry measurements in combination with drug self-administration are needed in order to identify possible subregions within the nucleus accumbens where increased dopamine may underlie self-administration behavior. In terms of addicted behavior, it is premature to conclude whether sensitized midbrain dopamine is critically involved in relapse behavior;[28,29,42,44] however, recent clinical data indicate that dopaminergic compounds may not be useful for relapse prevention. The outcome of these studies, however, could be confounded by the fact that relatively unspecific dopaminergic compounds were used.

WHAT IS CRAVING? DO WE NEED A CONCEPT OF CRAVING TO UNDERSTAND RELAPSE?

There are opposing views in the field regarding the term "craving," whether it describes a physiological, subjective, or behavioral state; if it is necessary at all to explain addictive behavior; or is it an epiphenomenon that is not necessary for the production of continued drug use in addicts. One should think the easiest way to find an answer to the question of the importance of craving would be to ask drug-dependent individuals who had not maintained abstinence, although they had wanted to, whether craving for the drug was a cause for their relapse. But one problem with self-report studies of craving is that this term carries many different connotations and different people might allocate different meanings to the term "craving." Thus, if one only asks about the experience of craving without defining the meaning of this term, varying answers might be given by the subjects although all of them might have experienced similar degrees of desire for alcohol. For example, an alcoholic might say she never consciously experienced a craving for alcohol because she always made sure she had enough alcohol in stock, because she could not bear the thought of running out of it, thus equating craving with unavailability of the drug. The same alcoholic would describe that her mouth would start watering in expectation of her first drink when the time of day she restricted her drinking to approached, and she would compare herself to a "Pavlovian dog." But she could not recall craving for alcohol. As a possible remedy to the problem of misunderstanding, it was proposed to use the term "urge" instead of the term "craving" because urge would be more understandable to lay persons and more unidimensional.[45]

However, there is still the need for a definition of what we are talking about. An Expert Committee gathered by the United Nations International Drug Control Programme (UNDCP) and the World Health Organization (WHO) agreed on the definition of craving as "the desire to experience the effect(s) of a previously experienced psychoactive substance."[46] Markou et al.[47] conceptualized craving within the framework of incentive motivational theories of behavior and modified the definition of craving as "incentive motivation to self-administer a psychoactive substance." Such an operational definition of craving has the advantage of making the phenomenon of craving accessible to experimental investigation and making it measurable. On the other hand, such a definition neglects the fact that craving also has a subjective dimension that is difficult, if at all possible, to assess in laboratory animals.

An important implication of the above-mentioned definitions of craving is that craving can occur independent of the development of drug dependence. Thus, anybody who has at least once experienced the effects of a psychoactive substance might eventually feel the desire (or incentive motivation) to take this drug again; the difference between a nondependent, occasional user and a drug-dependent individual lies only in the strength of the desire. In terms of the incentive motivational definition of craving, it is assumed that the incentive-motivational value of the drug is much higher for dependent than for nondependent individuals. This difference can be measured experimentally in the amount of effort that the dependent and the nondependent individuals are willing to exert to gain access to the drug.[47]

This concept of craving is more parsimonious than the hypothesis proposed by Ludwig and Wikler:[48] "craving for alcohol represents a psychological or cognitive correlate of a subclinical conditioned withdrawal syndrome which may be evoked by any state of physiological arousal resembling the syndrome." The latter description of craving implies that, first, craving only develops with prolonged, eventually chronic alcohol intake and the occurrence of withdrawal symptoms and, second, that craving is an important and necessary, but not sufficient, contributory factor to relapse.[48] The marked difference between these two concepts of craving is that the definition by Markou et al.[47] does not make any further assumptions about a putative cognitive nature of craving, the relation between craving and dependence and between craving and relapse, but leaves these questions open to experimental investigation. In contrast, the definition by Ludwig and Wikler[48] is a far-reaching hypothesis that needs to be tested. But also, the incentive-motivational concept of craving has been embedded in a theory about addiction, in which craving is a necessary component that drives drug-seeking and drug-taking behavior.[29] Both concepts of craving have in common that they assume that either drug-withdrawal or drug-incentive effects become conditioned to cues or situations reliably associated with drug administration and that these conditioned stimuli trigger drug craving and drug use. But is craving necessary to trigger drug use?

Thus far, there is only limited evidence that the occurrence of craving does predict future drug use or relapse. In an alcohol-cued context (i.e., when a detoxified alcoholic's preferred liquor was within easy reach and view), craving could predict subsequent alcohol consumption, but not in a context without the alcohol cue (i.e., when only water was visible).[49] However, this study also showed the importance of the alcohol cue to induce craving, so that possibly the alcohol cue might have been sufficient to predict alcohol consumption independent of the occurrence of craving. Cue-reactivity studies show that relative to neutral-cue control conditions, presentations of drug-related cues to addicts produce robust increases in craving reports in smokers, alcoholics, and heroin and cocaine addicts.[50] But this only shows that craving is highly stimulus-bound. A strong case against the importance of craving as a trigger for drug use comes from research that explicitly asked addicts about their level of craving just prior to a relapse. In these studies, a large percentage of relapsed addicts reported that craving did not play a primary role in their return to drug use.[51,52] Instead, relapse was often reported to occur as an impulsive action. One might argue that drug craving is such a prominent feature in an addict's life that the addict may take craving as a given and might not recognize it as a reason for relapse. But if craving was a necessary precedent to subsequent drug use, then measures of self-reported cravings should highly correlate with actual drug-use behavior. However, in several studies examining the relationship between craving and subsequent drug use in either alcoholics or smokers, the correlation between measures of craving and actual drug consumption was not particularly high (for review see Reference 53), indicating that the degree of craving does not precisely predict the level of subsequent drug intake.

Because of the lack of direct evidence that craving drives drug use, it was suggested that craving is not necessary to initiate renewed drug intake, but that relapse can also occur in an absent-minded, unintended way without the conscious perception of craving for the drug. It was hypothesized that in the course of the development of addiction, drug use becomes an automatized behavior that is relatively fast and efficient, stimulus controlled, initiated and completed without intention, difficult to impede, cognitively effortless, and capable of being enacted in the absence of awareness.[53] Craving, however, is viewed by Tiffany[53] as a nonautomatic cognitive process, which is activated in parallel with "drug use action schemata," either in support of drug taking or in support of attempts to impede drug taking. According to this view, as long as no external condition, such as unavailability of the drug, or no internal condition, such as a decision to abstain from drug taking, impedes the execution of the drug use action plan, craving does not necessarily have to be perceived. On the other hand, craving is presumably always perceived whenever drug use is hindered. The consequence of this concept of craving is that both craving and drug use are triggered in parallel by conditioned drug cues, but that craving is not necessary to drive drug-taking behavior.

Within this framework, the example at the beginning of this chapter of the alcoholic not recalling the experience of craving during the course of her drug-taking years could be interpreted in a different way and would not necessarily serve as an example of a misunderstanding of the term "craving." According to Tiffany's theory, she did not experience craving *because* she always made sure she had enough alcohol available, so that no impediment to her drug-taking plan could occur. Her physiological responses prior to her daily alcohol intake just describe conditioned effects in response to her drug cue, which was the time of day when she allowed herself to drink. The conscious experience of craving was not necessary to drive the execution of her drug-taking plan.

In comparison, an important recent finding should be mentioned; it indicated that opiate addicts process craving-related information differently from alcoholics.[54] This evidence supports the idea that cognitive and neural mechanisms involved in craving might be different in users of different drugs. In other words, for example, craving for a cigarette or for cocaine might have different origins and different consequences from craving for alcohol. Therefore, it may still be possible that drug craving might play different roles in relapse to different drugs.

How can a behavioral pharmacologist find an animal model that is relevant for research on alcoholism and what can he conclude from the above-mentioned considerations? Whether craving is necessary to induce drug-taking behavior or not, the prevention or reduction of drug taking and relapse are the primary goals of treatment. Thus, as long as the concept and the importance of craving are not undisputed, the most direct approach to promote the development of better treatment seems to be to concentrate on studying the mechanisms of drug-seeking and relapse behavior. A promising animal model to study relapse behavior and to test the efficacy of putative anti-relapse drugs is the so-called "alcohol deprivation effect" (ADE). Alcohol-experienced animals show a transient increase in alcohol consumption and alcohol preference after a period of forced abstinence (alcohol deprivation), which was termed "alcohol deprivation effect."[55] The ADE is regarded as an animal model of relapse drinking. It can be seen in long-term alcohol drinking rats that have developed a behavioral alcohol dependence[56-58] as well as in nondependent rats,[55,59,60] both under home-cage drinking and under operant self-administration conditions; and in monkeys[61] and man.[62] The ADE in long-term alcohol self-administering rats has interesting characteristics: during an ADE, these animals consume large amounts of highly concentrated alcohol solutions, even at unusual times (e.g., during the light phase when activity is usually minimal).[58] Furthermore, alcohol-drinking behavior during an ADE cannot be modified by taste adulteration with quinine or the additional choice of a highly palatable sucrose solution.[58,63] These findings suggest that the observed alcohol-drinking behavior is pharmacologically and not nutritionally motivated. In conclusion, alcohol drinking during the ADE seems to consist of an uncontrolled incentive motivation to self-administer the drug. This statement is fully compatible with the operational definition of craving by Markou et al.[47] However, the measurement of an ADE in long-term alcohol drinking rats assesses only a behavioral outcome and cannot tell us anything about a subjective state associated with an incentive motivation to drink alcohol. Nevertheless, the fact that clinically effective anti-relapse drugs also reduce the ADE[63-66] lends predictive value to this animal model for the development of new and better drugs for the treatment of alcoholism.[67] However, the lack of assessability of the subjective dimension in laboratory animals is a clear limitation of such an approach in the attempt to increase our understanding of the nature of craving and the relationship between craving and relapse behavior.

IS THERE A LINK BETWEEN ANXIETY AND ALCOHOL DRINKING?

Apart from the reinforcing and discriminative stimulus effects of alcohol,[68,69] its anxiolytic effects may also play a role in the motivation to take this drug, at least in individuals who are susceptible to an anxiolytic action of alcohol.[70,71] Studies in alcoholic patients suggest a positive correlation between the level of alcohol consumption and the severity of anxiety.[72,73] Based on the so-called "tension reduction hypothesis" by Conger[74] in which he argued that in situations where alcohol consumption is fear-reducing, this effect reinforces alcohol consumption and may therefore promote future alcohol intake, particularly in similar situations, it is asked whether the ingestion of alcohol may be an attempt at self-medication of anxiety symptoms.

All of these findings and arguments suggest that anxiety furthers alcohol intake. On the other hand, alcohol intake might also further the occurrence of anxiety symptoms. Indeed, clinical observations show that increased quantities of alcohol consumed per drinking occasion are associated with increased symptoms of anxiety in the sober state[75] and withdrawal from alcohol, which can be conceptualized as a rebound phenomenon of the central nervous system from recent alcohol consumption,[76] has been shown to be anxiogenic in humans[77] and in rats.[78] Furthermore, repeated alcohol withdrawal episodes potentiate subsequent withdrawal symptoms,[79-81] indicating a sensitizing effect of the repeated experience of withdrawal. Long-term alcohol self-administering rats exhibit a more pronounced anxiogenic response after repeated withdrawal episodes than after the first withdrawal experience.[56] It is argued that these enhanced anxiety levels might contribute to the relapse behavior observed in these animals.[56] Coinciding with these findings, clinical observations also suggest that avoidance of the negative affective state during withdrawal (i.e., anxiety, craving, and dysphoria) can contribute to the continuation of alcohol drinking. As shown in the aforementioned animal studies, in humans repeated alcohol withdrawal episodes might also sensitize the negative affective state experienced during withdrawal.[72,82] The similarity in symptoms and in neurochemical perturbations involved in both panic attacks and alcohol withdrawal has led to the hypothesis that chemical and cognitive changes occurring as the result of repeated withdrawals may condition panic attacks in susceptible individuals, through a "kindling" process,[72] which further underlines the concept of a causal relationship between alcohol withdrawal and anxiety. In conclusion, one link between alcohol intake and anxiety levels is suggested in the way that the anxiety experienced during alcohol withdrawal, which may be intensified after repeated experiences of alcohol withdrawal, furthers relapse to alcohol intake.[83] The observation that alcoholic subjects with a coexisting anxiety disorder have more frequent and more severe relapses[84] fits in well with this conclusion.

Because of the mutual interaction between anxiety and alcohol, it is both possible that anxiety disorders promote the development of alcoholism and that alcoholism promotes the development of anxiety disorders. Thus far, epidemiological investigations addressing the issue of identification of primary vs. secondary onset have yielded inconsistent results, which led to the demand for longitudinal prospective studies and, in retrospective studies, for the control of the withdrawal state of the probands, because the high rate of comorbidity in some studies might reflect a mixture of true anxiety disorders among alcoholics along with alcohol-induced anxiety syndromes.[85] Recent investigations that differentiated subtypes of anxiety disorders did not observe a consistent temporal pattern for alcoholism relative to these disorders.[86,87] Only for phobic disorders (agoraphobia, simple phobia, and social phobia) did epidemiological data indicate a temporal relationship underlying alcoholism comorbidity with phobic disorders.[73,87] Thus, phobic disorders rather preceded the onset of alcoholism and rarely occurred after the onset of alcoholism. Furthermore, alcoholism had little or no impact on the symptoms of phobic disorders, suggesting a unidirectional causal relationship whereby phobic disorders increase the risk of alcoholism, but not the reverse. These findings are consistent with the notion that alcohol drinking may be used to self-medicate phobic anxiety and indicate that phobic states may, therefore, serve as a salient risk factor for the subsequent onset of problem-drinking behavior. In addition, these findings suggest that it is necessary to differentiate between subtypes of anxiety disorders in future studies, since alcohol may interact differently with each anxiety disorder. Such differences, if verified, might explain previous inconsistent results when the relationship between alcoholism and "anxiety disorders" in general was considered. The role of gender is another issue that should be considered in future studies, because gender differences have been observed in alcohol intake and preference in rats,[88] and a higher comorbidity between alcoholism and anxiety disorders has been reported in women compared to men.[89] A positive family history of anxiety disorders alone can lead to stress response dampening effects of alcohol in women, but not in men, although it cannot be excluded that this finding may have been attributable to differences in drinking histories.[90]

What can animal models tell us about the relationship between anxiety and alcohol intake? The results in the literature concerning this issue are contradictory. At least in male heterogenous

Wistar rats, elevated measures of anxiety correlate with high voluntary alcohol consumption during the initiation of alcohol-drinking behavior.[71] In this study, the alcohol-drinking animals reached blood alcohol levels that were apparently capable of inducing anxiolytic-like effects in these animals.[71] These findings are supported by another study showing that central amygdala lesions reduce both experimental anxiety and voluntary alcohol intake in male Wistar rats, indicating a role of the central amygdala in the link between anxiety and alcohol drinking.[91] Therefore, one would predict, according to the above-mentioned findings and according to the "tension reduction hypothesis," that alcohol-preferring animals are more anxious than non-preferring ones. However, investigations in several rat lines that have been selectively bred for high or low voluntary alcohol drinking, the so-called alcohol-preferring and non-preferring lines, produced contradictory results. In the sP (sardinian alcohol-preferring) and sNP (sardinian nonpreferring) rats, the alcohol-preferring ones are more anxious basally, and this is true for male rats.[92] In contrast, in the Indianapolis P (preferring) and NP (non-preferring) rats, the male alcohol-preferring rats are less anxious than the non-preferring, but the females are more anxious, indicating that there can be a gender difference.[93,94] In the Finnish alcohol-preferring AA (Alko Alcohol) and ANA (Alko Non Alcohol) rats, all possible results have been obtained: alcohol-preferring rats are more anxious, are less anxious, or do not differ from nonpreferring rats.[95-97]

This just shows that it is not wise to try to deduce global conclusions from the comparison of a single pair of rat lines. If one looks at studies comparing the behaviors of several of these alcohol-preferring and non-preferring lines, one finds that most of the behavioral variables related to emotionality are not consistently related to alcohol drinking.[98-101] A factor analysis showed that in those few behavioral variables that are consistently related to alcohol drinking, alcohol-preferring rats exhibit less anxious behavior.[102] Thus, the overall analysis of alcohol-preferring rat lines suggests that if there is any relationship between basal anxiety levels and voluntary alcohol drinking, then it is a negative correlation instead of a positive one.[102] This conclusion is supported by yet another experimental approach. Recently, the establishment of two Wistar rat lines selectively bred for differing behavioral performances on the elevated plus-maze was reported.[103,104] The selective breeding resulted in animals with high-anxiety-related behavior (HAB) and low-anxiety-related behavior (LAB). Both lines were submitted to an alcohol preference test. Male animals differed neither in the initiation of alcohol drinking nor in relapse-like drinking following an alcohol deprivation phase. In contrast, female LAB rats initially showed a higher alcohol consumption and preference than female HAB rats. During the maintenance phase of alcohol self-administration, however, no more differences could be detected between both lines. During the relapse phase following alcohol deprivation, female LAB rats again consumed more alcohol than female HAB rats.[105] These experiments show that in rats, innate increased levels of anxiety can be negatively correlated with alcohol drinking and that gender can play a role in these behavioral patterns.

In summary, it is likely that differences in experimental parameters contributed to the contradictory results obtained by different laboratories concerning alcohol-preferring rat lines, but it must also be considered that at least in some of these rat lines, alcohol preference may be unrelated to anxiety levels.

This puzzling picture leaves us to conclude, as have many researchers before us, that the interaction between alcohol drinking and anxiety is complex. The quest for animal models relevant to clinical findings is not yet complete, and future clinical as well as animal studies could both profit from careful considerations of experimental design, gender differences, alcohol drinking history and withdrawal state of the subjects, the kind of "anxiety" under investigation, and perhaps also its intensity. Hopefully, such differentiated approaches might shed more light on the nature of the interaction between alcohol and anxiety.

REFERENCES

1. Olds, J. and Millner, P., Positive reinforcement produced by electrical stimulation of septal area and other regions of the rat brain, *J. Comp. Physiol. Psychol.*, 47, 419, 1954.
2. Wise, R.A. and Rompre, P.P., Brain dopamine and reward, *Annu. Rev. Psychol.*, 40, 191, 1989.
3. Di Chiara, G. and Imperato, A., Drugs abused by humans preferentially increase synaptic dopamine concentrations in the mesolimbic system of freely moving rats, *Proc. Natl. Acad. Sci. U.S.A.*, 85, 5274, 1988.
4. Imperato, A. and Di Chiara, G., Preferential stimulation of dopamine release in the nucleus accumbens of freely moving rats by ethanol, *J. Pharmacol. Exp. Ther.*, 239, 219, 1986.
5. Pontieri, F.E., Tanda, G., and Di Chiara, G., Intravenous cocaine, morphine, and amphetamine preferentially increase extracellular dopamine in the "shell" as compared with the "core" of the rat nucleus accumbens, *Proc. Natl. Acad. Sci. U.S.A.*, 92, 12304, 1995.
6. Brodie, M.S., Shefner, S.A., and Dunwiddie, T.V., Ethanol increases the firing rate of dopamine neurons of the rat, *Brain Res.*, 508, 65, 1990.
7. Gessa, G.L., Muntoni, F., Collu, M., Vargiu, L., and Mereu, G., Low doses of ethanol activate dopaminergic neurons of the ventral tegmental area, *Brain Res.*, 348, 201, 1985.
8. Kohl, R.R., Katner, J.S., Chernet, E., and McBride, W.J., Ethanol and negative feedback regulation of mesolimbic dopamine release in rats, *Psychopharmacology*, 139, 79, 1998.
9. Kalivas, P.W., Neurotransmitter regulation of dopamine neurons in the ventral tegmental area, *Brain Res. Rev.*, 18, 75, 1993.
10. Gatto, G.J., McBride, W.J., Murphy, J.M., Lumeng, L., and Li, T.-K., Ethanol self-infusion into the ventral tegmental area by alcohol-preferring rats, *Alcohol,* 11, 557, 1994.
11. Rassnick, S., Stinus, L., and Koob, G.F., The effects of 6-hydroxydopamine lesions of the nucleus accumbens and the mesolimbic dopamine system on oral self-administration of ethanol in the rat, *Brain Res.*, 623, 16, 1993.
12. Ikemoto, S., McBride, W.J., Murphy, J.M., Lumeng, L., and Li, T.-K., 6-OHDA lesions of the nucleus accumbens disrupt the acquisition but not the maintenance of ethanol consumption in the alcohol-preferring P line of rats, *Alcohol. Clin. Exp. Res.*, 21, 1042, 1997.
13. Samson, H.H., Tolliver, G.A. Haraguchi, M., and Hodge, C.W., Alcohol self-administration: role of mesolimbic dopamine, *Ann. N.Y. Acad. Sci.*, 654, 242, 1992.
14. Hodge, C.W., Samson, H.H., and Chappelle, A.M., Alcohol self-administration: further examination of the role of dopamine receptors in the nucleus accumbens, *Alcohol. Clin. Exp. Res.*, 21, 1083, 1997.
15. Phillips, T.J., Brown, K.J., Burkhart-Kasch, S., Wenger, C.D., Kelly, M.A., Rubinstein, M., Grandy, D.K., and Low, M.J., Alcohol preference and sensitivity are markedly reduced in mice lacking dopamine D2 receptors, *Nature Neurosci.*, 1, 610, 1998.
16. Tarantino, L.M., McClearn, G.E., Rodrigues, L.A., and Plomin, R., Confirmation of quantitative trait loci for alcohol preference in mice, *Alcohol. Clin. Exp. Res.*, 22, 1099, 1998.
17. Blum, K., Noble, E.P., Sheridan, P.J., Montgomery, A., Ritchie, T., Jagadeeswaran, P., Nogami, H., Briggs, A.H., and Cohn, J.B., Allelic association of human dopamine D2 receptor gene in alcoholism, *JAMA*, 263, 2055, 1990.
18. Begleiter, H., Reich, T., Hesselbrock, V., Porjesz, B., Li, T.-K., Schuckit, M.A., Edenberg, H.J., and Rice, J.P., The collaborative study on the genetics of alcoholism, *Alcohol Health Res. World*, 19, 228, 1995.
19. Edenberg, H.J., Foroud, T., Koller, D.L., Goate, A., Rice, J., Van Eerdewegh, P., Reich, T., Cloninger, C.R., Nurnberger Jr., J.I., Kowalczuk, M., Wu Bo, Li, T.-K., Conneally, P.M., Tischfield, J.A., Su, W., Shears, S., Crowe, R., Hesselbrock, V., Schuckit, M., Porjesz, B., and Begleiter, H., A family-based analysis of the association of the dopamine D2 receptor (DRD2) with alcoholism, *Alcohol. Clin. Exp. Res.*, 22, 505, 1998.
20. Weiss, F., Lorang, M.T., Bloom, F.E., and Koob, G.F., Ethanol self-administration stimulates dopamine release in the rat nucleus accumbens: genetic and motivational determinants, *J. Pharmacol. Exp. Ther.*, 267, 250, 1993.
21. Katner, S.N., Kerr, T.M., and Weiss, F., Ethanol anticipation enhances dopamine efflux in the nucleus accumbens of alcohol-preferring (P) but not Wistar rats, *Behav. Pharmacol.*, 7, 669, 1996.

22. Kiianmaa, K., Nurmi, M., Nykanen, I., and Sinclair, J.D., Effect of ethanol on extracellular dopamine in the nucleus accumbens of alcohol-preferring AA and alcohol-avoiding ANA rats, *Pharmacol. Biochem. Behav.,* 52, 29, 1995.

23. Nurmi, M., Ashizawa, T., Sinclair, J.D., and Kiianmaa, K., Effect of prior ethanol experience on dopamine overflow in accumbens of AA and ANA rats, *Eur. J. Pharmacol.,* 315, 277, 1996.

24. Yoshimoto, K., McBride, W.J., Lumeng, L., and Li, T-.K., Ethanol enhances the release of dopamine and serotonin in the nucleus accumbens of HAD and LAD lines of rats, *Alcohol. Clin. Exp. Res.,* 16, 781, 1992.

25. Kalivas, P.W. and Stewart, J., Dopamine transmission in the initiation and expression of drug- and stress-induced sensitization of motor activity, *Brain Res. Rev.,* 16, 223, 1991.

26. Spanagel, R., Modulation of drug-induced sensitization processes by endogenous opioid systems, *Behav. Brain Res.,* 70, 37, 1995.

27. Rossetti, Z.L., Hmaidan, Y., Diana, M., and Gessa, G.L., Lack of tolerance to ethanol-induced dopamine release in the rat ventral striatum, *Eur. J. Pharmacol.,* 231, 203, 1993.

28. Nestby, P., Vanderschuren, L.J.M.J., De Vries, T.J., Hogenboom, F., Wardeh, G., Mulder, A.H., and Schoffelmeer, A.N.M., Ethanol, like psychostimulants and morphine, causes long-lasting hyperreactivity of dopamine and acetylcholine neurons of rat nucleus accumbens: possible role in behavioural sensitization, *Psychopharmacology,* 133, 69, 1997.

29. Robinson, T.E. and Berridge, K.C., The neural basis of drug craving: an incentive-sensitization theory of addiction, *Brain Res. Rev.,* 18, 247, 1993.

30. May, T., Wolf, U., and Wolffgramm, J., Striatal dopamine receptors and adenylyl cyclase activity in a rat model of alcohol addiction: effects of ethanol and lisuride treatment, *J. Pharmacol. Exp. Ther.,* 275, 1195, 1995.

31. Boening, J., Drug-supported prevention of relapse in alcoholism — 72 results of controlled, double blind studies using anti-craving drugs, *Nervenheilkunde,* 15, 72, 1996.

32. Soyka, M., Relapse prevention in alcoholism, *CNS Drugs,* 4, 313, 1997.

33. Schmidt, L.G., Kuhn, S., and Rommelspacher, H., Pharmacological effects of lisuride shorten, expectations to receive the drug prolong the latency of relapse in cleaned alcoholics, *Pharmacopsychiatry,* 30, 219, 1997.

34. Boening, J., personal communication, 1999.

35. Heinz, A., Dufeu, P., Kuhn, S., Dettling, M., Graef, K.J., Kuerten, I., Rommelspacher, H., and Schmidt, L.G., Psychopathological and behavioral correlates of dopaminergic sensitivity in alcohol-dependent pateients, *Arch. Gen. Psychiatry,* 53, 1123, 1996.

36. Civelli, O., Bunzow, J.R., and Grandy, D.K, Molecular diversity of dopamine receptors, *Annu. Rev. Pharmacol. Toxicol.,* 32, 281, 1993.

37. Lévesque, D., Diaz, J., Pilon, C., Martres, M.-P., Giros, B., Souil, E., Schott, D., Morgat, J.-L., Schwartz, J.-C., and Sokoloff, P., Identification, characterization, and localization of the dopamine D_3 receptor in rat brain using 7-[^{3}H]hydroxy-N,N-di-n-propyl-2-aminotetralin, *Proc. Natl. Acad. Sci. U.S.A.,* 89, 8155, 1992.

38. Murray, A.M., Ryoo, H.L., Gurevich, E., and Joyce, J.N., Localization of dopamine D_3 receptors to mesolimbic and D_2 receptors to mesostriatal regions of human forebrain, *Proc. Natl. Acad. Sci. U.S.A.,* 91, 11271, 1994.

39. Shafer, R.A. and Levant, B., The D_3 dopamine receptor in cellular and organismal function, *Psychopharmacology,* 135, 1, 1998.

40. Eravci, M., Großpietsch, T., Pinna, G., Schulz, O., Kley, S., Bachmann, M., Wolffgramm, J., Goetz, E., Heyne, A., Meinhold, H., and Baumgartner, A., Dopamine receptor gene expression in an animal model of behavioral dependence on ethanol, *Mol. Brain Res.,* 50, 221, 1997.

41. Schultz, W., Predictive reward signals of dopamine neurons, *J. Neurophysiol.,* 80, 1, 1998.

42. Spanagel, R. and Weiss, F., The dopamine hypothesis of reward: past and current status, *Trends Neurosci.,* 22, 521, 1999.

43. Heidbreder, C. and Feldon, J., Amphetamine-induced neurochemical and locomotor responses are expressed differentially across the anteroposterior axis of the core and shell subterritories of the nucleus accumbens, *Synapse,* 29, 310, 1998.

44. Berridge, K.C. and Robinson, T.E., What is the role of dopamine in reward: hedonic impact, reward learning, or incentive salience? *Brain Res. Rev.,* 28, 309, 1998.

45. Hughes, J.R., Craving as a psychological construct, *Br. J. Addict.*, 82, 31, 1987.

46. UNDCP and WHO Informal Expert Committee on the Craving Mechanism: Report (1992) United Nations International Drug Control Programme and World Health Organization technical report series (No. V. 92-54439T), 1992.

47. Markou, A., Weiss, F., Gold, L.H., Caine, B., Schulteis, G., and Koob, G.F., Animal models of drug craving, *Psychopharmacology*, 112, 163, 1993.

48. Ludwig, A.M. and Wikler, A., "Craving" and relapse to drink, *Q. J. Stud. Alcohol,* 35, 108, 1974.

49. Ludwig, A.M., Wikler, A., and Stark, L.H., The first drink, *Arch. Gen. Psychiatry,* 30, 539, 1974.

50. Tiffany, S.T. and Carter, B.L., Is craving the source of compulsive drug use? *J. Psychopharmacol.,* 12, 23, 1998.

51. Baer, J.S., Kamark, T., Lichtenstein, E., and Ransom, C.C., Prediction of smoking relapse: analyses of temptations and transgressions after initial cessation, *J. Consult. Clin. Psychol.,* 57, 623, 1998.

52. Miller, N.S. and Gold, M.S., Dissociation of 'conscious desire' (craving) from and relapse in alcohol and cocaine dependence, *Ann. Clin. Psychiatry,* 6, 99, 1994.

53. Tiffany, S.T., A cognitive model of drug urges and drug-use behavior: role of automatic and nonautomatic processes, *Psychol. Rev.,* 97, 147, 1990.

54. Weinstein, A., Feldtkeller, B., Malizia, A., Wilson, S., Bailey, J., and Nutt, D.J., Integrating the cognitive and physiological aspects of craving, *J. Psychopharmacol.,* 12, 31, 1998.

55. Sinclair, J.D. and Senter, R.J., Increased preference for ethanol in rats following alcohol deprivation, *Psychonom. Sci.,* 8, 11, 1967.

56. Hoelter, S.M., Engelmann, M., Kirschke, C., Liebsch, G., Landgraf, R., and Spanagel, R., Long-term ethanol self-administration with repeated withdrawal episodes changes ethanol drinking pattern and increases anxiety during withdrawal in rats, *Behav. Pharmacol.,* 9, 41, 1998.

57. Hoelter, S.M., Linthorst, A.C.E., Reul, J.M.H.M., and Spanagel, R., Withdrawal symptoms in a long-term model of alcohol self-administration in unselected Wistar rats, *Alcohol. Clin. Exp. Res.,* 22, 92, 1998.

58. Spanagel, R. and Hoelter, S.M., Long-term alcohol self-administration with repeated alcohol depri-vation phases: an animal model of alcoholism? *Alcohol Alcohol.,* 34, 231, 1999.

59. Heyser, J.C., Schulteis, G., and Koob, G.F., Increased ethanol self-administration after a period of imposed ethanol deprivation in rats trained in a limited access paradigm, *Alcohol. Clin. Exp. Res.,* 21, 784, 1997.

60. Sinclair, J.D. and Li, T.-K., Long and short alcohol deprivation: effects on AA and P alcohol-preferring rats, *Alcohol,* 6, 505, 1989.

61. Sinclair, J.D., The alcohol-deprivation effect in monkeys, *Psychonom. Sci.,* 25, 21, 1971.

62. Burish, T.G., Maistro, S.A., Cooper, A.M., and Sobell, M.B., Effects of voluntary short-term abstinence from alcohol on subsequent drinking patterns of college students, *J. Stud. Alcohol,* 42, 1013, 1981.

63. Spanagel, R., Hoelter, S.M., Allingham, A., Landgraf, R., and Zieglgaensberger, W., Acamprosate and alcohol: I. Effects on alcohol intake following alcohol deprivation in the rat, *Eur. J. Pharmacol.,* 305, 39, 1996.

64. Hoelter, S.M., Landgraf, R., Zieglgaensberger, W., and Spanagel, R., Time course of acamprosate action on operant self-administration following ethanol deprivation, *Alcohol. Clin. Exp. Res.,* 21, 862, 1997.

65. Heyser, C.J., Schulteis, G., Durbin, P., and Koob, G.F., Chronic acamprosate treatment eliminates the alcohol deprivation effect while having limited effects on baseline responding for ethanol in rats, *Neuropsychopharmacology,* 18, 125, 1998.

66. Hoelter, S.M. and Spanagel, R., The effects of opiate antagonist treatment on the alcohol deprivation effect in long-term ethanol-experienced rats, *Psychopharmacology*, 145, 360, 1999.

67. Spanagel, R. and Zieglgaensberger, W., Anti-craving compounds: new pharmacological tools to study addictive processes, *Trends Phamacol. Sci.,* 18, 54, 1997.

68. Samson, H.H. and Harris, R.A., Neurobiology of alcohol abuse, *Trends Pharmacol. Sci.,* 13, 206, 1992.

69. Stolerman, I., Drugs of abuse: behavioural principles, methods and terms, *Trends Pharmacol. Sci.,* 13, 170, 1992.

70. Pohorecky, L.A., The interaction of alcohol and stress. A review, *Neurosci. Biobehav. Rev.,* 5, 209, 1981.

71. Spanagel, R., Montkowski, A., Allingham, K., Stoehr, T., Shoaib, M., Holsboer, F., and Landgraf, R., Anxiety: a potential predictor of vulnerability to the initiation of ethanol self-administration in rats, *Psychopharmacology,* 122, 369, 1995.

72. George, D.T., Nutt, D.J., Dwyer, B.A., and Linnoila, M., Alcoholism and panic disorder: is the comorbidity more than coincidence? *Acta Psychiatr. Scand.,* 81, 97, 1990.

73. Kushner, M.G., Sher, K.J., and Beitman, B.D., The relation between alcohol problems and the anxiety disorders, *Am. J. Psychiatry,* 147, 685, 1990.

74. Conger, J.J., Reinforcement theory and the dynamics of alcoholism, *Q. J. Stud. Alcohol,* 18, 296, 1956.

75. Haack, M.R., Harford, T.C., and Parker, D.A., Alcohol use and depression symptoms among female nursing students, *Alcohol. Clin. Exp. Res.,* 12, 365, 1988.

76. Castaneda, R., Sussman, N., Westreich, L., Levy, R., and O'Malley, M., A review of the effects of moderate alcohol intake on the treatment of anxiety and mood disorders, *J. Clin. Psychiatry,* 57, 207, 1996.

77. Roelofs, S.M.G.J., Hyperventilation, anxiety, craving for alcohol: a subacute alcohol withdrawal syndrome, *Alcohol,* 2, 501, 1985.

78. Lal, H., Harris, C.M., Benjamin, D., Springfield, A.C., Bhadra, S., and Emmett-Oglesby, M.W., Characterization of a pentylentetrazol-like interoceptive stimulus produced by ethanol withdrawal, *J. Pharmacol. Exp. Ther.,* 247, 508, 1988.

79. Maier, D.M. and Pohorecky, L.A., The effect of repeated withdrawal episodes on subsequent withdrawal severity in ethanol-treated rats, *Drug Alcohol Depend.,* 23, 103, 1989.

80. Becker, H.C. and Hale, R.L., Repeated episodes of ethanol withdrawal potentiate the severity of subsequent withdrawal seizures: an animal model of alcohol withdrawal "kindling," *Alcohol. Clin. Exp. Res.,* 17, 94, 1993.

81. Becker, H.C., Positive relationship between the number of prior ethanol withdrawal episodes and the severity of subsequent withdrawal seizures, *Psychopharmacology,* 116, 26, 1994.

82. Lepola, U., Alcohol and depression in panic disorder, *Acta Psychiatr. Scand. Suppl.,* 377, 33, 1994.

83. Adinoff, B., O'Neill, H.K., and Ballenger, J.C., Alcohol withdrawal and limbic kindling, *Am. J. Addict.,* 4, 5, 1995.

84. Baving, L. and Olbrich, H., Angst bei Alkoholabhaengigen, *Fortschr. Neurol. Psychiat.,* 64, 83, 1996.

85. Schuckit, M.A. and Hesselbrock, V., Alcohol dependence and anxiety disorders: What is the relationship? *Am. J. Psychiatry,* 151, 1723, 1994.

86. Merikangas, K., Stevens, D., and Fenton, B., Comorbidity of alcoholism and anxiety disorders: the role of family studies, *Alcohol Health Res. World,* 20, 100, 1996.

87. Swendsen, J.D., Merikangas, K.R., Canino, G.J., Kessler, R.C., Rubio-Stipec, M., and Angst, J., The comorbidity of alcoholism with anxiety and depressive disorders in four geographic communities, *Compr. Psychiatry,* 39, 176, 1998.

88. Almeida, O.F.X., Shoaib, M., Deicke, J., Fischer, D., Darwish, M.H., and Patchev, V.K., Gender differences in ethanol preference and ingestion in rats — the role of the gonadal steroid environment, *J. Clin. Invest.,* 101, 2677, 1998.

89. Ross, H.E., Glaser, F.B., and Stiasny, S., Sex differences in prevalence of psychiatric disorders in patients with alcohol and drug problems, *Br. J. Addict.,* 83, 1179, 1988.

90. Sinha, R., Robinson, J., and O'Malley, S., Stress response dampening: effects of gender and family history of alcoholism and anxiety disorders, *Psychopharmacology,* 137, 311, 1998.

91. Moeller, C., Wiklund, L., Sommer, W., Thorsell, A., and Heilig, M., Decreased experimental anxiety and voluntary ethanol consumption in rats following central but not basolateral amygdala lesions, *Brain Res.,* 760, 94, 1997.

92. Colombo, G., Agabio, R., Lobina, C., Reali, R., Zocchi, A., Fadda, F., and Gessa, G.L., Sardinian alcohol-preferring rats: a genetic animal model of anxiety, *Physiol. Behav.,* 57, 1181, 1995.

93. Baldwin, H.A., Wall, T.L., Schuckit, M.A., and Koob, G.F., Differential effects of ethanol on punished responding in the P and NP rats, *Alcohol. Clin. Exp. Res.,* 15, 700, 1991.

94. Stewart, R.B., Gatto, G.J., Lumeng, L., Li, T.-K., and Murphy, J.M., Comparison of alcohol-preferring (P) and nonpreferring (NP) rats on tests of anxiety and for the anxiolytic effects of ethanol, *Alcohol,* 10, 1, 1993.

95. Tuominen, K., Hilakivi, L.A., Paeivaerinta, P., and Korpi, E.R., Behavior of alcohol-preferring AA and alcohol-avoiding ANA rat lines in tests of anxiety and aggression, *Alcohol,* 7, 349, 1990.

96. Fahlke, C., Eriksson, C.J., and Hard, E., Audiogenic immobility reaction and open-field behavior in AA and ANA rat lines, *Alcohol,* 10, 311, 1993.

97. Moeller, C., Wiklund, L., Thorsell, A., Hyytiae, P., and Heilig, M., Decreased measures of experimental anxiety in rats bred for high alcohol preference, *Alcohol. Clin. Exp. Res.,* 21, 656, 1997.

98. Viglinskaya, I.V., Overstreet, D.H., Kashevskaya, O.P., Badishtov, B.A., Kampov-Polevoy, A.B., Seredenin, S.B., and Halikas, J.A., To drink or not to drink: tests of anxiety and immobility in alcohol-preferring and -nonpreferring rat strains, *Physiol. Behav.,* 57, 937, 1995.

99. Badishtov, B.A., Overstreet, D.H., Kashevskaya, O.P., Viglinskaya, I.V., Kampov-Polevoy, A.V., Seredenin, S.B., and Halikas, J.A., To drink or not to drink: open field behavior in alcohol-preferring and -nonpreferring rat strains, *Physiol. Behav.,* 57, 585, 1995.

100. Kampov-Polevoy, A.B., Kasheffskaya, O.P., Overstreet, D.H., Viglinskaya, I.V., Badishtov, B.A., Seredenin, S.B., Rezvani, A.H., Halikas, J.A., and Sinclair, J.D., Pain sensitivity and saccharin intake in alcohol-preferring and -nonpreferring rat strains, *Physiol. Behav.,* 59, 683, 1996.

101. Knapp, D.J., Kampov-Polevoy, A.B., Overstreet, D.H., Breese, G.R., and Rezvani, A.H., Ultrasonic vocalization behavior differs between lines of ethanol-preferring and nonpreferring rats, *Alcohol. Clin. Exp. Res.,* 21, 1232, 1997.

102. Overstreet, D.H., Halikas, J.A., Seredenin, S.B., Kampov-Polevoy, A.B., Viglinskaya, I.V., Kashevskaya, O., Badishtov, B.A., Knapp, D.J., Mormede, P., Kiianmaa, K., Li, T.-K., and Rezvani, A.H., Behavioral similarities and differences among alcohol-preferring and -nonpreferring rats: confirmation by factor analysis and extension to additional groups, *Alcohol. Clin. Exp. Res.,* 21, 40, 1997.

103. Liebsch, G., Montkowski, A., Holsboer, F., and Landgraf, R., Behavioral profiles of two Wistar rat lines selectively bred for high or low anxiety-related behavior, *Behav. Brain Res.,* 94, 301, 1998.

104. Liebsch, G., Linthorst, A.C.E., Neumann, I.D., Reul, J.M.H.M., Holsboer, F., and Landgraf, R., Behavioral, physiological, and neuroendocrine stress responses and differential sensitivity to diazepam in two Wistar rat lines selectively bred for high- and low-anxiety-related behavior, *Neuropsychopharmacology,* 19, 381, 1998.

105. Henniger, M.S.H., Hoelter, S.M., Wigger, A., Landgraf, R., and Spanagel, R., Alcohol self-administration in two Wistar rat lines selectively bred for high and low anxiety-related behaviour, submitted.

Section III

Useful Data and Definitions

37 Physicochemical Properties of Ethanol

Ethanol (ethyl alcohol)	C_2H_5OH
Molecular weight	46.07 g mol^{-1}
Melting point	−117.3°C
Boiling point	78.5°C
Density	0.7893 g ml^{-1} (20/4)

1 ml 100% alcohol = 0.7893 g alcohol

1 liter 100% alcohol = 17 mol

REFERENCE

1. Lide, D.R., *Handbook of Chemistry and Physics,* 79th ed., CRC Press, Boca Raton, FL, 1998.

38 How to Calculate Maximum Blood Alcohol Levels after a Drinking Event

Gerald Zernig and Hans J. Battista

Most countries impose an upper limit on allowable blood alcohol levels for drivers. It might therefore prove useful to estimate the maximum possible blood levels after a drinking event. Keep in mind that for most people, deterioration of driving skills begins at 50 mg dl^{-1}, and that 100 mg dl^{-1} is the legal level of intoxication in most of the U.S.[1,2] Maximum blood alcohol levels after a drinking event can be calculated by using Widmark's Formula,[3] named in honor of the pioneering studies by Erik M.P. Widmark of Sweden.[4,5]

For men with normal body weight (i.e., body length in centimeters minus 100 should correspond to weight in kg), the formula is:

$$\text{Maximum blood level in \textperthousand\ for men} = \frac{\text{Grams alcohol consumed}}{\text{Kilograms body weight} * 0.7}$$

An example: After downing half a liter of beer (20 g alcohol), the blood alcohol level of a man weighing 88 kg should not exceed 0.32 ‰ (or 340 mg%); that is, 20/(88 * 0.7) = 20/62 = 0.32.

Widmark's rho factor of 0.7 is a dimensionless constant that was empirically arrived at by relating administered alcohol dose, body weight, and measured blood alcohol level (all given in mass units). Widmark's rho factor (sometimes given as Widmark's "r" factor) corresponds to the volume of distribution (V_d, unit: 1 kg^{-1}, i.e., volume/mass) for alcohol in the following way: rho = 1.055 * V_d (1 ml whole blood weighs 1.055 g).[5] Alcohol is distributed almost exclusively in the body water. Men have 60% body water (i.e., 0.6 kg kg^{-1}). Women have, on average, a higher percentage of body fat and thus a lower lower percentage of body water (i.e., 0.5 kg kg^{-1}).[5] Hence, the respective formula for women is:

$$\text{Maximum blood level in \textperthousand\ for women} = \frac{\text{Grams alcohol consumed}}{\text{Kilograms body weight} * 0.6}$$

Thus, a woman weighing 88 kg would show a maximum blood alcohol level of 0.38‰ (400 mg%) after drinking half a liter of beer (20 g alcohol). The respective calculation is: 20/(88 * 0.6) = 20/53 = 0.38.

Differences in body fat should also be taken into account even when staying within the same gender. Accordingly, the factor 0.7 should be changed to 0.6 for distinctly obese men and to 0.8 for very lean men. In women, a factor of 0.5 should be used when calculating maximum blood levels for a distinctly obese woman, and a factor of 0.7 when doing the calculation for a distinctly lean woman.

One kilogram corresponds to 2.2 pounds, 1‰ to 105.5 mg% (see the conversion chart on the back inside cover). Thus, the above equations convert to:

$$\text{Maximum blood level in mg\% or mg dl}^{-1} \text{ for men} = \frac{\text{Grams alcohol consumed}}{\text{Pounds body weight}} * 3297$$

Thus, a 193-pound man downing half a liter of beer (i.e., 20 g alcohol) risks a maximum blood alcohol level of 342 mg%. The calculation runs as follows: (20/193) * 3297 = 342.

$$\text{Maximum blood level in mg\% or mg dl}^{-1} \text{ for women} = \frac{\text{Grams alcohol consumed}}{\text{Pounds body weight}} * 3868$$

Thus, a 193-pound woman would show a maximum blood alcohol level of 401 mg dl^{-1} after drinking half a liter of beer (20 g alcohol). The respective calculation is: (20/193) * 3868 = 401.

The multiplication factors vary according to nutritional status as follows: obese man, 3907; lean man, 2931; obese woman, 4587; and lean woman, 3297.

Note that the maximum blood alcohol levels calculated above will, in the overwhelming majority of cases, never be reached because alcohol is usually not consumed instantaneously and because elimination and distribution across body compartments are not taken into account in Widmark's formula, which was empirically derived by letting moderate drinkers consume low (0.5 to 1 g kg^{-1}) amounts of alcohol fast (within 20 to 30 min) on an empty stomach.[3] Under real-life (i.e., non-laboratory) drinking conditions, the maximum blood alcohol levels were, on average, found to be 10 to 30% lower than those obtained with Widmark's formula.[3] Thus, the maximum values derived with the formulae given above can be safely used when one tries to determine what to drink without violating the local legal limits of blood-alcohol concentration.

REFERENCES

1. National Institute on Alcohol Abuse and Alcoholism, Alcohol metabolism, *Alcohol Alert*, 35, 1, 1997.
2. Council on Scientific Affairs, Alcohol and the driver. Council on Scientific Affairs, *JAMA*, 255, 522, 1986.
3. Gilg, T., Alkohol (Ethanol): Pharmakologie, BAK-Berechnung und forensische Begutachtung, *Die Alkoholkrankheit — Diagnose und Therapie*, M. Soyka, Ed., Chapman & Hall, Weinheim, 1995, 18.
4. Gullberg, R.G. and Jones, A.W., Guidelines for estimating the amount of alcohol consumed from a single measurement of blood alcohol concentration: re-evaluation of Widmark's equation, *Forensic Sci. Int.*, 69, 119, 1994.
5. Jones, A.W. and Pounder, D.J., Measuring blood-alcohol concentration for clinical and forensic purposes, *Drug Abuse Handbook*, S.B. Karch, Ed., CRC Press, Boca Raton, FL, 1998, 327.

39 Basic Pharmacokinetics of Alcohol

Gerald Zernig and Hans J. Battista

After oral consumption, 10 to 20% of alcohol is absorbed in the the stomach and 80 to 90% in the small intestine, especially in the duodenum.[1] Absorption from the oral cavity is negligible; even keeping alcohol in the mouth for over 1 hour (!) results in blood alcohol levels of only 100 to 150 mg dl^{-1}.[2] Alcohol can be inhaled, taken up through the skin, the rectal mucosa, or it can be administered intravenously (concentrations exceeding 8 vol% damage veins).

The rate of absorption varies greatly, peak BAL times ranging from 10 to 100 min after the downing of 0.7 g kg^{-1} neat whiskey on an empty stomach by male volunteers.[3] For forensic purposes, absorption is considered to be complete 90 min after the end of a drinking bout.[1] As the major locus of absorption is the small intestine, quick passage through the stomach and a large surface area seem to be major determinants of the rate of absorption. Table 39.1 lists factors that speed up or slow down absorption.

Maximum blood alcohol levels can be calculated using Widmark's formula (see Chapter 38). However, due to distribution and redistribution within body compartments as well as elimination, actual maximum blood levels are about 10 to 30% lower than the calculated ones (resorption deficit). Alcohol penetrates the CNS well; estimated CNS levels are at least as high as those determined in plasma. Alcohol increases the permeability of the blood/brain barrier for other drugs.[1]

Blood vessels from the stomach and the small intestine drain into the portal vein and transport the absorbed alcohol to its main locus of elimination, the metabolic enzyme machinery of the liver ("first-pass" in the stricter sense, hepatic first-pass) before being further distributed in the body. Only a small fraction of alcohol might already be metabolized in the mucosa of the stomach (gastric first-pass). Overall, 95 to 98% of ingested alcohol is eliminated by being metabolized to acetaldehyde. The remaining 2 to 5% alcohol are conjugated with glucuronic acid and excreted in the urine and bile, or excreted unchanged in urine, breath, and sweat. Nonmetabolized alcohol readily crosses cell membranes and distributes almost exclusively within the aqueous compartments, both intracellular and extracellular, of the body (96%). Only 4% of the alcohol diffuses into body fat.

TABLE 39.1
Factors Affecting Alcohol Absorption

Absorption Speeded Up By:	Absorption Slowed Down By:
Empty stomach	Bulk of fatty food
Moderately concentrated alcohol	Highly concentrated alcohol (pylorospasm)
Large volumes	Spicy food (irritated mucosa)
Warm or hot drinks	Gastritis
Increased sympathetic tone (stress)	Increased vagal tone (nausea, anxiety)
Drinking before noon	Cigarettes (slowed gastric emptying)
Carbonated beverages	

TABLE 39.2
Alcohol-Metabolizing Enzymes

Feature	Alcohol Dehydrogenase (ADH), class I	Microsomal Ethanol-Oxidizing System (MEOS)	Catalase
Percent of alcohol bulk oxidized under normal conditions	90%	10% (at blood alcohol levels ≥ 100 mg dl^{-1})	1%
K_m for alcohol	1.2–2 mmol l^{-1} 5–9 mg dl^{-1}	10–15 mmol l^{-1} 45–68 mg dl^{-1}	
Cytochrome P450-dependent	No	Yes (CYP2E1)	No
Stimulated by chronic alcohol intake	No	Yes: increased susceptibility to environmental toxins	No
Stimulated by *chronic* administration of some drugs	No	Yes	No
Stimulated by *acute* administration of drugs	100–200 g fructose/h (*not* recommended; considerable side effects)		
Intracellular localization	Cytosol	Endoplasmic reticulum	Peroxisomes

Alcohol metabolism takes place almost exclusively in the liver. First, alcohol is oxidized mainly by the enzyme alcohol dehydrogenase (ADH), to varying degrees by the microsomal ethanol oxidizing system (MEOS), and, to a very small degree, by catalase. Table 39.2 compares the characteristics of the three oxidizing systems. Alcohol dehydrogenase shows considerable genetic polymorphism; five gene loci encode three classes of ADH enzymes, of which only class-I-ADH is of clinical importance (90% of whole body ADH in the liver, 10% in the stomach). Class-I-ADH has a higher affinity for alcohol ("low-K_m ADH") and is more sensitive to the experimentally used reversible inhibitor 4-methylpyrazol than the other ADH classes. Preliminary clinical investigations on the usefulness of 4-methylpyrazol as an antidote in ethylene glycol and methanol poisoning have been performed.[4,5]

K_m is the Michaelis-Menten constant, that is, the substrate concentration at which an enzyme runs at half-maximum speed. If the K_m for ADH is 9 mg dl^{-1} alcohol, this means that at $4 * K_m$ (i.e., at 36 mg dl^{-1} alcohol), ADH runs at 80% maximum speed. At $9 * K_m$ (i.e., at 81 mg dl^{-1}) ADH metabolizes alcohol at 90% maximum speed. This also means that at blood alcohol levels exceeding 100 mg dl^{-1}, the metabolic elimination of alcohol is essentially independent of the alcohol blood level; elimination becomes linear (zero-order kinetics). The rates of elimination for alcohol vary from 10 to 20 mg dl^{-1} per hour, with a mean value around 15 mg dl^{-1} h^{-1}.[1,2] Most likely because of the induction of MEOS activity, alcoholics show elimination rates up to 22 to 36 mg dl^{-1} h^{-1}.[1,2,6,7]

ADH has a 5- to 100-fold lower affinity for methanol and ethylene glycol than for ethanol. Thus, the best way to acutely block the accumulation of toxic metabolites after ingestion of methanol or ethylene glycol is the administration of ethanol with target blood alcohol levels of 50 to 100 mg dl^{-1}. Because of its higher affinity for the enzyme binding site, alcohol displaces methanol or methylene glycol, thus effectively blocking their conversion to toxic metabolites.

The actual activity state of MEOS is highly variable and almost unpredictable in the individual patient. Although chronic alcohol use induces MEOS and the associated cytochrome P450 CYP2E1, activity levels quickly return to baseline upon abstinence.[8] When considerable amounts of alcohol are in the body (e.g., after a drinking binge), metabolism of drugs that are substrates for CYP2E1 (e.g., barbiturates, phenytoin, warfarin, N-demethylated, and/or hydroxlated benzodiazepines such as diazepam) is *inhibited* due to direct competition for the enzyme. However, in chronic drinkers between binges (i.e., when no or very little alcohol is in the body), metabolism of these enzymes is actually *enhanced*. Induction of CYP2E1 also leads to an increased oxidative generation of a number of toxins stemming from environmental (e.g., industrial solvents, cigarette smoke) or drug (e.g., acetaminophen [paracetamol], pyrazole, isoniazid, phenylbutazone).[6,8-10] This may be the mechanism for the increased susceptibility of chronic alcohol abusers to liver injury.

The second step in the metabolic elimination of alcohol is the conversion of acetaldehyde to acetate by the enzyme aldehyde dehydrogenase (ALDH as compared to ADH, the alcohol dehydrogenase). There are two main classes of ALDH that are distinguished by their different affinity for acetaldehyde (ALDH$_2$, $K_m \approx 1$ to 3 mmol l^{-1}, located in mitochondria; vs. ALDH$_1$, $K_m \geq$ 30 mmol l^{-1}, located in the cytosol). About 50 to 80% of people of Asian descent, up to 43% of South American Indians, and about 20% Finns lack the high-affinity ALDH form. Disulfiram (Antabuse®) irreversibly inactivates ALDH, and calcium carbimide acts as a reversible inhibitor of ALDH. Lack of high-affinity enzyme or pharmacologic inhibition leads to accumulation of acetaldehyde after a drinking binge, resulting in facial flushing, headache, nausea, and, in more severe cases, in a sometimes life-threatening fall in blood pressure and elevated pulse rate. When induced by disulfiram, this syndrome is called disulfiram-alcohol reaction (DAR) or disulfiram-ethanol reaction (DER).

REFERENCES

1. Gilg, T., Alkohol (Ethanol): Pharmakologie, BAK-Berechnung und forensische Begutachtung, *Die Alkoholkrankheit — Diagnose und Therapie*, M. Soyka, Ed., Chapman & Hall, Weinheim, 1995, 18.
2. Jones, A.W., Forensic aspects of ethanol metabolism, *Forensic Sci. Prog.*, 5, 31, 1991.
3. Jones, A.W. and Pounder, D.J., Measuring blood-alcohol concentration for clinical and forensic purposes, *Drug Abuse Handbook*, S.B. Karch, Ed., CRC Press, Boca Raton, FL, 1998, 327.
4. Baud, F.J., Galliot, M., Astier, A., Bien, D.V., Garnier, R., Likforman, J., and Bismuth, C., Treatment of ethylene glycol poisoning with intravenous 4-methylpyrazole, *N. Engl. J. Med.,* 319, 97, 1988.
5. Harry, P., Turcant, A., Bouachour, G., Houze, P., Alquier, P., and Allain, P., Efficacy of 4-methylpyrazole in ethylene glycol poisoning: clinical and toxicokinetic aspects. *Hum. Exp. Toxicol.*, 13, 61, 1994.
6. Lieber, C.S., Ethanol metabolism, cirrhosis and alcoholism, *Clin. Chim. Acta*, 257, 59, 1997.
7. Seitz, H.K., Lieber, C.S., and Simanowski, U.A., *Handbuch Alkohol, Alkoholismus, alkoholbedingte Organschaeden,* Leipzig, Barth, 1995.
8. Fraser, A.G., Pharmacokinetic interactions between alcohol and other drugs, *Clin. Pharmacokinet.*, 33, 79, 1997.
9. Koop, D.R., Oxidative and reductive metabolism by cytochrome P450 2E1, *FASEB J.*, 6, 724, 1992.
10. Lieber, C.S., Biochemical and molecular basis of alcohol-induced injury to liver and other tissues, *N. Engl. J. Med.*, 319, 1639, 1988.

40 Drug Interactions

Gerald Zernig and Hans J. Battista

Alcohol is a sedative at high doses; it also increases the sedative effects of other sedatives (e.g., opioid analgesics or benzodiazepines). A number of drugs are substrates for the cytochrome P450 CYP2E1, the activity of which is induced by alcohol (see Chapter 39 on the basic pharmacokinetics of alcohol). Note that the effect of alcohol is dual: when a person is intoxicated with alcohol, the metabolic elimination of these drugs is *inhibited*. However, in chronic alcohol abusers between binges (i.e., when no or little alcohol is in the body), metabolic elimination of these drugs is *enhanced*. Table 40.1 was compiled from a variety of sources.[1-9] Individual references are given only for those cases in which the above references clearly differed from each other.

TABLE 40.1
Drug Interactions

Drug or Drug Class	Type of Interaction
Acetaminophen (paracetamol)	Increased susceptibility to hepatic injury after ingestion of nontoxic doses (CYP2E1 induction)
Acitretin	Increased formation of teratogenic metabolite etretinate
Aflatoxin B_1	Increased hepatic injury (CYP2E1 induction)
Anesthetics	Increased sedation
Aspirin (acetylsalicylic acid)	Gastrointestinal bleeding
Barbiturates	Increased levels during alcohol intoxication, decreased levels in chronic alcohol abusers (CYP2E1 induction)
Benzodiazepines	Increased sedation and psychomotor impairment
	Lorazepam: enhanced hypotension and bradycardia
	Diazepam and other *N*-demethylated and/or hydroxylated benzodiazepines: increased levels during alcohol intoxication, decreased levels in chronic alcohol abusers (CYP2E1 induction)
Carbamazepine	Increased levels during alcohol intoxication, decreased levels in chronic alcohol abusers (CYP2E1 induction)
Carbon tetrachloride (CCl_4)	Increased hepatic injury (CYP2E1 induction)
Cefamandole	Disulfiram-like reaction
Cefoperazone	Disulfiram-like reaction
Cigarette smoke	Increased mutagenicity (CYP2E1 induction)
Cimetidine	Conflicting data; most studies show no effect at alcohol doses > 0.15 g kg^{-1}. Drug may increase alcohol level by increasing gastric emptying after meal
Cisapride	Increased blood alcohol levels (increased gastric emptying)
Cocaine	Increased hepatic injury (CYP2E1 induction)
Erythromycin	Increased blood alcohol levels (increased gastric emptying)
Estradiol	Increased levels (3-fold) in substituted postmenopausal women
	No effect on estradiol in women not taking treatment
Ethylene glycol	Alcohol blocks metabolism (useful in ethylene glycol intoxication)
Griseofulvin	Disulfiram-like reaction
Guanethidine	Hypotension

TABLE 40.1 (continued)
Drug Interactions

Drug or Drug Class	Type of Interaction
H_1 receptor antagonists (antihistamines)	Increased sedation and psychomotor impairment
H_2 receptor antagonists (antiulcer medication)	Conflicting data; most studies show no effect at alcohol doses > 0.15 Hg/kg⁻¹; drug may increase alcohol level by increasing gastric emptying after meal
Hydralazine	Hypoglycemia and hypotension
Hypoglycemics (oral, long-acting)	Hypoglycemia and hypotension
Meprobamate	Increased levels during alcohol intoxication, decreased levels in chronic alcohol abusers (CYP2E1 induction)
Methadone	Increased levels during alcohol intoxication, decreased levels in chronic alcohol abusers (CYP2E1 induction)
Methanol	Alcohol blocks metabolism (useful in methanol intoxication)
Methotrexate	Increased hepatic injury (see chapter on immunological problems for details)
MethylDOPA	Hypoglycemia and hypotension
Metronidazole	Disulfiram-like reaction
Monoamine oxidase inhibitors (MAOI)	Severe hypertension (tyramine-containing beverages such as some wines or beers)
Narcotics (opioid analgesics)	Increased sedation, decreased metabolism
Neuroleptics (antipsychotics)	Increased sedation and psychomotor impairment
Nitroglycerin	Hypoglycemia and hypotension
NSAIDs (nonsteroidal anti-inflammatory drugs)	Gastrointestinal bleeding
Omeprazol (gastric proton pump inhibitor)	No effect
Opioid analgesics (narcotics)	Increased sedation, decreased metabolism
Paracetamol (acetaminophen)	Increased susceptibility to hepatic injury after ingestion of nontoxic doses (CYP2E1 induction)
Phenylbutazone	Increased susceptibility to hepatic injury after ingestion of nontoxic doses (CYP2E1 induction)
Phenytoin	Increased levels during alcohol intoxication, decreased levels in chronic alcohol abusers (CYP2E1 induction)
Propranolol	Decreased levels
Ranitidine	Conflicting data; most studies show no effect at alcohol doses > 0.15 g kg⁻¹; drug may increase alcohol level by increasing gastric emptying after meal
Reserpine	Hypotension
Rifampicin	Increased levels during alcohol intoxication, decreased levels in chronic alcohol abusers (CYP2E1 induction)
Sulfonamides	Disulfiram-like reaction
Tetracyclines	Increased levels
Tobacco smoke	Increased mutagenicity (CYP2E1 induction)
Tolbutamide	Disulfiram-like reaction
Tricyclic antidepressants	Increased sedation and psychomotor impairment
Warfarin	Increased levels during alcohol intoxication, decreased levels in chronic alcohol abusers (CYP2E1 induction)

REFERENCES

1. Fraser, A.G., Pharmacokinetic interactions between alcohol and other drugs. *Clin. Pharmacokinet.*, 33, 79, 1997.
2. Jonsson, K.A., Jones, A.W., Bostrom, H., and Andersson, T., Lack of effect of omeprazole, cimetidine, and ranitidine on the pharmacokinetics of ethanol in fasting male volunteers, *Eur. J. Clin. Pharmacol.*, 42, 209, 1992.
3. National Institute on Alcohol Abuse and Alcoholism, Alcohol-medication interactions, *Alcohol Alert*, 27, 1, 1995.
4. Koop, D.R., Oxidative and reductive metabolism by cytochrome P450 2E1, *FASEB J.*, 6, 724, 1992.
5. Lieber, C.S., Ethanol metabolism, cirrhosis and alcoholism, *Clin. Chim. Acta*, 257, 59, 1997.
6. Lieber, C.S., Interaction of alcohol with other drugs and nutrients. Implication for the therapy of alcoholic liver disease, *Drugs*, 40 (Suppl. 3), 23, 1990.
7. Whiting-O'Keefe, Q.E., Fye, K.H., and Sack, K.D., Methotrexate and histologic hepatic abnormalities: a meta-analysis, *Am. J. Med.*, 90, 711, 1991.
8. Zachariae, H., Methotrexate side-effects [see comments], *Br. J. Dermatol.*, 122 (Suppl. 36), 127, 1990.
9. Larsen, F.G., Jakobsen, P., Knudsen, J., Weismann, K., Kragballe, K., and Nielsen, K.F., Conversion of acitretin to etretinate in psoriatic patients is influenced by ethanol, *J. Invest. Dermatol.*, 100, 623, 1993.

41 Definitions of a "Standard Drink"

Definitions of a standard drink vary across countries and studies. Here is an incomplete list of "standard drinks" expressed in terms of grams alcohol. For the alcohol contents of typical alcoholic beverage types, see back inside cover.

Country	Gram Alcohol per Standard Drink (or "unit")	Ref.
Austria	20	1
U.K.	8	2,3
	9	4
	10	5
U.S.	14	National Institute on Alcohol Abuse and Alcoholism (NIAAA)
	Beer 12 oz (5 vol.%)	www.niaaa.nih.gov
	Wine 5 oz (12 vol.%)	
	Hard liquor 1.5 oz (80-proof = 40 vol.%)	6
	12	7

REFERENCES

1. Uhl, A. and Springer, A., *Studie ueber den Konsum von Alkohol und psychoaktiven Stoffen in Oesterreich unter Beruecksichtigung problematischer Gebrauchsmuster*, Austrian Federal Ministry of Health (Bundesministerium fuer Gesundheit und Konsumentenschutz), Vienna, 1996.
2. Royal College of General Practitioners, *Alcohol — A Balanced View*, 1986.
3. Anderson, P., Self-administered questionnaires for diagnosis of alcohol abuse, *Diagnosis of Alcohol Abuse*, R.R. Watson, Ed., CRC Press, Boca Raton, FL, 1989, 2321.
4. Tilley, S., Alcohol, other drugs and tobacco use and anxiolytic effectiveness. A comparison of anxious patients and psychiatric nurses, *Br. J. Psychiatry*, 151, 389, 1987.
5. Day, C.P., Gilvarry, E., Butler, T.J., and James, O.F., Moderate alcohol intake is not deleterious in patients with alcoholic liver disease, *Hepatology*, 24, 443A, 1996.
6. Dongier, M., Vachon, L., and Schwartz, G., Bromocriptine in the treatment of alcohol dependence, *Alcohol. Clin. Exp. Res.*, 15, 970, 1991.
7. Miller, W.R., Leckman, L., Delaney, H.D., and Tinkcom, M., Long-term follow-up of behavioral self-control training, *J. Stud. Alcohol*, 53, 249, 1992.

42 Harmful Daily Alcohol Consumption

Based on the epidemiological studies reviewed by Fleming and Baier Manwell (see Chapter 29 on harmful alcohol consumption) and by Stoschitzky (see Chapter 18 on the cardiovascular system), we suggest that any alcohol consumption

- Exceeding 30 to 60 g per day (i.e., 2 to 4 standard drinks) in men
- Exceeding 20 to 40 g per day (i.e., 1 to 3 standard drinks) in women

(for alcohol contents of typical drinks, please see the back inside cover)

must be considered harmful with respect to possible organ damage. Different organ systems show various sensitivities to alcohol's harmful effects. It has also been shown that the risk for suicide — which might be taken as a very coarse indicator of psychological problems — significantly increases with the first daily drink.[1] Thus, although very moderate alcohol drinking might not affect other organ systems adversely, it might already compromise the mental health and psychosocial functioning of the patient.

REFERENCE

1. Boffetta, P. and Garfinkel, L., Alcohol drinking and mortality among men enrolled in an American Cancer Society prospective study, *Epidemiology*, 1, 342, 1990.

43 DSM-IV and ICD-10 Definitions of Alcohol Intoxication, Abuse, Dependence, and Withdrawal

Worldwide, the diagnostic criteria for alcohol abuse and dependence of two institutions, the World Health Organization (WHO) and the American Psychiatric Association (APA), are the most widely accepted. The WHO issues the *International Classification of Diseases* (ICD),[1] which contains a numbering system frequently used by hospital administrations when processing patient data.

ICD-10 CODES

These ICD-10 codes (source: World Health Organization, reproduced with permission) are:

F10.0	Alcohol intoxication
F10.03	Alcohol intoxication delirium
F10.1	Alcohol abuse
F10.2	Alcohol dependence
F10.3	Alcohol withdrawal
F10.4	Alcohol withdrawal delirium
F10.51	Alcohol-induced psychotic disorder, with delusions
F10.52	Alcohol-induced psychotic disorder, with hallucinations
F10.6	Alcohol-induced persisting amnestic disorder
F10.72	Alcohol-induced mood disorder
F10.73	Alcohol-induced persisting dementia
F10.8	Alcohol-induced anxiety disorder
F10.8	Alcohol-induced sexual dysfunction
F10.8	Alcohol-induced sleeping disorder
F10.9	Alcohol-related disorder not otherwise specified

The APA issues the *Diagnostic and Statistical Manual of Mental Disorders* (DSM).[2] Both institutions regularly update their classification systems; ICD is in its 10th version (ICD-10), DSM in its 4th (DSM-IV). Unfortunately, we could not find ICD-10- nor DSM-IV-definitions listed for public use on the Internet (one site, www.mental-health.com/icd/ has disappeared). Both the WHO (www.who.int/whosis/icd10/) and the American Psychiatric Association (APA: www.psych.org) sell print and electronic versions of their classification systems. A lower-cost way to obtain the DSM criteria is to purchase a little booklet, *Quick Reference to the Diagnostic Criteria from DSM-IV™*, ISBN 0-89042-063-7. The APA cautions against using this little condensed companion book to the bigger DSM-IV tome as the only source of information; however, it might serve well as a first introduction. ICD-10 does not seem to separate alcohol abuse and dependence into separate diagnostic entities. For the WHO definition of harmful drinking, see Chapter 42. DSM-IV does give separate definitions of substance abuse and substance dependence (which of course, apply to alcohol as well), and a host of definitions for alcohol-related psychiatric disorders, some of which are listed in the respective chapters of this handbook.

0-8493-7801-X/00/$0.00+$.50
© 2000 by CRC Press LLC

DSM-IV CRITERIA FOR ALCOHOL INTOXICATION[2]

A. Recent ingestion of alcohol.
B. Clinically significant maladaptive behavioral or psychological changes (e.g., inappropriate sexual or aggressive behavior, mood lability, impaired judgment, impaired social or occupational functioning) that devleoped during, or shortly after alcohol ingestion.
C. One (or more) of the following signs, developing during, or shortly after, alcohol use:
    1. Slurred speach
    2. Incoordination
    3. Unsteady gait
    4. Nystagmus
    5. Impairment in attention or memory
    6. Stupor or coma
D. The symptoms are not due to a general medical condition and are not better accounted for by another mental disorder.

DSM-IV CRITERIA FOR SUBSTANCE ABUSE[2]

A. A maladaptive pattern of substance use leading to clinically significant impairment or distress, as manifested by one (or more) of the following, occurring within a 12-month period:
    1. Recurrent substance use resulting in a failure to fulfill major role obligations at work, school, or home (e.g., repeated absences or poor work performance related to substance use; substance-related absences, suspensions, or expulsions from school; neglect of children or household)
    2. Recurrent substance use in situations in which it is physically hazardous (e.g., driving an automobile or operating a machine when impaired by substance use)
    3. Recurrent substance-related legal problems (e.g., arrests for substance-related disorderly conduct)
    4. Continued substance use despite having persistent or recurrent social or interpersonal problems caused or exacerbated by the effects of the substance (e.g., arguments with spouse about consequences of intoxication, physical fights)
B. The symptoms have never met the criteria for Substance Dependence for this class of substance.

DSM-IV CRITERIA FOR SUBSTANCE DEPENDENCE[2]

A maladaptive pattern of substance use, leading to clinically significant impairment or distress, as manifested by three (or more) of the following, occurring at any time in the same 12-month period:

1. Tolerance, as defined by either of the following:
    a. A need for markedly increased amounts of the substance to achieve intoxication or desired effect
    b. Markedly diminished effect with continued use of the same amount of the substance
2. Withdrawal, as manifested by either of the following:
    a. The characteristic withdrawal syndrome for the substance (refer to Criteria A and B or the criteria sets for withdrawal from the specific substances)
    b. The same (or a closely related) substance is taken to relieve or avoid withdrawal symptoms
3. The substance is often taken in larger amounts of over a longer period than was intended
4. There is a persistent desire or unsuccessful efforts to cut down or control substance use

5. A great deal of time is spent in activities necessary to obtain the substance (e.g., visiting multiple doctors or driving long distances), use the substance (e.g., chain-smoking), or recover from its effects

6. Important social, occupational, or recreational activities are given up or reduced because of substance use

7. The substance is continued despite knowledge of having a persistent or recurring problem that is likely to have been caused or exacerbated by the substance (e.g., current cocaine use despite recognition of cocaine-induced depression, or continued drinking despite recognition that an ulcer was made worse by alcohol consumption)

Specify if:

With Physiological Dependence: evidence of tolerance or withdrawal (i.e., either Item 1 or 2 is present)

Without Physiological Dependence: no evidence of tolerance or withdrawal (i.e., neither Item 1 nor 2 is present)

DSM-IV CRITERIA FOR ALCOHOL WITHDRAWAL

A. Cessation of (or reduction in) alcohol use that has been heavy and prolonged.

B. Two (or more) of the following, developing within several hours to a few days after criterion A:
   1. Autonomic hyperactivity (e.g., sweating or pulse rate greater than 100)
   2. Increased hand tremor
   3. Insomnia
   4. Nausea or vomiting
   5. Transient visual, tactile, or auditory hallucinations or illusions
   6. Psychomotor agitation
   7. Anxiety
   8. Grand-mal seizures

C. The symptoms in criterion B cause clinically significant distress or impairment in social, occupational, or other important areas of functioning.

D. The symptoms are not due to a general medical condition and are not better accounted for by another mental disorder.

ICD-10 DIAGNOSTIC CRITERIA FOR ALCOHOL ABUSE, DEPENDENCE, AND WITHDRAWAL,[1] U.S. VERSION

A. **Alcohol abuse:** A destructive pattern of alcohol use, leading to significant social, occupational, or medical impairment.

B. Must have three (or more) of the following, occurring when the alcohol use was at its worst:
   1. **Alcohol tolerance:** Either need for markedly increased amounts of alcohol to achieve intoxication, or markedly diminished effect with continued use of the same amount of alcohol.
   2. Alcohol withdrawal symptoms: Either (a) or (b).
      a. Two (or more) of the following, developing within several hours to a few days of reduction in heavy or prolonged alcohol use:
         • Sweating or rapid pulse
         • Increased hand tremor

- Insomnia
- Nausea or vomiting
- Physical agitation
- Anxiety
- Transient visual, tactile, or auditory hallucinations or illusions
- Grand-mal seizures

   b. Alcohol is taken to relieve or avoid withdrawal symptoms.
3. Alcohol was often taken in larger amounts or over a longer period than was intended
4. Persistent desire or unsuccessful efforts to cut down or control alcohol use
5. Great deal of time spent in using alcohol, or recovering from hangovers
6. Important social, occupational, or recreational activities given up or reduced because of alcohol use
7. Continued alcohol use is continued despite knowledge of having a persistent or recurrent physical or psychological problem that is likely to have been worsened by alcohol (e.g., continued drinking despite knowing that an ulcer was made worse by drinking alcohol)

ICD-10 DIAGNOSTIC CRITERIA FOR ALCOHOL DEPENDENCE, EUROPEAN VERSION

F10.2 ALCOHOL DEPENDENCE SYNDROME

A cluster of physiological, behavioral, and cognitive phenomena in which the use of alcohol takes on a much higher priority for a given individual than other behaviors that once had greater value. A central descriptive characteristic of the dependence syndrome is the desire (often strong, sometimes overpowering) to take alcohol. There may be evidence that return to alcohol use after a period of abstinence leads to a more rapid reappearance of other features of the syndrome than occurs with nondependent individuals.

DIAGNOSTIC GUIDELINES

A definite diagnosis of dependence should usually be made only if three or more of the following have been experienced or exhibited at some time during the previous year:

a. A strong desire or sense of compulsion to take alcohol;
b. Difficulties in controlling alcohol-taking behaviour in terms of its onset, termination, or levels of use;
c. A physiological withdrawal state when alcohol use has ceased or been reduced, as evidenced by: the characteristic withdrawal syndrome for alcohol; or use of the alcohol with the intention of relieving or avoiding withdrawal symptoms;
d. Evidence of tolerance, such that increased doses of alcohol are required in order to achieve effects originally produced by lower doses (clear examples of this are found in alcohol-dependent individuals who may take daily doses sufficient to incapacitate or kill nontolerant users);
e. Progressive neglect of alternative pleasures or interests because of alcohol use, increased amount of time necessary to obtain or take alcohol or to recover from its effects;
f. Persisting with alcohol use despite clear evidence of overtly harmful consequences, such as harm to the liver through excessive drinking; efforts should be made to determine that the user was actually, or could be expected to be, aware of the nature and extent of the harm.

Narrowing of the personal repertoire of patterns of alcohol use has also been described as a characteristic feature (e.g., a tendency to drink alcoholic drinks in the same way on weekdays and weekends, regardless of social constraints that determine appropriate drinking behavior). It is an essential characteristic of the dependence syndrome that either alcohol taking or a desire to take alcohol should be present; the subjective awareness of compulsion to use alcohol is most commonly seen during attempts to stop or control alcohol use.

Includes:

* chronic alcoholism

REFERENCES

1. World Health Organization, *Tenth Revision of the International Classification of Diseases (ICD-10)*, World Health Organisation, Geneva, 1992.
2. American Psychiatric Association, *Diagnostic and Statistical Manual of Mental Disorders, Fourth Edition (DSM-IV)*, American Psychiatric Association, Washington, D.C., 1994.

44 Alphabetical List of Psychometric Test Instruments

- *ADS©*
- *AUDIT©* (free test form and manual)
- **CAGE**
- **CIWA-Ar**
- *MALT©*
- **MAST** and **Brief MAST**
- *OCDS©*
- **QF**
- *RTCQ©*
- **sMAST**
- *T-ACE©*
- *TLFB©* (free test form)
- **TWEAK**

The sources of these tests are given in:

- Psychometric Screening Instruments, Chapter 4
- Alcohol Withdrawal Syndrome, Chapter 6
- Psychometric Instruments to Evaluate Outcome in Alcoholism Treatment, Chapter 30

ALCOHOL DEPENDENCE SCALE© (ADS)©

INSTRUCTIONS:

1. Carefully read each question and the possible answers provided. Answer each question by circling the ONE choice that is most true for you.
2. The word "drinking" in a question refers to "drinking of alcoholic beverages."
3. Take as much time as you need. Work carefully, and try to finish as soon as possible. Please answer ALL questions.

These questions refer to the past 12 months*

1. How much did you drink the last time you drank?
   a. Enough to get high or less
   b. Enough to get drunk
   c. Enough to pass out
2. Do you often have hangovers on Sunday or Monday mornings?
   a. No
   b. Yes
3. Have you had the "shakes" when sobering up (hands tremble, shake inside)?
   a. No
   b. Sometimes
   c. Often
4. Do you get physically sick (e.g., vomit, stomach cramps) as a result of drinking?
   a. No
   b. Sometimes
   c. Almost every time I drink
5. Have you had the "DT's" (delirium tremens) — that is, seen, felt or heard things not really there; felt very anxious, restless, and over excited?
   a. No
   b. Sometimes
   c. Several times
6. When you drink, do you stumble about, stagger, and weave?
   a. No
   b. Sometimes
   c. Often
7. As a result of drinking, have you felt overly hot and sweaty (feverish)?
   a. No
   b. Once
   c. Several times
8. As a result of drinking, have you seen things that were not really there?
   a. No
   b. Once
   c. Several times
9. Do you panic because you fear you may not have a drink when you need it?
   a. No
   b. Yes
10. Have you had blackout ("loss of memory" without passing out) as a result of drinking?
    a. No, never
    b. Sometimes
    c. Often
    d. Almost every time I drink
11. Do you carry a bottle with you or keep one close at hand?
    a. No
    b. Some of the time
    c. Most of the time
12. After a period of abstinence (not drinking), do you end up drinking heavily again?
    a. No
    b. Sometimes
    c. Almost every time I drink
13. In the past 12 months, have you passed out as a result of drinking?
    a. No
    b. Once
    c. More than once

---

* Instructions can be altered for use as an outcome measure at selected intervals (e.g., 6, 12, 24 months) during or following treatment.

14. Have you had a convulsion (fit) following a period of drinking?
    a. No
    b. Yes
    c. Several times
15. Do you drink throughout the day?
    a. No
    b. Yes
16. After drinking heavily, has your thinking been fuzzy or unclear?
    a. No
    b. Yes, but only for a few hours
    c. Yes, for one or two days
    d. Yes, for many days
17. As a result of drinking, have you felt your heart beating rapidly?
    a. No
    b. Yes
    c. Several times
18. Do you almost constantly think about drinking and alcohol?
    a. No
    b. Yes
19. As a result of drinking, have you heard "things" that were really not there?
    a. No
    b. Yes
    c. Several times
20. Have you had weird and frightening sensations when drinking?

    a. No
    b. Once or twice
    c. Often
21. As a result of drinking have you "felt things" crawling on you that were not really there (e.g., bugs, spiders)?
    a. No
    b. Yes
    c. Several times
22. With respect to blackouts (loss of memory):
    a. Have never had a blackout
    b. Have had blackouts that last less than an hour
    c. Have had blackouts that last for several hours
    d. Have had blackouts that last a day or more
23. Have you tried to cut down on your drinking and failed?
    a. No
    b. Once
    c. Several times
24. Do you gulp drinks (drink quickly?)
    a. No
    b. Yes
25. After taking one or two drinks, can you usually stop?
    a. Yes
    b. No

Scoring

Dichotomous items are scored 0, 1; three-choice items are scored 0, 1, 2; and four-choice items are scored 0, 1, 2, 3. In each case, the higher the value the greater the dependence. Total scores can range from 0 to 47.

ALCOHOL USE DISORDERS IDENTIFICATION TEST© (AUDIT)©

Please circle the answer that is correct for you.

1. How often do you have a drink containing alcohol?

   Never   Monthly   Two to four   Two to three   Four or more
                or less   times a month   times a week   times a week

2. How many drinks containing alcohol do you have on a typical day when you are drinking?

   1 or 2   3 or 4   5 or 6   7 to 9   10 or more

3. How often do you have six or more drinks on one occasion?

   Never   Less than monthly   Monthly   Weekly   Daily or almost daily

4. How often during the last year have you found that you were not able to stop drinking once you had started?

   Never   Less than monthly   Monthly   Weekly   Daily or almost daily

5. How often during the last year have you failed to do what was normally expected from you because of drinking?

   Never   Less than monthly   Monthly   Weekly   Daily or almost daily

6. How often during the last year have you needed a first drink in the morning to get yourself going after a heavy drinking session?

   Never   Less than monthly   Monthly   Weekly   Daily or almost daily

7. How often during the last year have you had a feeling of guilt or remorse after drinking?

   Never   Less than monthly   Monthly   Weekly   Daily or almost daily

8. How often during the last year have you been unable to remember what happened the night before because you had been drinking?

   Never   Less than monthly   Monthly   Weekly   Daily or almost daily

9. Have you or someone else been injured as a result of your drinking?

   No   Yes, but not in the last year   Yes, during the last year

10. Has a relative or friend, or a doctor or other health care worker been concerned about your drinking or suggested you cut down?

    No   Yes, but not in the last year   Yes, during the last year

PROCEDURE FOR SCORING THE AUDIT©

Questions 1 to 8 are scored 0, 1, 2, 3, or 4. Questions 9 and 10 are scored 0, 2, or 4 only. The response is as follows:

	0	1	2	3	4
Question 1	Never	Monthly	Two to four times per month	Two to three times per week	Four or more times per week
Question 2	1 or 2	3 or 4	5 or 6	7 to 9	10 or more
Questions 3–8	Never	Less than monthly	Monthly	Weekly	Daily or almost daily
Questions 9–10	No		Yes, but not in the last year		Yes, during the last year

The minimum score (for non-drinkers) is 0 and the maximum possible score is 40.

A score of 8 or more indicates a strong likelihood of hazardous or harmful alcohol consumption.

THE CAGE TEST

Cut down	1. Have you ever felt that you ought to cut down on your drinking?
Annoyed	2. Have people annoyed you by criticizing your drinking?
Guilty	3. Have you ever felt bad or guilty about your drinking?
Eye opener	4. Have you ever had a drink first thing in the morning to steady your nerves or get rid of a hangover?

Two or more positive responses on the CAGE indicates a strong likelihood that a patient has experienced significant alcohol-related problems or is alcohol-dependent.

CLINICAL INSTITUTE WITHDRAWAL ASSESSMENT SCALE FOR ALCOHOL, REVISED (CIWA-Ar)

Nausea and vomiting — Ask "Do you feel sick to your stomach? Have you vomited?"

Observation
0 No nausea with no vomiting
1
2
3
4 Intermittent nausea with dry heaves
5
6
7 Constant nausea, frequent dry heaves and vomiting

Paroxysmal sweats — Observation

0 No sweats visible
1
2
3
4 Beads of sweat obvious on forehead
5
6
7 Drenching sweats

Agitation — Observation

0 Normal activity
1
2
3
4 Moderately fidgety and restless
5
6
7 Paces back and forth during most of the interview or constantly thrashes about

Headache, fullness in head — Ask "Does your head feel different? Does it feel like there is a band around your head?" Do not rate for dizziness or light-headedness. Otherwise rate severity.

0 Not present
1 Very mild
2 Mild
3 Moderate
4 Moderately severe
5 Severe
6 Very severe

7 Extremely severe

Anxiety — Ask "Do you feel nervous?"

Observation
1 No anxiety, at ease
1
2
3
4 Moderately anxious, or guarded, so anxiety is inferred
5
6
7 Equivalent to acute panic states as seen in severe delirium or acute schizophrenic reactions

Tremor — Arms extended and fingers spread apart

Observation
0 No tremor
1 Not visible, but can be felt fingertip to fingertip
2
3
4 Moderate, with patient's arm extended
5
6
7 Severe, even with arms not extended

Visual disturbances — Ask "Does the light appear to be too bright? Is its color different? Does it hurt your eyes? Are you seeing anything that is disturbing to you? Are you seeing things you know are not there?"

Observation
1 Not present
1 Very mild sensitivity
2 Mild sensitivity
3 Moderate sensitivity
4 Moderately severe hallucinations
5 Severe hallucinations
6 Extremely severe hallucinations
7 Continuous hallucinations

Tactile disturbances — Ask "Have you any itching, pins and needles sensations, any burning, any numbness or do you feel bugs crawling on or under your skin?"

Observation
0 None
1 Very mild itching, pins and needles, burning, or numbness
2 Mild itching, pins and needles, burning, or numbness
3 Moderate itching, pins and needles, burning, or numbness
4 Moderately severe hallucinations
5 Severe hallucinations
6 Extremely severe hallucinations
7 Continuous hallucinations

Auditory disturbances — Ask "Are you more aware of sounds around you? Are they harsh? Do they frighten you? Are you hearing anything that is disturbing you? Are you hearing things you know are not there?"

Observation
0 None present
1 Very mild harshness or ability to frighten
2 Mild harshness or ability to frighten
3 Moderate harshness or ability to frighten
4 Moderately severe hallucinations
5 Severe hallucinations
6 Extremely severe hallucinations
7 Continuous hallucinations

Orientation and clouding of sensorium — Ask "What day is this? Where are you? Who am I?"

0 Oriented and can do serial additions
1 Cannot do serial additions
2 Disoriented for date by no more than 2 calendar days
3 Disoriented for date by more than 2 calendar days
4 Disoriented for place and/or person

Total score is a simple sum of each item score (maximum score, 67)

THE MUNICH ALCOHOLISM TEST© (MALT)©

(cannot be reproduced without permission)

Items To Be Assessed by the Physician

1. Diseases of the liver (at least one symptom found on physical examination in addition to one positive laboratory test)
2. Polyneuropathy (only if no other cause is known, e.g., diabetes mellitus)
3. Delirium tremens (on the present examination or previously)
4. Alcohol consumption of more than 150 ml (women 120 ml) of pure alcohol a day at least continued over several months
5. Alcohol consumption of more than 300 ml (women 240 ml) of pure alcohol at least once a month (alcoholic benders)
6. Foetor alcoholicus (at the time of medical examination)
7. Spouse, family members, or good friends have sought help because of alcohol-related problems of the patient (e.g., from a physician, social worker, or other appropriate source)

Items To Be Assessed by the Patient as Being "True" or "Not True"

1. My hands have been trembling a lot recently.
2. In the morning, I sometimes have the feeling of nausea.
3. I have sometimes tried to get rid of my trembling and nausea with alcohol.
4. At the moment, I feel miserable because of my problems and difficulties.
5. It is not uncommon that I drink alcohol before lunch.
6. After the first glass or two of alcohol, I feel a craving for more.
7. I think about alcohol a lot.
8. I have sometimes drunk alcohol even against my doctor's advice.
9. When I drink a lot of alcohol, I tend to eat too little.
10. At work I have been criticized because of my drinking.
11. I prefer drinking alone.
12. Since I have started drinking I have been in worse shape.
13. I have often had a guilty conscience about drinking.
14. I have tried to limit my drinking to certain occasions or to certain times of the day.
15. I think I ought to drink less.
16. Without alcohol I would have fewer problems.
17. When I am upset I drink alcohol to calm down.
18. I think alcohol is destroying my life.
19. Sometimes I want to stop drinking, and sometimes I don't.
20. Other people can't understand why I drink.
21. I would get along better with my spouse if I didn't drink.
22. I have sometimes tried to get along without any alcohol at all.
23. I'd be content if I didn't drink.
24. People have often told me that they could smell alcohol on my breath.

SCORING

Each affirmative response on the seven-item physician-rating section is given a weighted score of 4, whereas each positive response on the self-report section is given a score of 1. Based on data gathered from the initial MALT validation study of 1335 German patients, the authors of the MALT recommend that patients who score 11 or above be considered alcoholic and patients scoring between 6 and 10 should be considered as "suspected" alcoholic.

MICHIGAN ALCOHOLISM SCREENING TEST (MAST)

Points   YES   NO

        0.   Do you enjoy a drink now and then?   ____ ____

(2)   *1.   Do you feel you are a normal drinker? (By normal we mean you drink less than or as much as most other people.)   ____ ____

(2)   2.   Have you ever awakened the morning after some drinking the night before and found that you could not remember a part of the evening?   ____ ____

(1)   3.   Does your wife, husband, a parent, or other near relative ever worry or complain about your drinking?   ____ ____

(2)   *4.   Can you stop drinking without a struggle after one or two drinks?   ____ ____

(1)   5.   Do you ever feel guilty about your drinking?   ____ ____

(2)   *6.   Do friends or relatives think you are a normal drinker?   ____ ____

(2)   *7.   Are you able to stop drinking when you want to?   ____ ____

(5)   8.   Have you ever attended a meeting of Alcoholics Anonymous (AA)?   ____ ____

(1)   9.   Have you gotten into physical fights when drinking?   ____ ____

(2)   10.   Has your drinking ever created problems between you and your wife, husband, a parent, or other relative?   ____ ____

(2)   11.   Has your wife, husband (or other family member) ever gone to anyone for help about your drinking?   ____ ____

(2)   12.   Have you ever lost friends because of your drinking?   ____ ____

(2)   13.   Have you ever gotten into trouble at work or school because of drinking?   ____ ____

(2)   14.   Have you ever lost a job because of drinking?   ____ ____

(2)   15.   Have you ever neglected your obligations, your family, or your work for two or more days in a row because you were drinking?   ____ ____

(1)   16.   Do you drink before noon fairly often?   ____ ____

(2)   17.   Have you ever been told you have liver trouble? Cirrhosis?   ____ ____

(2)   **18.   After heavy drinking have you ever had delirium tremens (DTs) or severe shaking, or heard voices or seen things that really weren't there?   ____ ____

(5)   19.   Have you ever gone to anyone for help about your drinking?   ____ ____

(5)   20.   Have you ever been in a hospital because of drinking?   ____ ____

(2)   21.   Have you ever been a patient in a psychiatric hospital or on a psychiatric ward of a general hospital where drinking was part of the problem that resulted in hospitalization?   ____ ____

(2)   22.   Have you ever been seen at a psychiatric or mental health clinic or gone to any doctor, social worker, or clergyman for help with any emotional problem, where drinking was part of the problem?   ____ ____

(2) ***23. Have you ever been arrested for drunk driving, driving while
intoxicated, or driving under the influence of alcoholic beverages?   ____   ____
(IF YES, How many times? _____)

(2)   24. Have you ever been arrested, or taken into custody, even for a few
hours, because of other drunk behavior?   ____   ____
(IF YES, How many times? _____)

SCORING SYSTEM

Use weighed values shown in parentheses to compute a patient's total score.
   * Alcoholic response is negative
   ** 5 points for *each* delirium tremens
   *** 2 points for *each* arrest

In general, five points or more would place the subject in an "alcoholic" category. Four points
would be suggestive of alcoholism, three points or less would indicate the subject was not alcoholic.

THE BRIEF MAST

QUESTIONS

1. Do you feel you are a normal drinker?   Yes (0) No (2)

2. Do friends or relatives think you are a normal drinker?   Yes (0) No (2)

3. Have you ever attended a meeting of Alcoholics Anonymous (AA)?   Yes (5) No (0)

4. Have you ever lost friends or girlfriends/boyfriends because of
   drinking?   Yes (2) No (0)

5. Have you ever gotten into trouble at work because of drinking?   Yes (2) No (0)

6. Have you ever neglected your obligations, your family, or your work
   for two or more days in a row because you were drinking?   Yes (2) No (0)

7. Have you ever had delirium tremens (DTs), severe shaking, heard voices
   or seen things that weren't there after heavy drinking?   Yes (2) No (0)

8. Have you ever gone to anyone for help about your drinking?   Yes (5) No (0)

9. Have you ever been in a hospital because of drinking?   Yes (5) No (0)

10. Have you ever been arrested for drunk driving or driving after drinking? Yes (2) No (0)

Scoring: Use weighted values shown in parentheses to compute total scores. Cut-off scores are the
same as for the full version of the MAST.

OBSESSIVE-COMPULSIVE DRINKING SCALE© (OCDS)©

Directions: The questions below ask you about your drinking alcohol and about your attempts to control your drinking. Please circle the number next to the statement that best applies to you.

1. How much of your time when you're not drinking is occupied by ideas, thoughts, impulses, or images related to drinking?

   (0) None
   (1) Less than 1 hour a day
   (2) 1–3 hours a day
   (3) 4–8 hours a day

2. How frequently do these thoughts occur?

   (0) Never
   (1) No more than 8 times a day
   (2) More than 8 times a day, but most hours of the day are free of these thoughts
   (3) More than 8 times a day and during most hours of the day
   (4) Thoughts are too numerous to count and an hour rarely passes without several such thoughts occurring

Insert the Higher Score of Questions 1 or 2 here _____

3. How much do these ideas, thoughts, impulses, or images related to drinking interfere with your social or work (or role) functioning? Is there anything you don't or can't do because of them? [If you are not currently working, how much of your performance would be affected if you were working?]

   (0) Thoughts of drinking never interfere. I can function normally.
   (1) Thoughts of drinking slightly interfere with my social or occupational activities, but my overall performance is not impaired.
   (2) Thoughts of drinking definitely interfere with my social or occupational performance, but I can still manage.
   (3) Thoughts of drinking cause substantial impairment in my social or occupational performance.
   (4) Thoughts of drinking interfere completely with my social or work performance.

4. How much distress or disturbance do these ideas, thoughts, impulses, or images related to drinking cause you when you're not drinking?

   (0) None
   (1) Mild, infrequent and not too disturbing
   (2) Moderate, frequent and disturbing, but still manageable
   (3) Severe, very frequent, and very disturbing
   (4) Extreme, nearly constant, and disabling distress

5. How much of an effort do you make to resist these thoughts or try to disregard or turn your attention away from these thoughts as they enter your mind when you're not drinking? (Rate *your efforts made to resist these thoughts*, not your success or failure in actually controlling them.)

   (0) My thoughts are so minimal, I don't need to actively resist. If I have thoughts, I make an effort to *always* resist.
   (1) I try to resist most of the time.
   (2) I make some effort to resist.

    (3) I give in to all such thoughts without attempting to control them, but I do so with some reluctance.

    (4) I completely and willingly give in to all such thoughts.

6. How successful are you in stopping or diverting these thoughts when you're not drinking?

    (0) I am completely successful in stopping or diverting such thoughts.

    (1) I am usually able to stop or divert such thoughts with some effort and concentration.

    (2) I am sometimes able to stop or divert such thoughts.

    (3) I am rarely successful in stopping such thoughts and can only divert such thoughts with difficulty.

    (4) I am rarely able to divert such thoughts, even momentarily.

7. How many drinks do you drink each day?

    (0) None

    (1) Less than one drink per day

    (2) 1–2 drinks per day

    (3) 3–7 drinks per day

    (4) 8 or more drinks per day

8. How many days each week do you drink?

    (0) None

    (1) No more than one day per week

    (2) 2–3 days per week

    (3) 4–5 days per week

    (4) 6–7 days per week

Insert the Higher Score of Questions 7 or 8 here _____

9. How much does your drinking interfere with your work functioning? Is there anything that you don't or can't do because of your drinking? [If you are not currently working, how much of your performance would be affected if you were working?]

    (0) Drinking never interferes — I can function normally.

    (1) Drinking slightly interferes with my occupational activities, but my overall performance is not impaired.

    (2) Drinking definitely interferes with my occupational performance, but I can still manage.

    (3) Drinking causes substantial impairment in my occupational performance.

    (4) Drinking problems interfere completely with my work performance.

10. How much does your drinking interfere with your social functioning? Is there anything that you don't or can't do because of your drinking?

    (0) Drinking never interferes — I can function normally.

    (1) Drinking slightly interferes with my social activities, but my overall performance is not impaired.

    (2) Drinking definitely interferes with my social performance, but I can still manage.

    (3) Drinking causes substantial impairment in my social performance.

    (4) Drinking problems interfere completely with my social performance

Insert the Higher Score of Questions 9 or 10 here _____

11. If you were prevented from drinking alcohol when you desired a drink, how anxious or upset would you become?

    (0) I would not experience any anxiety or irritation.
    (1) I would become only slightly anxious or irritated.
    (2) The anxiety or irritation would mount, but remain manageable.
    (3) I would experience a prominent and very disturbing increase in anxiety or irritation.
    (4) I would experience incapacitating anxiety or irritation.

12. How much of an effort do you make to resist consumption of alcoholic beverages? (Only rate *your effort to resist*, not your success or failure in actually controlling the drinking.)

    (0) My drinking is so minimal, I don't need to actively resist. If I drink, I make an effort to always resist.
    (1) I try to resist most of the time.
    (2) I make some effort to resist.
    (3) I give in to almost all drinking without attempting to control it, but I do so with some reluctance.
    (4) I completely and willingly give in to all drinking.

13. How strong is the drive to consume alcoholic beverages?

    (0) No drive
    (1) Some pressure to drink
    (2) Strong pressure to drink
    (3) Very strong drive to drink
    (4) The drive to drink is completely involuntary and overpowering.

14. How much control do you have over the drinking?

    (0) I have complete control.
    (1) I am usually able to exercise voluntary control over it.
    (2) I can control it only with difficulty.
    (3) I must drink and can only delay drinking with difficulty.
    (4) I am rarely able to delay drinking, even momentarily.

Insert the Higher Score of Questions 13 or 14 here_____

QUANTITY-FREQUENCY (QF) MEASURES — EXAMPLE

DQ1. **During the past 6 months, how often did you have WINE?**   __.____

Code for Jessor Weights: *Notes:*
1. Daily = 1.00
2. Five or six days a week = 0.80
3. Three or four days a week = 0.50
4. One or two days a week = 0.20
5. Three times a month or fewer = 0.05
6. No wine in the last six months = 0.00

DQ2. **During the past 6 months, about how much wine did you drink on a typical day in which you drank wine?**   ____.____

Key for the number of ounces: *Notes:*
A gallon = 128 oz
A liter = 33.8 oz.
A fifth = 25.6 oz
1 wine glass = 4 oz, 1 water glass = 8 oz.

DQ3. Ounces of ethanol for wine consumed: [# oz × 0.15 (or 0.20 if fortified)]   ___.____

DQ4. QF-Wine: Multiply ounces of EtOH by Jessor wt.   ___.__

DQ5. **During the past 6 months, how often did you have BEER?**   __.____

Code for Jessor Weights: *Notes:*
1. Daily = 1.00
2. Five or six days a week = 0.80
3. Three or four days a week = 0.50
4. One or two days a week = 0.20
5. Three times a month or fewer = 0.05
6. No wine in the last six months = 0.00

DQ6. **During the past 6 months, about how much beer did you drink on a typical day in which you drank beer?**   ____.____

Key for the number of ounces: *Notes:*
A case = 288 oz.
A forty = 40 oz.
A quart = 32 oz
1 beer = 12 or 16 oz.

DQ7. Ounces of ethanol for beer consumed: [# oz × 0.05 (for reg Penna beer]
[if other type beer, specify]   ___.____

DQ8. QF-Beer: Multiply ounces of EtOH by Jessor wt.   ___.____

DQ9. **During the past 6 months, how often did you have drinks containing WHISKEY or LIQUOR?**   __.____

Code for Jessor Weights: *Notes:*
1. Daily = 1.00
2. Five or six days a week = 0.80
3. Three or four days a week = 0.50
4. One or two days a week = 0.20
5. Three times a month or fewer = 0.05
6. No wine in the last six months = 0.00

**DQ10. During the past 6 months, on the days that you would drink whiskey
or liquor, about how much did you typically drink?** ＿＿＿.＿＿

Key for the number of ounces: *Notes:*
A quart = 32 oz.
A fifth = 25.6 oz.
A pint = 16 oz.
1 shot = 1.5 oz.

DQ11. Ounces of ethanol for liquor consumed: [# oz × 0.45 (for 80 proof)]   ＿＿.＿＿
OR: [0.50 for 100 proof, 0.75 for 151 proof, 0.95 for 190 proof]

DQ12. QF-Liquor: Multiply ounces of EtOH by Jessor wt.   ＿＿.＿＿

DQ13. *During the past 6 months, how often have you had any kind of beverage
containing alcohol (any kind of alcohol)? [review info already said]*   ＿.＿＿

Daily = 1.00
Five or six days a week = 0.80
Three or four days a week = 0.50
One or two days a week = 0.20
Three times a month or fewer = 0.05
No alcohol in the last six months = 0.00

QFI.   Add together QFs for wine, beer, and liquor for total quantity frequency index:
[DQ4 + DQ8 + DQ12]   ＿＿.＿＿

ADDITIONAL ITEMS SUCH AS THE FOLLOWING CAN BE INCLUDED:

TQ. Typical Quantity:

**During the past 6 months, on the days that you drink, how much do you typically
drink?**
[review info already said]

Wine: ＿＿＿＿＿＿＿
Beer: ＿＿＿＿＿＿＿
Liquor: ＿＿＿＿＿＿(include type and proof)   ＿＿.＿＿

MQ: Maximum Quantity:

During the past 6 months, what is the MOST you drank in any 24-hour period?

Wine: ＿＿＿＿＿＿＿
Beer: ＿＿＿＿＿＿＿
Liquor: ＿＿＿＿＿＿(include type and proof)   ＿＿.＿＿

5+: **How many times in the last 6 months have you had five or more drinks
on one occasion?**   ＿＿＿.

READINESS TO CHANGE QUESTIONNAIRE© (RTCQ)©

The following questionnaire is designed to identify how you personally feel about your drinking right now. Please read each of the questions below carefully, and then decide whether you agree or disagree with the statements. Please tick the answer of your choice to each question. **Your answers are completely private and confidential.**

	Strongly Disagree	Disagree	Unsure	Agree	Strongly Agree
1. I don't think I drink too much.					
2. I am trying to drink less than I used to.					
3. I enjoy my drinking, but sometimes I drink too much.					
4. Sometimes I think I should cut down on my drinking.					
5. It's a waste of time thinking about my drinking.					
6. I have just recently changed my drinking habits.					
7. Anyone can talk about wanting to do something about drinking, but I am actually doing something about it.					
8. I am at the stage where I should think about drinking less alcohol.					
9. My drinking is a problem sometimes.					
10. There is no need for me to think about changing my drinking.					
11. I am actually changing my drinking habits right now.					
12. Drinking less alcohol would be pointless for me.					

SCORING

The Precontemplation items are numbers 1, 5, 10, and 12; the Contemplation items are numbers 3, 4, 8, and 9; and the Action items are numbers 2, 6, 7, and 11. All items are to be scored on a 5-point rating scale ranging from:

-2 Strongly Disagree   +1 Agree
-1 Disagree   +2 Strongly Agree
 0 Unsure

To calculate the score for each scale, simply add the item scores for the scale in question. The range of each scale is -8 through 0 to +8. A negative scale score reflects an overall disagreement with items measuring the stage of change, whereas a positive score represents overall agreement. The highest scale score represents the Stage of Change Designation.

Note: If two scale scores are equal, then the scale farther along the continuum of change (Precontemplation — Contemplation — Action) represents the subject's Stage of Change Designation. For example, if a subject scores 6 on the Precontemplation scale, 6 on the Contemplation scale, and -2 on the Action scale, then the subject is assigned to the Contemplation stage. Note that positive scores on the Precontemplation scale signify a *lack* of readiness to change. To obtain a score for Precontemplation that represents the subject's degree of readiness to change, directly comparable to scores on the Contemplation and Action scales, simply reverse the sign of the Precontemplation score (see below).

Scale Scores   **Readiness to change**

Precontemplation Score_____   Precontemplation_____(reverse score)
Contemplation Score_____   Contemplation_____(same score)
Action Score_____   Action_____ (same score)

Stage of Change Designation (P, C, or A)_____

SHORT MICHIGAN ALCOHOLISM SCREENING TEST (sMAST)

	NO	YES

1. Do you feel you are a normal drinker? (By normal, we mean you drink less than or as much as most other people.)

2. Does your wife, husband, a parent, or other near relative ever worry or complain about your drinking?

3. Do you ever feel guilty about your drinking?

4. Do friends or relatives think you are a normal drinker?

5. Are you able to stop drinking when you want to?

6. Have you ever attended a meeting of Alcoholics Anonymous (AA)?

7. Has your drinking ever created problems between you and your wife, husband, a parent, or other relative?

8. Have you ever gotten into trouble at work or school because of drinking?

9. Have you ever neglected your obligations, your family, or your work for two or more days in a row because you were drinking?

10. Have you ever gone to anyone for help about your drinking? If YES, was this other than Alcoholics Anonymous or a hospital? (If YES, code as YES; if NO, code as NO.)

11. Have you ever been in a hospital because of drinking?

    If YES, was this for (a) detox; (b) alcoholism treatment; (c) alcohol-related injuries or medical problems, e.g., cirrhosis or physical injury incurred while under the influence of alcohol (car accident, fight, etc.).

12. Have you ever been arrested for drunk driving, driving while intoxicated, or driving under the influence of alcoholic beverages?

13. Have you ever been arrested, or taken into custody, even for a few hours, because of other drunk behavior?

SCORING

Sum across the items that are endorsed. Use the same cut-offs as the full version of the MAST.

T-ACE© QUESTIONS AND SCORING

T How many drinks does it take to make you feel high (TOLERANCE)?
A Have people ANNOYED you by criticizing your drinking?
C Have you felt you ought to CUT DOWN on your drinking?
E Have you ever had a drink first thing in the morning to steady your nerves or get rid of a hangover (EYE OPENER)?

SCORING

Question 1: Patient is considered tolerant if it took greater than two drinks to make her feel high; 2 points are assigned for this question.

Questions 2–4: 1 point is assigned to each question.

Sum all points (0–5 max). A total score of 2 or greater is considered positive for risk-drinking

TLFB©: ALCOHOL TIMELINE FOLLOW-BACK©

Start Calendar with Respondent

- Let's begin! As I said before, what we want you to do is use the calendar to record your drinking over the past ## days.
- Let's start with yesterday (date) and go back ## days — Those days are (date) through (date). **(Interviewer marks these dates on the calendar and shows the respondent.)**
- Do you have any special holidays or dates you want to mark on the calendar to help you better recall your drinking during the past ## days? **(Respondent replies and fills in calendar if appropriate.)**
- When did you last drink in this ## day period? **(Respondent replies with a date.)**
- How much did you drink on this day? **(Respondent replies with an amount and interviewer puts that number in on the calendar for the appropriate date.)**
- What was the greatest amount you consumed on any given day during this period? Do you recall when this occurred? **(Respondent replies with an amount and a date.)**
- What was the least amount of drinking during this period? **(Respondent replies with an amount.)**
- As mentioned earlier, some people will have patterns to their drinking that can help them recall their use. Do you have any notable patterns to your drinking? **(Respondent replies.)**

One Standard Drink is equal to:	
One 12-oz. regular beer	*which is equal to*
One 5-oz. glass of regular wine	*which is equal to*
1.5 oz. of spirits such as vodka or whiskey	

Your Best Estimate

- In filling out the calendar, we want you to be as accurate as possible.
- We realize that it is hard for anyone to recall things with 100% accuracy, whether it is drinking or anything else.
- If you can't recall whether you drank on a Monday or a Thursday of a certain week, or whether it was the week of November 9th or November 16th, **GIVE IT YOUR BEST GUESS.**

Probing Extended Abstinent or Drinking Periods

- During this period of time, did you have any extended periods of abstinence of 7 days or more when you did not drink any alcohol at all, not even a drop? **(Respondent replies.)**
  - What was the longest period of total abstinence during this time?
  - What was the next longest period of total abstinence?
- During this period of time, did you have any extended periods of heavy drinking of 7 days or more?
  (Respondent replies.)
  - What was the longest number of continuous days in a row you were drinking during this period? **(Determine dates and amounts of alcohol consumed on each day.)**
  - What was the next longest period of continuous drinking days?

- You appear ready to fill in the rest of the calendar. Do you have any questions?
- If not, let's begin. If you have any questions, I will be **(wherever interviewer will be).**

Example of TLFB Calendar: March 1999

Sunday	Monday	Tuesday	Wednesday	Thursday	Friday	Saturday
	1	2	3	4	5	6
7	8	9	10	11	12	13
14	15	16	17	18	19	20
21	22	23	24	25	26	27
28	29	30	31			

TWEAK QUESTIONS AND SCORING

T How many drinks can you hold ("hold" version: 5+ drinks indicates tolerance), or how many drinks does it take before you begin to feel the first effects of alcohol? ("high" version: 3+ drinks indicates tolerance).

W Have close friends or relatives WORRIED or complained about your drinking in the past year?

E Do you sometimes take a drink in the morning when you first get up?

A Has a friend or family member ever told you about things you said or did while you were drinking that you could not remember?

K Do you sometimes feel the need to cut down on your drinking?

SCORING

2 points each for T and W and 1 point each for E, A, and K. Sum all points (total 0–7 max). A total score of 3 or more is considered positive for at-risk drinking.

45 Useful (Internet) Addresses

Alcoholics Anonymous (AA)
A.A. General Service Office
Adrienne M. Brown
Coordinator, Cooperation with the Professional Community
475 Riverside Drive (between 119th and 120th Streets)
New York, NY 10115

or:

Grand Central Station
P.O. Box 459
New York, NY 10163
Tel: direct (212) 870-3107
Tel: AA operator (212) 870-3400
Fax: (212) 870-3003
coop_pc@compuserve.com
www.aa.org

National Clearinghouse for Alcohol and Drug Information
P.O. Box 2345
Rockville, MD 20847-2345
www.health.org/pubs/catalog/ordering.htm

National Institute on Alcohol Abuse and Alcoholism (NIAAA)
Parklawn Building
5600 Fishers Lane
Rockville, MD 20857
Tel: (301) 443-4223
www.niaaa.nih.gov
list of psychometric tests:
silk.nih.gov/silk/niaaa1/publication/instable.htm

Research Society on Alcoholism
4314 Medical Parkway
Suite 300
Austin, TX 78756-3332
Debra Sharp, Director
Tel: (512) 454-0022
Fax: (512) 454-0022
debbyrsa@bga.com
www.rsa.am

46 Abbreviations Used

Abbreviations for psychometric tests are sometimes followed by the © sign to indicate that the respective test is copyrighted. As there are other excellent non-copyrighted psychometric tests in the public domain, we strongly suggest use of the non-copyrighted tests rather than the copyrighted ones (please consult Chapter 44 for details and test forms).

5-HIAA	5-hydroxyindoleacetic acid, a 5HT metabolite
5HT	5-hydroxytryptamine = serotonin
A10	dopamine-neuron containing area 10, ventral tegmental area
AA	Alcoholics Anonymous
AA rat	Alko rat, alcohol-preferring
AC	adenylyl cyclase
ACE	angiotensin converting enzyme
ACM	alcoholic cardiomyopathy
ACTH	adrenocorticotrophic hormone, corticotropin
ADE	alcohol deprivation effect
ADH	antidiuretic hormone, vasopressin
ADHD	attention deficit hyperactivity disorder
ADS©	Alcohol Dependence Scale©
AE	alcoholic embryopathy
AG	anion gap
AH	alcoholic hepatitis
AKA	alcoholic ketoacidosis
ALAT	alanine aminotransferase
ALD	alcoholic liver disease
ALP	alkaline phosphatase
ALT	alanine aminotransferase
ANA rat	Alko rat, non-alcohol-preferring
ASAT	aspartate aminotransferase
ASI	Addiction Severity Index
ASPD	antisocial personality disorder
AST	aspartate aminotransferase
ATN	acute tubular necrosis
AUDIT©	Alcohol Use Disorders Identification Test©
AV	atrioventricular
AWS	alcohol withdrawal syndrome
b.i.d., BID	*bis in die* (two times a day)
BAC	blood alcohol concentration
BAL	blood alcohol level
bMAST	brief Michigan Alcoholism Screening Test
BRFSS	Behavioral Risk Factor Surveillance System
BUN	blood urea nitrogen
CAGE	Cut down-Annoyed-Guilty-Eye opener (i.e., a short psychometric test)
cAMP	cyclic adenosine monophosphate
CBT	cognitive behavioral therapy
CCK	cholecystokinin
CD4+	helper (T-cells)
CD8+	suppressor (T-cells)

CDT	carbohydrate-deficient transferrin
CHD	coronary heart disease
CIWA-Ar	Clinical Institute Withdrawal Assessment Scale for Alcohol, Revised
CK	creatine kinase
COGA	Collaborative Study on the Genetics of Alcoholism
ConA	concanavalin A
COPD	chronic obstructive pulmonary disorder
COX-2	cyclooxygenase type 2
CRH	corticotropin-releasing hormone
CRP	C-reactive protein
CT	computed tomography
CV	coefficient of variation
CYP2E1	isoform E1 of family 2 of the cytochrome P450-associated enzyme system
D_1, D_2, D_3, D_4, D_5	Dopamine receptor subtypes: Dopamine 1 receptor, etc.
DA	dopamine
DAR	disulfiram-alcohol reaction
DAT	dopamine transporter
DER	disulfiram-ethanol reaction
DOPA	dihydroxyphenylalanine
DOPAC	dihydroxyphenylacetic acid
DSM DSM-IV	Diagnostic and Statistical Manual (of Mental Disorders); currently in version IV (DSM-IV)
DUI	driving under the influence of alcohol
DWI	driving while intoxicated
ECA	Epidemiological Catchment Area (study)
ECG	electrocardiogram
ECT	electroconvulsive therapy
EEG	electroencephalogram
ERCP	Endoscopic retrograde cholangiopancreatography
FAE	fetal alcohol effects
FAS	fetal alcohol syndrome
FHM	negative family history of alcoholism
FHP	positive family history of alcoholism
FRAMES	six elements of brief intervention: Feedback – Responsibility – Advice – Menu – Empathy – Self-efficacy
FSH	follicle stimulating hormone
GABA	gamma-aminobutyric acid
GAD	generalized anxiety disorder
GGT	gamma-glutamyl transferase
GH	growth hormone
GHB	gamma-hydroxybutyric acid
GOT	glutamic-oxaloacetic transaminase (= AST)
GPT	glutamic-pyruvic transaminase (= ALT)
H, H_1, H_2	histamine, histamine$_1$ (receptor), histamine$_2$ (receptor)
HAB	High-anxiety-related behavior (rats)
HAM-D	Hamilton Depression (scale)
HDL	high density lipoprotein (cholesterol)
HFE	hemochromatosis (gene)
HLA	human leukocyte antigen
HPA	hypothalamic-pituitary-gonadal
HRS	hepatorenal syndrome
HVA	homovanillic acid
ICD ICD-10	International Classification of Diseases, currently in version 10 (ICD-10)
IFN	interferon

IL	interleukin
IQ	intelligence quotient
ITT	intention-to-treat
IUGR	intrauterine growth retardation
JNC	Joint National Committee on prevention, detection, evaluation, and treatment of high blood pressure
K_m	Michaelis-Menten constant
LAB	Low-anxiety-related behavior (rats)
LDH	lactate dehydrogenase
LDL	low density lipoprotein (cholesterol)
LH	luteinizing hormone
LPA	liters pure alcohol
μM	micromolar, *see* M
M	molar, mol per liter (mol/l)
MALT©	Munich Alcoholism Test©
MAO	monoamine oxidase
MAST	Michigan Alcoholism Screening Test
MCH	mean corpuscular hemoglobin
MCV	mean corpuscular volume (of erythrocytes)
MET	Motivational Enhancement Therapy
MHC	major histocompatibility complex
mM	millimolar, see M
mol	6×10^{23} molecules
MRCP	Magnetic resonance cholangiopancreatography
MRI	magnetic resonance imaging
NAC	nucleus accumbens
NASH	non-alcoholic steatohepatitis
NCS	National Comorbidity Survey
NIAAA	National Institute on Alcohol Abuse and Alcoholism
N_{ITT}	number of patients included on an intention-to-treat basis
NMDA	N-methyl-D-aspartate
NP rat	alcohol-non-preferring rat
NSAID	nonsteroidal antiinflammatory drug
OCD	obsessive compulsive disorder
OCDS©	Obsessive-Compulsive Drinking Scale©
OPRM1	allele 1 for the mu opioid receptor
OR	odds ratio
P rat	alcohol-preferring rat
P300	positive EEG wave 300ms after an event
PAOD	peripheral arterial occlusive disease
PB	peripheral blood
PCT	Porphyria cutanea tarda
PDYN	Pro-dynorphin
PENK	Pro-enkephalin
pg	picogram, 10^{-12} grams
PHA	phytohemagglutinin
PKC	protein kinase C
POMC	Pro-opiomelanocortin
PPI	proton pump inhibitor
PT	prothrombin time
PTH	parathyroid hormone
PTSD	posttraumatic stress disorder
PUVA	Psoralen and UV-A-irradiation
PWM	pokeweed mitogen
q.i.d., QID	*quater in die* (four times a day)

QF	Quantity-Frequency measures
QTL	quantitative trait locus (analysis)
RA	rheumatoid arthritis
RIA	radioimmunoassay
ROC	receiver operating characteristic
RSA	Research Society on Alcoholism
RTCQ©	Readiness to Change Questionnaire©
SAM	S-adenosyl-L-methionine
SCD	sudden cardiac death
SCID	Structured Clinical Interview (for DSM-IV disorders)
SLE	systemic lupus erythematosus
sMAST	Short Michigan Alcoholism Screening Test
SOCRATES	Stages of Change Readiness and Treatment Eagerness Scale
SSRI	selective serotonin reuptake inhibitor
t.i.d., TID	*tres in die* (three times a day)
T_3	triiodothyronine
T_4	tetraiodothyronine, thyroxine
T-ACE©	Tolerance-Annoyed-Cut Down-Eye opener (i.e., a short psychometric test)©
Th-1	a certain type of differentiated T cell
TIA	turbidimetric immunoassay
TIPS	transjugular intrahepatic portasystemic shunt
TLFB©	alcohol Timeline Follow-Back©
TNF	tumor necrosis factor
TPH	tryptophan hydroxylase
TSF	Twelve-Step Facilitation
TWEAK	Tolerance-Worried-Eye opener-Amnesia –Kutdown (i.e., a short psychometric test)
UNDCP	United Nations International Drug Control Programme
UV-A	ultraviolet radiation of lower energy and higher wavelength (315–400 nm) than UV-B
VTA	ventral tegmental area, A10 area

Index

Note: When several page numbers are given, bold face type indicates that the term is discussed in most detail on that page. Often, the terms "alcohol," "ethanol," "alcoholism," "alcoholic," and "alcoholics" are not explicitly used as they are an inherent part of many terms. For example, "alcoholism typology" or "types of alcoholics" can by found under "typology." Similarly, "drug interactions" refer to "alcohol-drug interactions." Treatment of any alcohol-related disorder can be found under the name of the disorder. Comentioning of two terms does not mean that a relationship actually exists; for example, a number of parameters have been claimed to be markers for a (hereditary) vulnerability to alcoholism; most of them are not. However, all *alleged* markers of a predisposition to alcoholism that are discussed in this handbook are listed as "marker." Similarly, the concept and factual basis for craving and the "anti-craving" effect of "anticraving drugs" is highly controversial (although some of these drugs significantly reduce alcohol consumption and are effective in the treatment of alcohol abuse and dependence). Still, these drugs are listed as "anticraving drugs" wherever this concept is discussed.

4-Methylpyrazol,
    in ethylene glycol and methanol poisoning, 421
5-HIAA, 372, 389–390
5HT, *see also* Serotonin
5HT system,
    and alcohol abuse and dependence, 372–373
    and SSRIs, 121
    as marker of vulnerability to alcoholism, 309
$5HT_{1A}$ agonists, 372
$5HT_{1A}$ receptor,
    and buspirone, 121
$5HT_{1B}$ receptor,
    knockout, 394
$5HT_3$ receptor,
    in ventral tegmental area (VTA) and nucleus accumbens (NAC), 373
    signal transfer, 373
$5HT_3$ receptor antagonists,
    anxiogenic properties, 373
    effect on neurochemical and behavioral alcohol effects, 372
    exacerbation of alcohol withdrawal-induced seizures, 373
8-OH-DPAT, 372

A

A_1 allele of the D_2 receptor gene,
    as marker of vulnerability to alcoholism, 310, 402
A10 area,
    is ventral tegmental area (VTA), 373
AA, *see* Alcoholics Anonymous
AA rat, 374, 377, 393–394, 402, 408
Abbreviations, 459

Abdominal pain,
    and alcoholic ketoacidosis, 209
Absorption,
    of alcohol, 421
    influencing factors, 421
Abstinence, 85, 105
    contented,
        as goal of psychotherapy, 6, 104
    continuous,
        as outcome criterion in clinical trials, 121, 122
    predictors, 23, 24
    reversibility of bodily disorders upon, *see* Reversibility
Abstinence violation effect, 115
Abuse,
    case study, 328
    in childhood,
        as risk factor for alcohol abuse in women, 153
    of adolescents, 129
Acamprosate,
    in alcohol abuse and dependence, 85, **121–125**, 170, 171, 343, 339–351, 356–360
    animal research, 395
    dosage, 123
    effect size, 345
    mechanism of action, 121, 395
    meta-analysis of published clinical trials, 356–360
    side effects and contraindications, 123
Accident rates,
    and alcohol consumption in the general population, data on 40 countries, 205, 273
Accumbens, *see* Nucleus accumbens
Accuracy,
    definition of, 29
ACE, *see* Angiotensin converting enzyme
Acetaldehyde, 309, 317

and gastric injury, 199
  role in flushing, 241
  toxic effects on endocrine system, 231
Acetaldehyde-protein adducts, 318
  and anaphylactic reactions, 241
Acetate,
    CNS effects in common with alcohol and adenosine,
      375
Acetylsalicylic acid,
    in chlorpropamide-alcohol flush, 241
Acid-base disturbances, 209–212
Acidosis, 209–211, *see also* individual acidotic disorders
  alcoholic ketoacidosis (AKA), 209–210
  lactic, 210–211
Acitretine, 246–247
Acne comedonica, 246
Acne conglobata, is Acne nodulocystica, 246
Acne rosacea, *see* Rosacea
Acneiform skin disorders, alcohol-induced, *see* Rosacea
Acoustic hallucinations, alcohol-induced, 74
Acrocyanosis, 249
Acrodermatitis enteropathica, 248
ACTH, *see* Adrenocorticotropic hormone
Action,
    in stage model of change, 99, 100
Action schemata,
    in drug use, 405
Activation of resources,
    as general effect factor in psychotherapy, 105
Actualization of the underlying psychological problem,
    as general effect factor in psychotherapy, 105
Acute alcohol intoxication, *see* Intoxication
Acute renal failure,
    in cirrhosis, 220
    secondary to rhabdomyolysis, 217
Acute tubular necrosis (ATN), 220
Addiction counseling, *see* Counseling
Addiction Severity Index (ASI), **332–333**, 366
Addiction,
    vs. dependence 92
Addresses,
    useful, 457
Adenocarcinomas,
    of esophagus and gastric carida, 198
Adenosine receptor,
    and alcohol abuse and dependence, 375
Adenosine reuptake inhibitor, 375, 376
Adenylyl cyclase (AC),
    activity,
        as marker of vulnerability to alcoholism, 308
    and adenosine receptor, 375, 376
Adolescents,
    consequences of alcohol abuse, 133
    special therapeutic considerations, 15, **129–136**
Adolescent alcohol abuse and dependence,
    differential diagnosis, 133
Adoption studies, 305
Adrenalin,
    in alcohol-related anaphylactic reactions, dosage, 241
Adrenoceptor, 174

Adrenoceptor antagonists, *see* Alpha blockers and Beta
      blockers
Adrenocorticotropic hormone (ACTH), 234
ADS©, *see* Alcohol Dependence Scale©
Adulthood,
    alcohol problems in, 17
Adverse effects of alcohol,
    vs. cultural factors,
        impact on alcohol consumption in Japanese and
          Caucasians, 274
Advice, *see* Psychotherapy and Motivational therapy
Affective disorders,
    and alcohol abuse and dependence, 291
Aftercare, 113–114
  in women, 156
Aggression,
    verbal,
        against women, 153
Agitation,
    in electrolyte disturbances, 212–215
    in hypokalemia, 214
    in withdrawal, 66
Agoraphobia, 407
Alanine aminotransferase (ALT), 32, 185
Al-Anon, www.alanon.org
Alcohol, *see* more specific terms
    as antidote in ethylene glycol and methanol poisoning,
      421
    inhibition of inhibitory GABA$_A$ interneurons in ventral
      tegmental area, 401
Alcohol competence,
    in stage model of change, 100
Alcohol consumption,
    per capita,
        Austria, 273,274
        USA, 273, 274
        data on 40 countries, 272–274
Alcohol contents of typical drinks, *see* back inside cover
Alcohol dehydrogenase (ADH), 309, 317
    activity in women, 152
    enzymatic parameters, 421
    gastric, 421
    gastric,
        generation of toxic alcohol metabolites 199
    polymorphism, 321
Alcohol Dependence Scale (ADS)©, 333
    test form, 440–441
Alcohol deprivation effect (ADE), 391, 406
Alcohol embryopathy (AE), 206, 251–267
    definition of stages I to III, 254
    degree of,
        correlation with degree of maternal alcohol
          consumption, 260–263
    diagnosis and classification, 253
    differential diagnosis, 260
    in twins, 263
Alcohol intolerance, 227–228, 240–241
    treatment,
        dosages, 241
Alcohol patch test, *see* Ethanol patch test
Alcohol serum levels, *see* Blood alcohol level

Alcohol Use Disorder Identification Test (AUDIT) ©, 43, 166
    in geriatric patients, 139
    test form, 167–168, 442–443
Alcohol withdrawal delirium, *see* Delirium and Withdrawal
Alcohol withdrawal syndrome (AWS), *see* Withdrawal
Alcohol-disulfiram reaction (DAR),
    definition and clinical signs, 423
Alcoholic cardiomyopathy (ACM), 203
Alcoholic ketoacidosis, *see* Acidosis
Alcoholic personality, 93, *see also* Typology
Alcoholic polyneuropathy, *see* Polyneuropathy
Alcoholics Anonymous (AA), 107, 110, 170, 365
    address and web site, 457, www.aa.org
    and women, 155
Alcoholics,
    types, *see* Typology
Alcoholism, *see* all alcohol-related disorders, especially Section 1 (Chapters 1–24)
Aldehyde dehydrogenase (ALDH), 309
    deficiency,
        in Finns, 423
        in people of Asian descent, 423
        in South-American indians, 423
    enzymatic parameters, 423
    isoforms,
        as marker of vulnerability to alcoholism, 310
Aldosterone, 206, 234
    level, 174
Alkaloses, 211–212
Alkalosis,
    metabolic, 211
    respiratory, 211
Alko® rat, 393
Alleles, 310, 402
Allergic reaction, type I,
    against alcohol, 241
Allergies,
    worsening by alcohol, 241
Alpha blockers,
    in alcohol-induced hypertension, 206
Alpha hypoactivity,
    as marker of vulnerability to alcoholism, 307
Alpha$_2$ receptor,
    and buspirone, 121
ALT, *see* Alanine aminotransferase
Alzheimer's disease, 138
Ambivalence,
    in stage model of change, 100
Amblyopy, 177
Amenorrhoea, 232, 233
American Psychiatric Association (APA), 170
American Society of Addiction Medicine,
    guidelines for treatment of withdrawal, 170
Ammonia, 66
Amnesia,
    in Korsakoff syndrome, 176
Amnestic syndrome, 7, *see also* Cognitive deficits
Amount of alcohol consumed,
    as outcome criterion in clinical trials, 122
    determination of,
        psychotherapeutic relevance, 8

Amygdala,
    reward pathways, 374
ANA rats, 374, 377, 393–394, 402, 408
Anabolic androgens,
    in alcoholic hepatitis, 188
Anaphylactic reactions,
    to alcohol 240–241
Androgen deficit,
    in alcohol dependence, 231
Androgens,
    anabolic,
        in alcoholic hepatitis, 187–188
Anemia, 7
    hyperchrome, 66
    megaloblastic, *see* Anemia, pernicious
    pernicious, 240
Angiotensin, 234
Angiotensin converting enzyme (ACE) inhbitors,
    in alcohol-induced hypertension, 206
Anhedonic components,
    of reinforcement, 403
Animal studies,
    relevance to human situation,
        criteria, 386–387
Anion gap, 60, 62, 210
    definition and normal range, 210
    in acute alcohol intoxication, 60, 62
Anorexia,
    and alcohol abuse and dependence, 293
Antabuse®, *see* Disulfiram
Antacids,
    in acute gastritis, 199
Anterior commissure, *see* Commissura anterior
Antibiotics,
    in acute pancreatitis, 197
Anticonvulsant prophylaxis,
    in withdrawing alcohol dependent patients, 67–68
Anticonvulsants,
    in alcohol withdrawal syndrome, 68
Anticraving drugs,
    concept of, 125
    in geriatric patients, 143
    meta-analysis of clinical trials with, 340
Antidiuretic hormone (ADH), *see* Vasopressin
Antihistamines,
    in alcohol intolerance, 228, 241
    in alcohol-related anaphylactic reactions,
        dosages 241
Antimongoloid slant,
    to palpebral fissures,
        in alcohol embryopathy, 254
Antioxidant effects,
    of wine, 226
Antipsychotics, *see* Neuroleptics
Antireflux surgery, 198
Antirheumatic drugs,
    drug interaction with alcohol, 228
Antisocial personality disorder (ASPD), 153, *see also* Personality disorder
    and alcohol abuse and dependence, 294
    definition of, 294

Anxiety,
   and alcohol dependence, 406–408
   as negative reinforcer maintaining alcohol abuse, 407
   as risk factor in adolescents, 133
   generalized and other, 7, 133, 288
   in geriatric patients, 138
   in withdrawal, 66
Apgar score,
   decrease after maternal alcohol consumption, 263
Apnea,
   during sleep, *see* Sleep apnea
   in hypokalemia, 214
Apomorphine,
   in the treatment of alcohol dependence, 96
Appetite,
   reduced, 7
Appetitive behavior,
   in eating disorders, 293
   naltrexone effects on, 395
Area tegmentalis ventralis (VTA), *see* Ventral tegmental
      area
Arrhythmias,
   in alcohol-induced hypokalemia, 214–215
   supraventricular or ventricular, 205
Arterial obliteration, *see* Coronary heart disease (CHD)
Arterial puncture,
   vs. venous sampling, 61
Arthropathy,
   psoriatic, 244–245
Ascites,
   detection limit in routine physical examination, 218
   pathophysiology, 218–219
Ascorbic acid,
   deficiency,
      in alcohol dependence, 240
   supplementation,
      dosage, 240
ASI, *see* Addiction Severity Index
Aspartate aminotransferase (AST), 32, 185
Aspirin®, *see* Acetylsalicylic acid
Assertiveness training, 96
Assessment,
   of alcohol abuse and dependence, in adolescents, 130,
      132
Asterixis (flapping tremor),
   in hepatic encephalopathy, 176
Asthma,
   in alcohol-related anaphylactic reactions, 241
Ataxia,
   in alcohol embryopathy, 258
   in myelinolysis, 176
Atenolol,
   effect size, 345
   in alcohol abuse and dependence, 123, 343
Atherosclerosis, 174
Atrial fibrillation,
   in alcohol-induced heart failure, 203
Atrioventricular block,
   alcohol-induced, 205
At-risk drinker, *see* Problem drinker

Attention,
   decrease in,
      in withdrawal, 66
Attention deficit,
   in alcohol embryopathy, 253
Attention deficit disorder,
   as risk factor,
      in adolescents, 132
Attention deficit hyperactivity disorder (ADHD), 297
Attitude,
   obtaining a helpful therapeutic one, 90
   towards alcohol,
      role in the development of alcohol dependence 95,
         see also Stage model of change
AUDIT©, *see* Alcohol Use Disorder Identification Test©
Authentic affective response,
   of psychotherapist, 99, 101
Authenticity,
   in client-centered therapy, 101
Authority,
   and adolescents, 130
Autoantibodies,
   in alcohol dependence, 227
Autogenic training, 102–103
Autoimmune diseases, 227
Autonomic disorders, 178
Auxiological data,
   in alcohol embryopathy, 259
AV block,
   alcohol-induced, 205
Aversion therapy, 96
Aversive states,
   induced by mu opioid receptor inhibition, 374
Avoidant personality disorder,
   and alcohol abuse and dependence 294
Awareness,
   importance for relapse prevention, 115
Azotemia, 219

B

B cells,
   reduced levels,
      in alcohol dependence, 226
Babinski sign, 50
Baboon, 388
Babor's classification, of alcoholism types, 297
BALB/cJ mouse, 393
Balint groups, 93
Barbiturates,
   and GABA$_A$ receptor, 369, 370
   drug interactions with alcohol, 422, 425–427
   in alcohol withdrawal syndrome and dependence,
      obsolete, 68
   in drug discrimination 371
Barrett's esophagus, 198
Beer, alcohol contents, *see* back inside cover
   as histamine-rich food,
      in alcohol intolerance, 241
   phytoestrogens in, 232
Beer drinker's syndrome 216

Behavioral pharmacology, 385–400

Behavioral therapy, *see* Cognitive behavioral therapy

Beliefs,
    alcohol-related, 95

Beneficial effect of some alcoholic beverages,
    in atherosclerosis,
        see Resveratrol

Benzodiazepines,
    and GABA$_A$ receptor,
    in alcohol abuse and dependence, 369, 370
    drug interactions with alcohol, 422, 425–427
    effective doses in chronic alcohol users, 67–68
    in agitation-induced respiratory alkalosis, 212
    in alcohol withdrawal syndrome, **67**, 169–170, 212
    in delirium tremens, 67
    risks in acute alcohol intoxication, 58

beriberi, 240

Beta blockers,
    in alcohol withdrawal syndrome, 68, 207
    in alcohol-induced arrhythmias, 206
    in alcohol-induced hypertension, 206

Beta hyperactivity,
    as marker of vulnerability to alcoholism, 307

Beta-endorphin, 373
    as agonist for mu opioid receptor, 373
    as marker of vulnerability to alcoholism, 309

Beverages,
    alcohol contents, *see* back inside cover
    rich in histamine, 241

Bilirubin, 66
    in alcoholic hepatitis, 187
    in cirrhosis, 189

Binge drinking,
    differences across countries, 276
    in adolescents, 278
    in primates, 397

Biofeedback, 102–103

Biopsy,
    of the liver, 186

Bipolar disorders,
    and alcohol abuse and dependence, 292

Birth, problems during, in alcohol abuse and dependence, 152

Birth weight, in alcohol embryopathy, 259

Blackouts, in adolescents, 134
    in the elderly, 141

Bladder,
    diverticula of,
        in alcohol embryopathy, 258

Bleeding,
    from esophageal varices, 189
    intracranial, *see* front inside cover, 55

Blepharophimosis,
    in alcohol embryopathy, 254

Blood alcohol concentration, *see* Blood alcohol level

Blood alcohol level,
    and GABA$_A$ receptor interaction, 369
    and NMDA receptor interaction, 371
    calculation of,
        after drinking event, 419
    in mild intoxication, 60, 173

in moderate intoxication, 60, 173
    in severe intoxication, 60, 173
    in women, 152
    lethal, 60, 173
    monkey, 387–390
    rat, 390–395
    time course after drinking, 31, 419
    units and conversion factors, *see* back inside cover

Blood gas analysis,
    in acute alcohol intoxication, 56
    normal range, 56

Blood presssure,
    see also Hypertension and Hypotension
    alcohol as secondmost prevalent risk factor for
        hypertension, 206
    dual effect of alcohol on, 206
    in alcohol withdrawal syndrome, 66

Blood tests,
    in acute alcohol intoxication, 56, 60
    normal values, 60

Blood vessels, 203–207
    enlargement of collaterals,
        in cirrhosis, 189

Blood-to-plasma level conversion, 462, *see* back inside
        cover

bMAST,
    test form, 41, 447, *see also* Michigan Alcoholism
        Screening Test, brief version

Bodily sensations,
    reattribution of,
        in psychotherapy, 102

Body fat,
    in the calculation of maximum blood alcohol level, 419

Body hair,
    loss of,
        in hypogonadism, 233

Body therapy, 102

Body water,
    percent,
        in men, 419
        in women, 419

Boiling point,
    of alcohol (ethanol), 417

Bone and mineral metabolism,
    impairment by alcohol, 232, 235

Bone,
    loss of,
        in alcohol dependence, 235

Borderline personality disorder, 153, *see also* Personality
        disorder
    and alcohol abuse and dependence, 294
    in psychoanalytic theory, 99

Bourbon whiskey,
    phytoestrogens in, 232

Brachyclinodactyly,
    in alcohol embryopathy, 252, 258

Brain areas,
    involved in alcohol reinforcement, 374

Brain morphology,
    in alcohol embryopathy, 258

Brain serotonin,
    upon acute alcohol administration, 372
Brain stimulation,
    electrical, 401
Breast milk,
    free passage of alcohol into,
        in alcohol-abusing nursing mothers, *see*
            Pharmacokinetics
British units,
    conversion to U.S. measures and SI units, *see* back
        inside cover, 61, 63
Bromocriptine,
    effect size, 345
    in alcohol abuse and dependence, 121, 343, 403
Bugs,
    in epizoonoses, 249
Bulimia,
    and alcohol abuse and dependence, 293
    in differential diagnosis of adolescent alcohol abuse,
        133
Bull's neck,
    in Pseudo-Cushing's syndrome, 233
Bundle branch block,
    alcohol-induced, 205
Buspirone,
    effect size, 345
    in alcohol abuse and dependence, 121–124, 343
    mechanism of action, 121
Butterfly skin eruption, 240

C

C57BL/6J mouse, 393
CAGE, 41, 42, 44, 157, 166
    test form, 167, 443
CAGE scores,
    in primary care setting, 280
    and probability of detecting alcohol dependence, 166
Calcitriol,
    active metabolite of vitamin D, *see* Vitamin D
Calcium,
    supplementation,
        dosage, 235
Calcium antagonists,
    in alcohol-induced hypertension, 206
Calcium carbimide, *see* Carbimide
Calcium channel blockers, *see* Calcium antagonists
Calcium channels/influx, 371, 395
Calcium influx,
    NMDA-mediated, 371
Calculation,
    of maximum blood alcohol level, after drinking event,
        419
    of meta-analysis, 353–362
cAMP,
    and adenosine receptor, 375
Cancer
    breast,
        prevalence in alcohol dependence, 227
    colorectal, 200

esophageal, 198
    prevalence in alcohol dependence, 227
    liver, *see* Liver, cancer of
    oral mucosa, 249
        prevalence in alcohol dependence, 227
    stomach, 198
Caput medusae,
    in cirrhosis, 189
Carbamazepine,
    in alcohol abuse and dependence, 123
    in alcohol withdrawal syndrome, 68
Carbimide, 423
Carbohydrate deficient transferrin (CDT), 7, 29, 32–34
        commercially available tests, description of, 33–34
        in geriatric patients, 139
        transferrin (CDT),
            sensitivity and specificity, 32, 34–35
Carbonated beverages,
    and alcohol absorption, 421
Carcinogenesis,
    of alcohol and smoking,
        of esophageal cancer, 198
Cardiomyopathy, alcoholic, 203
Cardiovascular system, 203–207
    harmful and beneficial alcohol effects on, 204
Carotid atherosclerosis, 174
Casal's necklace, 240
Case manager,
    and women, 157
Case studies,
    of natural recovery, 283–284
Catabolic conditions, 248
Catalase,
    enzymatic parameters, 421
Caudate,
    reward pathways, 374
Causal attribution,
    in alcohol dependence, 96
Caveats,
    when performing a meta-analysis, 360
CBT, *see* Cognitive Behavioral Therapy
CD4+ T cells,
    and alcohol, 225
CD8+ T cells,
    and alcohol, 225
CDT, *see* Carbohydrate deficient transferrin
Cefuroxime,
    in acute pancreatitis, 197
Cerebellum,
    atrophy, 175
    hypoplasia,
        in alcohol embryopathy, 258
    vermis, 175
Cerebral atrophy, alcoholic,
    greater risk for women, 152
Cerebral vascular diseases, 174
Cerebrospinal fluid (CSF), 389
Cetirizine,
    in alcohol-related anaphylactic reactions, dosage, 241
Chain of seemingly minor decisions,
    leading to relapse, 115

Champagne,
    alcohol contents, *see* back inside cover
    as histamine-rich food, in alcohol intolerance, 241
Change,
    of attitude toward alcohol, *see* Stage model of change
Cheese,
    as histamine-rich food, in alcohol intolerance, 241
Cheilitis, 246
Chemical structure and properties,
    of alcohol (ethanol), 417
Child-Pugh classification,
    of chronic liver diseases,
        definition of 190
Children,
    as beneficial factor,
        in women, 155
    of alcohol dependent parents,
        risk of alcohol abuse and dependence, *see*
            Adolescents
    of alcohol dependent parents,
        risk of malformations, *see* Alcohol embryopathy
Chlordiazepoxide,
    in withdrawal, 169
Chloroquine, 244
Chlorpheniramine,
    in alcohol-related anaphylactic reactions, dosage, 241
Chlorpropamide-alcohol-flush, 241
Choice of psychotherapeutic approach, 106
Cholecystokinin (CCK) test,
    in chronic pancreatitits, 197
Cholecystolithiasis,
    in erythropoetic proptoporphyria, 244
Cholestasis, 186
    pathophysiology, 320
Cholesterol,
    and alcohol, 205
Choreiform dyskinesia,
    see Dyskinesia, choreiform
Choreoathetotis,
    in hepatic encephalopathy, 176
Chromosome 11, 402
Chronic obstructive pulmonary disease (COPD), 53
Chvostek sign,
    in hypocalcemia or hypomagnesemia, 213, 214
Cimicosis, 249
Cinnarizine,
    in perniones, 249
Cirrhosis, 218, 321
    and immune function, 226
    associated renal disturbances, 218
    clinical signs, 189, 218
    definition of, 189
    differential diagnosis, 189
    diuretic therapy, 218–219
Cirrhosis rate, and alcohol consumption, data on 40
        countries, 273
    and alcohol consumption,
        dose-cirrhosis rate-relationship, 183–184, 326
    beneficial effect of Prohibition on, 183
Citalopram,
    effect size, 345

in alcohol abuse and dependence, 121, 123, 343
    mechanism of action, 121
CIWA-Ar, *see* Clinical Institute Withdrawal Assessment
        Scale for Alcohol, Revised
Clarification,
    as general effect factor in psychotherapy, 105
    definition of, in psychoanalysis, 98
Class-I-ADH, 421
Cleft palate,
    in alcohol embryopathy, 258
Client-centered therapy, 101
Clinical Institute Withdrawal Assessment Scale for
        Alcohol, Revised (CIWA-Ar), 66
    score,
        as criterion for therapy of withdrawal, 67
    test form, 444
Clinical interview technique, 9–10, 107
Clinical setting, *see* Setting
Clinical signs,
    in geriatric patients, 140–141
    of alcohol-disulfiram-reaction, 423
    of alcohol-induced gastrointestinal disorders, 196
    of chronic alcohol consumption, 7,8,107
Clinical trials,
    criteria for inclusion in meta-analysis, 354, 360
    criteria of quality, 354, 360
    on pharmacotherapy of alcoholism, 121–127, 339–351,
        356–360
    on psychotherapy of alcoholism, 111
Clinodactyly,
    in alcohol embryopathy, 252, 258
Clomethiazol,
    is obsolete in alcohol withdrawal syndrome and
        dependence, 68
Clonidine,
    in alcohol withdrawal syndrome, 68
Cloninger's classification,
    of alcoholism types, *see* Typology, Clonininger
        classification
Clouding of consciousness,
    in alcohol withdrawal syndrome, 66
Coabuse,
    of other drugs of abuse with alcohol, *see*
        Polytoxicomania
Coarctation,
    of the aorta, 206
Cocaine,
    in acute alcohol intoxication, 59
Codependence,
    definition of, 108–109
COGA, *see* Collaborative Study on the Genetics of
        Alcoholism
Cognitive behavioral therapy (CBT), 83, 94–97, 105, 365
    brief definition of theoretical concept, 94
Cognitive deficits,
    in alcohol dependence, 6, 175
Cognitive distortions,
    leading to relapse, 115
Cognitive premises,
    change of,
        in social skills training, 96

Colchicine,
in cirrhosis, 190
Collaborative Study on the Genetics of Alcoholism
(COGA), 289, 290, 292, 293, 311, 402
Collateral reports, 8, 39–40, 332–335, *see also*
Psychometric test instruments and Denial
Collateral vessels,
enlargement of,
in cirrhosis, 189
Colorectal cancer, 200
Colorectal polyps, 200
Coma,
in acute alcohol intoxication, 54
in hepatic encephalopathy, 176
COMBINE,
clinical trial combining acamprosate and naltrexone,
125
Comedication,
in alcohol users, *see* Drug interactions
Commissura anterior,
reward pathways, 374
Commitment,
in stage model of change, 99, 100
Comorbidity,
definition of, 287
Comorbidity of alcohol abuse and dependence,
and abuse of other drugs, 290, *see also* Polytoxicomania
and affective disorders, 291
and anxiety, 271, 288, 406–408
and bipolar disorders, 292
and depression (major), 271, **291**
and diabetes mellitus, 271
and eating disorders, 293
and hypertension, 206, 271
and mania, 292
and personality disorders, 293
and phobic disorders, 407
and posttraumatic stress disorder (PTSD), 289
and psychiatric disorders, 271, 287–303
and schizophrenia, 271, 295
and smoking, 271, 295, 307
and suicidal behavior, 295
and thought disorders, 271
and violence, 271
in geriatric patients, 138
in women, 153
Complaints,
of alcohol-abusing and dependent patients, 7–8
Complications,
in intoxication, 58
Concanavalin A (ConA), 225
Concentrated alcohol,
and alcohol absorption, 421
Concentration,
loss of, *see* Cognitive deficits
Concentration of alcohol,
maximum,
in intravenous administration, 395
Conditioned place preference, 373
Conditioning, *see* Operant or Respondent conditioning
Conflicts,

definition of,
in psychoanalysis, 98
leading to relapse, 115
Confrontation,
definition of,
in psychoanalysis, 98
Confusion,
in electrolyte disturbances, 212–215
Congenital malformations,
in alcohol embryopathy, 251–260
Congestive heart failure,
alcohol-induced, 203
Conjunctivitis, 246
Consciousness,
clouding of,
in withdrawal, 66
Consequences,
of alcohol abuse, *see* Chapters 3–24
in adolescents, 133
Consumption,
monkey, 387–390
rat, 390–395
Contemplation,
in stage model of change, 99, 100
Contents,
of alcoholic drinks, *see* back inside cover
Continuous variable,
definition of, 355, 356
Controlled drinking,
as goal of psychotherapy, 104
predictors of success of, 23
vs. abstinence, 85, 345, 347
Controversial research areas, 401–413
Conversion table, *see* back inside cover
Coping deficits, 96
Coronary heart disease (CHD),
alcohol as benefical factor against, 204
Corpus callosum,
agenesis of,
in alcohol embryopathy, 258
Correlation coefficient,
as a measure of effect size, 356
Cortex,
cerebellar, 175
increase in NMDA receptor,
after chronic alcohol exposure, 371
(pre)frontal,
reward pathways, 374
Corticosteroids, 206, 245
effects on alcohol consumption, 234
in alcoholic hepatitis, 188
in alcohol-related anaphylactic reactions,
dosage, 241
role in cerebral vascular disease, 174
Corticotropin releasing hormone (CRH), 234
Cortisol, *see* Corticosteroids
Counseling, 110
short,
efficacy of, 105
Countertransference, 93, 99
definition of, 97

Country,
    differences in drinking across, 271–286
Couples therapy, *see* Systemic therapy
Cramps,
    in alcohol-induced myopathy, 179
Craving, 114, 403, 404–406
    and drugs used in alcohol abuse and dependence, 125
    as negative reinforcer maintaining alcohol abuse, 407
    definition by Tiffany, 405
    definition by World Health Organization (WHO), 404
    definition by Wikler, 404
    drug-specific, 406
    lack of correlation with alcohol/drug use, 125, 405
C-reactive protein (CRP),
    in acute pancreatitis, 195
Creatine kinase (CK),
    in myopathy, 179
    risk of not detecting renal failure, 217
Crime,
    and alcohol, *see* Violence, or Aggression, or Accident
            rates, or Injury rates
Cross-sensitization,
    to psychostimulants and morphine, after alcohol, 403
Cryptorchism,
    in alcohol embryopathy, 258
Cue exposure, 96
Cue reactivity, 96
Cultural, *see* Sociocultural background
Curative factors,
    in psychotherapy, *see* Effect factors
Cutaneous vessels,
    dilation,
        by alcohol, 249
Cutis vagantium, 249
Cutoff point,
    definition of, 30
Cyanamide, *see* Carbimide
Cyanides,
    in amblyopy,
        caused by tobacco and alcohol, 177
Cyanocobalamin,
    is Vitamin B_{12}, 240
Cyclooxygenase-2 (COX-2) inhibitors,
    as analgesics in patients with liver damage, 228
Cytochrome P450,
    CYP2E1 isoform, 421
    induction,
        and esophageal cancer, 198
Cytokeratin intermediate filament cytoskeleton, 320
Cytokines,
    in alcohol dependence, 226

D

D_2 gene,
    as marker of vulnerability to alcoholism, 310, 402
D_2 receptor,
    and buspirone, 121, *see also* Dopamine receptor
D_2 receptor knockout mice,
    and alcohol consumption, 402

D_3 receptor, 403, *see also* Dopamine receptor
Daily alcohol consumption,
    harmful,
        as proposed in this handbook, 431
Death of significant other,
    leading to relapse, 115
Death rate in young men,
    and amount of alcohol consumed, 327
Decision,
    in stage model of change, 99, 100
Defeat,
    feelings of, 8
Defeminization,
    by alcohol, 232
Defense mechanisms,
    in alcohol dependence,
        as encountered in psychotherapy, 8, 110
Deficiency,
    in endogeneous opioids,
        thought to cause alcohol abuse, 373–374
Definitions of alcohol-related disorders,
    according to DSM-IV, 433–435
    according to ICD-10, 433, 435–437
Degeneration, *see* respective organ
Dehydration,
    by alcohol as risk factor for cerebral vascular diseases,
            174
    clinical signs, 209
    in alcoholic ketoacidosis, 209
    therapy by hydration via saline infusion, 51
Delinquency,
    and alcohol, *see* Violence, or Aggression, or Violence,
            or Accident rates, or Injury rates
Delirium tremens, 65, 67, 174
    definition of, 65
Delta hypoactivity,
    as marker of vulnerability to alcoholism, 307
Delta opioid receptor, *see* Opioid receptor, delta
Delusions, in alcohol-induced psychotic disorders, 74
Dementia,
    alcoholic, 175
    vascular, 138
Demodex folliculorum,
    in rosacea, 247
Demyelination, *see* Myelinolysis
Denial, 8, 110, 166
Density,
    of alcohol (ethanol), 417
    of whole blood, 419
Dental status,
    deterioration in,
        as clinical sign of alcohol dependence, 7
Dependence,
    case study, 329
    on family,
        of adolescents, 129
    rate of development,
        in adolescents, 129
    treatment in primary care, 169
Dependent personality disorder,
    and alcohol abuse and dependence 293

Depression,
    and alcohol abuse and dependence, 7, 271, **291**
    and self-medication hypothesis of alcoholism, 291
    as risk factor,
        in adolescents, 133
    clinical signs, 291
    in geriatric patients, 138
    in women, 153
Dermatitis,
    acral, 248
Desipramine,
    in alcohol abuse and dependence, 123
Detection,
    of alcohol in blood, *see* Blood alcohol level
Detoxi(fi)cation, 110
    in geriatric patients, 142
Developmental arrest,
    induced by alcohol abuse and dependence, 129
Diabetes mellitus,
    alcohol is not a risk factor for, 235
Diagnostic and Statistical Manual of Mental Disorders
        (DSM), *see* DSM-IV
Diagnostic efficacy,
    definition of, 30
Diagnostic tests, *see* Laboratory parameters
    in acute intoxication, 56
Diamine oxidase deficiency,
    and alcohol intolerance, 228, 241
    in alcohol dependence, 228
Diarrhea,
    alcohol-induced, 199
    in alcohol intolerance, 227, 241
Diazepam,
    in alcohol withdrawal syndrome, 67–68, 169
    in delirium tremens, dosage, 67–68
Dichotomous variable,
    definition of, 354, 356, 358
Diet,
    enteral,
        in cirrhosis, 190
    in alcoholic hepatitis, 189
    in alcoholic liver disease, 189
Dietary fat, 321
Dietary problems, *see* Malnutrition
Diffuse unpleasant emotions, alcohol as self-medication
        against, 98
Dihydroxyphenylacetic acid (DOPAC), 378
Dilazep, 375
Dimetinden,
    in alcohol-related anaphylactic reactions, dosage, 241
Discriminant function,
    in alcoholic hepatitis,
        formula, 187
Disorientation,
    in withdrawal, 66
Distribution,
    of alcohol in body, 421
Disulfiram, 105, 121, 122, 123, 124, 170
    mechanism of action,
        is irreversible inhibition of aldehyde
            dehydrogenase, 423

Disulfiram-alcohol reaction,
    clinical signs, 423
Diuretics,
    in cirrhosis, 218–219
Divorce,
    leading to relapse, 115
    of parents,
        as risk factor in adolescents, 132
Dizocilpine,
    is MK-801, 371
Dizygotic (DZ) twins, 306
DNA damage,
    by alcohol-induced free radicals, 318
Domestic disputes, *see* Codependence, or Systemic therapy,
        or Adolescents
Dopamine,
    in acute alcohol intoxication, 51
    in drug reward, 401–403
    in reinforcement, 401–403
Dopamine hypothesis,
    of alcohol reward, 377, 378, 401
Dopamine overflow,
    in nucleus accumbens, 371, 372, 373, 374, 377, 403
        alcohol-stimulated one inhibited by opioid
            antagonists, 374
        and lack of correlation to reinforcement 403
        in mice, 403
        stimulation by alcohol, 377, 378, 401
    in the ventral tegmental area, 373, 377
Dopamine receptor, 121
    and alcohol abuse and dependence, 375–378
Dopamine system,
    mesolimbic/mesocorticolimbic, and alcohol
        reinforcement 374
Drink sizes, *see* back inside cover
Drinking before noon,
    and alcohol absorption, 421
Drinking patterns, *see* Binge drinking or Natural history or
        Psychometric instruments
Drinking statistics, 271–286
Drinking unit,
    definitions, 429
Driver's license,
    loss of, 8, 419
Driving,
    legal alcohol limits for, 419
Dropouts,
    from clinical trials, 341
Drug abuse,
    and alcohol abuse and dependence,
        comorbidity, 290, *see also* Polytoxicomania
    other than alcohol, *see* Polytoxicomania
Drug discrimination,
    definition of, 370
    $GABA_A$ receptor agonists in, 371
Drug interactions,
    with alcohol, 425–427, *see also* individual chapters
    with retinoids, 247
Drug use action schemata, 405
Drunk driving, *see* Driving
DSM-IV definition,

of alcohol abuse, 434
of alcohol dependence, 434
of alcohol intoxication, 434
of alcohol withdrawal, 435
Dual effect on drug metabolism,
    by alcohol, 422
Dupuytren's disease,
    in alcohol dependence, 7
Duration,
    of inpatient treatment,
        relation to outcome, 105
Dynorphins, 373
Dysarthria,
    in hepatic encephalopathy, 176
Dysfunctional family,
    as risk factor,
        in adolescents, 132
Dyskinesia,
    choreiform, 176
Dysmotility,
    of small intestine, 199
Dysphoria,
    alcohol as self-medication against, 98
    as negative reinforcer maintaining alcohol abuse, 407
Dyspnea,
    in alcohol intolerance, 227, 241
    in alcohol-induced heart failure, 203

E

Early intervention, **5–11**, 165, *see also* First contact
Early start of drinking,
    as risk factor,
        in adolescents, 132
Eating disorders,
    and alcohol abuse and dependence, 293
ECA Study, *see* Epidemiological Catchment Area Study
ECG,
    in acute alcohol intoxication, 59, 205–206
    in electrolyte disturbances, 212–215
Eclectic therapies,
    in psychotherapy, 106
Ecthymata, 249
Edema,
    in cirrhosis, 218
    peripheral,
        in alcohol-induced heart failure, 203
Edinburgh Dependence Scale, 366
EEG,
    in alcohol-related neurological diseases, 173–181
    in seizures, 174
EEG abnormalities,
    as marker of vulnerability to alcoholism, 307
Effect factors,
    in psychotherapy, 104–105
    general,
        in psychotherapy, 105
    nonspecific,
        in psychotherapy, 104
Effect size,
    definition of, 341, 354–356

Effect size measures,
    comparison and definitions, 356
Effects,
    of psychotherapy, 104
Efficacy,
    clinical trials on,
        in pharmacotherapy, 121–127, 339–351, 356–360
        in psychotherapy, 104–106, 111
    of motivational therapy,
        clinical trials on, 111
Ego defects,
    structural,
        in psychoanalytical theory, 99
Ego functions and dysfunctions, 98
Ejection fraction,
    in alcoholic cardiomyopathy, 203
Elderly, *see* Geriatric patients, Young Elderly, and Older
        Elderly
Electrical brain stimulation, 401
Electrocardiogram, *see* ECG
Electrolyte disturbances, 212–216
Elimination kinetics,
    of alcohol, 422
Emergency management,
    of acute alcohol intoxication,
        see front inside cover, 49–64
Emotions,
    negative,
        leading to relapse, 114
    positive,
        leading to relapse, 114
Empathy,
    how to obtain, 90
    in client-centered therapy, 101
Empty stomach,
    and alcohol absorption, 421
Encephalopathy,
    hepatic, 176, 189
    Wernicke, *see* Wernicke encephalopathy
Endocardial cushion defect, 206
Endocrine system, 231–237
    effects of alcohol on,
        summary tables, 232–233
Endorphin, *see* Beta-endorphin
Endoscopic retrograde cholangiopancreatography (ERCP),
    in chronic pancreatitis, 197
Enkephalins,
    and reinforcing effect of alcohol, 373
    as agonists for delta opioid receptor, 373
Enteral tube feeding,
    in cirrhosis, 190
Environment,
    role in development of alcohol abuse and dependence,
        see Heritability, or Adolescents, or
        Psychotherapy
Environmental toxins,
    drug interaction with alcohol, 423
Enzyme induction,
    by alcohol, 422
Epidemiological Catchment Area (ECA) Study, 289, 290,
        292, 294

Epidemiology,
    of alcohol abuse and dependence, 271–286
Epileptic fits, *see* Seizures
Epizoonoses, 249
Erythema,
    acral, 248
    palmar, 7, 189
Erythropoiesis, 322
Esophageal varices,
    in cirrhosis, 189
Esophagitis, 198
Esophagus, 189, 198
    cancer of, 198
    chronic inflammation, 198
    varices in, 189
Estradiol, 232–233
Estrogen deficit,
    in alcohol dependence, 233
Estrone, 232
Ethanol patch test, 241
Ethanol, *see* Alcohol
Ethanol-disulfiram reaction (DER),
    definition and clinical signs, 423
Ethnic differences, *see* Epidemiology
Ethylene glycol poisoning,
    and 4-methylpyrazol, 421
Etretinate, 247
Euphoria,
    leading to relapse, 114
Evidence-based pharmacotherapy, 121–127, 339–351
Evidence-based psychotherapy, 105
Excitability,
    as clinical sign of alcohol abuse and dependence, *see*
        Hyperexcitability
Expectations,
    alcohol-related, 95
    wishful, of children, 130
Extremities,
    skin lesions, 249
Eyelids,
    in alcohol embryopathy, 254

F

Face,
    alcoholic, 247, *see* Rosacea
    in alcohol embryopathy, 251, 254
Facies ethylica, 247, *see* Rosacea
Fainting, *see* Orthostatic hypotension
Fallot's tetra/pentalogy,
    in alcohol embryopathy, 206, 258
False negative rate,
    definition of, 30
False positive rate,
    definition of, 30
Family,
    as beneficial factor,
        in women, 155
    dysfunctional,

    as risk factor for alcohol abuse and dependence in
        adolescents, 132
    involvement of,
        in general psychotherapy, 101, 134–135
        in psychotherapy of adolescents, 134–135
Family physician, *see* Primary care physician
Family problems,
    typical for alcohol dependent patients, *see*
        Codependence
Family setting,
    and adolescents, 129
    role in alcohol dependence, 7, 108, 132
Family studies, 305
Family therapy, *see* Systemic therapy
Fasciculations, *see* Muscle fasciculations
Fasting,
    risk of alcoholic ketoacidosis, 209
Fat,
    dietary, 321
    of body,
        in calculation of maximum blood alcohol level, 419
Fatty acids,
    unsaturated, 321
Fatty food,
    and alcohol absorption, 421
Fatty liver, 185, 317
Favre-Racouchot syndrome, 244
Female patients,
    special therapeutic considerations, *see* Women
Feminization,
    of alcohol dependent men, clinical signs, 232
Fenfluramine,
    effect size, 345
    in alcohol abuse and dependence, 343
Ferritin, 322
Fetal alcohol effects (FAE),
    definition of, 251
Fetal alcohol syndrome (FAS), *see* Alcohol Embryopathy
Fibrillation,
    atrial or ventricular, 205
Fibrogenesis,
    in cirrhosis, 319
Financial status,
    in alcohol dependence, 7
Fingers,
    malformations,
        in alcohol embryopathy, 252, 258
Firing rate,
    of dopamine neurons in the ventral tegmental area,
        increase by alcohol, 374, 375, 376, 377
First aid,
    in acute alcohol intoxication, *see* **front inside cover,**
        49–64
First contact, **5–11**, 107
    with adolescents, 134
    with geriatric patients, 141
First impression, *see* First contact
First-pass of alcohol,
    gastric, 421
    hepatic, 421
Fixed-effect models,

in meta-analysis, 356

Flapping tremor, *see* Asterixis

Flavonoids,
    in cirrhosis, 190

Flavor, *see* Taste

Fleas,
    in epizoonoses, 249

Fluid disturbances, 215–216

Flunitrazepam,
    binding,
        antagonism by 5HT$_3$ receptor antagonists, 373

Fluoxetine,
    in alcohol abuse and dependence, 121, 123, 124, 343
    mechanism of action, 121

Flupenthixol,
    in alcohol dependence, 403

Flushing,
    after alcohol,
        in people of Asian descent, 240, 274, 309
    in alcohol intolerance, 227, 241, 274
        effect on alcohol consumption, 274
    in disulfiram-alcohol reaction, 423

Flutter,
    atrial, 205

Focusing,
    in psychotherapy, 102

Folate deficiency,
    is folic acid deficiency, 322

Follicle stimulating hormone (FSH),
    blunting of response by alcohol, 231

Food,
    rich in histamine, 241

Food allergies,
    worsening by alcohol, 241

Food and Drug Administration (FDA), 170

Forgetfulness, *see* Cognitive deficits

Fortified wine,
    alcohol contents, *see* back inside cover

FRAMES,
    six elements of brief intervention, 367

Framingham Study, 227

Fraternal twins, 306

Free radicals, 317, 318

Free radical scavengers,
    in cirrhosis, 190

French Paradox, 205, *see also* Resveratrol

Front loading strategy,
    of diazepam,
        in treatment of alcohol withdrawal syndromes, 68

Frontal cortex,
    reward pathways, 374

Functionality,
    of alcohol abuse, 98

Furosemide,
    in cirrhosis, 218–219

G

GABA receptor, 121, 395
    and gammahydroxybutyrate, 121

and seizures, 174

GABA system,
    and alcohol abuse and dependence, 369–371
    as marker of vulnerability to alcoholism, 309

GABA$_A$ receptor,
    and acamprosate, 121
    structure, 370
    subunits,
        stoichiometry, 370

GABA$_A$ receptor interaction,
    at different blood alcohol levels, 369

Gabexate mesilate,
    in acute pancreatitis, 197

Gait ataxia, *see* Ataxia

Gall stones, *see* Cholecystolithiasis

Gallop sounds,
    in alcohol-induced heart failure, 203

Gammaglutamyltransferase (GGT), 7, 29, 32, 34–35, 185
    in geriatric patients, 139
    sensitivity and specificity, 32

Gammahydroxybutyrate (GHB),
    adverse effects and possible abuse liability, 124
    and firing rate of dopamine neurons in the ventral
        tegmental area, 377
    effect size, 345
    Food and Drug Administration (FDA) guidelines on
        use, 124
    in alcohol abuse and dependence, 121–124, 343
    mechanism of action, 121, 377

Gammahydroxybutyrate (GHB) receptor,
    and gammahydroxybutyrate, 121

Gastritis,
    acute, 199
    hemorrhagic, 199

Gastrointestinal system, 195–202

Gateway drugs, *see* Adolescents and Natural history

GBR12909, 401

Gender differences, 151–164

Gender gap, in problem drinking, 151

Genes, as markers of vulnerability to alcoholism, 310, 402
    for opioid receptor,
        and vulnerability to alcoholism, 311

Genetics,
    of alcohol dependence, *see* Heritability

Genital tract malformations,
    in alcohol embryopathy, 258

Geriatric patients,
    special therapeutic considerations, 137–147

GHB, *see* Gammahydroxybutyrate

Glasgow Coma Scale (GCS),
    definition and scoring, 63

Glomerular filtration rate,
    false-normal creatine kinase levels in, 217

Glomerulonephritis,
    in cirrhosis, 221

Glossitis,
    in alcohol-related niacin deficiency, 240

Glucagon,
    in alcoholic hepatitis, 188

Gluconeogenesis,
    impairment by alcohol, 235

Glucose,
  normal range, *see* front inside cover, 210
  supplementation,
    dosage, 210
Glucose intolerance, 235
Glutamate,
  and seizures, 174
Glutamate system,
  and alcohol abuse and dependence, 371
Glutamic oxaloacetic transaminase (GOT), *see* Aspartate
    aminotransferase (AST)
Glutamic pyruvic transaminase (GPT), *see* Alanine
    aminotransferase (ALT)
Goals,
  in treatment, *see* Treatment, goals
Gonadal atrophy,
  male and female, 218, 232, 233
Gout,
  in alcohol dependence, 227
Gram alcohol per standard drink, **429,** *see* **back inside
    cover**
Grand mal seizures,
  in alcohol withdrawal syndrome, 66
  in the elderly, 141
Grandparents,
  and adolescents, 130
Group therapy,
  vs. single therapy, 106
Growth hormone (GH),
  and alcohol-induced hypoglycemia, 235
Growth retardation,
  in alcohol embryopathy, 259
Guilt,
  feelings of, 8
Gynecomastia,
  in alcohol dependent men, 232

H

H$_1$ receptor antagonists, *see* Antihistamines
H$_2$ receptor antagonists,
  in acute gastritis, 199
  in metabolic alkalosis, 211
Hair,
  increased growth in eyebrows and on cheeks,
    in porphyria cutanea tarda, 244
  loss of body hair,
    in hypogonadism, 233
Hallucinations,
  in alcohol withdrawal syndrome, 66
  alcohol-induced, 74
Haloperidol,
  in alcohol withdrawal syndrome, 68
  in alcohol-induced psychotic disorders, 75
  in excited intoxicated patients, 173
Hamilton Depression Scale scores,
  in alcohol dependence, 292
Hard liquor,
  alcohol contents of, *see* back inside cover
Harm reduction paradigm,

  in the treatment of alcohol abuse and dependence, 272
Harmful alcohol consumption, 166, 281, 325–329, *see also*
    Abuse
  as proposed in this handbook, 431
  case studies, 325, 328–329
  definition of, 326–328
  for alcohol embryopathy, 253, 260
  for cardiovascular diseases, 203–204
  for cirrhosis, 273
  for the central nervous system, 174
Headache,
  in alcohol withdrawal syndrome, 66
Heart, 203–207
Heart defects,
  in alcohol embryopathy, 258
Heart failure,
  alcohol-induced, 203
Hedonic components,
  of reinforcement, 403
Helicobacter pylori,
  in gastritis, 199
Helper T cells,
  and alcohol, 225
Helpful advice, *see* Psychotherapy and Motivational
    therapy
Helpful attitude,
  how to obtain, 90
Hemochromatosis,
  hereditary 321
Hemoconcentration, 174
Hemoglobin,
  normal range, *see* front inside cover
Hemorrhage,
  intracerebral, 174, 204, 206
Hepatic encephalopathy, *see* Encephalopathy, hepatic
Hepatitis,
  alcoholic, **186,** 234, 317
    and TNF-alpha, 226
Hepatitis B, 322
Hepatitis C, 322
Hepatocellular carcinoma, *see* Liver, cancer of
Hepatomegaly, *See* Liver, enlargement of
Hepatoprotective drugs, 183, 186–188, 191
Hepatorenal syndrome (HRS), 220–221
Hepatotoxicity,
  of alcohol, 183, **317–323**
Heritability,
  of alcohol dependence, 305–315
Heterogeneity,
  of clinical studies sample, in meta-analysis, 360
Hexachlorocyclohexane,
  in epizoonoses, 249
HFE gene, 322
Hiding alcohol problems, *see* Denial
High density lipoprotein (HDL) cholesterol,
  increase by alcohol, 205
High-anxiety-related behavior (HAB) rat, 408
Hippocampus,
  reward pathways, 374
His-Purkinje system,
  alcohol-induced conduction disturbances in, 205

Histamine,
    role in alcohol intolerance, 228, 241
Histamine degradation,
    impairment of,
        in alcohol dependence, 228
Histamine intolerance,
    in alcohol intolerance, 227–228, 241
Histamine release,
    by alcohol, 241
Histamine-rich beverages and food, 241
Histrionic personality disorder,
    and alcohol abuse and dependence, 294
Holiday heart syndrome, 205
Homeless, 7, 249
Homogeneity,
    of clinical studies sample,
        in meta-analysis, 360
Homovanillic acid (HVA), 378
Hope,
    mobilization of,
        as general effect factor in psychotherapy, 105
Hormone levels,
    and alcohol, 233
Humanistic psychotherapy, 101
Hydration,
    by drinking water, 216
    by saline infusion, 51
Hydrocephalus internus,
    in alcohol embryopathy, 258
Hydrocortisone,
    in alcohol-related anaphylactic reactions,
        dosage, 241
Hygiene,
    deterioration in alcohol dependence, 7
Hyperactivity,
    in alcohol embryopathy, 251, 258
Hyperaldosteronism,
    secondary,
        alcohol-induced, 234
Hyperbilirubinemia, 187
Hypercapnia,
    in acute alcohol intoxication, 53
Hyperestrogenization,
    of alcohol dependent men, 232
Hyperexcitability,
    in alcohol embryopathy, 258
    in alcohol withdrawal, 66
Hyperhidrosis,
    in alcohol withdrawal syndrome, 66
    risk factor for perniones, 249
Hypernatremia,
    role in myelinolysis, 176
Hypertension,
    chronic alcohol abuse as secondmost prevalent risk
        factor for, 206
    in alcohol dependence, 174, 206, 271
    in alcohol withdrawal syndrome, 66
    portal, 189
Hyperthermia,
    in alcohol withdrawal syndrome, 66
Hyperthyroidism, 234

Hypertrichosis, 244
Hyperuricemia, 216–217
Hyperventilation,
    in withdrawal leading to respiratory alkalosis, 211
Hypnosis,
    graduated active, 103
    relaxing, 102–103
Hypoandrogenization,
    by alcohol, 231, 232
Hypocalcemia,
    in alcohol dependence,
        and hypoparathyroidism, **214**, 234
    secondary to magnesium depletion, 214
    treatment,
        dosage, 212
Hypoglycemia,
    alcohol-induced, 59, **210**, 231, 233, 235
    blood glucose level in, 210
    in acute alcohol intoxication, 59
Hypogonadism,
    female, 233
    male, 231, 233
Hypokalemia, 212, 214–215
    and arrhythmias, 205
    and myopathy, 179
    and risk of rhabdomyolysis after seizures, 217
    in acute intoxication, 66
Hypomagnesemia, 212, 213, 234
    and myopathy, 179
    and secondary hypocalcemia, 213
    in alcohol withdrawal syndrome, 66
Hyponatremia, 212, 214, 215–216
    in acute alcohol intoxication, 59
    in alcohol withdrawal syndrome, 66
Hypoparathyroidism, 214, **234**
Hypophosphatemia, 212–213
    increased risk of rhabdomyolysis, 213, 217
Hypospadia,
    in alcohol embryopathy, 258
Hypotension,
    in acute alcohol intoxication, **51**, 206
    in alcoholic ketoacidosis, 209
Hypothalamic-pituitary-gonadal (HPA) axis,
    and alcohol, 231, 233
Hypothalamus,
    lateral,
        reward pathways, 374
Hypothermia,
    in acute alcohol intoxication, 59
Hypoxia,
    centrolobular (liver), 317
    in acute alcohol intoxication, 53

I

ICD-10 codes,
    for alcohol-related psychiatric disorders, 433
ICD-10 definition,
    of alcohol abuse, 435–436
    of alcohol dependence, 435–436

of alcohol intoxication, 435–436
of alcohol withdrawal, 435–436
European version, 436
ICS 205–930, 372
Icterus, 186–187
pathophysiology, 320
Imagery,
in psychotherapy, 102
Imipenem,
in acute pancreatitis, 197
Immune system, 225–229
Immunodeficiency,
alcohol-induced, 225, 227
Immunoglobulin A (IgA) deposition,
in alcohol-induced glomerulonephritis, 221
Immunoglobulin E,
against acetaldehyde-protein adducts,
in anaphylactic reactions against alcohol, 241
Immunoglobulins,
elevated levels, in alcohol dependence, 225
Important Persons and Activities Interview, 366
Impotence,
erectile, 6, **232**
Impression,
first, *see* First contact
In vitro alcohol effects,
under laboratory conditions, 121, **369–384**, 401–409
In vivo alcohol effects,
under laboratory conditions, **385–400**, 401–409
In vivo microdialysis,
and dopamine transmission, *see* Dopamine overflow
Infarction,
myocardial, 204
Infections,
incidence,
in alcohol dependence, 225
Infertility, 233
Information,
as general effect factor in psychotherapy, 105
Injury rates,
and alcohol consumption in the general population,
data on 40 countries, 273
Inotropic effect,
negative,
of alcohol, 203
Inpatient treatment,
vs. outpatient treatment,
efficacy of, 105
Insect bites, 249
Insomnia,
alcohol as self-medication against, 177
and chronic alcohol consumption, 7
in alcohol withdrawal syndrome, 66
treatment of,
with benzodiazepines, 67
Instrumental conditioning, *see* Operant conditioning
Instrumentalization,
definition of,
in psychoanalysis, 99
Insulin,
drug interaction with alcohol, 235
in alcoholic hepatitis, 188

Intake,
of alcohol, *see* Alcohol consumption
Intelligence Quotient (IQ),
in alcohol embryopathy, 251, 252, 253, 258
Interferon-gamma (IFN-γ)increase 226
Interleukins, 319
Interleukin-2 (IL-2), 226
Interleukin-6 (IL-6), 245
Interleukin-12 (IL-12), 226
International Classification of Diseases (ICD), *see* ICD
Internet addresses,
useful, 457
Interpersonal focus,
in psychotherapy, 101
Interpersonal relationships, *see* Codependence and Family
and Systemic Therapy
Interview technique, 9–10, 107
Intestinal dysmotility, 199
Intolerance,
of alcohol, 227–228, 240–241
treatment, 241
Intoxication,
alcohol consumption leading to,
in man, 419
in monkey, 390
in mouse, 393
in rat, 391
and alcoholic ketoacidosis, 209
blood alcohol level,
in man 173
in monkey, 385
clinical signs, *see* **front inside cover, 49–64, 173**
clinical signs at different severity levels, 173
complications, 58
differential diagnosis 56–57
ECG, 59, 205–206
Glasgow Coma Scale (GCS), 55
in monkey, 387–390
in mouse, 393
in rat, 391–392
methanol intoxication,
treatment, 59
risk of alcoholic ketoacidosis, 209
treatment, *see* **front inside cover, 49–64**
Intracranial bleeding, *see* front inside cover, 55
Intracranial self-stimulation (ICSS), 401
Intrauterine growth retardation (IUGR),
in alcohol embryopathy, 251
Intravenous administration,
maximum alcohol concentration,
in animal research, 395
Intubation, 54
IQ, *see* Intelligence quotient
Iritis, 248
Iron, effect on oxidation-reduction reactions and liver
damage, 322
therapeutic depletion in porphyria cutanea tarda, 244
Iron deficiency,
not a problem in chronic alcohol users, *see* Iron
overload
Iron overload, 321

Irreversibility,
    of alcoholic pancreatitis, 195
Irreversible blockade,
    of aldehyde dehydrogenase (ALDH), *see* Alcohol-
        disulfiram reaction
Ischemia, cerebral, 174
Isotretinoin, 247, 248
Itching skin,
    in alcohol intolerance, 227, 241

J

J-shaped curve,
    of alcohol-induced risk of cardiovascular diseases,
        203–205
Jaundice, *see* Icterus
Jealousy,
    delusional, 74

K

Kava,
    and niacin deficiency, 240
Keratitis, 248
Ketamine, 371
Ketoacidosis, *see* Acidosis
Kidney,
    alcohol-related disorders of, 209–224
Kidney malformations,
    in alcohol embryopathy, 258
Kindling,
    of panic attacks in withdrawal, 407
Klinodactyly, *see* Clinodactyly
K_m, definition of, 421
Kupffer cell, 319, 321
Kupffer cell impairment,
    and glomerulonephritis, 221

L

Labia minora,
    hypoplasia of,
        in alcohol embryopathy, 258
Laboratory parameters,
    accuracy in alcoholic liver disease, 186
    as outcome criterion in clinical trials, 122, 343
    in acute alcohol intoxication, *see* front inside cover, 56,
        212
    in alcohol dependence, 31
    in geriatric patients, 139
    normal range, *see* front inside cover, 56, 212
Lack of role model, *see* Role model
Lactate dehydrogenase (LDH),
    in acute pancreatitis, 196
    in alcohol-induced myopathies, 179
Lactic acidosis, *see* Acidosis
Laennec's cirrhosis, 189
Lansoprazole,
    proton pump inhibitor, 211

Lapse,
    as outcome criterion in clinical trials, 122
    leading to relapse, 114
Latent actions,
    definition of,
        in psychoanalysis, 97
Lateral hypothalamus,
    reward pathways, 374
Lavage,
    in acute pancreatitis, 197
Learning disorder,
    as risk factor,
        in adolescents, 132
Left lateral decubitus, *see* front inside cover
Legal problems, 8
    in adolescents, 131–132
Lethal alcohol blood level, 60, 173, *see also* Blood alcohol
        level
Leu-enkephalin, *see* Enkephalins
Leukocytes,
    normal range, *see* front inside cover
Leukopenia,
    as a consequence of splenomegaly in portal
        hypertension, 189
Libido,
    loss of, 6, **233**
Lice,
    in epizoonoses, 249
Lidocaine,
    in liver function test, 190
Lies, *see* Collateral reports
Life,
    meaning of, *see* Psychotherapy
Limb-girdle weakness,
    in hypokalemia, 214
Limits,
    of "safe" alcohol consumption, *see* Harmful alcohol
        consumption
Lipid peroxidation, 317–318
    role in cancer of the oral mucosa, 249
Lipopolysaccharides, 319
Lipotropic factors, 321
Liquor (drinks),
    alcohol contents of, *see* back inside cover
List of abbreviations, 459
Listeriosis,
    incidence,
        in alcohol dependence, 225
Lithium,
    in alcohol abuse and dependence, 121, 124
Liver, 183–193, 317–323
    cancer of, 322
    enlargement of, 7, 10, 186
    protection of, *see* Hepatoprotective drugs
Liver biopsy, *see* Biopsy
Liver cirrhosis, *see* Cirrhosis
Liver damage,
    in immunosuppressed alcohol dependent patients, 228
Liver diet, 189
Liver diseases,
    alcoholic, 183–193

differential diagnosis, 186
laboratory parameters in, 185–186
Liver transplantation, 190
Living conditions,
in alcohol dependence, 7
Locus coeruleus,
reward pathways, 374
Long-Evans rats, 393
Long-sleep mice, 375
Loratadine,
in alcohol-related anaphylactic reactions,
dosage, 241
Lorazepam,
in withdrawal, 169
Low density lipoprotein (LDL), 205
Low-anxiety-related behavior (LAB) rats, 408
Low-K_m alcohol dehydrogenase (ADH), 421
Low-T_3 syndrome, 231, 233
LS mice, 371, 375
Luteinizing hormone (LH),
blunting of response by alcohol, 232, 233
Lying, *see* Collateral reports

M

Macrophage,
hepatic, *see* Kupffer cell
Magnetic resonance cholangiopancreatography (MRCP)
in chronic pancreatitits, 197
Magnetic Resonance Imaging (MRI),
in Wernicke encephalopathy, 176
Maintenance,
in stage model of change, 99, 100
of drug abuse, 95
Major depression, *see* Depression
Malabsorption,
alcohol-induced, 200
Maladaptive behaviors,
in alcohol embryopathy, 259
Male patients,
and alcohol-induced hypogonadism, 231–233
typical subject in clinical studies on alcoholism, 121
Malformations,
in alcohol embryopathy, 251
Malignancies, *see* Cancer
Mallory body (MB), 319
Mallory-Weiss tears,
in acute gastritis, 199
Malnutrition, 189, 321
and immunoglobulin formation, 226
MALT©, *see* Munich Alcoholism Test©
Malt liquor,
alcohol contents, *see* back inside cover
Mamillar body,
atrophy,
in Wernicke encephalopathy, 176
Management,
of acute intoxication, *see* front inside cover, 49–64
Mandible,
hypoplasia of,
in alcohol embryopathy, 254

Mania,
and alcohol abuse and dependence, 292
definition of, 292
Manifest actions,
definition of,
in psychoanalysis, 97
Marchiafava-Bignami syndrome, 177
Marital problems,
typical for alcohol dependent patients, *see*
Codependence
Marital status,
as risk factor,
in women, 155
Marital therapy, *see* Systemic therapy
Markers,
of vulnerability to alcoholism, 307–311
MAST, *see* Michigan Alcoholism Screening Test
Mast cell degranulation,
alcohol-induced, 241
MATCH, *see* Project MATCH
Maternal alcohol consumption,
and risk of malformations in offspring, 260–263, *see*
also Apgar score
Maturation,
of adolescents, 130
MDL 72222, 373
Mean corpuscular hemoglobin (MCH), 66
Mean corpuscular volume (MCV), 7, 32, 185
in geriatric patients, 139
Meaning of life, *see* Psychotherapy
Mechanism of action,
of drugs used in alcohol abuse and dependence, **121**,
124–125
Menstrual cycle,
disturbances, 152
Mental retardation,
in alcohol embryopathy, 254, 258
Meprobamate,
in alcohol withdrawal syndrome and dependence,
obsolete, 68
Mesolimbic dopamine system, 377, *see also* Dopamine
system
Meta-analysis,
introduction to the calculation of, 353–362
of pharmacotherapeutic trials, 339–351
Metabolic alkalosis, *see* Alkalosis
Metabolism of alcohol,
in women, 152
Met-enkephalin, *see* Enkephalins
**Methanol intoxication,
treatment, 59**
Methionine,
S-Adenosyl-L-methionine, 191
Methotrexate (MTX),
drug interaction with alcohol, 228
Methylpyrazol,
in ethylene glycol and methanol poisoning, 421
mg%,
definition of, *see* back inside cover
MHC II proteins, 226

Michaelis-Menten constant,
    definition of, 421
Michigan Alcoholism Screening Test (MAST), 41
      test form, 446
    brief version (bMAST), 41
      test form, 447
    in geriatric patients (MAST G), 139
    short version (sMAST) 41
      test form, 454
Microcephaly,
    in alcohol embryopathy, 251, 254
Microdialysis, *see* Dopamine overflow
Microsomal ethanol oxidizing system (MEOS), 317
    enzymatic parameters, 421
Mid-face hypoplasia,
    in alcohol embryopathy, 254
Milk,
    mother's, *see* Breast milk
Milk thistle extracts,
    in cirrhosis, 190
Miscarriage, 152
Mites, 249
Mitral regurgitation,
    in alcohol-induced heart failure, 203
MK-801, *see* Dizocilpine
Moderate drinking, 23–24
Molecular pharmacology,
    of alcohol abuse and dependence, 121, 124–125,
      369–384
Molecular weight,
    of alcohol (ethanol), 417
Money problems,
    in alcohol dependence, 7
Monkey, 387–390
Monoamino oxidase (MAO) activity,
    as marker of vulnerability to alcoholism, 308
Monoethylglicinexylidide (MEGX),
    in liver function test, 190
Mononuclear cells,
    responsiveness, and alcohol, 225
Monozygotic (MZ) twins, 306
Moon face,
    in Pseudo-Cushing's syndrome, 234
Morbid jealousy,
    in alcohol dependence, *see* Jealousy, delusional
Morbidity, *see* Harmful alcohol consumption and
      Comorbidity
Morell's laminar sclerosis, 177
Morning sickness,
    in acute gastritis, 199
Morphine,
    and dopamine overflow in the nucleus accumbens, 374
    inhibition of inhibitory $GABA_A$ interneurons in the
      ventral tegmental area, 374
Mortality,
    and amount of alcohol consumed, 328
Mother's milk, *see* Breast milk
Motivational Enhancement Therapy (MET), 365
Motivational therapy, 9, 100, 109
    goals of, 9
Mouse, 393–395

Movement disorders, *see* Dyskinesia
MR monkey, 389
Mu opioid receptor, *see* Opioid receptor, mu
Munich Alcoholism Test (MALT)©, 43
    in geriatric patients, 139
    test form, 445
Muscimol, 371
Muscle cramps,
    in alcohol necrotizing myopathy, 179
    in alcoholic ketoacidosis, 209
    in hypokalemia, 212, 214
Muscle fasciculations,
    in hypocalcemia or hypomagnesemia, 213, 214
Muscle tenderness,
    in myopathies, 179
Muscle weakness, in hypomagnesemia and hypocalcemia,
    213
    in hypophosphatemia, 212, 213
    in myopathy, 179
Muscular hypotonia,
    in alcohol embryopathy, 258
Myelinolysis,
    central pontine, 176
    extrapontine, 176
Myelopathy, 177
Myocardial infarction, 204
Myocardial ischemia,
    in alcohol withdrawal syndrome, 207
Myocardium,
    in alcoholic cardiomyopathy, 203
Myopathy, 179
    acute, 179
    and rhabdomyolysis, 179
    associated with hypokalemia, 179, 214
    chronic, 179

N

Nalmefene,
    animal research, 395
    effect size, 345
    in alcohol abuse and dependence, 121–125, 343
    mechanism of action, 121
Naloxone,
    animal research, 395
    inhibition of alcohol-induced dopamine overflow in
      nucleus accumbens, 374
Naltrexone,
    and appetitive factors, 395
    animal research, 395
    dosage, 123
    effect size, 345
    in alcohol abuse and dependence, 85, **121–125**, 170,
      343, 373
    mechanism of action, 373, 395
    side effects and contraindications, 123
Naltrindole, 375
    inhibition of alcohol-induced overflow in nucleus
      accumbens, 374
National Alcohol and Drug Survey, 325

National Comorbidity Survey (NCS), 287, 289, 290, 292
National Institute on Alcohol Abuse and Alcoholism
      (NIAAA), 82, 125, 311, 327, 389, 398
  address and web site, 457,   www.niaaa.nih.gov
Natural history, 13–28
Natural recovery, 19–24, 85, 271
  case studies, 283
  from alcohol problems, 19–24
  predictors, 23, 24
  prevalence, 283
Nature vs. nurture,
  in Japanese and Caucasian flushers and non-flushers,
     277
  testing with twin/family designs, 307
Nausea,
  and alcohol absorption, 421
  in alcoholic ketoacidosis, 209
  in withdrawal, 66
Neck,
  bull's, *see* Bull's neck
Necrosectomy,
  in acute pancreatitits, 197
Negative attitudes,
  of therapist, 92
Negative emotions, *see also* Emotions, negative
  alcohol as self-medication against, 98
Negative reinforcement,
  in maintenance of alcohol dependence, 96, 102
  of negative emotions,
     in alcohol dependence, 407
Nervous system,
  treatment of alcohol-induced disorders, 173–181
Nervousness, *see* Tension, Diffuse unpleasant emotions,
     and Hyperexcitability
Neuroanatomy,
  of alcohol abuse and dependence, 369–384
Neuroleptics,
  in alcohol withdrawal syndrome, 68
  in alcohol-induced psychotic disorders, 74–76
Neuropathy,
  alcohol-induced, *see* Polyneuropathy
Neurotransmitter systems,
  mediating alcohol reinforcement, 121, **369–384**,
     401–404
Neutrophil dysfunction,
  in alcohol dependence, 226
NG 108–15 cells, 375
NIAAA, *see* National Institute on Alcohol Abuse and
     Alcoholism (NIAAA)
Niacin,
  name given to nicotinic acid=Vitamin B_3 to avoid
     confusion with the alkaloid nicotine, 240
  supplementation,
    dosage 240
Nicotinamide,
  the amide of nicotinic acid, *see* Niacin
Nicotine, *see also* Smoking
Nicotine abuse,
  and alcohol abuse and dependence, comorbidity, 295
Nissen fundoplication,
  in reflux esophagitis, 198

NMDA receptor, 395
  and acamprosate, 121, 124
  increase in cortex,
    after chronic alcohol exposure, 374
NMDA receptor antagonists, 371
NMDA receptor interaction
  at different blood alcohol levels, 371
NMDA system,
  and alcohol abuse and dependence, 371
Non-alcoholic steatohepatitis (NASH), 187
Non-directive therapy, *see* Client-centered therapy
Nonsteroidal antiinflammatory drugs (NSAIDs),
  drug interaction with alcohol, 209, 228
Nontherapeutic attitudes, 92
Noradrenaline,
  in acute alcohol intoxication, 51
  in alcohol-related anaphylactic reactions,
    dosage, 241, *see also* Adrenalin
Nose,
  red, *see* Rosacea
  short and upturned,
    in alcohol embryopathy, 254
NP rat, 391–392, 408
NR_1 receptor, 371
NR_{2A} receptor, 371
Nuclear factor-kappa-B (NF-κB), 319, 320
Nucleus accumbens (NAC), 371, 372, 373, 374, 403
  heterogeneity, 403
  reward pathways, 374
  subregions, 403
Nucleus arcuatus paraventricularis,
  opioid system, 373
  reward pathways, 374
Nursing, *see* Breast-feeding
Nystagmus, 176

O

Obesity, and hypertension, 206
  truncal, in Pseudo-Cushing's syndrome, 234
Obsessive compulsive disorder, 133
Obsessive-compulsive drinking scale (OCDS)©, 333
  test form, 448–450
Obstetric disorders, in alcohol abuse and dependence, 152
Occult head injury, 55, 59
  and seizures, 174
Odds ratio (OR), definition of, 354
Oesophagus or oesophageal, *see* Esophagus or esophageal
Offering,
  of a psychological theory of alcohol abuse and
     dependence,
     as general effect factor in psychotherapy, 105
Older elderly, 142
Olfactory tubercle,
  reward pathways, 374
Oligomenorrhea, 232, 233
Omeprazole,
  proton pump inhibitor, 211
Onset,
  of alcohol use and abuse, 15–17

Ontario Alcohol and Drug Opinion Survey, 325

Operant conditioning,
   role in alcohol dependence, 95, 385–400

Ophthalmoplegia,
   in Wernicke-Korsakoff syndrome, 175

Opioid deficiency hypothesis,
   of alcohol abuse, 373–374

Opioid receptor,
   and dopamine overflow in the nucleus accumbens, 395
   delta, 121, 373, 395
   kappa, 395
   mu, 121, 373, 395

Opioid receptor blockade,
   and alcohol consumption, 373

Opioid receptor genes,
   and vulnerability to alcoholism, 311

Opioid system,
   and alcohol abuse and dependence, 373–376
   as marker of vulnerability to alcoholism, 309

Opposite effects on drug metabolism,
   by alcohol, 422

Organ damage,
   underestimation of,
      by adolescents, 130

Organic brain syndrome,
   alcohol-induced, 175

Orthostatic hypotension,
   in alcoholic ketoacidosis, 209
   in Wernicke encephalopathy, 179

Osmolal gap, see Anion gap

Osteopenia,
   alcohol-induced, 231, 233

Other drugs,
   abuse of,
      in alcohol dependence, 290, see also
         Polytoxicomania

Outcome criteria,
   of clinical trials, 121–124, 343, 348

Outcome studies,
   of pharmacotherapy of alcohol dependence, 121–127,
      339–351, 356–360
   of psychotherapy of alcohol dependence, 104–106, 111

Outpatient setting,
   and choice of psychotherapy, 107

Outpatient treatment,
   vs. inpatient treatment,
      efficacy of, 105

Ovarian atrophy, 232

Overconsumption,
   of alcohol as measured in animal research, 385–400

Overflow hypothesis,
   of edema formation in cirrhosis, 218

Oxazepam,
   in agitation-induced respiratory alkalosis,
      dosage, 212
   in alcohol withdrawal syndrome, 169, 212

Oxidation,
   of alcohol,
      by colon bacteria, 200

Oxidative stress, 318

P

P rat, 391–393, 408
   and 5HT$_3$ receptor antagonists, 372

P300 amplitude,
   as marker of vulnerability to alcoholism, 308

Pain,
   abdominal,
      in alcoholic ketoacidosis, 209
   in alcohol-induced polyneuropathy, 178

Pair therapy, see Systemic therapy

Palate malformations, in alcohol embryopathy, 258

Palmar erythema, see Erythema, palmar

Palpebral fissure,
   length of,
      in alcohol embryopathy, 254

Palpitations,
   in alcohol-induced arrhythmias, 205

Pancreas, 195–198

Pancreatitis,
   acute, 195
   chronic calcifying, 197

Pancreolauryl test,
   in chronic pancreatitis, 197

Panic disorder,
   in alcohol dependence, 7

Pantoprazole,
   proton pump inhibitor, 211

Paralysis,
   in hypokalemia, 214
   of eye muscles,
      in Wernicke-Korsakoff syndrome, 175

Paranoid personality disorder,
   and alcohol abuse and dependence 294

Parathormone resistance,
   in alcohol dependence, 234

Parathyroid glands, 234

Parathyroid hormone (PTH), 234
   and hypocalcemia, 214

Parents,
   as drinking role models,
      for adolescents, 134

Parkinson-like symptoms,
   in alcohol withdrawal syndrome, 176

Paronychia, 248

Parotid gland, 198

Partner,
   typical problems of alcoholics with, see Codependence

Patient treatment matching, 82, 106, 363–368
   for women, 155

Patterns, of alcohol consumption, see Drinking patterns

Pavlovian dog, 404

Pectus carinatum,
   in alcohol embryopathy, 258

Pectus excavatum,
   in alcohol embryopathy, 258

Pediculosis, 249

Peer group,
   as risk factor,
      in adolescents, 15, 133

Peer pressure,

in adolescents, 15, 133
on women, 154
Pellagra, 240, 243
Pentalogy of Fallot, *see* Fallot's tetra/pentalogy
Pentoxifyllin,
in perniones, 249
Percent abstinent days,
as outcome criterion in clinical trials, 122, 344
Periaqueductal grey,
reward pathways, 374
Peripheral arterial occlusive disease (PAOD),
alcohol as benefical factor against, *see also* Coronary
heart disease (CHD),
Peristalsis, *see* Diarrhea
Perleche, 248
Permeability,
of intestinal mucosa,
alcohol effect on, 200
Perniones, 249
Personal relationships,
in alcohol dependence, 7
Personal therapist, 111, 112
Personality,
alcoholic, 93, *see* Typology
Personality disorder,
antisocial, 7, 293
borderline, 7, 293
other, 293
Person-centered therapy, *see* Client-centered therapy
Pharmacodynamics,
of drugs used in alcohol abuse and dependence, 121
Pharmacokinetics,
of alcohol, 421–423
Pharmacology,
of drugs used in alcohol abuse and dependence,
121–127, 369–384
Pharmacotherapy, for women, 161
of alcohol abuse and dependence, 121–127
Phases,
of alcohol abuse and dependence, *see* Stage model of
change and Natural history
Phenytoin,
drug interactions with alcohol, 422, 425–427
Philtrum,
flatness of,
in alcohol embryopathy, 254
Phlebotomy,
in porphyria cutanea tarda, 244
Phobic disorders,
and alcohol abuse and dependence, 407
Physicochemical properties,
of alcohol (ethanol), 417
Physiological responses,
as marker of vulnerability to alcoholism, 309
Phytoestrogens,
in some alcoholic beverages, 232
Phytohemagglutinin (PHA), 225
Pit cells, 319
Placebo, 340
efficacy of, 105
Placenta,

free passage of alcohol through, *see* Alcohol
embryopathy or Pharmacokinetics
Plasma-to-whole blood level conversion, 462, *see* back
inside cover
Platelets,
normal range, *see* front inside cover
Platelet reactivity,
and alcohol, 205
Pneumonia,
increased vulnerability to,
in alcohol dependence, 227
Poisoning rates,
and alcohol consumption in the general population,
data on 40 countries, 273
Poisons,
co-ingested in acute alcohol intoxication, 57, 59
Pokeweed mitogen (PWM), 225
Polioencephalitis hemorrhagica superior, *see* Wernicke
encephalopathy
Polydipsia,
schedule-induced, 387
Polydrug abuse, 290, *see also* Polytoxicomania
Polyneuropathy, 178
amount of alcohol consumption leading to, 178
Polyphenols,
in wine,
antioxidant effect, 205, 226, *see also* Resveratrol
Polytoxicomania, 7, 59
in adolescents, 130
Pontine myelinolysis, *see* Myelinolysis
Populations,
differences in drinking across, 271–286
Porphyria cutanea tarda (PCT), 243
Porphyria,
intermittent, 243
Porphyrias, 243–244
Portal hypertension, *see* Hypertension, portal
Portasystemic shunt, 232
Position,
obtaining a clear and unequivocal one, 93
Positive emotions, *see* Emotions, positive
Positive reinforcer,
alcohol as,
in humans, 95
Posttraumatic stress disorder (PTSD),
and alcohol abuse and dependence, 289
Postural hypotension, *see* Orthostatic hypotension
in Wernicke encephalopathy, 179
Potassium,
in acute alcohol intoxication, 56, 61
normal range, 56
supplementation, in alcohol withdrawal syndrome, 69,
207
supplementation, in alcohol-induced arrhythmias, 206
PR monkey, 389
Precision,
definition of, 29
Precontemplation,
in stage model of change, 99, 100
likelihood of,
upon first contact, 108

Preference procedure,
    two-bottle, 393
Prefrontal cortex,
    reward pathways, 374
Pregnancy, 206
    and alcohol withdrawal syndrome, 69
    of alcohol abusing mothers,
        and risk of malformations in offspring, 260–263
Preparation,
    in stage model of change, 99, 100
Prerenal azotemia,
    in cirrhosis, 219–220
Preterm birth, 152
Prevalence,
    of alcohol abuse and dependence,
        and of comorbid psychiatric disorders, 282, 283
        in adolesents, 15, **130–131**, 278
        in ambulatory care settings, 39
        in emergency care setting, 281
        in geriatric population, 137, 279
        in hospital populations, 281
        in pregnant women, 278
        in primary care setting, 279
        in university students, 279
        in USA 15, 385
        in women, 151
        worldwide, 125, 276
        in German inpatient settings, 92
    of alcohol embryopathy, 264
    of alcohol-induced acid-base disorders, 209, 210
    of alcohol-induced electrolyte disorders 212–215
    of alcohol-induced polyneuropathy, 178
    of alcohol-induced psychotic disorders, 73
    of birth defects, in offspring of alcohol abusing mothers,
        264
    of harmful drinking,
        worldwide, 276
    of infectious diseases,
        in alcohol dependence, 227
    of kidney and electrolyte disturbances,
        in alcohol dependence, 213, 214
    of natural recovery, 283
Prevention,
    in adolescents, 130
    of relapse, *see* Relapse prevention
Prick test, *see* Skin prick test
Primary care,
    implications of Project MATCH for, 367
Primary care physician,
    choice of psychotherapy for, 106
Primary care setting,
    special therapeutic considerations in, 165–172
Problem drinker,
    and brief intervention, 169
    and controlled drinking, 104
    diagnosis of, 166
    vs. alcohol dependent patients, ratio, 325
Problem drinking, *see also* Abuse
Problem solution,
    active help in,
        as general effect factor in psychotherapy, 105

Prochaska and DiClemente model, *see* Stage model of
        change
Pro-enkephalin (PENK), 373
Prognosis,
    in adolescents, 129
    in geriatric patients, 143
    in women, 156
    of alcohol-related disorders under therapy, *see also*
        Efficacy
    of controlled drinking, 23, 345, 347
    of pharmacotherapy, 121–127
    of quitting on one's own, 23, 24, 283
Progression,
    of alcohol abuse and dependence, in women, 152, 156
Progressive relaxation, 102–103
Prohibition,
    beneficial effect on cirrhosis rate in the general
        population, 183
Project MATCH, 83, 106, 107, **363–368**
    outcome criteria, and outcome, 367
Projection,
    as defense mechanism in alcohol dependent patients, 8
Promille,
    definition of, *see* back inside cover
    conversion to mg% or mg dl-1 *see* back inside cover,
        61, 63
Pro-opiomelanocortin (POMC), 373
Prooxidant effect,
    of alcohol, 226
Prophylaxis,
    of alcohol withdrawal syndrome, 67, 68
Propylthiouracil, in alcoholic hepatitis, 187–188
Protease inhibitors,
    in acute pancreatitis, 197
Protection of liver, *see* Hepatoprotective drugs
Protein kinase C (PKC),
    and $GABA_A$ receptor, 369–370
    gamma isoform knockout,
        behavioral effects, 369–370
Prothrombin time (PT), 187
Proton pump inhibitors (PPIs),
    in acute gastritis, 199
    in metabolic alkalosis, 211
Protoporphyria,
    erythropoetic, 244
Providing,
    of a psychological theory of alcohol abuse and
        dependence,
        as general effect factor in psychotherapy, 105
Pruritus, in alcohol intolerance, 227, 241
Pseudo-Cushing's syndrome, 231, 233, 234
Pseudohyponatremia, 215
Psoralen, 246
Psoriases, 228, 244–245
Psoriasis guttata, 245
Psoriasis inversa, 245
Psoriasis pustulosa, 245
Psoriasis vulgaris, 244
Psychoanalysis, 94, 97–99
    brief definition of theoretical concept, 94
Psychoanalytic-interactional therapy, 99

Psychodrama, 101

Psychometric instruments, 39–46, 331–338, 439–456
    criteria for choice of, 40
    for evaluation of treatment outcome, 331–338
    for screening, 39–46
    in women, 157
    test forms, 439–456

Psychotherapeutic approach,
    choice of, 106

Psychotherapy, 89–120
    adaptation to clinical/therapeutic setting, 106
    in clinical trials on pharmacotherapy, 135
    in geriatric patients, 142–143

Psychotic disorders,
    treatment, 75–76

Psychotic disorders induced by alcohol, 73–77
    differential diagnosis, 74–75
    pathophysiology, 75

Puberty, see Adolescents

Publication bias, 360

Pulicosis, 249

Purkinje cell degeneration, 175

Putamen,
    reward pathways, 374

PUVA, 246

Pyramidal signs,
    in Encephalopathy,
        hepatic, 176

Q

QF, see Quantity-Frequency measures

Quality,
    of clinical trials,
        criteria of, 354, 360

Quantification,
    of alcohol in blood, see Blood alcohol level

Quantitative trait locus (QTL) analysis, 402

Quantity-Frequency measures (QF), 334
    test form, 451–452

Questionnaires, 39–46, 331–338, 439–456, see also
            Psychometric instruments

Quitting,
    on one's own, 19–24, 85, 271, 283, see also Natural
        recovery

R

R factor, 419

Racial differences, see Epidemiology

Radical formation,
    in hepatotoxic effect of alcohol, 317, 318

RAND report, 105

Ranson's criteria,
    for estimation of mortality and complications in acute
        pancreatitis, 196

Rat, 390–395

Rationalization, 8

Readiness to Change Questionnaire (RTCQ)©, 333

test form, 453

Reality testing,
    as ego function, 98

Reattribution,
    of bodily sensation,
        in psychotherapy, 102

Receiver operating characteristic (ROC) curve, 30

Recovery position,
    in emergency medicine, see front inside cover

Rectum,
    cancer of, 200

Red nose, see Rosacea

Red wine,
    and risk for developing alcoholic liver disease, 321
    as histamine-rich food,
        in alcohol intolerance, 241

Reflexes,
    in alcohol-induced neurological disorders, 171–183

Reflux esophagitis, 198

Reframing, of cognitive premises, 96

Rehydration, see Hydration

Reinforcement, 385–400
    definition of, 385
    negative, see Negative reinforcement

Reinforcer, see Reinforcement

Reinforcing effect, see Reinforcement

Relapse,
    as outcome criterion in clinical trials, 122

Relapse prevention, 113–115, 339

Relapse rates, 347

Relationships, see Codependence and Systemic Therapy

Relative risk,
    definition of, 354

Relatives, see Family and Adolescents

Relaxation techniques, 96, 102

Renal disorders, 209–224

Renal dysfunction,
    in cirrhosis, 218–224

Renal failure,
    problems with creatine kinase as indicator, 217

Renal tubular dysfunction, 216–217

Renin, 174, 206, 234
    normal level, 174

Repeal of Prohibition,
    and rise in cirrhosis rate, 183

Research design issues,
    in prospective designs, 14
    in retrospective designs, 13–14

Research Society on Alcoholism (RSA),
    adddress and web site, 457, www.sci.sdsu.edu/RSA/

Resources,
    activation of,
        as general effect factor in psychotherapy, 105

Respect, unconditional,
    in client-centered psychotherapy, 101

Respiration, 52
    in acute alcohol intoxication, see front inside cover,
        49–64

Respiratory alkalosis, see Alkalosis

Respiratory failure,
    in acute alcohol intoxication,

treatment, *see* **front inside cover, 52**
  in hypokalemia, 214
  in hypophosphatemia, 212
Respondent conditioning,
  role in alcohol dependence, 95
Restlessness,
  in alcohol embryopathy, 254
  in alcohol abuse and dependence, 7
Resveratrol,
  as beneficial factor in atherosclerosis, 205, 226, *see also*
      French Paradox and Polyphenols
Retardation,
  mental,
      in alcohol embryopathy, 258
Retinoids, 246
Reversibility,
  of alcoholic fatty liver, 186
  of alcoholic gastritis, 199
  of alcoholic hepatitis, 186–187
  of alcohol-induced immunodeficiency, 227
  of alcohol-induced psychotic disorders, 74, 76
  of electrolyte disturbances, 209–217
  of esophageal varices only after portal shunt surgery
      including TIPS, 189, 219, **220**
  of gout attacks, 217
  of hypogonadism, 233
  of liver function impairment, 190
  of low T_3 syndrome, 234
  of pseudo-Cushing's syndrome, 234
  of reflux esophagitis, 198
  of seizures in acute alcohol intoxication, 174
  of seizures in withdrawal, 174
  partial (initial)
      of cerebellar atrophy, 175
      of polyneuropathy, 178
  partial, of movement disorders, 176
      of myopathy 179
      of sleep disorders, 177
      of Wernicke-Korsakoff syndrome, 176
Reward, *see also* Reinforcement
Reward pathways,
  schematic drawing of, 374
Reward system, *see* Reward pathways
Rhabdomyolysis, 59, 179, 217
  alcohol as the drug most frequently causing it, 179
  and renal failure, 217
  in myopathy, 179
  increased risk in hypophosphatemia, 212, 217
Rhesus monkey, 387–390
Rheumatoid arthritis,
  in alcohol dependence, 227
Rhinophyma, 246
Rho factor, 419
Risk, *see also* Prevalence
Risk factors,
  for alcohol abuse and dependence,
      in adolescents, 132
      in general, *see* Psychotherapy, or Heritability, or
          Comorbidity
      in women, 151–164
Risperidone,

  in alcohol-induced psychotic disorders, 76
Role model,
  lack of,
      as risk factor in adolescents, 132
Role play,
  in psychotherapy, 96, 101, 112
Rosacea, 6, **247**
Routines, *see* Structured daily routines
RSA, *see* Research Society on Alcoholism

S

S49 cells, 375
Sacral dimple,
  in alcohol embryopathy, 258
S-Adenosyl-L-methionine (SAM),
  possible hepatoprotective effect of, 191
Safe alcohol consumption, *see* Harmful alcohol
      consumption
Salivary glands, 198
Satiation,
  animal research, 395
Scabies, 249
Scavengers,
  in cirrhosis, 190
Schizophrenia,
  and alcohol abuse and dependence, 295
Sclera,
  yellow *see* Icterus
Screening,
  for alcohol abuse and dependence, 166
Seafood,
  as histamine-rich food,
      in alcohol intolerance, 241
Sebaceous glands,
  hyperplasia, 247
Secretin-cholecystokinin test,
  in chronic pancreatitis, 197
Sedation,
  in acute alcohol intoxication, 54
Seizures, 173–174
  and risk of rhabdomyolysis, 217
  differential diagnosis, 174
  in withdrawal, 66
      treatment, 67–68
Selection of clinical studies,
  for meta-analysis, 354
Selective serotonin reuptake inhibitors (SSRIs),
  effect size, 345
  in alcohol abuse and dependence, 121, 123, 343
  mechanism of action, 121
Selenium deficiency, 321
Self-administration, 385–400
  intravenous,
      primates, 390
      rodents, 394–395
  monkey 387–390
  oral,
      primates, 387–390
      rodents, 390–394

rat 390–395
Self-destruction,
    in adolescents, 133
Self-esteem,
    in women, 153
Self-help groups, 10, 104–105, 110, 112, *see also*
        Alcoholics Anonymous and Al-Anon
    and women, 155
Self-management,
    as goal in cognitive behavioral therapy, 97
    for women, 155
Self-medication hypothesis, 98, 133, 288, 291, 339
Self-medication with alcohol,
    in adolescents, 133
    of depression, 271, **291**
    of essential tremor, 177
    of sleep disorders, 177
    of tension, 98, 102
Sensation,
    loss of,
        in alcohol-induced polyneuropathy, 178
Sensations,
    reattribution of,
        in psychotherapy, 102
Sensibility,
    in alcohol-induced neurological disorders, 171–183
Sensitivity,
    of laboratory tests,
        definition of, 29
Sensitization,
    behavioral,
        to alcohol, 403
Separation,
    of adolescents, 130
Serotonin, *see also* 5HT
    brain levels,
        upon acute alcohol administration, 372
Serotonin system,
    as marker of vulnerability to alcoholism, 309
Serum-to-whole blood lever conversion, 462, *see* back
        inside cover
Setting,
    and choice of psychotherapeutic approach, 106
Settings,
    benefecial for women, 158
Sexual dysfunctions,
    in alcohol dependence 6
Sexuality,
    development,
        in adolescence, 129, 130
Shame,
    feelings of, 8
Shared environment,
    in twin studies of alcohol heritability, 306
Short counseling, *see* Counseling
Shortness of breath,
    in alcohol intolerance, 227, 241
Short-sleep mice, 375
SI units,
    conversion to U.S. units, *see* back inside cover, 61, 63
Sideroblastic abnormalities, 322

Sign,
    definition of,
        in psychoanalysis, 97
Significant others,
    of adolescents, 130
    self-help groups of, 113, *see also* Al-Anon
Silymarin,
    in cirrhosis, 190
Situations,
    leading to alcohol abuse, *see* Social situations
Sizes of drinks, *see* back inside cover
Skills training, 96
Skin,
    alcohol-related disorders, 239–241, 243–250
    brownish-grey / bronze, *see* Hemochromatosis
    hyperpigmentations in sunlight-exposed areas, *see*
        Pellagra
    red, *see* Rosacea and 239–241, 243–250
    yellow, *see* Icterus
Skin prick test,
    in diagnosis of type I allergic reaction to alcohol, 241
Sleep apnea,
    and alcohol-induced cardiovascular diseases, 205
Sleep disorders, 177
Slip, *see* Lapse
sMAST, 454, *see also* Michigan Alcoholism Screening
        Test, short version
Smoking,
    and alcohol absorption, 421
    and alcohol abuse and dependence, comorbidity, 295,
        307
    and cerebral vascular diseases, 174
    as risk factor in esophageal cancer, 198
Snoring,
    worsening by alcohol, 177
Social abnormalities,
    as clinical signs of alcohol abuse and dependence, 107
Social cognitive therapy, 96
Social drinker, *see* Peer pressure
Social roles,
    of women, 154
Social situations,
    leading to relapse, 96, 115
Social skills training, 96
    for women, 159, 161
Social therapy,
    for adolescents, 135
    for women, 161
Sociocultural background,
    as risk factor,
        in adolescents, 133
Sociophobia, 7
Socratic dialogue,
    as psychotherapeutic technique, 96
Sodium,
    normal range, 56
    supplementation, 176
Somatic signs and frequent complaints,
    by alcohol-abusing and dependent patients, 7–8
Somatostatin,
    in acute pancreatitis, 197

Somnolence,
in electrolyte disturbances, 212
Specific weight,
of alcohol (ethanol), 417
of whole blood, 419
Specificity,
definition of, 30
Speech disturbances, *see* Dysarthria
Spermatogenesis,
cessation of,
alcohol-induced, 231–232
Spices,
as histamine-rich food,
in alcohol intolerance, 241
Spider naevi, 7, 10, 232
Spielberger State-Trait Anxiety Scale, 366
Spina bifida,
in alcohol embryopathy, 258
Spironolactone,
in cirrhosis, 218–219
risk in feminized alcohol dependent men, 219, 232
Spleen,
enlargement of, *see* Splenomegaly
Splenomegaly, 189
Spontaneous remission, *see* Natural recovery
Spouse pressure,
on women, 154
Squamous cell carcinoma,
esophageal, 198
SS mice, 371, 375
SSRIs, *see* Selective serotonin reuptake inhibitors
Stage model of change, 94, **99–101**, 333
Stages of Change Readiness and Treatment Eagerness Scale
(SOCRATES), 333
Stages,
of alcohol abuse and dependence, *see* Stage model of
change and Natural history
Standard drink,
definitions of, 429
Standardized difference,
as a measure of effect size, 355, 356
Statistics,
of alcohol consumption, 271–286
Status epilepticus, 174, *see also* Seizures
Steatosis,
pathophysiology, 320
Step-by-step instruction in meta-analysis, 353–362
Still birth, 152
Stoichiometry,
of GABA$_A$ receptor, 370
Stomach,
cancer of, 198
empty,
and alcohol absorption, 421
gastritis, 199
Stomatitis,
in alcohol-related niacin deficiency, 240
Stool fat excretion,
in chronic pancreatitis, 197
Streptococcus,
role in ecthymata, 249

Stress,
and alcohol absorption, 421
Stressful life events,
leading to relapse, 115
Stroke,
hemorrhagic, 174
alcohol as risk factor 206
ischemic, 174
beneficial and harmful effects of alcohol on, 206
Structure,
of alcohol (ethanol), 417
Structured Clinical Interview for DSM-IV disorders
(SCID), 332
Structured daily routines,
importance for inpatient psychotherapy, 112
lack of,
leading to relapse 115
Students,
prevalence of alcohol abuse and dependence in,
278–279
Study selection,
for meta-analysis, 354
Subarachnoidal hemorrhage, 204
Subdural hematoma,
chronic, 174
Subjection,
feelings of, 8
Substance abuse, *see* Drug abuse
Substantia nigra,
pars compacta,
reward pathways, 374
pars reticulata,
reward pathways, 374
Sucralfate,
in acute gastritis, 199
Sucrose-fading procedure, 392
Sudden cardiac death (SCD),
alcohol-induced, 205–206
Suicidal behavior, 133, 295
Sulfite sensitivity,
in alcohol intolerance, 227
Superego functions, 98
Superoxide anion, 318–319
Supination,
limited,
in alcohol embryopathy, 258
Supportive psychotherapy, 98, 108
Suppressor T cells,
and alcohol, *see* T cells, suppressor
Suspecting,
acute alcohol intoxication, 49
Sweating,
in withdrawal, 7, 66, *see also* Hyperhidrosis
Symbol,
definition of,
in psychoanalysis, 97
Sympathetic tone,
and alcohol absorption, 421
Sympatholytics,
in alcohol withdrawal syndrome, 68
Symptoms, *see* individual disorders and Clinical signs

Syncope, *see* Orthostatic hypotension
Systemic lupus erythematosus (SLE),
    in alcohol dependence, 227
Systemic therapy, 101
Systolic murmur,
    in alcohol-induced heart failure, 203

T

T cells,
    suppressor, 225
T_4, *see* Thyroxine
Tablespoon,
    definition of, *see* back inside cover
T-ACE©, 44, 157
Tachycardia, alcohol-induced, 203
    in alcohol withdrawal syndrome, 66
    in alcoholic ketoacidosis, 209
    in withdrawal, 66
Tachymeningeosis hemorrhagica interna, *see* Subdural
            hematoma, chronic
Taste,
    of alcoholic beverage,
        and alcohol intake in aminal studies, 388
Teleangiectasias, 7, 248
Telescoping,
    of negative consequences of alcohol consumption in
            women, 152
Tenderness, *see* Muscle tenderness
Tension,
    alcohol as self-medication against, 98, 102
Tension reduction hypothesis,
    definition of, 102, 288, 406, *see also* Self-medication
    and comorbidity data on alcohol dependence and
            anxiety, 288, *see also* Self-medication
Teratogenic effects,
    of alcohol on other than the cardiovascular system,
            251–259
    of alcohol on the cardiovascular system, 206, 252
Termination,
    of treatment,
        criteria for, 104
Test forms,
    of psychometric tests, 167, 439–456, *see also* individual
            psychometric tests
Testicular atrophy,
    alcohol-induced, 231
Testosterone,
    decrease by alcohol, 231
Tetracyclines,
    in treatment of rosacea, 248
Tetralogy of Fallot, *see* Fallot's tetra/pentalogy
Th-1 cells, 226
Thalamus,
    dorsal medial,
        reward pathways, 374
Therapeutic attitude,
    in the treatment of adolescents, 133–135
Therapeutic settings,
    beneficial for women, 158

Therapies,
    psychotherapy and pharmacotherapy combined, 83
    sequencing, 84
Therapist attitude,
    obtaining a helpful therapeutic one, 90
Therapist effect,
    in psychotherapy, 91
Therapy, *see also* Treatment, Psychotherapy,
            Pharmacotherapy, and individual chapters
    goals of, *see* Treatment goals
Thermoregulation,
    impairment, 249
Theta hypoactivity,
    as marker of vulnerability to alcoholism, 307
Thiamine contents,
    of beer, 241
Thiamine,
    in cerebellar atrophy, 175
    supplementation,
        dosage, 176, 210, 240
Thiamine deficiency, 175, 210, 239
    laboratory diagnosis of, 178
Third spacing,
    leading to hypovolemia, 52
Thistle extracts,
    in cirrhosis, 190
Thrombo(cyto)penia, 7, 66
    as a consequence of splenomegaly in portal
            hypertension, 189
Thyroid gland, 231, 232, 234
Thyroxine levels, estrogen-induced,
    in feminized alcohol dependent men, 234
Tiapride,
    effect size, 345
    in alcohol abuse and dependence, 121–124, 343, 403
Timeline Follow-Back (TLFB), 334
    test form, 455–456
Tobacco, *see* Smoking
Tobacco-alcohol-amblyopy, *see* Amblyopy
Tolerance,
    to alcohol, 50, 434, 435
    to diazepam (benzodiazepine), 67–68
Total enteral nutrition,
    in cirrhosis, 190
Toxins,
    drug interaction with alcohol, 423
Traditions,
    clinical,
        transatlantic differences, 94
trans-3, 4, 5-trihydroxystilbene
    is resveratrol, *see* Polyphenols
Transference,
    definition of, 97
Transferrin, 322
Transjugular intrahepatic portasystemic shunt (TIPS), 219,
            220
Transketalose activity,
    in thiamine deficiency, 178
Transplantation,
    of the liver, 190
Traumatization,

of adolescents, 129
Treatment,
  setting-oriented, 81–87
Treatment goals, 23–24, 85, 104
  in psychotherapy, 104
Treatment seeking, 18
  of women, 155
Tremor,
  essential,
    alcohol as self-medication against, 177
  flapping (Asterixis),
    in hepatic encephalopathy, 176
  in withdrawal, 66
Trial, *see* Clinical trials
Triggers,
  for alcohol abuse, *see* Psychotherapy and Social
    situations
    specific for women, 159
Trousseau sign,
  in hypocalcemia or hypomagnesemia, 213, 214
Truthful reporting,
  of alcohol consumption, *see* Collateral reports
Tuberculosis,
  incidence,
    in alcohol dependence, 225, 227
Tuberculum olfactorium,
  reward pathways, 374
Tumor necrosis factor alpha (TNF-alpha),
  effects on liver, 319
  increased levels,
    in alcohol dependence, 226
Tumor promotion,
  role in cancer of the oral mucosa, 249
TWEAK, 44, 157
  test form, 456
Twelve-Step Facilitation (TSF), 365
Twin studies, 305
Twin/family designs, 307
Type I allergic reaction,
  against alcohol, 241
Types of alcoholic beverages,
  alcohol contents, *see* back inside cover
Typology, 93, 139–140, 294, 297
  Babor classification, 297
  Cloninger classification, 294, 297, 306
    animal research on, 389
    definition of, 294

U

Ulcer,
  duodenal,
    alcohol no risk factor for duodenal, *see also*
      Cirrhosis
  gastric, 7, *see* Gastritis, hemorrhagic
Unconditional respect,
  in client-centered therapy, 101
Underfilling hypothesis,
  of edema formation in cirrhosis, 218
Unemployment,

in alcohol dependence, 7
  as risk factor,
    in women, 155
Unit conversion table, *see* back inside cover, 61, 63
Unit drink,
  definitions of, 429
United Nations International Drug Control Programme
    (UNDCP), 404
Unpleasant emotions,
  alcohol as self-medication against, 98
Unsaturated fatty acids, 321
Ureter malformations,
  in alcohol embryopathy, 258
Urine,
  red-brown, *see* Porphyrias
Urogenital tract malformations,
  in alcohol embryopathy, 258
Ursodeoxycholic acid,
  possible hepatoprotective effect of, 191
Urticaria,
  in alcohol-related anaphylactic reactions, 241
U.S. units, conversion to SI units, *see* back inside cover,
    61, 63
Useful (internet) addresses, 457
UV-A irradiation, 246, 274

V

Vagabond's Skin, 249
Vagal tone,
  and alcohol absorption, 421
Valsalva maneuver,
  in diagnosis of autonomic disorders, 179
Variable, *see* Continous variable and Dichotomous variable
Varices,
  esophageal, 189
Vasodilation,
  of cutaneous vessels by alcohol, 249
  of peripheral vessels by alcohol, 206
Vasopressin, 174, 220
  suppression of release by alcohol, 216
Vasospasm,
  cerebral, 174
Ventral pallidum (VP),
  reward pathways, 374
Ventral tegmental area (VTA),
  reward pathways, 373, 374
Vermis,
  cerebellar, 175
Violence,
  and alcohol, 271
    dose-mortality relationship 328
Vital functions,
  assessment in acute alcohol intoxication, *see* front
      inside cover, 49–64
Vitamin B deficiencies, 239–240
Vitamin B, in alcohol withdrawal syndrome, 69
Vitamin B_1, *see* Thiamine
Vitamin B_3, *see* Niacin
Vitamin B_{12}, *see* Cyanocobalamin

Vitamin C, *see* Ascorbic acid
Vitamin D, *see also* Calcitriol
    supplementation,
        dosage, 235
Vitamin D deficiency,
    and hypophosphatemia, 212
Vitamin deficiencies,
    in alcohol dependence, 212, 239–240, 321
Voices,
    in alcohol hallucinosis, 74
Voltammetry,
    of drug-induced dopamine overflow in various brain
            areas, 403
Volume depletion, *see* Dehydration
Volume of distribution,
    of alcohol, 419
Voluntary associations, *see* Self-help groups or Alcoholics
            Anonymous or Al-Anon
Volunteer groups, *see* Self-help groups or Alcoholics
            Anonymous or Al-Anon
Vomiting,
    in withdrawal, 66
    risk of metabolic alkalosis, 211
Vomitus matutinus,
    in acute gastritis, 199
Vulnerability for alcoholism,
    markers of, 307–311
    of women, 152
Vulvitis,
    in alcohol-related niacin deficiency, 240

W

Warfarin,
    drug interactions with alcohol, 422, 425–427
Water intoxication, 216
Weakness, *see* Muscle weakness
Weight at birth,
    in alcohol embryopathy, 259
Wernicke encephalopathy, 54, 59, 69, 175–176
    definition of, 175
Wernicke-Korsakoff syndrome,
    definition of, 175
Wheezing,
    in alcohol-related anaphylactic reactions, 241
Widmark's formula, 419
Widmark's rho factor, 419
Wine,
    alcohol contents of, *see* back inside cover
    red, *see* Red wine
Withdrawal,
    alcohol consumption leading to,
        in man, 65
        in monkey, 387
        in rat, 387
    and respiratory alkalosis, 211
    cardiovascular symptoms, 207
    clinical signs, 66
    common mistakes in the treatment of, 70
    depression of VTA firing and DA release in, 377

    in geriatric patients, 140–141
    in pregnancy, 69
    laboratory parameters in, 66
    mycocaridal ischemia in, 207
    prophylaxis of,
        with benzodiazepines, 67
        with carbamazepine, 68
    psychotherapy during, 109–112
        inpatient setting, 111
        outpatient setting, 112
    symptoms,
        in rat, 392
    treatment, 65–71
    in primary care, 169–170
Wolffgramm and Heyne model,
    in laboratory animals, 391
Women,
    alcohol effects on hormonal functions of the
            reproductive system, 232–233
    breast-feeding and alcohol abuse, *see* Breast milk
    higher comorbidity of phobic disorders and alcoholism,
            407
    increased vulnerability for alcoholic cardiomyopathy,
            203
    special therapeutic considerations, 151–164
    specific therapies, 156–161
Workaholic,
    risk of relapse, 115
World Health Organization (WHO), 43, 272, 404, 433,

Y

Yellow skin and sclera, *see* Icterus
Young elderly, 142
Youths, *see* Adolescents

Z

Zero-order kinetics,
    of alcohol metabolism, 422
Zieve's syndrome, 185
Zinc deficiency syndrome,
    acquired, 239, 246, 321
    false normal levels in hypoalbuminemia, 239
    normal range, 246
    supplementation,
        dosage, 239, 246

ALCOHOL CONTENTS OF TYPICAL DRINKS

The alcohol concentration of types of drinks (usually given in vol.%) may vary (e.g., beers range from 4 to 6 vol.%, wines from 10 to 20 vol.%, hard liquors from 36 to 73 vol.%). For the following table, the most common vol.% have been assumed.

$$1 \text{ vol.\% corresponds to } 0.79 \text{ wt/vol.\% or } 0.0079 \text{ g ml}^{-1} \text{ or } 7.9 \text{ g l}^{-1}.$$

One-proof corresponds to 0.5 vol.%, for example, the usual 80-proof beverage is a 40 vol.% solution of alcohol. Colloquial Austrian and German measures (e.g., shot, Kruegel, Pfiff, Stamperl, simple Schnaps) are given in parenthesis.

DRINK (type, size)	Grams Alcohol per Drink
Beer (5 vol.%), 1 liter	40
0.2 liter (A: Pfiff; Stifterl)	8
0.33 liter (A,D: small beer; Seidel; European can)	13
12 fl. oz. (U.S. can; 0.355 liter)	14
Pint (0.47 liter; "tall boy" U.S. can)	19
0.5 liter (A,D: large beer, Kruegel; Halbe; can)	20
1 liter (Maβ)	40
Malt Liquor (7 vol.%) (e.g., Colt45®, Elephant Beer®, Bockbier, Starkbier), 1l	55
12 fl. oz. (U.S. can, 0.355 l)	20
0.5 l (A,D: large beer, Kruegel)	28
Wine (12 vol.%), 1 liter	95
0.1 liter (small glass, sampling glass)	10
0.125 liter (A,D: Achterl)	12
0.175 liter (U.K.: glass)	17
0.2 liter	19
8 fl. oz. (U.S.: 0.24 l; glass)	23
0.25 liter (A,D: Vierterl)	24
0.7 liter (A,D: bottle)	67
0.75 liter (F: bottle)	71
Fortified Wine (20 vol.%) (e.g., MadDog®, Thunderbird®, Port), 1 liter	158
Liqueur (30 vol.%) (e.g., highballs, Cassis, Jaegermeister®), 1 liter	237
0.02 liter	5
0.04 liter	9
(Hard) liquor (40 vol.%), 1 liter	316
0.02 liter (Stamperl, single Schnaps)	6
0.025 liter (shot, U.K.)	8
0.04 liter (double Schnaps; sample bottles)	13
0.044 liter (shot, U.S.; 1.5 fl. oz.)	14
0.1 (Flachmann)	32
Other alcoholic beverages	
"Alcohol-free" beer (0.5 vol%), 1 liter	4
Beer light (3.7 vol%), 1 liter	29
Champagne (12.5 vol%), 1 liter	99
Cider (cidre; Most; 5 vol%), 1 liter	40
Met (honey wine; 11.5 vol%), 1 liter	91
Port (20 vol%), 1 liter	16
Sherry (18 vol%), 1 liter	14

BLOOD ALCOHOL LEVEL: UNITS AND CONVERSION FACTORS

Clinical blood alcohol levels (BALs; blood alcohol concentration, BAC) are usually reported in terms of mass/volume unit (i.e., mg dl^{-1}) in English-speaking countries and in terms of mass/mass unit (i.e., g kg^{-1} or ‰) in Europe. Because 1 ml whole blood has, on average, a specific weight of 1.055, the mass/mass unit has a higher numerical value.

$$100 \text{ mg\%} = 100 \text{ mg dl}^{-1} = 95 \text{ mg/100 g} = 0.95 \text{ g kg}^{-1} = 0.95‰$$